Health Dynamics

Attitudes and Behaviors

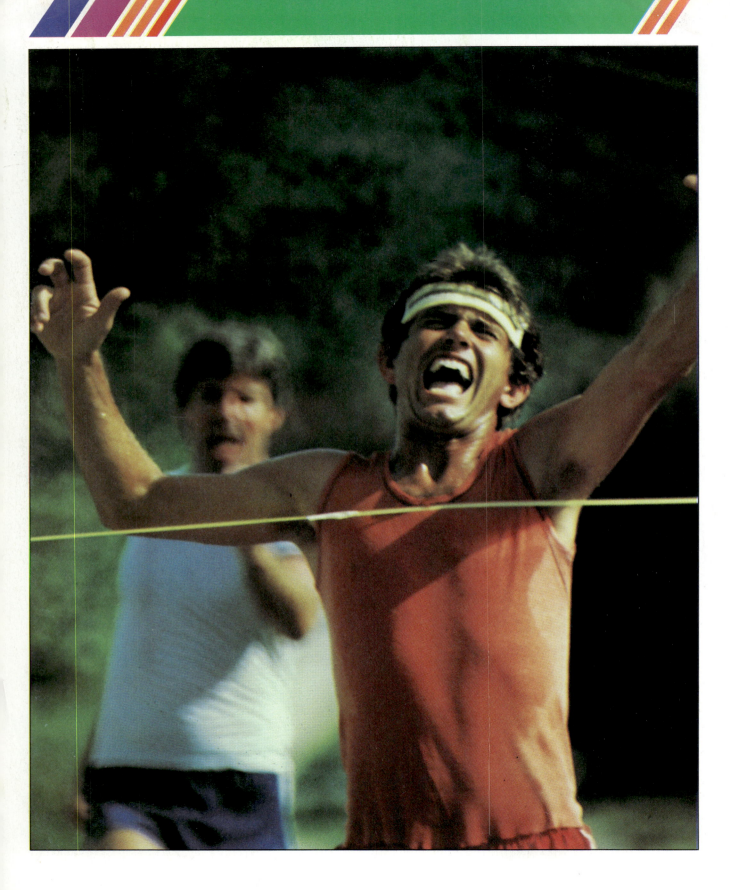

Health Dynamics

Attitudes and Behaviors

Warren Boskin, Ed.D.
SAN DIEGO STATE UNIVERSITY

Department of Health Science

Gerald Graf, M.A., R.Ph.
SAN DIEGO STATE UNIVERSITY

Department of Health Science

Virginia Kreisworth, Ph.D.
SAN DIEGO STATE UNIVERSITY

Department of Health Science

WEST PUBLISHING COMPANY

Saint Paul New York Los Angeles San Francisco

Copyeditor: Judith Lary
Composition: Parkwood Composition
Text Design: Kristen M. Weber
Cover Image: Mitchell Funk, Image Bank
Artwork: Rolin Graphics

COPYRIGHT © 1990   By WEST PUBLISHING COMPANY
50 West Kellogg Boulevard
P. O. Box 64526
St. Paul, MN 55164-1003

All rights reserved

Printed in the United States of America

97 96 95 94 93 92 91 90   8 7 6 5 4 3 2 1 0

Library of Congress Cataloging-in-Publication Data

Boskin, Warren D.
   Health dynamics, attitudes, and behaviors / Warren D. Boskin, Gerald Graf, Virginia Kreisworth.
       p.   cm.
   ISBN 0-314-66787-3
   1. Health.   2. Mind and body.   I. Graf, Gerald.
II. Kreisworth, Virginia.   III. Title
RA776.B668 1990   89-48512
613-dc20   CIP

About the Authors

Warren Boskin has taught health education at the college level for the past 27 years and two years prior to that at the high school level. He received his Doctorate from West Virginia University, Masters Degree from the University of Illinois, and Baccalaureate from Brooklyn College. A professor at San Diego State University since 1965, he is a former chairperson of the University's Department of Health Science and was twice selected as the department's "Most Influential Professor." He has been active in numerous local, state, and national health education organizations. His areas of specialty in health education are death education, mental health, spirituality, safety, international health, self-care, and professional preparation. His avocations include running, cycling, music (playing folk rock guitar), camping and hiking, international travel, gardening, and spending time with his granddaughter, Molly.

Gerald Graf has taught health education courses for 23 years. He is currently teaching in the Department of Health Science at San Diego State University, and also has taught at the high school level. As a registered pharmacist in New York and California, he has done extensive research in the field of drug-drug interactions among the elderly, and has served as a consultant pharmacist for several nursing homes. Gerald has worked with community clinics in the San Diego area, primarily with a clinic which has one of only two local programs involved in screening high-risk individuals for HIV infection and other sexually transmitted diseases. He earned certification in New York as an emergency medical technician and pre-hospital critical care technician, and served as a basic life support instructor-trainer and an advanced life support instructor for the New York affiliate of the American Heart Association. He has taught cardiopulmonary resuscitation in New York, Massachusetts, and Georgia.

Virginia Kreisworth received her Ph.D from Purdue University. Her Bachelor's and Master's degrees are in health science, which she obtained from New York University. As part of her Master's Degree, she received specialized education in human sexuality at Uppsala University in Uppsala, Sweden. In 1983, she was bestowed the honor of being selected "Professor of the Year" at the University of Miami. She is currently a faculty member in the department of Health Science at San Diego State University where she teaches courses in human sexuality, health and lifestyle, and consumer health. In 1989, she received an "Outstanding Faculty Award" at San Diego State University. She has experience teaching health education at both the junior and senior high school levels, as well as being a K–9 coordinator of health education.

Contents In Brief

SECTION I — Health and the Mind 1

Chapter 1 Wellness and Health Actions 3
Chapter 2 Mental Well-Being 31
Chapter 3 Managing Stress 57

SECTION II — Body Dynamics 83

Chapter 4 Food Facts 85
Chapter 5 Eating Behaviors 119
Chapter 6 Getting Physical 145

SECTION III — Understanding Sexuality 175

Chapter 7 Relationships 177
Chapter 8 Sexual Bodyworks 197
Chapter 9 Family Planning 221
Chapter 10 Conception Through Birth 257

SECTION IV — Drugs and Your Body 275

Chapter 11 The Tobacco Road 277
Chapter 12 Alcohol Awareness 303
Chapter 13 Psychoactive Drugs 327

SECTION V — Coping With Disease 349

Chapter 14 Understanding the Disease Process and Infectious Diseases 351
Chapter 15 Sexually Transmitted Disease 373
Chapter 16 Becoming Heart Smart 399
Chapter 17 Dealing With Chronic Disease 415

SECTION VI — Taking Control of Your Health 441

Chapter 18 Consumer Health 443
Chapter 19 Occupational and Environmental Risks 473

SECTION VII — The Final Transition 503

Chapter 20 Maturing Gracefully 505
Chapter 21 The Ultimate Loss 527

APPENDIX A — First Aid 547

APPENDIX B — Classification of Mental Disorders and Illness 555

GLOSSARY 557

INDEX 567

Contents

SECTION I Health and the Mind 1

Chapter 1 Wellness and Health Actions 3
Defining Health and Wellness 5
  Dimensions of Health and Wellness 6
  Guidelines to Your Good Health: Achieving Self-Responsibility 7
Holistic Health 10
Factors Affecting Health and Wellness 10
  How Healthy Do I Have To Be? 13
  Quality of Life/Quantity of Life 13
Motivation and Health Behavior 15
  Some General Principles of Motivation 16
  Maslow's Hierarchy of Needs 17
Behavior As a Learned Trait 18
  Personal Perceptions of Health 18
Behavior-Change Strategies 19
  Problem Solving 19
  Analyzing Problem Situations 20
  Guidelines to Your Good Health: Achieving Self Control 21
  Self-Management and Change 22
  Behavioral-Change Contracts 23
Self-Inventory 1.1 Healthful Lifestyle 24
  Guidelines to Your Good Health: Developing Contracts 26
Positive Behaviors 26
Positive Behaviors 27
Now You Know 28
Summary 28
References 29
Suggested Readings 29

Chapter 2 Mental Well-Being 31
What Is Mental Wellness? 32
  Normality 33
Self Esteem 33
  The True or Accurate Self 33
  Guidelines to Your Good Health: Fulfilling Your "Self" 34
  Self-Concept 34
Spiritual Well-Being 36
  Aspects of Spiritual Awareness 36
  Guidelines to Your Good Health: Spiritual Awareness 36
Self-Inventory 2.1 Spiritual Wellness Assessment 38
Enhancing Mental Wellness 40
  Your Good Listener/Friend 41
Expressing Emotions 41
  Joy/Sadness 42
  Depression 42
  Anger 44
  Guilt 44
  Anxiety and Fear 45
  Loneliness 45
  Shyness 46
Suicide 46
Self-Inventory 2.2 Mental Health Assessment 47
Mental Ill Health 49
  Mental Illness Defined 49
Caring For Mental Health Problems 49
  Types of Psychotherapies 50
  Mental Health Practitioners 50
Issues in Mental Health 52
Positive Behaviors 53
Now You Know 54
Summary 54
References 55
Suggested Readings 56

Chapter 3 Managing Stress 57
What Is Stress? 58
  Physiology of Stress 59
  Patterns of Stress 59
Sources of Stress 61
  Life Events and Change 61
Self-Inventory 3.1 The Social Readjustment Rating Scale 63
Self-Inventory 3.2 A Social Readjustment Rating Scale for College Students 64
  Managing Crises 66
Manifestations Of Stress 69
Managing Your Stress 70
  Coping Strategies 70
  Guidelines to Your Good Health: Positive Thinking 71
  Relaxation Techniques 72

CONTENTS

Guidelines to Your Good Health: Meditative Technique 73
Keeping a Journal 74
Social Well-Being And Stress 75
Guidelines to Your Good Health: Personal Journals 75
Social Support and Health 76
How Social Supports Help 77
Positive Behaviors 79
Now You Know 80
Summary 80
References 81
Suggested Readings 81

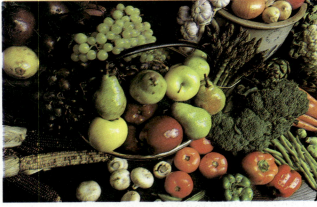

SECTION II   Body Dynamics 83

Chapter 4   Food Facts   85
Dietary Guidelines for Americans 88
What Are Nutrients 88
Calorie Awareness 90
Carbohydrates: The Total Picture 91
Simple Carbohydrates or Sugars 92
Guidelines to Your Good Health: Minimizing Sugar 93
Complex Carbohydrates or Starches 93
Fiber 94
Guidelines to Your Good Health: Increasing Fiber 95
Protein 95
Protein for the Vegetarian 97
Fats 98
Triglycerides 99
Cholesterol 100
Vitamins 102
Minerals 104
Guidelines to Your Good Health: Vitamins and Minerals 106
Electrolytes 106
The Trace Mineral Iron 107

Vitamin and Mineral Supplements 109
Water 110
Health Foods 111
An Anti-Cancer Diet 112
Self-Inventory 4.1   Are You a Healthy Eater? 114
Positive Behaviors 115
Now You Know 116
Summary 116
References 117
Suggested Readings 117

Chapter 5   Eating Behaviors   119
Body Weight 120
Body Composition 121
The Body Fat Component 122
The Lean Body Mass Component 122
The Decision to Lose Weight 122
Assessment of Eating Habits 124
Understanding the Labels 125
The Decision to Gain Weight 126
Theories of Weight Control 127
Genetic Predisposition Theory 128
Fat-Cell Theory 129
White Fat versus Brown Fat Activity Theory 129
The Setpoint Theory 130
Weight Reduction 131
Guidelines to Your Good Health: Weight-Reduction Diets 132
Popular Diets 132
Prescription Diet Pills 134
Over-the-Counter Diet Preparations 134
Surgical Procedures 135
Self-Help Groups 136
Self-Inventory 5.1   Are You in Control of Your Weight? 137
Eating Disorders 138
Anorexia Nervosa 138
Bulimia 139
Positive Behaviors 141
Now You Know 142
Summary 142
References 143
Suggested Readings 143

Chapter 6   Getting Physical   145
Definition of Physical Fitness 146
Components of Physical Fitness 147
Benefits of Exercise 148
Disease Prevention 149
Physiological Benefits 149
Psychological Benefits 151
Principles of a Fitness Program 152
Controversy over Activity Level 153
Guidelines to Your Good Health: Planning an Exercise Program 155

Self-Inventory 6.1 ■ How Physically Fit
    Are You? 156
Developing Your Exercise Program 158
    Evaluation of Current Physical Fitness Level 158
    Defining Your Goals 159
    Choosing Your Exercise Activities 159
    Guidelines to Your Good Health: Choosing Exercise
        Shoes 162
    Reviewing Your Resources 167
    Designing Your Plan 167
Athletic Training 169
    Concepts of Training 169
    Carbohydrate Loading 170
    Steroids 170
Positive Behaviors 171
Now You Know 172
Summary 172
References 173
Suggested Readings 173

SECTION III ■ Understanding Sexuality 175

Chapter 7 Relationships 177
Foundations for a Healthy Relationship 178
Healthy versus Unhealthy Love in Adult
    Relationships 180
Exploitive Behavior 181
    Guidelines to Your Good Health: Helping a Rape
        Victim 181
Love and Physical Intimacy 182
The Romantic Love Cycle 183
Communication Skills 186
    Guidelines to Your Good Health: Contact and the Four
        "Cs" 188
Effective Communication in a Relationship 188
When Love Blooms: Getting Married 189
When Love Fades: Getting Divorced 190
Picking Up the Pieces 191
Self-Inventory 7.1 ■ How Confident Are You in
    Social Situations? 192
Positive Behaviors 194
Now You Know 195
Summary 195
References 196
Suggested Readings 196

Chapter 8 Sexual Bodyworks 197
Sexual Anatomy and Physiology: Male 198
    External Genitals 198
    Internal Organs 200
    Genital Ducts 200
    Fluid-Producing Glands 200

Sexual Anatomy and Physiology: Female 201
    External Genitals 201
    Internal Organs 202
Hormones and Sexual Functioning 205
The Major Sex Hormones 206
    Testosterone 206
    Estrogen 207
    Progesterone 207
Sexual Preferences and Behaviors 207
The Sexual Response Cycle 208
The Menstrual Cycle 210
    Follicular Phase 212
    Ovulation 212
    Luteal Phase 212
    Menstruation 212
Menstrual Synchrony 213
Menstrual Myths 213
Toxic Shock Syndrome 214
Premenstrual Syndrome 214
    Guidelines to Your Good Health: Using Tampons 215
Positive Behaviors for Males 216
Positive Behaviors for Females 217
Now You Know 218
Summary 218
References 219
Suggested Readings 219

Chapter 9 Family Planning 221
Responsible Sexual Behavior 222
Birth Control versus Contraception 223
Birth-Control Options 223
Self-Inventory 9.1 ■ What Is Your Attitude about
    Birth Control? 224
    Guidelines to Your Good Health: Using
        Contraceptives 228
    Guidelines to Your Good Health: Oral Contraceptive
        Risks 231
Abortive Procedures 246
    Postcoital Methods 247
    First-Trimester Methods 248
    Second-Trimester Methods 249
    The Abortion Pill 249
Future Trends 250
Self-Inventory 9.2 ■ Which Method of Birth Control
    Should You Use? 252
Positive Behaviors 253
Now You Know 254
Summary 254
References 255
Suggested Readings 255

Chapter 10 Conception Through Birth 257
The Sexual Beginning 258
Sperm Production 258
Egg Production 258

xii CONTENTS

The Process of Fertilization and Implementation 258
Gender Differentiation: Prenatal Variables 260
  Genetic Gender 260
  Gonadal Gender 260
  Hormonal Gender 260
  Genital Gender 261
Determining Your Child's Sex 261
The Question of Parenthood 262
  Guidelines to Your Good Health: Choosing to Have a Child 263
Pregnancy 264
  Pregnancy Testing 264
  Pregnancy and Diet 264
  Pregnancy and Activity 266
Fetal Development 267
  First Trimester 267
  Second Trimester 268
  Third Trimester 268
Childbirth 268
  First Stage of Labor 268
  Second Stage of Labor 269
  Third Stage of Labor 269
Gender Differentiation: Postnatal Variables 270
Positive Behaviors 271
Now You Know 272
Summary 272
References 273
Suggested Readings 273

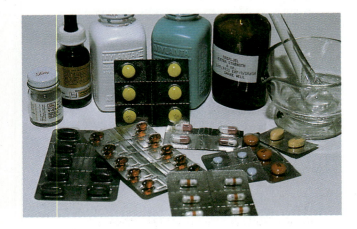

SECTION IV ■ Drugs and Your Body 275

Chapter 11 The Tobacco Road 277
The Nervous System 278
Basic Facts About Smoking 279
  Smoking and Life-Style 279
  Economics of Tobacco 281
Nicotine Addiction 282
The Major Constituents of Cigarette Smoke 282

Self-Inventory 11.1 ■ Why Do You Smoke? 283
  Nicotine 284
  Carbon Monoxide 284
  Tars 285
Smoking and Health 285
  Smoking and Cancer 285
  Smoking and Respiratory Disease 285
  Smoking and Cardiovascular Disease 286
  Smoking and Other Diseases 287
  Smoking and Pregnancy 287
  Smoking and Aging 288
  Guidelines to Your Good Health: Reducing Smoking 289
  Smoking and Life Expectancy 290
Smoking-Cessation Programs 290
The Benefits of Quitting Smoking 295
Involuntary Smoking 295
Smokeless Tobacco 296
  Guidelines to Your Good Health: Avoiding Second-Hand Smoke 296
Clove Cigarettes 297
Tobacco and the Law 297
Positive Behaviors 299
Now You Know 300
Summary 300
References 301
Suggested Readings 301

Chapter 12 Alcohol Awareness 303
Basic Facts about Alcohol 304
Pharmacology 305
  Absorption and Elimination 305
  Physiological Effects 306
  Tolerance 308
  Dependence 309
  Synergism 309
  Alcohol and Other Drugs 311
  Psychological Effects 311
Alcohol and Disease 311
  Alcohol and the Liver 311
  Alcohol and Circulation 312
  Alcohol and Cancer 312
  Alcohol and Nutrition 312
Alcohol and the Law 312
  Learn The Law 312
  Drinking and Driving 312
Fetal Alcohol Syndrome 316
Alcoholism 318
  Why People Drink 318
  Alcohol and Teenagers 318
  Guidelines to Your Good Health: Responsible Alcohol Use 319
  What is Alcoholism? 319
Self-Inventory 12.1 ■ Do You Have A Drinking Problem? 320
  Alcoholics Anonymous 322

Guidelines to Your Good Health: Coping with an Alcoholic 323
Positive Behaviors 324
Now You Know 325
Summary 325
References 326
Suggested Readings 326

Chapter 13 Psychoactive Drugs 327
Deliriants 328
  Volatile Solvents 328
  Poppers 328
Depressants 328
  Barbiturates 328
  Minor Tranquilizers 330
  Other Sedative-Hypnotics 330
  Opiates 331
Stimulants 332
  Cocaine 332
  Amphetamines 335
Hallucinogens 335
  LSD 336
  Peyote 336
  Mescaline 337
  Psilocybin 337
  Ololiuqui 337
  PCP 337
Marijuana 338
  Guidelines to Your Good Health: Avoiding Illegal Drug Use 339
Designer Drugs 340
  MDMA 340
  MDEA 341
  China White 341
  MPPP 341
  A Final Note 341
  Guidelines to Your Good Health: Responsible Drug Use 341
The Xanthines 342
Self-Inventory 13.1 ■ Responsible Drug Use 343
Positive Behaviors 345
Now You Know 346
Summary 346
References 347
Suggested Readings 347

SECTION V ■ Coping With Disease 349

Chapter 14 Understanding the Disease Process and Infectious Diseases 351
Disease Organisms 352
  Viruses 352
  Bacteria 353
  Rickettsia 354
  Protozoa 354
  Fungi 355
  Parasitic Worms 355
Disease Transmission 356
Stages of Communicable Disease 357
Prevention of Communicable Disease 358
  The Body's Defense Mechanisms 358
  Immunizations 359
  Guidelines to Your Good Health: Reducing Risks of Communicable Diseases 359
Miscellaneous Communicable Diseases 361
  Viral Diseases 361
  Guidelines to Your Good Health: Speedier Recovery from Communicable Diseases 366
  Bacterial Diseases 367
Positive Behaviors 369
Now You Know 370
Summary 370
References 371
Suggested Readings 371

Chapter 15 Sexually Transmitted Disease 373
The Scope of the Problem 374
  Sexually Transmitted Diseases Defined 374
  Factors Affecting Disease Transmission 374
Bacterial Diseases 376
  Syphilis 376
  Gonorrhea 379
  Nongonococcal Urethritis 380
  Chlamydia Infection 380
  Pelvic Inflammatory Disease 380
  Bacterial Vaginosis 381
  Chancroid 382
  Granuloma Inguinale 382
  Lymphogranuloma Venereum 382
Viral Diseases 383
  Acquired Immunodeficiency Syndrome (AIDS) 383
  Guidelines to Your Good Health: Reducing STD Risks 383
  Herpes Simplex 388
  Hepatitis B 390
  Human Papilloma Virus, or HPV (Venereal Warts) 390
  Guidelines to Your Good Health: Maintaining a Strong Immune System 391
  Molluscum Contagiosum 391
Other Sexually Transmitted Diseases 391
  Candida Albicans 391
  Trichomonas Vaginalis 392
  Pubic Lice 392
  Guidelines to Your Good Health: Reducing STD Complications 393
  Scabies 393

Prevention of Sexually Transmitted Disease 394
Positive Behaviors 395
Now You Know 396
Summary 396
References 397
Suggested Readings 397

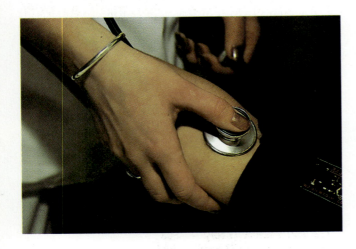

Chapter 16 Becoming Heart Smart 399
Risk Factors and Their Relationship to Chronic Disease 400
Cardiovascular Disease 403
 Some Physiology 403
 Hypertension 403
 Arteriosclerosis 407
 Guidelines to Your Good Health: Reducing Risk of Cardiovascular Diseases 408
 Guidelines to Your Good Health: Symptoms of a Heart Attack 410
 Atherosclerosis 410
Self-Inventory 16.1 ■ **Your Risk for Cardiovascular Disease** 411
Positive Behaviors 412
Now You Know 413
Summary 413
References 413
Suggested Readings 414

Chapter 17 Dealing With Chronic Disease 415
Cancer 416
 General Information about Cancer 416
 Terminology 416
 Benign versus Malignant Growths 418
 Risk Factors 418
 Cancer Cures 420

 Guidelines to Your Good Health: Reducing Cancer Risks 420
 Signs and Symptoms 421
 Types of Cancer 421
Self-Inventory 17.1 ■ **How Can I Protect Myself from Cancer** 427
Arthritis 427
 Rheumatoid Arthritis 428
 Guidelines to Your Good Health: Reducing Arthritis Risks 430
 Juvenile Arthritis 430
 Osteoarthritis 430
 A Few Final Thoughts 430
 Gout 431
 Ankylosing Spondylitis 431
 Systemic Lupus Erythematosus (SLE) 431
Diabetes Mellitus 432
Other Chronic Diseases 434
 Chronic Obstructive Pulmonary Disease 434
 Epilepsy 435
Genetic Disorders 435
 Sickle-Cell Anemia 435
 Cystic Fibrosis 436
 Tay-Sachs Disease 436
 Phenylketonuria (PKU) 437
Positive Behaviors 437
Now You Know 438
Summary 438
References 439
Suggested Readings 439

SECTION VI ■ Taking Control of Your Health 441

Chapter 18 Consumer Health 443
Consumer Protection Agencies 444
The Power of Advertising 445
Consumer Protection Skills 448
Self-Inventory 18.1 ■ **What Kind of Shopper Are You** 449
Accuracy of Health Information 451
 Guidelines to Your Good Health: When to Contact Your Primary Care Physician 452
Health Care 452
 Guidelines to Your Good Health: How to Find Physicians 454
Health Insurance 456
 Traditional Health Insurance 456
 Health Maintenance Organizations (HMO's) 458
Over-the-Counter Drugs and the Consumer 460
 Analgesics 460
 Cold and Allergy Preparations 462
 Guidelines to Your Good Health: Questions to Answer Before Taking Medications 463

CONTENTS

xv

Understanding Your Prescription   464
Generic Drugs   464
Drug Laws   467
   Legend Drugs   468
   Controlled Substances   469
Positive Behaviors   470
Now You Know   471
Summary   471
References   472
Suggested Readings   472

Chapter 19   Occupational and Environmental Risks   473
Sources of Toxic Waste and the Chemical Industry   475
The Hazardous Materials in Our Environment   475
   Household Hazardous Waste   475
   There Are Large Information Gaps   476
   Hazardous Wastes   478
The Nature and Extent of the Problem   478
   Human Health Effects   479
   Environmental Health Effects   480
   The Threat of Nuclear War—The Last Epidemic   482
   Guidelines to Your Good Health: Minimizing Hazardous Substance Injuries   484
Toxic Substances: Who Is at Risk?   484
   Workers   484
   Neighbors and Communities   484
DBCP: A Case Study   486
   What Is an Occupational Disease? Who Is at Risk?   486
   Sterility Is an Occupational Hazard   487
   Environmental Exposures Occur via Air, Drinking Water, and Food   487
   Who Diagnoses Occupational Health Problems?   488
   What Are the Health Problems?   489
   Could the DBCP-Related Sterility Have Been Prevented?   490
   The Right to Know   490
Community Health Protection   491
   Where Do We Go from Here?   492
Accidental Injury: The Number-One Health Problem   494
   Analyzing Accidents   495
   Motor-Vehicle Accidents   496
   Nonmotor-Vehicle Accidents   497
   Fires   497
   Guidelines to Your Good Health: Using a Fire Extinguisher Safely   498
Positive Behaviors   499
Now You Know   500
Summary   500
References   501
Suggested Readings   501

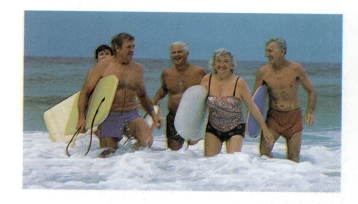

SECTION VII   The Final Transition   503

Chapter 20   Maturing Gracefully   505
Aging versus Being Old   506
The Process of Aging   507
Theories of Aging   508
   The Error Hypothesis   508
   The Free Radical Theory   508
   The Cross-linkage Theory   508
   The Brain Hypothesis   509
   The Autoimmune Theory   509
Ageism   509
Overcoming the Stereotypes of Aging   510
Self-Inventory 20.1   What Are Your Attitudes Regarding the Elderly?   511
Physiological Changes of Aging   514
   Wrinkles   514
   Changes in Hair   515
   Changes in Vision   515
   Changes in Hearing   516
   Changes in Bones   517
Alzheimer's Disease and Aging   518
Sexuality and Aging   520
Successful Retirement   521
Caregiving: Taking Care of an Elderly Parent   521
   Guidelines to Your Good Health: Seeking Help from Others   522
Positive Behaviors   524
Now You Know   525
Summary   525
References   526
Suggested Readings   526

Chapter 21   Ultimate Loss   527
The Role of Death in Life   528
Concepts of Death and Dying   530
Fears of Death and Dying   531
The Process of Dying   533

Self-Inventory 21.1 ■ **Hardt Death Attitude Scale** 535
    Guidelines to Your Good Health: How to Speak with a Dying Person 536
Dying with Dignity 537
Funerals 539
Handling Grief 541
Positive Behaviors 543
Now You Know 544
Summary 544
Suggested Readings 544
References 545

APPENDIX A ■ **First Aid** 547

APPENDIX B ■ **Classification of Mental Disorders and Illness** 555

GLOSSARY ■ 557

INDEX ■ 567

Preface

When the three of us were first approached by West Educational Publishing Company about the possibility of writing a personal health book, we were somewhat skeptical. Although we have a combined seventy years of experience teaching personal health courses as well as complementary areas of expertise, we wondered how we would be able to transfer our successes in the classroom to the pages between the two covers of a book. We decide to go on the premise that if we just wrote the way we conducted lectures and discussions in class, our book would be interesting to read and the material would be relevant to students' needs. This book, therefore, communicates with students, on their level, information about topics that are of most interest to them.

There is no more exciting and interesting subject to study than personal health and well-being. It is part of every aspect of our lives. We see health and wellness as a dynamic state of being rather than a static, precisely measurable entity—hence the book's title, *Health Dynamics*. Wellness is a holistic concept that connotes an everchanging condition of growth and development moving in a positive direction. With these parameters in mind, we have chosen an approach that has an overwhelming positive tone and that assumes a philosophy of self-responsibility.

This book has also been structured to reflect a relative balance among the following:

1. The presentation of information and concepts that enable one to make sound decisions.
2. An approach that helps students develop self-awareness and clarify attitudes and values that influence their behaviors.
3. An emphasis on the acquisition and refinement of skills that are necessary for the achievement of high-level wellness.

Most of the pedagogical features are aimed at achieving the last two objectives, as are the majority of learning activities described in the Instructor's Manual. The bulk of the material covered in the text and in-class lectures presumably focuses on the cognitive domain.

Organization

Although every instructor presents course content differently, we have attempted to arrange this book so that it reflects the most commonly used and logical organization. Each section (with the exception of Chapter 1) is freestanding enough to be covered in an sequence that best suits your situation.

Section I, *Health and the Mind,* covers three of the four dimensions of personal health—mental, social, and spiritual well-being. The book begins with a strong focus on personal behavior and the ways in which the individual can affect control over his or her life and health. The social and spiritual dimensions, although recognized as being just as important as the mental and physical dimensions, are not usually covered to any great extent in personal-health textbooks. We have gone into somewhat greater detail than most, but you may want to spend even more time on these topics. Chapter 1 lays the groundwork for the entire course. It not only defines the basic terms of health and wellness, but it also explains health-related behavior and gives concrete suggestions for controlling health actions that can be applied to all topics covered in the rest of the book.

Section II, *Body Dynamics,* basically deals with eating and exercising. These topics are presented early in the book because they are the two areas most frequently chosen by students when implementing a semester long personal-health behavior-change project. If such a health behavior-change activity is undertaken, the contract approach in Chapter 1 and journal keeping as presented in Chapter 2 will be particularly helpful.

Understanding Sexuality, as presented in Section III, emphasizes the positive nature of our sexuality. It follows a sequence beginning with presentation of the development of healthy relationships (Chapter 7) and continues through childbirth and responsible parenthood.

Section IV, *Drugs and Your Body,* looks at commonly used, abused, and potentially habit-forming substances. The topics are covered here in a nonjudgmental, straightforward manner, with the expectation that values and behaviors related to substance use and misuse will be explored in the classroom. Some of the pedagogical features in this section will be particularly useful in this regard.

Although the leading causes of death in the United States have changed in this century from communicable to chronic diseases, the control of both is equally important to our health and well-being. In Section V, *Coping with Disease,* the basics of infectious-disease control are first presented, followed by a discussion of sexually transmitted diseases (STDs), including up-to-date coverage of AIDS. The last section in Chapter 15 deals with the prevention of STDs. This chapter also includes material on life-styles and their effect on the development of such killers as cancer and heart disease.

Section VI, *Taking Control of Your Health,* focuses on citizenship issues related to health (i.e., consumer and environmental responsibilities). We have taken the liberty of including injury control within the framework of environmental threats. After all, accidents take more college students' lives than all other causes combined.

The book closes with a section on *The Final Transition,* which includes the topics of aging and dying. It was with some trepidation that we put these two topics together, because aging should be looked on positively as a fruitful time of life rather than merely as a stage before dying. Even the topic of death should be seen in a positive light, since it is a normal and expected part of life and questions about it address many of the concerns of spirituality.

Pedagogy, and Special Features

To make the information presented in the text more applicable and personally meaningful, the following pedagogical features have been integrated throughout the book.

What Do You Know?/Now You Know. Each chapter begins with ten statements, related to the content of that chapter, to be determined True or False. They are meant to stimulate the reader's curiosity about what's to come. The answers are given at the end of the chapter in annotated form in the *Now You Know* section.

Problem Situations. As a means of developing critical thinking and problem-solving skills, problem situations have been interspersed throughout each chapter. These are mostly open-ended situations that are geared toward the college-age population and require an application of the information contained in the chapter.

Guidelines to Your Good Health. These are practical suggestions that can be applied to one's life, giving students concrete actions that can be taken to improve their health and well-being.

Self-Inventories. Self-assessment instruments (many were originally created for this book) are useful for evaluating one's health and life-style. Although these will not provide a definite diagnosis, they do give feedback about desirable traits that the individual possesses and behavioral changes that may be needed.

Fast Facts. Up-to-date facts are scattered in the margins of the book to make the reading light and interesting.

Summary. At the end of each chapter is a summary of the major points presented in that chapter. This may be helpful as a study guide, particularly for essay questions.

Positive Behaviors. Because the bottom line to personal well-being lies in individual actions, a section has been included after each chapter that asks students which major positive health behaviors they practice. It is then up to each individual to decide whether or not the behavior is important enough to make any life-style changes. Keep in mind that none of us is a perfect paragon of good health behavior, but we can all improve our current health actions. If a major change is attempted, it is suggested that the contract approach presented in Chapter 1 be used.

Glossary. All boldfaced key terms are defined and listed alphabetically at the end of the book.

References. References listed at the end of each chapter include all sources that were used to gather information for the book. For the sake of readability, we decided not to use a formal footnoting system. Be assured, however, that we were scrupulous in our attention to detail and scholarship.

Suggested Readings. The most current and interesting literature available that relates to the material covered in each chapter is listed for those who care to read further about a topic. These sources would be a good starting point for gathering information for a paper.

Supplements

An extensive array of backup materials have been put together to assist in the teaching-learning process.

1. A "state of the art" instructor's manual with test bank has been prepared by Dr. Rebecca Banks of Mankato State University. It includes the following:

Overall course strategies that give suggestions for semester-long activities and approaches; *Learning objectives* to guide students and instructors; *Extensive chapter outlines* on which lectures can be built; *Discussion topics* aimed at stimulating class discussion; *Teaching ideas* that are pedagogically sound and fun; *Suggested readings* to accompany each chapter; *Video and film titles* that are available for purchase or loan; *Health-related software* that is currently available for purchase; a *listing of national health organizations and agencies* along with their functions. A *test bank* of multiple-choice, true-false, fill-in, and essay questions, which is also available on WESTEST software for IBM-PC and APPLE II microcomputers.

2. Videos on a variety of topics, some created just for *Health Dynamics,* are available to qualified adopters.

3. Transparencies, including many of the figures presented in the text, are available.

Acknowledgments

At various stages in the development of this book, numerous people contributed in a variety of ways. *Health Dynamics* became a stronger book with the contributions of each of these people. We thank all of them for their time and assistance.

- Adele Andres
- Dean A. Chiasson, MD.
- Ruth Heifetz, M.D., Department of Community Medicine, University of California at San Diego
- Christina S. Kinney, California State University, Dominguez Hills
- Marc Robin, Family Nurse Practitioner
- Diane Takvorian, M.S.W., Executive Director, San Diego Environmental Health Coalition

We are also grateful to the people who reviewed the manuscript at different stages of the project. Many of their recommendations have found their way into the final text.

Lou Albert
Los Angeles Valley College

Carolyn M. Allred
Central Piedmont Community College, NC

Pamela Andresen
Loyola University, IL

Rick Barnes
East Carolina University, NC

PREFACE

Bud Belnap
Weber State College, UT

Henry Baughman
Western Kentucky University

Robert Bowers
Tallahassee Community College, FL

Kenneth Briggs
Central Washington University

James Brown
University of Missouri

Donald L. Calitri
Eastern Kentucky University

David Diaz
Cuesta College, CA

William G. Dinsmoor
Shoreline Community College, WA

Frank Egan
Queensborough Community College, NY

Carlton Fancher
Central Michigan University

Sally Friend
Gavilan College, CA

Erwin Goldbloom
Los Angeles Pierce College

Ralph Grawunder
San Diego State University

Christopher Gussis
Montclair State College, NJ

James A. Herauf
Northwest Missouri University State

Marsha Hoagland
Modesto Jr. College, CA

Frank Hostetler
Northeastern Illinois University

Herbert Jones
Ball State University, IN

Mark J. Kittleson
Youngstown State University, OH

Vera Konig
Nassau Community College, NY

Warren L. McNab
University of Nevada–Las Vegas

Judith A. Nevin
University of Arizona

Judy Riggs
University of Southern Florida

Steve Sansone
Chemeketa Community College, OR

John Savage
New Mexico State University

Victor Schramske
Normandale Community College, MN

Albert Simon
University of Southwest Louisiana

Sherman K. Sowby
California State University–Fresno

David Wilkie
Cedar Valley College, TX

Barbara Wilks
University of Georgia

Janice Clark Young
Iowa State University

Virginia Kreisworth
Gerald Graf
Warren Boskin

SECTION I

Health and the Mind

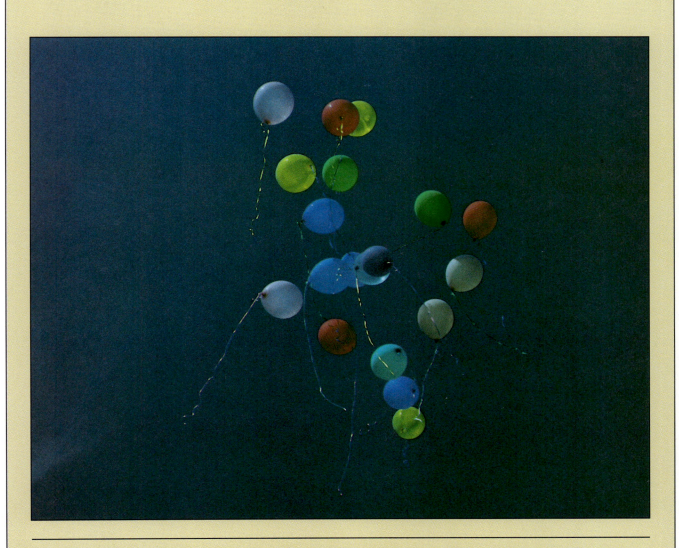

Chapter 1: Wellness and Health Actions
Defining Health and Wellness
Holistic Health
Factors Affecting Health and Wellness
Motivation and Health Behavior
Behavior as a Learned Trait
Behavior Change Strategies

Chapter 2: Mental Well Being
What is Mental Wellness?
Self Esteem
Spiritual Well Being
Enhancing Mental Wellness
Expressing Emotions
Suicide
Mental Ill-Health
Caring for Mental Health Problems
Issues in Mental Health

Chapter 3: Managing Stress
What is Stress?
Sources of Stress
Manifestations of Stress
Managing Your Stress
Social Well-Being and Stress

CHAPTER 1

Wellness and Health Actions

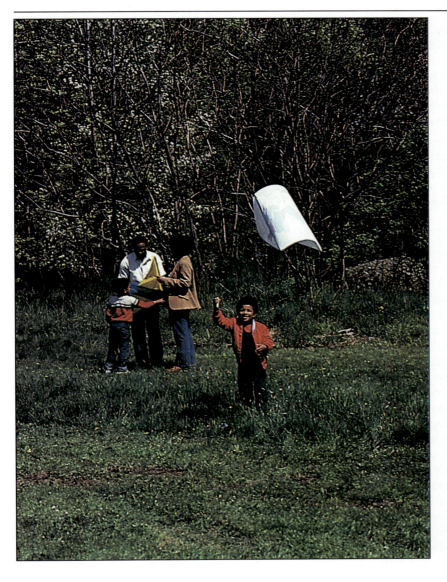

////// ⁄
What Do You Know?

Are the following statements true or false?

1. The greatest threat to human health and wellness in the United States today comes from chronic rather than acute conditions.
2. The concept of high-level wellness is dynamic, positively directed, and open-ended in nature.
3. Only two basic factors influence the health and well-being of members of a community—heredity and environment.
4. Physical fitness includes all of the following aspects: organic soundness, functional capabilities, *and* psychomotor coordination.
5. The synergistic integration of the physical, mental, spiritual, and social dimensions of wellness is known as holistic health.
6. The greatest motivational force in health behavior is the maintenance of one's self-esteem.
7. Overall, our peers exert the most influence over our health behaviors.
8. Even though people may be informed that certain behaviors are unhealthy, they may still act in a seemingly irrational manner because they are trying to satisfy two or more inconsistent or conflicting motivators.
9. Health behavior is based on whether or not similar previous experiences have been satisfactory. We tend to act consistently according to how our responses have been reinforced in the past.
10. A good approach to problem solving is to list all driving and restraining forces that bear upon a problem, evaluate the strength of each force, and choose to work on those forces that can be most easily changed and have the biggest payoff.

Consider this! On a typical day in the United States:

- 9,000 babies are born (1,300 are born out of wedlock).
- 5,200 people die.
- 5,000 people reach their 65th birthday.
- 6,000 couples wed (2,000 couples divorce).
- 1,370 men undergo vasectomies.
- 3,200 women have abortions.
- 2,700 teenagers become pregnant.
- Someone is raped every 8 minutes, murdered every 27 minutes, and robbed every 78 seconds.
- People drink 90 million cans of beer.
- People smoke 1.4 billion cigarettes.

Why do people do the things they do regarding health matters? Why do people jog, eat healthful foods, protect themselves from the sun's harmful rays, take mental health breaks, and engage in other health-promoting activities? Why do they smoke, eat junk foods, commit homicides, and engage in other negative health behaviors? The answers to these questions are based on a complex set of psychological and sociological principles.

The understanding of health behavior is particularly important today because in the western world, **morbidity** and **mortality** can be controlled more by lifestyle factors than by medical technology. According to Joseph A. Califano, former U.S. Secretary of Health and Human Services:

We are killing ourselves by our own careless habits.

We are killing ourselves by carelessly polluting the environment.

We are killing ourselves by permitting harmful social conditions to persist—conditions like poverty, hunger, and ignorance—which destroy health, especially for infants and children.

. . . You, the individual, can do more for your own health and well-being than any doctor, any hospital, any drug, any exotic medical device.

Just look at the leading causes of death in the United States today, and you'll see that they can be controlled, to a large extent, by human behavior. Table 1–1 shows that in 1900, the chief causes of death were infectious or acute diseases (influenza, pneumonia, tuberculosis, and gastroenteritis), but by 1950 and continuing today, the major killers are chronic diseases, particularly heart disease, cancer, cerebrovascular disease (stroke), and accidents.

Glancing at Table 1–2, you will notice that the risk of heart disease, for example, can be reduced by eliminating such habits as smoking, improving diet, exercising and managing stress. Alteration of your behavior will lead to control of both hypertension (high blood pressure) and elevated serum cholesterol (fatty deposits in the blood). There isn't much you can do about your family history except be aware of your inherited risks and take additional precautions if there is a high incidence of heart disease in your ancestry. Table 1–2 also shows that for communicable diseases such as influenza and pneumonia, you can lower your susceptibility by not smoking and by maintaining recommended vaccinations. The leading causes of death in the United States are mostly noncommunicable diseases. This means that by controlling your lifestyle and healthful behavior, *you* can probably prolong your life.

In this book, you will read about major aspects of your well-being with particular emphasis on understanding how you can intentionally influence your own health in a positive way.

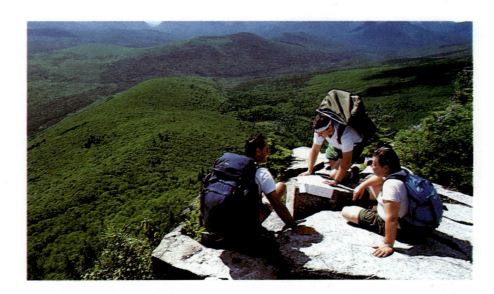

Health involves physical, social, spiritual and mental well-being.

■ Defining Health and Wellness

Health is defined as the achievement of spiritual, social, mental, and physical fitness that enables one to live life to the fullest. It is a state of being rather than an action leading to good or poor health. **Wellness** is defined as the optimal functioning of each individual at the present time within genetic limits and

TABLE 1–1 ■ The Ten Leading Causes of Death in the United States

1900	1950	1988
1. Influenza and pneumonia	Heart disease	Heart disease
2. Tuberculosis	Cancer	Cancer
3. Gastroenteritis/ Diarrhea	Cerebrovascular disease	Cerebrovascular disease
4. Heart disease	Accidents	Accidents
5. Cerebrovascular disease	Influenza and pneumonia	Chronic obstructive pulmonary disease
6. Nephritis	Diseases of early infancy	Influenza and pneumonia
7. Accidents	Diabetes	Diabetes
8. Cancer	Suicide	Suicide
9. Diseases of early infancy	Chronic liver disease and cirrhosis	Chronic liver disease and cirrhosis
10. Diphtheria	Homicide	Atherosclerosis

SOURCE: National Center for Health Statistics, 1989.

TABLE 1–2 ■ Major Causes of Death and Selected Risk Factors, 1988

Cause	Percentage of All Deaths	Selected Risk Factors
1. Heart disease	35.8	Smoking, hypertension, elevated serum cholesterol, diet, lack of exercise, stress, family history
2. Cancer	22.5	Smoking, worksite and environmental carcinogens, alcohol, diet
3. Cerebrovascular disease	7.1	Hypertension, smoking, stress, elevated serum cholesterol
4. Chronic obstructive pulmonary disease	3.7	Smoking, air pollution
5. Influenza and pneumonia	3.3	Smoking, vaccination status
6. Motor vehicle accidents	2.3	Alcohol, failure to use seatbelt, speed, roadway and automobile engineering
7. Accidents other than motor vehicle	2.2	Alcohol, smoking (fires), drug abuse, product design, handgun availability
8. Diabetes	1.8	Obesity, alcohol, poor diet
9. Suicide	1.5	Stress, alcohol and drug abuse, gun availability
10. Chronic liver disease and cirrhosis	1.2	Alcohol abuse

SOURCE: National Center for Health Statistics, 1989.

environmental conditions. High-level wellness connotes an individual's positive progress toward a higher potential level of functioning. The future of a well individual is expanding so that what is possible tomorrow may not even have been conceived of today; in other words, well people are in a constant state of becoming more than who they are.

Dimensions of Health and Wellness

Each of the four dimensions of health—physical, mental, social, and spiritual well-being—will be defined here and discussed in greater detail throughout the book. Each dimension affects and is affected by every other.

Physical Well-Being. When you think of a physically fit person, what do you envision? Someone with well-defined muscles? An expanded lung capacity? Good coordination? Actually, all of these characteristics, and more, are parts of physical fitness. Physical well-being involves having the energy to perform necessary daily tasks plus enough reserve for physically active play and for emergencies, if necessary. It means having healthy organs as well as functional abilities. Even if our bodies are not completely disease-free, we can achieve high levels of wellness by adapting to, compensating for, or correcting pathologic disorders. Use Figure 1–1 to record your medical history.

Mental Well-Being. We can all agree that health is more than merely being physically fit. A sound mind (including the emotions and intellect) is also vital for high-level functioning. Mental well-being involves the entire person and includes a positive body self-image, a constructive personal philosophy of living, and supportive social relationships. It also involves satisfying work, enjoyable and worthwhile leisure activities, a happy family life, enriching aesthetic experiences, good personal relationships, and love.

Social Well-Being. Human beings are social animals. We live together and we depend on each other for meeting our survival needs. Those individuals who have strong social support systems are more likely to be in good health. A socially healthy person has a network of family members, friends, and others who can be called on in times of need and who are continually available to learn from. This is a two-way street, however, as we must give similar support to those around us.

Spiritual Well-Being. How can you get someplace unless you know where you're going? What good is it to achieve a high level of physical, mental, and social well-being unless there is some purpose to attach it to? The spiritual dimension is that part of ourselves that seeks to discover personal meaning in life. It is not synonymous with religion, although for many people this purpose is ascertained through religion. Spiritual well-being is the understanding of who we are in relation to the broadest concepts of being. It considers our changing

FAST FACTS

Experts are now agreeing that mental well-being, including a low-stress environment, is an important factor in the health of expectant mothers and their developing fetuses.

GUIDELINES TO YOUR GOOD HEALTH

Achieving Self-Responsibility Responsibility for the ultimate care of your mind, body, and spirit lies largely within yourself. Here are some guidelines to keep you on the path to optimal medical self-care.

1. Keep a copy of your own medical chart and a personal health history. (See Figure 1–1 for an example.)
2. Know when and how to self-diagnose and self-treat for minor illnesses and when to see a professional health practitioner.
3. Choose a medical practitioner who will work for and with *you*.
4. Have a basic home medical kit with medicines on hand to meet your daily and emergency needs.
5. Keep up with current health and medical information.
6. Keep a few basic health references, including a good first-aid manual, on hand.
7. Take a basic course in first-aid and cardiopulmonary resuscitation (CPR).

FIGURE 1–1 ■ Personal Medical Record

Important Telephone Numbers

Medical Practitioners:
_____   _____
_____   _____
_____   _____
_____   _____

Dentist and Dental Hygienist:
_____   _____
_____   _____

Pharmacist:
_____   _____

Therapists:
_____   _____
_____   _____

Family Health History

Name	Relationship	Birth Date	Blood Type & Rh	Occupation	Major Accidents, Diseases, Disabilities	Age and Cause of Death

Birth Records of Self, Children, and Siblings

Name	Date	Sex	Wt.	Blood Type & Rh	Apgar Score	Where Born	Attending Physician	Circumstances

Immunization Record (Enter month and year of completed series, boosters, and single immunizations.)

Immunization	Date Completed
Diphtheria, Pertussis, Tetanus (DPT) completed boosters	
Polio completed boosters	
Tuberculin test	
Rubeola (measles)	
Rubella (German measles)	
Mumps	
Tetanus boosters	
Others	

Periodic Physical Examinations

Date	Physician/Clinic	Ht.	Wt.	Blood Pressure	Findings and Advice

Individual Problems, Medications, Allergies

Condition	Special Instructions, Treatment, or Medication

Record of Illnesses and Injuries

Date	Nature of Illness, Injury, Surgery, etc.	Practitioner/Clinic	Treatment

nature, helps us define what the good life is, and concerns the establishment of long-range goals. It is, therefore, a core and unifying component of wellness.

Because spirituality is subjective and intuitive in nature, it addresses questions for which there may not be **empirical** answers. Each person develops his or her own spiritual identity in an entirely unique and individual manner.

> ■ *PROBLEM SITUATION* Your sister doesn't exercise, has no apparent purpose in her life, seems depressed most of the time, and has few, if any, close friends. What could you tell her about what's lacking in her life and how she might improve the quality of her life? Besides talking, what else could you do to help her start growing toward achieving high-level wellness?

■ Holistic Health

Continued growth and development are crucial to the achievement of high-level wellness and so is the integration of the four dimensions of health and wellness. The integrated functioning of the total self is called **holistic health.** Health is multidimensional, interrelated, interdependent, balanced, and harmonious. *Holistic* means to consider the "whole" person in his or her environment, not merely as the accumulation of parts operating in isolation but as a total functioning unit, with the whole being greater than its parts. Such an effect, where two or more factors acting together increase each other's effectiveness is called **synergism.**

Instead of concentrating only on disease processes and treatment, holistic medicine emphasizes prevention of disease and promotion of good health. The philosophy of holistic practitioners is not to treat diseases that happen to exist in people but to treat people who happen to have a disease. Doctors practicing holistic medicine consider the social and physical environments in which their patients live as these factors affect the disease process and the treatment regimen prescribed. They look at illness not as something to be overcome but as a positive opportunity for growth and understanding. As a matter of fact, the philosophy underlining holistic medicine emphasizes moving in a positive direction, because positivism nurtures the will to survive and be well whereas negative thinking causes fatigue and defeatism and inhibits the healing process.

■ Factors Affecting Health And Wellness

What affects the level of health and wellness that you will achieve? The usual way of looking at determinants of health is to break them down into categories

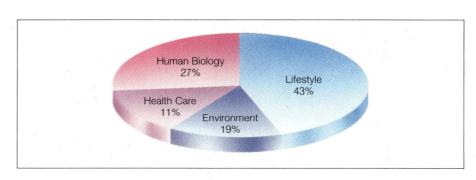

FIGURE 1–2 ■ **The Canadian Concept of Determinants of Health** Percentages indicate the relative allocation of mortality attributed to each factor.

SOURCE: Based on G. E. Alan Dever, *Community Health Analysis: An Holistic Approach* (Rockville, Md.: Aspen Systems Corporation, 1980).

of elements that interact in a health-enhancing manner. In 1974, Marc LaLonde, Canada's Minister of Health, identified four such categories—human biology, environment, lifestyle, and health-care organization (see Figure 1–2).

Human Biology. This element has to do with an individual's inherited capacities, the aging process, and the organic systems of the body. People possess a genetically endowed range of capacities that contain the potential for illness as well as for high-level wellness.

Environment. The environment's effect on our health is much more global and less parochial today than it once was. For example, the radiation emitted from the 1986 nuclear energy plant disaster at Chernobyl in the Soviet Union affected the health of people in countries thousands of miles away. Maintaining a safe and secure ecosystem involves controlling environmental factors to ensure clean air, water, and food supplies; safe sanitary and waste management; avoidance of noise pollution; a safe public-transportation system; secure social surroundings; and an aesthetically pleasing landscape.

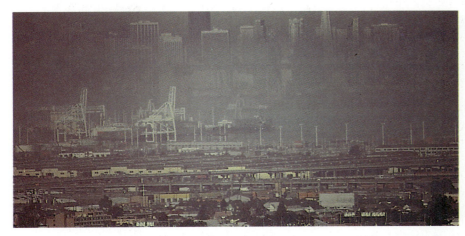

Environmental influences can be positive or negative.

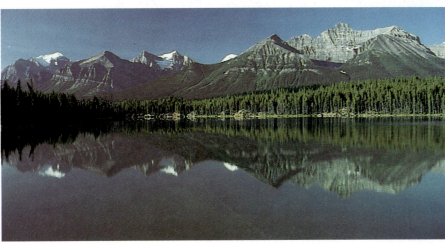

FAST FACTS

Approximately one-half of all the deaths in the United States have been attributed to lifestyle factors such as smoking, alcohol abuse, failure to use safety belts, improper diet, and lack of regular exercise.

FIGURE 1–3 ■ **The Healthiest Couple**
By William Carlyon

Lifestyle. Every minute of every day, we make decisions to act or not act in ways that will influence our well-being. The aggregate of these behaviors composes what we call our lifestyle. Personal health habits have become more important to longevity and quality of life, as we have overcome many of the communicable diseases and are increasingly threatened with chronic diseases.

Health-Care Organization. The provision of health care (by doctors, clinics, hospitals, and so on) is often taken for granted in the United States, Canada, and most of the developed world. Nevertheless, it is not always adequate for the achievement of wellness for all people. In a country in which the medical system is based mainly on fee-for-service payment for treatment, the poor and

---

"They brush and they floss
with care every day,
but not before breakfast
of both curds and whey.

He jogs for his heart
she bikes for her nerves;
They assert themselves daily
with appropriate verse.

He is loving and tender
and caring and kind,
Not one chauvinist thought
is allowed in his mind.

They are slim and attractive
well-dressed and just fun.
They are strong and well-immunized
against everything under the sun.

They are sparkling and lively
and having a ball.
Their diet? High fiber
and low cholesterol.

Cocktails are avoided
in favor of juice;
Cigarettes are shunned
as one would the noose;

They drive their car safely
with belts well in place;
at home not one hazard
ever will they face.

1.2 children they raise,
both sharing the job.
One is named Betty,
.2 is named Bob.

And when at the age of
two hundred and three
they jog from this life
to one still more free,

They'll pass through those portals
to claim their reward
and St. Peter will stop them
"JUST FOR A WORD."

"What Ho" he will say,
"You cannot go in.
This place is reserved
for those without sin."

"But we've followed the rules"
She'll say with a fright.
"We're healthy"—
"Near perfect"—
"And incredibly bright."

"But that's it" will say Peter,
drawing himself tall.
"You've missed the point of living
By thinking so small."

"Life is more than health habits.
Though useful they be,
it is purpose and meaning,
the grand mystery."

"You've discovered a part
of what makes humans whole
and mistaken that part
for the shape of the soul."

"You are fitter than fiddles
and sound as a bell.
Self-righteous, intolerant
and boring as hell."

W. H. Carlyon, Director, Department of Health Education, American Medical Association, Chicago. Given to "Promoting Health Through the Schools, A National Conference," August 25–26, 1980, Denver, Colorado.
SOURCE: Larry S. Chapman, "Developing a Useful Perspective on Spiritual Health: Love, Joy, Peace and Fulfillment," *American Journal of Health Promotion* (Fall 1987).

unemployed often find medical care to be inaccessible and unaffordable. A health-care system that is responsive to the needs of all people is necessary for achieving good health. In addition, economic and political factors must be considered, because they determine how much money will be allotted for health resources and where it will go.

How Healthy Do I Have To Be?

If you read the newspaper, you'll notice that there's a health-related article on page one of the main section almost every day. Most of these articles tell us what we need to do to improve our lot in life—as if anything but a paragon of healthful virtue is unacceptable. The poem, *The Healthiest Couple* (see Figure 1–3), satirizes playing it too safe. Enjoying ourselves, taking meaningful risks, and being healthy should go together. How healthy each of us chooses to be depends on what our goals are and how easily we can overcome any barriers that may prevent the achievement of those goals.

How do you feel right now? Okay? Not so good? On top of the world? How is your physical status? How about your spiritual, social, or emotional well-being? On a scale of one to ten, how would you rate each component? Taken as a whole, where would you place your health on a continuum of levels of health? If you were to create such a continuum, how would it look? What conditions would be at the top and what would be at the bottom?

Figure 1–4 is an example of a health continuum. Although this represents what most people think of as degrees of good and poor health, it may vary as values and cultural beliefs vary. For example, we usually think of death as being at the bottom of the ladder, but some people see death as the beginning of a new existence. Furthermore, definitions of what is functional or limiting and what is major or minor in the way of a disability or illness vary according to individual values and perspectives.

Quality of Life/Quantity of Life

How good is your life, anyway? What do you mean by "the good life"? Does it mean living for a long time? Does it mean being happy? How do *you* define

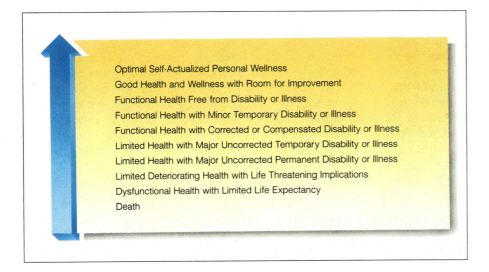

FIGURE 1–4 ■ **A Comprehensive Continuum of Health Levels**

SOURCE: Adapted from Howard S. Hoyman, "Rethinking an Ecologic System of Man's Health, Disease, Aging, Death," *Journal of School Health*.

FIGURE 1–5 ■ Selected Social and Personal Indicators of Quality of Life

Social	Personal
Illegitimacy	Self-Esteem
Population	Meaningful Employment
Welfare	Physical Well-Being
Unemployment	Meaning in Life
Absenteeism	Safety
Alienation	Love
Hostility	Relationships
Discrimination	Recreational Opportunity
Votes	Creative Outlets
Riots	
Crime	
Crowding	

SOURCE: Based on Lawrence Green, et al, *Health Education Planning: A Diagnostic Approach* (Palo Alto, Calif.: Mayfield Publishing Company, 1980).

happiness? Are there universal criteria for happiness? Where does wealth enter into the health picture? We're now going to look at some ideas about standards of quality of life and length of life.

Figure 1–5 presents a partial list of the social and personal indicators that may bear on the quality of life in a community. It's up to both the individual and society to define quality of life, but the definition differs according to circumstances of time, place, and person. Quality of life involves all of the dimensions of health and wellness discussed previously and is determined by the factors of a clean and safe environment, sound heredity, a healthful lifestyle, and the availability of good health care.

How long do you think you will live? What is your possible maximum **life span?** The *Guinness Book of World Records* lists the oldest person as having been more than 120 years of age when he died in 1986. Others have claimed to have been older, including Charlie Smith, a former slave who was reported to be 137 when he died in 1979. The Russian press reported in 1970 that the oldest citizens in the U.S.S.R. were a man aged 165 years and a woman aged 195 years. These claims have never been authenticated, and maximum life span for humans today is probably about 120 years of age. Do you think that with new technologies, it may be possible to increase life span by replacing body parts and using genetic manipulation?

Length of life, which is the same as **longevity,** refers to the average number of years lived by persons in a particular group. A more useful concept, however, is that of **life expectancy,** which is the average remaining lifetime for persons at any given age. Average length of life, therefore, is the same as life expectancy at birth. If you look at Table 1–3, you'll see that in 1987, life expectancy at birth was 74.9 years and at age 65 it was 16.8 years. That means that a person who was 65 years old in 1987 could expect, on the average, to live past 81 years of age.

Examining Table 1–3 further, we see that in 1900, life expectancy at birth was only 47.3 years. It rose to 68.2 years in 1950 and to 75.0 years in 1988. (To what factors do you attribute this gain in longevity?) When you look at the factors of sex and race, you'll notice that life expectancy is greatest for

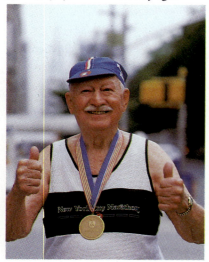

Quality of life is not limited by age.

TABLE 1-3 ■ Life Expectancy at Birth and at 65 Years of Age, According to Race and Sex

	1900 At Birth	1900 At 65 Years	1950 At Birth	1950 At 65 Years	1988 At Birth	1988 At 65 Years
All Races						
Both sexes	47.3	11.9	68.2	13.9	75.0	16.8
Male	46.3	11.5	65.6	12.8	71.5	14.5
Female	48.3	12.2	71.1	15.0	78.4	18.7
White						
Both sexes	47.6	—	69.1	—	75.6	16.9
Male	46.6	11.5	66.5	12.8	72.2	14.6
Female	48.7	12.2	72.2	15.1	78.9	18.8
Black						
Both sexes	33.0	—	60.7	13.9	69.4	15.6
Male	37.5	10.4	58.9	12.9	65.2	13.4
Female	33.5	11.4	62.7	14.9	73.6	17.5

SOURCE: National Center for Health Statistics, 1989.

FAST FACTS

For the 1.1 billion people (20 percent of the world's population) who live in the 40 poorest countries, life expectancy at birth is only 46 years.

females and whites. Relatively speaking, the differences in longevity between the races was much greater at the turn of the century, but average length of life is still significantly shorter for blacks in the United States than it is for whites. This difference is not due to genetics, so why is it that blacks have a shorter life expectancy than whites? (Incidentally, vital statistics have not always been kept separately for other races, so we can only compare blacks and whites.) Why do you think women live longer than men?

■ Motivation And Health Behavior

To what extent do you identify with the following scenario? You receive a notice from your dentist saying that it's been more than six months since your last visit and advising you to make an appointment for a cleaning and check up. You tell yourself that you'll call as soon as possible to set up an appointment, but you're so busy that day that you never get around to it. As a matter of fact, for the next week—what with school, studying, work, band practice, and social events—the dentist doesn't even enter your mind. On Sunday you see the notice from the dentist and promise yourself to call. You even jot a reminder down on a piece of paper, but for the next week you forget to look at the note that you wrote to yourself. Finally, after a three-week delay, you call for an appointment, which is scheduled for you in a month's time. When the appointment day arrives, you have two mid-term exams and tickets for a concert that night, and you forget all about going to the dentist. A week later you call to reschedule, and by the time you finally get to the dentist, three months have passed. Despite your good intentions, you have delayed needed health care by a substantial period of time, during which tooth decay may have begun.

We may have good intentions regarding our health practices, but we don't always follow them. In the preceding scenario, other priorities came before dental health. Why? What other factors might have been involved?

Some General Principles of Motivation

We've already seen that physical well-being is not always the major motivating factor in behavior. We choose those behaviors that we perceive to be in our best interests. By "best interests," we mean those actions that help us cope with living and especially those that maintain our self-esteem. We are motivated to do what makes us feel good about who we are now. Generally speaking, we seek pleasure and avoid displeasure. If the thought of visiting the dentist makes us break out in cold sweats and have other severe anxiety reactions, our internal defense mechanisms may tell us to postpone seeing the dentist. Time is important when considering the strength of a motivator, because we are most likely to satisfy the needs of the present. The further away from the present, the weaker the motivator.

On the other hand, if our intellect intervenes by telling us that delayed treatment may cause greater physical and mental pain, we may be motivated to prompt action. It is not easy to deal with these conflicting motives. The psychologist Leon Festinger used the term **cognitive dissonance** to explain how people are motivated to reduce conflict by seeking pleasure and avoiding displeasure. When two or more inconsistent cognitions (beliefs, concepts, directions, and even feelings) occur simultaneously, we are uncomfortable with the dissonance that is created. We deal with this dissonance by attempting to make the ideas or events be consistent with each other—that is, to fit psychologically. Reducing our dissonance helps us maintain positive self-esteem and keeps our ego strong. For example, people who smoke despite knowing the potential harmful effects of tobacco may reduce their dissonance by rationalizing that they have to die sooner or later, or they may simply ignore its illness-causing properties.

Along the same lines, we are motivated by a host of related and unrelated factors. We often think that single factors cause us to behave in one way or another when actually our brain considers multiple factors, consciously and unconsciously, in making decisions. For example, we are influenced by the expectations of our family and friends, the desire for sensory pleasure, the fulfillment of self-esteem needs, the avoidance of pain, and many other motivating forces that work simultaneously. Some of these forces are stronger than others, depending on the time and circumstances. In general, the desire for fulfillment of self-esteem needs tends to be a stronger motivating force than other needs, such as the wish for pleasure, as long as basic survival needs are being met.

On the social level, health behavior is strongly influenced by *cultural and class background*. Everyone belongs to a variety of cultural or subcultural groups simultaneously, and the combination of these groups determines the roles that you assume and your predilection towards certain behaviors. For example, as a member of the "student" group, you may be expected to "act as students normally do." You also have an ethnic heritage with which you may identify, whether it be Irish, Hispanic, Jewish, Moslem, Oriental, African, and so on.

The influence of certain vital people in our lives cannot be overlooked. The term **significant others** has been coined to identify those people to whom we are closest and who mean the most to us. Obviously, people such as our parents, lovers/spouses, close friends, and even teachers exert a tremendous pressure on us to behave in certain ways. We model much of our behavior after those people whose opinions we value.

Maslow's Hierarchy of Needs

The theory of human motivation developed by Abraham Maslow is a good example of a holistic and dynamic model. It states that motivation is based on the attempt to fulfill certain basic needs, which are met in a hierarchical order. These needs include the following.

Physiological Needs. If we "listen to" our bodies, they will usually let us know what they need. Persons who lack the basics are likely to first be motivated to meet their physiological or survival needs for air, water, food, and warmth.

Safety Needs. If our physiological needs are being met, we become motivated to meet the needs for security, stability, dependency, structure, order, and freedom from fear and anxiety. As with any other category of needs, people may dwell on the satisfaction of safety needs to the exclusion of meeting other needs. For example, some people never marry or move away from their parents because of an overdependency or unmet security need.

Belongingness and Love Needs. These needs are social in nature and point out the human quality that drives us to seek a bond with other human beings. The failure to give and receive love and attention results in loneliness and alienation and their concomitant negative effects. Families and other support groups exist for us, to a large degree, as a means of fulfilling the needs for belongingness and love.

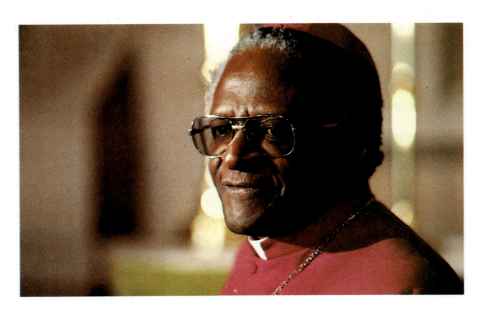

Someone such as Bishop Tutu of South Africa exemplifies a self-actualized person.

FIGURE 1–6 ■ **Characteristics of Self-Actualized Individuals**

- Have accurate perception of reality
- Accept their own real nature
- Are spontaneous
- Are centered on broader, more eternal matters rather than on trivia
- Are comfortable with solitude
- Are autonomous and independent
- Have fresh appreciation of basic good in life
- Are able to have mystical or peak experiences
- Feel love and kinship for humankind
- Are democratic, possessing qualities of respect and humility
- Have deep, profound interpersonal relationships
- Have strong ethical and moral sense
- Can clearly distinguish means and ends but can appreciate the means for its own sake
- Have sense of humor that doesn't poke fun at others
- Are creative and original
- Are resistant to enculturation
- Fully use talents and capabilities
- Are not perfect!

SOURCE: Adapted from Abraham H. Maslow, *Motivation and Personality* (New York: Harper and Row, 1987).

Esteem Needs. Most people have a strong desire to feel good about who they are. Much of our health-related behavior stems from the need to see ourselves as worthwhile, capable, and lovable people. Our behaviors are usually based on wanting to make more of what we are rather than wanting to change our self-image completely.

Self-Actualization Needs. Maslow identified our need to expand our potential and to become even more of what we are in all dimensions of our lives. In reality, few people are fully self-actualized, but it is a worthy goal for which to strive. Figure 1–6 lists the characteristics of a self-actualized individual. To what extent do you think you possess these qualities? Which ones do you think best describe you?

■ Behavior As a Learned Trait

Our capacity to respond to stimuli, which we call behavior, is innate, but the way in which we respond or act is mostly a learned trait. If, therefore, a behavior is unhealthful, it is possible to unlearn it and replace it with a more healthful behavior. Keep in mind, however, that it is usually more difficult to change a poor health habit than it is to learn good health behaviors in the first place. As a learned trait, behavior is largely dependent on one's **cognitive ability,** which consists, among other things, of accumulating knowledge (facts), understanding what these facts and concepts mean, and being able to apply them to real-life situations.

Personal Perceptions of Health

Your likelihood of engaging in health-enhancing behavior has been expressed in what is called the *Health Belief Model*. This model is based on your personal

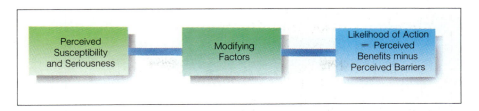

FIGURE 1–7 ■ **Simplified Health Belief Model**

perception and acceptance of the threat of a disease and consists of three components (see Figure 1–7).

First, how *serious* do you perceive a disease to be and how personally *susceptible* do you believe you are to contracting that disease? Individual perception is based on knowledge of the disease and its related consequences. For example, some people may know about the harmful effects of smoking but may deny that they themselves could actually get a disease such as lung cancer or emphysema. They may not even be aware of such denial.

Second, *modifying factors* refer to characteristics of an individual and the groups to which the individual belongs. It includes such factors as age, sex, ethnicity, socioeconomic status, and personality, as well as previous experience with and knowledge about the disease. It also includes information and advice obtained from health professionals, the media, and other sources.

Third, the *likelihood of taking action* is a result of the perceived benefits of a disease-prevention or health-promotion behavior minus the perceived barriers to effectively taking that action. Even if someone perceives a particular behavior to be desirable, that person might not take action if he or she has to give up too much to take it.

> ■ *PROBLEM SITUATION* Your friend confides in you that he has some symptoms of a sexually transmitted disease but denies that he could actually have such a disease because he has had sex with only one woman and she claims that she has not had another sexual partner. How could you increase his knowledge and improve his perception of the situation, help him to overcome his denial, and get him to go to health services for testing? How would you involve the woman who was his exclusive sexual partner?

■ Behavior-Change Strategies

Problem Solving

Can you think of some major problems that have come into your life? They probably took a good deal of effort, time, and emotional involvement to handle. Sometimes you were able to solve them adequately. Other times they seemed to defy solution; eventually they worked themselves out but not until you went through more suffering than necessary. Actually, if a problem is big enough and important enough, it would be to your advantage to use an organized, systematic approach to solving it.

The following are suggested steps to solving health-related (or any other) problems.

1. Determine the precise *problem*. When defining a problem, you need to consider its salient aspects and identify those people who are involved in both the problem and its solution. It is sometimes helpful to chart your behavior related

Doctors often diagnose patient complaints by following the common problem-solving steps including gathering information about the patient.

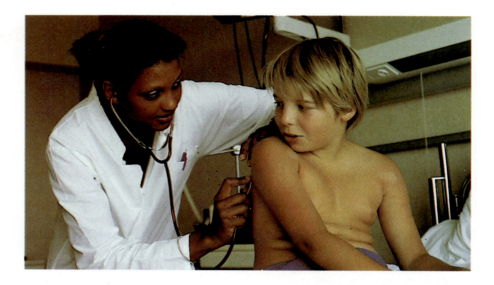

to the problem for a week or so. Include in this analysis where the behavior occurs, when, with whom, and other circumstances.

2. Define your specific *objectives* regarding the stated problem. These objectives should be stated in terms so that you can actually see or measure whether or not you've achieved them.

3. Decide on the realistic *steps to be taken* in reaching your objectives. Consider as many possible alternative strategies as you can, keeping in mind the limitations and availability of resources at your disposal (including time and money, if relevant) and the people who will be affected by your actions. The eventual strategy you choose should be feasible and aimed at reaching your stated objectives. Avoid putting forth more time, energy, money, and emotions than the problem warrants.

4. Now, *implement* these steps! If your plan is feasible and it's important to you to accomplish your objectives, you'll be more likely to carry it out.

5. Keep a journal or other *records* showing the effort and progress made toward achieving your objectives. At this point you may want to modify your strategies to make them more effective.

6. *Evaluate* whether or not you achieved your objectives. If you stated your objectives clearly and precisely, it will be simple to observe whether they have been achieved. This kind of personal evaluation is helpful as a reference when facing similar circumstances or problems in the future.

Analyzing Problem Solutions

Think of a health behavior that you want to change. It needn't be a major behavioral change, although the use of a special technique like the **force-field analysis** described here takes a little time, so you won't want to use it for every little change you want to adopt. If you follow the steps outlined here and apply it to the change you have in mind, you'll learn how to plan and implement changes in your life in an organized, rather than haphazard, manner.

The basic procedure in conducting a force-field analysis is to list all of the pertinent and important forces affecting the problem and determine their strengths. These forces are divided into two categories: *driving* (+) and *restraining* (−) forces. Driving forces are those that move or drive us toward a solution to the

GUIDELINES TO YOUR GOOD HEALTH

Achieving Self-Control Here are some steps for developing a healthy feeling of self-control and mastery.

1. Engage in as many tasks as you can in which you're likely to succeed. Repeated success raises feelings of mastery.
2. Become aware of the performance attainment of others with whom you identify (vicarious experience).
3. Listen to the *positive* things that others say about you, especially those whose judgments you value.
4. Listen to your body by observing your physiological states in various situations.
5. Finally, list those positive attributes based on past-performance successes, vicarious experiences, feedback from significant others, and observations of your physiological reactions.

problem, whereas restraining forces are those that act as barriers to achieving a problem solution.

When driving and restraining forces are essentially equal, there's a status quo, and behavior remains the same. When the forces are unbalanced, however, the behavior will move in the direction of the unbalanced force. By assigning a relative weight to each of the forces, we can determine which forces, when acted upon, will most likely cause a change and in which direction. Then we can, for example, remove or lessen one of the restraining forces, thus enabling the desired change to take place.

Figure 1–8 is an example of a force-field analysis applied to a hypothetical situation. As you can see, the strongest driving force operating here is that this person's friends jog. Couple this with "can't get motivated" as a restraining force of fairly high magnitude, and this person might come up with a strategy

Driving Forces	Value	Restraining Forces	Value
1. Weight loss	7	1. Heavy academic load	8
2. Cardiovascular fitness	5	2. Work 20 hours per week	8
3. Friends jog	9	3. Can't get motivated	6
4. Get into shape for hiking	4	4. No running shoes	4
5. Will feel good	5	5. Gets dark early in winter	5
6. Emotional stress outlet	8	6. Fear of injury	2
7. Was on high-school track team	6		

Weighted values: Use a scale of 1 to 10, with 10 being the strongest force.

FIGURE 1–8 ■ **Force-Field Analysis**
Behavioral Goal: To jog three miles per day four days per week

to get her friends to call her at a prearranged time so that they can run together. The heavy work and school loads are strong restraining forces that she might not be able to eliminate, but they can be lessened through careful scheduling and disciplined use of time. Restraining forces 4 and 5 can be eliminated fairly easily, and restraining force 6 is not a major factor, so it can be ignored.

Take the health-behavior change that you thought about at the beginning of this section and perform a force-field analysis on it. Although you can affect change by either increasing driving forces or decreasing restraining forces, long-range goals are usually better met by removing restraining forces. Nevertheless, you may choose to work on both simultaneously.

> ■ PROBLEM SITUATION   Your group of friends go out for beer every Friday after classes are over. The drinking lasts into the evening and is usually repeated on Saturday as well. You are afraid that you and your friends are overindulging in alcohol, but they don't agree with you. Nevertheless, you resolve to reverse this tradition of heavy drinking on weekends. Analyze this problem using a force-field approach, keeping in mind that your goal is to maintain your friendships but curtail your drinking. You may make any assumption about this situation that isn't implicitly stated.

Self-Management and Change

How easy is it for you to change your way of living? If you're like most people, it will be relatively easy to change small, rather inconsequential behaviors merely through the exertion of will. However, when it comes to major, deeply ingrained health habits, you must usually resort to other techniques. Because people's habits are not easy to change, the social and physical environment must be altered to help change long-established behaviors. Few dieters, for example, can say to themselves, "I'm going to cut out 500 to 1,000 calories from my daily diet," and just do it!

Furthermore, change (even a small change) can be traumatic. Change almost always involves the need for other people to adjust their lives to accommodate our new behaviors. Also, a change in one aspect of our lives requires adaptations in other areas. If you were to begin an exercise program for an hour a day, you would have to give up whatever else you would have been doing during that hour. Even if it meant foregoing goofing-off time, you might miss that hour of doing "nothing."

Let's consider a program that you can use for your own behavioral management. It was developed by psychologist Carl Thoresen at Stanford University. Although it is best applied under the direction of a trained psychologist, you can adapt this approach for simple personal health-behavior changes. Once you have identified the specific problem you face and the objectives you wish to achieve, follow this four-step approach to successfully managing the identified behavior. To help you remember these steps, the acronym CARE has been coined.

Commitment involves identifying your beliefs about why the problem exists for you and why it's personally important to change your behavior. Unless you can see the relevance of changing your behavior, it's not likely that you'll put forth much effort to change it.

Awareness means understanding exactly what the problem is and all that it entails. This is why it is vital to state the problem and all of its pertinent aspects as accurately and fully as possible.

Restructuring of the environment is a key to behavioral conditioning. If environmental stimuli lead to an unwanted response, such as eating cookies and candy, you can get the responses you want by providing an environment that will most likely elicit the desired responses. If eating sweets is the problem, not keeping sweets around the house may help you to cut down on these unwanted calories. If other members of the household insist on having cookies and candy in the house, you can at least store them in a place where they can't be seen or are hard to get to. You can also ask significant others in the household not to eat these foods in your presence. You can place a sign on the cupboard where cookies and other sweets are kept that reads "THINK TWICE!" Besides these steps to avoid sweets, you can also buy low-calorie foods to snack on.

Evaluation of the consequences (and personal standards) is, as usual, the final step in this process. You must judge whether or not you affected the desired behavioral change both immediately and in the long term.

> ■ **PROBLEM SITUATION** You strongly believe that you are overindulging in junk foods, both at mealtimes and for snacks. Using the CARE approach to behavioral self-management, outline a program that will help you overcome this excessive, unhealthful behavior.

Behavioral-Change Contracts

A tried and true approach to formalizing any health-behavior change that you've deemed important is to draw up a contract, such as the one in Figure 1–9,

---

I, Florence Smith, snack on too many sweets. My roommate, Lucinda Jones, keeps cookies and cake in the kitchen but she is able to resist overindulging in these foods.

My target behavior is to eat at least two servings of fresh fruit between meals or as dessert and to have no sweets for snacks. As a result, I expect to have a slight weight loss and an improved self-image.

My sister, Amanda Smith, will give me a $25 gift certificate for Henderson's Department Store if I have eaten two separate servings of fresh fruit and no sweets for 30 consecutive days, beginning tomorrow.

Lucinda Jones has agreed not to keep cookies or other sweets in the kitchen or in any other visible place in the house. I will know that I have achieved my target goal when I have had only fresh-fruit snacks twice a day for 30 days. My roommate, Lucinda, will sign the daily record that I will keep verifying that I have snacked only on fresh fruits each day. My long-term intention is to continue to eat fresh-fruit snacks as part of my diet.

Signed _____   _____
            Florence Smith   Date

         _____   _____
            Amanda Smith   Lucinda Jones

FIGURE 1–9 ■ **A Sample Health-Behavior Contract**

SELF-INVENTORY 1.1

Healthful Lifestyle

There are six sections to this inventory: smoking, alcohol and drugs, nutrition, exercise and fitness, stress management, and safety. Complete each section by circling the number corresponding to the answer that best describes your behavior. Then add the numbers you have circled to determine your score for that section. Write the score at the bottom of each section. The highest score that you can earn for each section is 10.

Cigarette Smoking

If you never smoke, enter a score of 10 for this section and go to the next section, Alcohol and Drugs.

1. I avoid smoking cigarettes. *Almost Always* (2), *Sometimes* (1), *Almost Never* (0).
2. I smoke only cigarettes low in tar and nicotine. *Almost Always* (2), *Sometimes* (1), *Almost Never* (0).

Smoking Score:_____

Alcohol and Drugs

1. I avoid drinking alcoholic beverages, or I drink no more than one or two drinks a day. *Almost Always* (4), *Sometimes* (1), *Almost Never* (0).
2. I avoid using alcohol or other drugs (especially illegal drugs) as a way of handling stressful situations or the problems in my life. *Almost Always* (2), *Sometimes* (1), *Almost Never* (0).
3. I am careful not to drink alcohol when taking certain medicines (for example, medicines for sleeping, pain, colds, or allergies) or when pregnant. *Almost Always* (2), *Sometimes* (1), *Almost Never* (0).
4. I read and follow the label directions when using prescribed and over-the-counter drugs. *Almost Always* (2), *Sometimes* (1), *Almost Never* (0).

Alcohol and Drugs Score:_____

Eating Habits

1. I eat a variety of foods each day, such as fruits and vegetables, whole grain breads and cereals, lean meats, dairy products, dried peas and beans, and nuts and seeds. *Almost Always* (4), *Sometimes* (1), *Almost Never* (0).
2. I limit the amount of fat, saturated fat, and cholesterol I eat (including fat on meats, eggs, butter, cream, shortenings, and organ meats such as liver). *Almost Always* (2), *Sometimes* (1), *Almost Never* (0).
3. I limit the amount of salt I eat by cooking with only small amounts, not adding salt at the table, and avoiding salty snacks. *Almost Always* (2), *Sometimes* (1), *Almost Never* (0).
4. I avoid eating too much sugar (especially frequent snacks of sticky candy or soft drinks). *Almost Always* (2), *Sometimes* (1), *Almost Never* (0).

Eating Habits Score:_____

Exercise/Fitness

1. I maintain a desired weight, avoiding overweight or underweight. *Almost Always* (3), *Sometimes* (1), *Almost Never* (0).
2. I do vigorous exercises for 15 to 30 minutes at least three times a week. *Almost Always* (3), *Sometimes* (1), *Almost Never* (0).
3. I do exercises that enhance my muscle tone for 15 to 30 minutes at least three times a week. *Almost Always* (2), *Sometimes* (1), *Almost Never* (0).
4. I use part of my leisure time participating in individual, family, or team activities that increase my level of fitness. *Almost Always* (2), *Sometimes* (1), *Almost Never* (0).

Exercise/Fitness Score:_____

---

with yourself that clearly spells out your precise objectives and delineates the agreed-upon contingencies or **reinforcements** involved in the behavior change. Reinforcements are any actions that support a behavior and can take the form of praise or material rewards. The reward must have a real incentive value to you personally and be contingent upon your actually doing the stated behavior. The sooner after the behavior that the reinforcement occurs, the more effective

Stress Management

1. I have a job (including school) or do other work that I enjoy. *Almost Always* (2), *Sometimes* (1), *Almost Never* (0).
2. I find it easy to relax and express my feelings freely. *Almost Always* (2), *Sometimes* (1), *Almost Never* (0).
3. I recognize ahead of time, and prepare for, events or situations that are likely to be stressful for me. *Almost Always* (2), *Sometimes* (1), *Almost Never* (0).
4. I have close friends, relatives, or others to whom I can talk about personal matters and on whom I can call for help when needed. *Almost Always* (2), *Sometimes* (1), *Almost Never* (0).
5. I participate in group activities or hobbies that I enjoy. *Almost Always* (2), *Sometimes* (1), *Almost Never* (0).

Stress Management Score:_____

Safety

1. I wear a safety belt while riding in a car. *Almost Always* (3), *Sometimes* (1), *Almost Never* (0).
2. I avoid driving in a car if the driver (which could be myself) is under the influence of alcohol or other drugs. *Almost Always* (3), *Sometimes* (1), *Almost Never* (0).
3. I obey traffic rules and the speed limit when driving. *Almost Always* (2), *Sometimes* (1), *Almost Never* (0).
4. I take precautions when using potentially hazardous products or substances around the house. *Almost Always* (2), *Sometimes* (1), *Almost Never* (0).

Safety Score:_____

Interpretation

There is no total score for this self-inventory. Consider each section separately. You are trying to identify aspects of your lifestyle that you can improve in order to achieve and maintain good health and wellness.

What Your Score Means to YOU

Scores of 9–10 Excellent! You are aware of this area's importance to your personal health and well-being. You are putting your knowledge to work for you by practicing healthful habits, and you are setting a good example. Keep up the good work!

Scores of 6–8 Your health practices in this area are good, but there is room for improvement. Look again at the items that you answered "Sometimes" or "Almost Never" and think about how you can improve. Even small changes can help you to achieve better health.

Scores of 3–5 Your health risks are higher than they should be. You need to take this health-education course seriously. Use the behavior-change contract form in this chapter to make important lifestyle changes.

Scores of 0–2 You are taking serious and unnecessary risks with your health. Perhaps you are not aware of the risks and what to do about them. Speak to your instructor about how to make the necessary changes in your lifestyle. Choose the most important and changeable behaviors, and make a contract that will enable you to implement these needed changes.

SOURCE: This self-inventory is based on *Health Style: A Self-Test* (Washington, D.C.: U. S. Department of Health and Human Services, 1981).

---

it will be, because it will then be clearly linked to that behavior. To establish a new behavior, it is far better to provide rewards or positive reinforcement than negative reinforcement.

If other people are directly involved in the new or desired behavior, their role should be clearly stated. You might designate a good friend to dole out your rewards when they are earned. The contract should be in written form and signed or witnessed by another person so that you will be accountable to someone besides yourself.

Finally, although you should seriously attempt to achieve the goals stated in your behavior-change contract, it will not be the end of the world if you don't reach the intended outcome. If you are unsuccessful at losing weight, if you are unable to stop smoking, or if you cannot implement an exercise regimen, you are still a good and worthwhile person!

Outline for a Health Behavior Contract. The following components should be included in drawing up any health-behavior contract for yourself:

A. I see the problem to be that _____ .
(Include what you do too little or too much of, who else is involved, and what the environment is like related to the problem.)
B. The target behavior that I am striving for is _____ .
(State the new behavior that will replace the old one, including short- and long-term goals, if appropriate.)
C. The results of the new behavior will be _____ .
(State the inherent positive results of the change.)
D. The conditions of the target behavior are _____ .
(Indicate the reinforcement that will be provided, other people who may be involved and how, the starting and ending dates, and the changes that will be made in your environment.)
E. I will know that I have achieved my behavioral-change objective when _____ .
(State a precise measurement that will tell you when and if your goal has been accomplished.)

GUIDELINES TO YOUR GOOD HEALTH

Some guidelines for developing contracts include the following:

1. Be fair. Don't make reinforcers too intense, although they should be motivational.
2. Be perfectly clear about the terms of the contract.
3. Be positive.
4. Be systematic and consistent in the terms of the contract and in the application of the reinforcers.
5. Have at least one other person participate in the contract.

■ POSITIVE BEHAVIORS

At the end of each chapter in this book, you will find a list of "Positive Behaviors" which represent the most important behaviors related to the topics discussed. It is an opportunity for you to assess which personal health actions you follow, which ones you don't, and which ones you'd like to change. Don't expect to engage in all of the behaviors listed; nor will you want to adopt every single positive health behavior in which you don't currently engage. Most behavior changes that you choose to implement, you'll probably be able to accomplish by making a commitment to yourself and using your willpower. For those you find more difficult to change, you may want to rely on the above outline for a health-behavior contract which can facilitate the achievement of your goals.

POSITIVE BEHAVIORS

I. *Place a check mark in front of each behavior that you now practice.*

_____ 1. My lifestyle is such that I have achieved optimal health and fitness in all four dimensions of physical, mental, social, and spiritual well-being. (LIFESTYLE)

_____ 2. I have attained a dynamic balance in my life so that I am functioning in an open-ended manner, integrating all aspects of my life in a positive direction. (BALANCE)

_____ 3. I take primary responsibility for my personal health and well-being. (SELF-RESPONSIBILITY)

_____ 4. I have a well-developed concept of personal meaning that gives direction to my life. (MEANING)

_____ 5. When I am faced with conflicting motivations or choices in making health-related decisions, I identify the negative and positive factors bearing upon the decision, take into consideration emotional aspects, and make rational decisions. (DECISIONS)

_____ 6. I am meeting all of my basic survival, safety, belonging, and esteem needs and even some self-actualization needs on occasion. (NEEDS)

_____ 7. When I implement a change in my health behavior, I am able to accomplish it by sheer willpower or by controlling my physical and social environment. (CONTROL)

II. *For each behavior that you DO NOT ENGAGE IN, write the KEY WORD(S) that is in parentheses at the end of the statement in the column below. Then put a check mark in the appropriate column to indicate whether you are going to keep or change that behavior.*

Behaviors I Don't Engage In   KEEP/CHANGE

_____ /_____
_____ /_____
_____ /_____
_____ /_____
_____ /_____
_____ /_____
_____ /_____

III. *For each of the preceding behaviors that you choose to KEEP, write a statement indicating why you are choosing to keep that behavior.*

I choose to keep behavior _____ because:
                                KEY WORD

For each of the preceding behaviors that you choose to CHANGE, write a statement indicating how you plan to implement that change.

I will change behavior _____ by:
                         KEY WORD

Now You Know

1. TRUE. The biggest killers today, heart disease and cancer, are long-term and chronic in nature and are best controlled by healthful lifestyles.
2. TRUE. High-level wellness is a dynamic state in which we are maximizing our potential within our environmental and genetic limits.
3. FALSE. Besides heredity and environment, lifestyles, the delivery of health care, and even economic and political factors influence health and well-being.
4. TRUE. Physical fitness doesn't depend merely on the amount of musculature we have or how we look outwardly but on how well our body functions in a dynamic way.
5. TRUE. Holistic health is not the use of alternative treatment modalities or adherence to organic living principles but an integration of mind, body, and spirit.
6. TRUE. The strongest motivating force is the acceptance of who we are and to like ourselves.
7. FALSE. Parents, because they are our first models and because of our life-long emotional attachments, are the most important and influential people in our lives.
8. TRUE. The tendency to try to restore psychological imbalances or inconsistencies is known as the balance theory of motivation. Cognitive dissonance theory states that we are motivated to reduce cognitive conflict in the easiest manner.
9. TRUE. Learned behavior stems from the interaction of individuals with their meaningful environments.
10. TRUE. This approach is called force-field analysis.

Summary

1. The leading causes of death in the United States today are chronic diseases, which can best be controlled through lifestyle-related behaviors.
2. Wellness may be defined as the optimal functioning of each individual at the present time.
3. Personal health and well-being comprise physical, mental, social, and spiritual dimensions.
4. The spiritual dimension of health and wellness is a core component because it deals with the search for meaning in life, which serves to unify all other dimensions in a meaningful way and gives direction to our morals, values, and behavior.
5. The concept of high-level wellness sees health as a dynamic, positively directed, and open-ended state of growth and development.
6. Holistic health is the synergistic functioning of the total self within which the physical, mental, spiritual, and social dimensions operate in an integrated manner.
7. The determinants of the health of a community's citizens are heredity or human biology, the environment, lifestyles, the health-care delivery system, and economic and political factors.
8. When making long-term health decisions, some questions to consider are: How healthy do I have to be? What are acceptable levels of health? What quality of life do I desire? and How long do I want to live?
9. Health behaviors are directed by many, often conflicting, motivating factors. The strongest motives are those that are directed towards maintaining one's self-esteem.
10. The needs theory developed by Maslow states that motivation is directed by the fulfillment of five basic types of needs—physiological, safety, love or belonging, self-esteem, and self-actualization needs—which are met in that hierarchical order.
11. The Health Belief Model explains the likelihood of people taking recommended health-enhancing actions according to (1) whether or not they perceive a disease as being a threat to them, (2) their individual and group characteristics, and (3) the balance of perceived benefits versus barriers.
12. There is a variety of behavior-change strategies available for us to use to control our health-related behaviors, including problem solving, force-field analysis, and self-management techniques.
13. Reinforcements necessary to maintain behavior change may consist of any actions that support that behavior. Whatever form they take, positive reinforcers usually work better than negative ones for the implementation of new behaviors.
14. Writing a contract with oneself is a helpful approach for controlling and changing personal health behavior.

References

1. Bandura, Albert. *Social Foundations of Thought and Action: A Social Cognitive Theory*. Englewood Cliffs, N.J.: Prentice-Hall, 1986.
2. Dunn, Halbert. *High-Level Wellness*. Arlington, Va.: R. W. Beatty, Ltd., 1961.
3. Festinger, Leon. *Conflict, Decision and Dissonance*. Stanford, Calif.: Stanford University Press, 1964.
4. *Healthy People: The Surgeon General's Report on Health Promotion and Disease Prevention*. Washington, D.C.: Department of Health, Education, and Welfare, 1979.
5. Hoyman, Howard S. "Rethinking an Ecologic System of Man's Health, Disease, Aging, Death." *Journal of School Health* 45 (1975): 509–518.
6. Lalonde, Marc. *A New Perspective on the Health of Canadians*. Ottawa: Information Canada, 1975.
7. Lewin, Kurt. *Field Theory in Social Sciences*. New York: Harper Torchbooks, 1964.
8. Maslow, Abraham. *Motivation and Personality*. New York: Harper and Row, 1970.
9. Rostenstock, Irwin M. "Historical Origins of the Health Belief Model." *Health Education Monographs* 2 (1974): 328–335.
10. Thoresen, Carl, and Michael Mahoney. *Behavioral Self-Control*. New York: Holt, Rinehart and Winston, 1974.

Suggested Readings

Ardell, Donald. *High-Level Wellness*. Berkeley, Calif.: Ten Speed Press, 1986.

Burns, David D. *The Feeling Good Workbook: Using New Mood Therapy in Everyday Life*. New York: New American Library, 1989.

Flynn, Patricia. *Holistic Health*. Bowie, Md.: Robert J. Brady Co., 1980.

Ornstein, Robert, and David Sobel. *Healthy Pleasures*. Reading, Mass.: Addison-Wesley, 1989.

Samuels, Mike, and Nancy Samuels. *The Well Adult Book*. Malibu, Calif.: Summit Books, 1988.

Sheehy, Gail. *Pathfinders*. New York: William Morrow, 1981.

Siegel, Bernie. *Peace, Love, and Healing*. New York: Harper and Row, 1989.

Weil, Andrew. *Health and Healing*. Boston: Houghton-Mifflin, 1988.

CHAPTER 2

Mental Well-Being

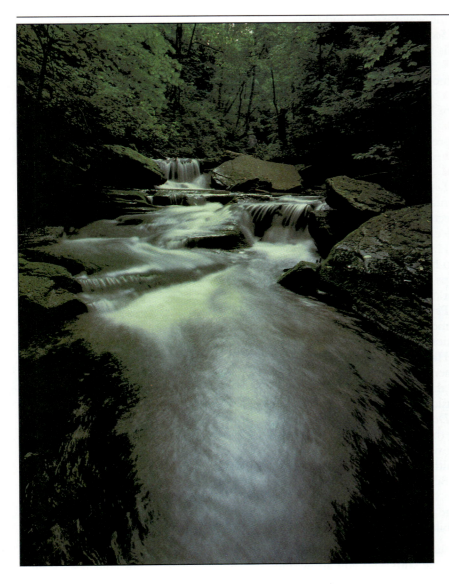

What Do You Know?

Are the following statements true or false?

1. The most frequently mentioned characteristic of mental well-being is love.
2. Your self consists of the roles you play, personal qualities you possess, and groups that you belong to.
3. You are a good person, lovable and capable.
4. Although spiritual wellness is a commendable goal, it is divorced from the world of science because of its vague and intangible qualities.
5. We learn about the meaning of life from painful as well as pleasurable experiences.
6. Depression is a state of mind that we all feel once in a while, and it usually doesn't require formal intervention.
7. Loneliness and solitude are synonymous terms used to describe alienation from society.
8. Three times as many women attempt suicide as men, but three times as many men successfully complete the suicide act.
9. Action therapy is the approach that acts directly on relief of symptoms rather than focusing on why people do the things they do.
10. Men and women are treated differently by the mental-health system.

What Is Mental Wellness?

This chapter emphasizes positive mental health and discusses what you can do to maintain a high level of mental health. In identifying what characterizes a mentally healthy person, we shall use the findings from various studies that define mental wellness as perceived by mental-health professionals. As you read through these findings, think about how well each characteristic describes you, which components you'd like to strengthen (none of us is a perfect paragon of mental wellness), and how you might accomplish personal change in these areas.

The components of mental wellness include the following:

- *Self-acceptance* connotes having a positive view of who you are. It means that you like yourself and have an inner harmony that comes from being comfortable with who you are.
- *Acceptance of others* is the ability to treat people as individual human beings, to see them as being more important than objects, and to respect differences in the way they feel and think.
- *Social responsibility* is perhaps more encompassing than acceptance of others. This includes a variety of characteristics:
  - showing appropriate social behavior by adjusting to social norms and mores
  - maintaining a social support system necessary to help cope with problems of living
  - having a special person or persons to talk to about intimate and difficult problems
  - associating with different kinds of people
  - contributing to the well-being of others
- *Love* has probably been mentioned most frequently as a characteristic of the mentally healthy individual. A loving person is able to give as well as receive affection. It is important to have a number of people to love in our lives, from objects of brotherly/sisterly love to parental love to erotic love.
- Having a *sense of purpose in life* not only makes living more meaningful but also has direct implications for mental wellness. Being guided by this purpose helps us to make sense of our perceptions of how things fit together in this world.
- Psychologists have consistently identified being *active and productive* as a trait of mental wellness. This means recognizing and accepting your assets and limitations and using the talents and resources at your disposal.
- Having a *variety of sources of gratification* enhances the quality of one's life in general and makes it easier to enjoy what one does. This means being able to do things alone or with others with equal pleasure in such areas as the arts, music, sport, writing, cooking, gardening, working with animals, and so on.
- *Dealing with stress* in a satisfactory, resourceful, and flexible manner is vital for the attainment of mental wellness. It requires adapting to changes in one's life when new information or new experiences are encountered. A mentally healthy person will deal with stress by using positive problem-solving skills.
- Being comfortable with the entire *range of emotions* that one experiences is also vital for high-level mental wellness. Mentally healthy individuals acknowledge anger, guilt, and fear as well as all of the positive emotions and maintain stability in expressing them.

In summary, you can be said to have attained mental wellness if you are comfortable with who you are within your environment, accept your roles in life, and have satisfying relationships with others. These abilities are not present at birth but gradually develop as you move through the complex stages from childhood to maturity.

Normality

Few people ever achieve all of the characteristics in the preceding list. How do you know, then, whether you are mentally healthy or not? Although there is no definite dividing line between optimal, normal, and abnormal mental health, it will help to examine the concept of **normality** and deviations from normal behavior.

Normality refers to a *range* of expected behavior and does not involve a precise measurement. In mental health, normality is limited by how most of society acts and how well individuals conform to role expectations. Although a certain degree of difference among individuals in our culture is expected and encouraged, people are generally rewarded for being close to the midline of the normal range and are sometimes mistrusted if they are too different.

Self-Esteem

Who am I? Why do I exist? What is the experience of living? Now that "I am," what am I going to do about it? How do I fit in with other human beings around me? Each of us is in the process of answering these questions every day as we make decisions and act. As humans, we continually grow and change in some respects, but we also stay the same as we strive to validate our current selves by being more of what we perceive ourselves to be.

The basis for healthful and positive self-esteem must begin with the awareness that you are good and worthy and lovable simply because you exist and that your worth is not a result of your belonging to a particular group, having been given a title, acquiring wealth, or achieving high status. You are a unique and beautiful individual with personal characteristics like no other. The perception of who you are is a function of the sum total of your experiences.

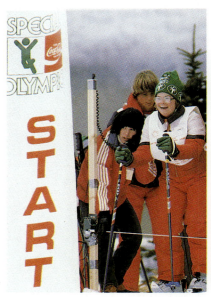

The Special Olympics allow for a wide range of competition so that everyone is able to perform at personally optimal levels.

> ■ **PROBLEM SITUATION** Members of your family have some strong expectations and perceptions about who you are, but they're not really consistent with who you think you are and would like to be. You've clearly communicated this to your family, but they continue to push their values and aspirations on you in areas that may include career, religion, marriage, and friendships. What can you do either to change the situation or to live with it?

The True or Accurate Self

Sometimes we perceive ourselves realistically, but at other times, for various reasons, our self-perception is inaccurate. We may think that we are better looking or have greater intelligence than we actually possess in order to gain self-esteem. Frequently we underestimate ourselves because we take other people's criticism of us too literally. Sometimes people try to elevate their own egos or relieve their self-doubts by putting someone else down.

There are times when we are unable to be our real selves for various compelling reasons. Imagine a little boy with a natural fear of animals who cries when approached by a barking dog. His parents may comment that grown men aren't afraid of such small animals. What a quandary that could present! The boy's true self wants to run from the dog, but his evolving self-concept, which also depends on what others will or will not allow him to be, prevents this.

How we interpret the reactions of others can be quite tricky. This is because they may not be responding directly to us as much as they are trying to cope with their own problems or self-esteem. Consider, for example, a person who is dying. This person is angry about his or her imminent death but doesn't know how to appropriately and directly express that anger. Frequently a nurse or orderly, being the most available person, will bear the brunt of this anger. It takes a strong and perceptive individual to recognize that he or she is not really the target and to react appropriately and constructively.

GUIDELINES TO YOUR GOOD HEALTH

The following checklist may help you in fulfilling the potentials of your "self."

- Develop an ability to perceive and judge others accurately.
- Accept yourself and others.
- Act simply and spontaneously.
- Focus on both your inner self and the outer world.
- Become comfortable with solitude.
- Seek and accept occasional peak experiences.
- Identify deeply with humankind.
- Possess a sense of humor that doesn't focus on others' differences or misfortune.
- Express your creativity in any appropriate manner.

Self-Concept

Who we perceive ourselves to be is a result of both **intrapersonal** (internal) and **interpersonal** (external) factors. Our uniqueness transcends traditional or typical behavior and is not limited by social expectation. Nevertheless, our true selves are not actually shown to the outside world. What is seen is that part of ourselves that develops in response to societal expectations. How we present ourselves is an attempt to appear as we think we should in fulfilling our roles. This means that others may initially react to us in terms of the way we look—how we carry ourselves, the clothes we wear, the way we fix our hair, and so on.

When you first come to a class, you present yourself to the professor as the person you are in your student's role. The professor forms a perception of who you are as a whole person, influenced by your dress, mannerisms, speech, age, attitudes, and so forth. He or she then responds to you, both verbally and nonverbally, in a way that reflects his or her perception. You, in turn, interpret that person's response and alter your future behavior accordingly. In essence, rather than showing the real you, you are putting on a "mask" that you want that person to see. To a large degree, people act as they think others want them to act.

There is, however, more to the self than we are aware of. There is an unconscious self, termed the **personal unconscious** by the famous psychiatrist Carl Jung, which can, through certain analytical techniques such as dream interpretation, be called to a conscious level. Jung also theorized that there is a **collective unconscious,** or deep unconscious shared by all. This collective unconscious is the result of all human experiences since the beginning of time.

In general, we act consistently within our prescribed roles, but occasionally we may seem to act out of character. As we continue to grow and develop, we need to alter our roles and try new ones. In order to promote high-level wellness, it is necessary to probe our potential, including all of our functional roles. Sometimes these changes are minor, involving such things are hairstyles, clothing, or friends. Yet at certain "seasons" of our lives, such as at the onset of adolescence, when graduating from college, upon getting married, when entering middle-age, or at retirement, we experience greater changes in our roles (which may be accompanied by increased stress). It is not always easy to readjust our expectations and responses, or those of others.

> ■ *PROBLEM SITUATION* You are about to undergo some major changes in your life involving new roles and relationships. You may be graduating, trading in your "student" role for a job title; or getting married, thus leaving the single scene; or perhaps buying your own home; or starting a family—parenthood! What changes in yourself and your self-concept can you expect to take place, both as you see yourself and as others see you? What are the potential positive and negative consequences? Should you take any overt steps to deal with this "new" self, and if so, what?

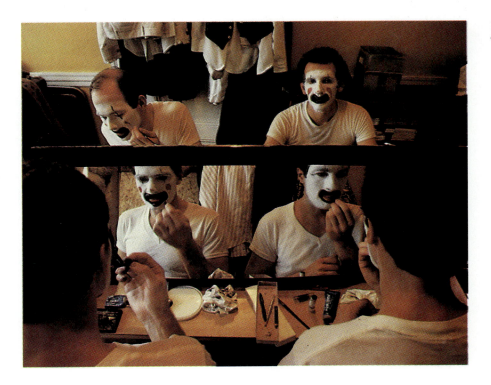

We play many roles and wear different "masks" in life.

Spiritual Well-Being

As important as it is to know who you are from a psychological standpoint, it is just as crucial to know yourself in relation to the total universe. This does not mean that you can expect to come up with clear and definite answers, but you should be able to at least gain some understanding of how your unique being fits into both the observable and the unexplainable world.

The very first issue of the *American Journal of Health Promotion* in 1986 contained an article by Larry Chapman, the spiritual-health editor, who defined optimal spiritual health as

> ... the ability to develop our spiritual nature to its fullest potential. This would include our ability to discover and articulate our own basic purpose in life, learn how to experience love, joy, peace and fulfillment, and how to help ourselves and others achieve their full potential.

The spiritual dimension gives direction and purpose to physical, mental, and social well-being. Having big muscles, a high IQ, and many friends can be meaningless unless it's considered from a greater perspective. From a societal point of view, the spiritual dimension is important because it provides us with basic values, standards, and codes of human decency.

Aspects of Spiritual Awareness

A survey of a group of health-education experts conducted by Dr. Rebecca Banks, a professor of health education, concluded that the most relevant aspects of spiritual awareness to personal health include the following components.

FAST FACTS

It has been found that qualities of hope, faith, love, determination (the will to live) and a good sense of humor can increase the rate of recovery from illness and injury.

GUIDELINES TO YOUR GOOD HEALTH

The following settings and activities can help nurture and intensify spiritual awareness:

Feelings of wonder and awe are often experienced when we are in touch with nature. This can be accomplished in the woods, on a mountain, at sea, or in some other natural setting.

Having "peak experiences," which are those special times in our lives when an event has occurred about which we feel so elated that words cannot adequately describe it. For some, a peak experience happens in a love relationship, when two people feel an intensely strong bond that seems to go beyond normal human interaction.

Solitary activities like spontaneous writing, reflective meditation, and even the reading of inspirational books help to expand spiritual awareness.

Those long philosophical rap sessions that you have with your friends and family are another vehicle for developing spiritual awareness. Don't avoid them, but try to remain objective.

Finding Meaning or Purpose in Life. The French philosopher and novelist Albert Camus said, "There is only one truly serious philosophical problem, and that is suicide. Judging whether life is or is not worth living amounts to answering the fundamental question of philosophy." Shakespeare said the same thing through Hamlet's words in his famous soliloquy, "To be or not to be." Our point is not that people should be considering suicide but that for life to be truly worthwhile, it must have some perceived purpose. There is purpose for everyone on earth, and it's up to each individual to seek that purpose. For this reason alone, the search is as important as the finding.

Establishing Moral Principles. In the process of searching for meaning in life, we are also determining what values to adopt and maintain as we carry out our daily lives. The moral code that we develop and live by represents our human dignity. It also provides us with some of the means by which we can create a meaningful life. For example, it is a woman's code of ethics and moral values that guide her if she has had an unwanted pregnancy to decide whether to carry her pregnancy to full term (with the options of keeping the baby or giving it up for adoption) or to have an abortion.

A Sense of Selflessness. The sense of selflessness and caring for others is that part of spirituality wherein we see ourselves as having a responsibility for the betterment of humankind because we see ourselves as an integral part of all humanity. In this respect, selflessness manifests itself as a willingness to do as much as possible for others while we continue to meet our own needs.

A Perception of the Cosmos. Have you ever wondered where the universe ends and if it does, what lies beyond space? Have you thought about the concepts of time or eternity? Does a reality exist outside of our abilities of comprehension? Human beings have always been driven to know what is currently unknown. There are some who claim to already have the answer, regardless of the faith they hold to. Others accept the unknown as something that can't be known in one's lifetime here on earth. Whatever you think about the nature of the universe, an important part of the spiritual dimension is to contemplate these eternal questions. We're not suggesting that you should spend inordinate amounts of time doing this, but you shouldn't avoid it, either. Recognition of your attitude toward the unknown influences your life decisions just as other aspects of spiritual awareness do.

Love. Once again, the phenomenon of love appears to be a necessity for achieving high-level wellness, this time in the spiritual domain. The giving and receiving of love is the essence of becoming self-actualized and of fulfilling our roles as human beings. In relation to spiritual awareness, love carries the connotation of humaneness and caring, which include justice, fairness, and com-

---

FAST FACTS

Experts are now agreeing that mental well-being is an important factor in the health of expectant mothers and their developing fetuses.

SELF-INVENTORY 2.1

Spiritual Wellness Assessment

For each of the following statements, circle the letter that best describes how frequently the statement is true for you. Use the following scale:

R = RARELY, if ever, true
S = SOMETIMES true
H = True approximately HALF the time
O = OFTEN true
A = ALWAYS, or nearly always, true

Sample Item

R Ⓢ H O A   I want to change but don't know how.
By circling the S, the respondent is indicating the statement is SOMETIMES true for him/her.

Questions

1. R S H O A   I find myself in a rut.
2. R S H O A   I'm confident in my ability to cope.
3. R S H O A   I live by my convictions.
4. R S H O A   My life has meaning and direction.
5. R S H O A   Self-improvement is important to me.
6. R S H O A   Life excites me.
7. R S H O A   I face situations I doubt I can handle.
8. R S H O A   When I confront choices, I am unsure what to do.
9. R S H O A   Life makes sense to me.
10. R S H O A   I lack the motivation I need to change.
11. R S H O A   I get bored.
12. R S H O A   I find myself at the end of my rope.
13. R S H O A   I know what I want from life.
14. R S H O A   I explore the why of life.
15. R S H O A   I achieve the goals I set for myself.

Score Sheet

Point Score 5 4 3 2 1

1. R S H O A _____
6. A O H S R _____
11. R S H O A _____

VITALITY TOTAL _____

Point Score 5 4 3 2 1

3. A O H S R _____
8. R S H O A _____
13. A O H S R _____

VALUES TOTAL _____

Point Score 5 4 3 2 1

5. A O H S R _____
10. R S H O A _____
15. A O H S R _____

OPENNESS TO CHANGE TOTAL _____

Point Score 5 4 3 2 1

2. A O H S R _____
7. R S H O A _____
12. R S H O A _____

RESILIENCE TOTAL _____

Point Score 5 4 3 2 1

4. A O H S R _____
9. A O H S R _____
14. A O H S R _____

MEANING TOTAL _____

Subtotals

Vitality _____
Resilience _____
Values _____
Meaning _____
Change _____

OVERALL SCORE _____

Interpreting Your Score

The Spiritual Wellness Assessment is intended as a simple tool to help you assess your level of spiritual wellness. Results provide scores on five different scales, plus an overall score.

The definition of the assessment scores follows:

- **VITALITY:** Provides feedback on your zest for life. High scores indicate vitality and enthusiasm. Low scores indicate boredom and stagnation.

- **RESILIENCE:** Provides feedback on your ability to cope with adversity. High scores reflect confidence in coping ability. Low scores indicate doubt about your ability to cope.

- **VALUES:** Provides feedback on clarity of life values and the ability to make choices. High scores indicate clear values and confidence in life choices. Low scores indicate uncertainty about life choices.

- **MEANING:** Provides feedback on your ability to find meaning in life. High scores indicate the presence of meaning. Low scores indicate life questions.

- **OPENNESS TO CHANGE:** Provides feedback on your motivation for change and your confidence in achieving the goals you set for yourself. High scores indicate enthusiasm for change. Low scores indicate potential difficulty in implementing planned change.

- **OVERALL SCORE:** A sum of five scales. Provides feedback on the overall level of spiritual wellness.

Scores on the individual scales and the overall score are meant to be sources of feedback. The following score ranges may be helpful in identifying areas that need attention:

If Your Score On Any Scale Is	And/Or Your Overall Score Is	Then You May Wish To
12 to 15	61 to 75	Examine ways that you can use your strengths to help you make desired lifestyle changes.
7 to 11	41 to 60	Review the questions on which you scored low. A goal of improvement might be called for.
3 to 6	Less than 40	Speak to your instructor about how to address your concerns.

SOURCE: Adapted from Larry Chapman, "Developing a Useful Perspective on Spiritual Health: Well-being, Spiritual Potential, and the Search for Meaning," *American Journal of Health Promotion* 1 (Winter 1987): 35–36.

---

how they reacted to our responses to psychological, cultural, physical, and other aspects of our environment. Did you grow up in a household in which free expression of feelings and emotions was fostered? When stressful situations arose, did a relaxed atmosphere prevail, or did people seem to be uptight about it? Chances are that the ways you handle emotions now were displayed in your family in the past. Your ability to cope now depends on these past influences as well as on the resources currently available to you, such as money and friends.

Achieving emotional health should be thought of as a positive concept. It includes, first, being aware of the emotions that you experience and, second, being able to freely communicate your feelings, both with yourself and others. The more direct and open you are in your expressions of emotions, the more likely you are to maintain a full range of emotional communications. This doesn't mean that you should let everyone know about every little feeling you have, but it does mean that you can express yourself when it is appropriate. When happy, laugh; when sad, cry.

Figure 2–1 shows a chain of reactions that occurs as emotions are elicited. First there is a situation, event, or object that we respond to. We perceive this

passion, all desirable traits for achieving a good world for all. It is with the quality of love that we are able to probe more fully the question of meaning in life.

> ■ *PROBLEM SITUATION* You are working part-time in an after-school recreation program for 13 to 16 year olds, and you've gotten to know some of the kids pretty well. One of them, with whom you've had some nice discussions in the past, asks you, "What is life all about, anyway?" He means: What is ultimate reality? Is there a god? What is my purpose in life? and How do I know what is moral behavior? You don't want to answer these questions directly, so you decide to ask him some questions that deal with spiritual awareness. Compile a list of five to ten questions that might elicit clarifying responses concerning personal spiritual awareness. Suggest some

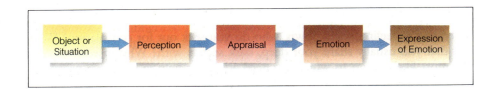

FIGURE 2–1 ■ Chain of Emotional Response

object or situation in such a way that we relate to it personally. We appraise that situation or object by giving it meaning so that we can evaluate it before an emotional response is elicited. The expression or action elicited may either attract us to or repel us from the object, depending on its appraised threat or worth.

In addition to recognizing the presence of various emotions, we need also to recognize their intensity. Sometimes an emotion becomes so intense that it can cause a tunnel vision that blocks out other emotions and that controls us rather than our controlling it. When this happens, it is time to touch base with our good listener/friend or a professional counselor. Even the positive emotion of love, when most intense, has prevented people from concentrating on their work or has interfered with other areas of their life. This negative aspect is expressed in the line in an old song that goes, "You're not sick, you're just in love."

It is desirable to feel and constructively express a full range of emotions. However, sometimes normal emotions are expressed, either verbally or by "acting out," in a destructive manner. This type of emotional expression is usually more harmful to the one expressing such feelings than to the intended object, a fact that is often unrecognized.

Joy/Sadness

Joy and *sadness* are emotions that represent the high and low points of daily living. They can be expressed either in a quiet, solitary, and contemplative manner or overtly and publicly. Joy brings an inward satisfaction, a good feeling that things have gone well. Objects of joy can be sensual, aesthetic, spiritual, or pastoral or they can involve any other events that bring about feelings of contentment and satisfaction. Joy is a sense of personal or global fulfillment and remains within us as part of our internal strength.

The experience of sadness, although often unwelcome, is necessary for a full range of living. It is the valleys that make possible the peaks of joy and happiness. When we are sad because of some loss, we must be aware that all things must eventually come to an end. Sometimes expressions of these losses and resultant sadness are inhibited for various cultural and personal reasons (e.g., "men don't cry" or "big girls don't cry"). It is as if people discourage expressions of sadness because they want to deny that sadness is part of everyday life.

Depression

When sadness is allowed to remain without resolution, a state of *depression* ensues. Although depression is sometimes considered to be an emotion, it is really a prolonged psychological state. Symptoms of depression may include a lowering of one's energy level, decreased appetite, feelings of being overwhelmed, negative self-concept, and a general lack of assertiveness. The depressed state is extremely draining and negative; in contrast, sadness is more

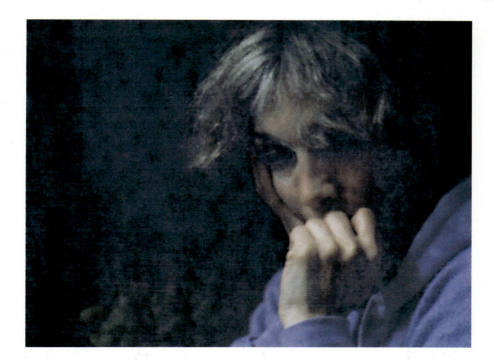

Depression can be temporary, such as when we experience loss, or it can be severe and long-lasting.

meaningful and more easily dealt with in a realistic manner. Whereas sadness is connected to a loss involving an event, person, or object, depression is linked to conditions of alienation and loneliness. Some forms of severe depression may have organic origins and require professional intervention.

Depression is something that we all experience at one time or another. For example, approximately three-fourths of all college students feel depressed during the school year. However, just saying that we are "bummed out" or "down in the dumps" doesn't tell how badly "bummed" we are. Sometimes it's not hard to cope with depression, but at other times it can seem overwhelming. If it becomes too difficult to overcome depression on our own, professionally trained helpers may be needed. We depend on their expertise to analyze the depression so that we can consciously cope with it.

Knowing that we have successfully coped with depression in the past or that everybody goes through it every once in a while helps us deal with it more easily. Experience is a wonderful teacher. Previous successful experiences also help with the spiritual aspect of wellness by showing that even in despair, life is not meaningless. It leads to the knowledge that in traversing hills and valleys, every depth will be followed by a peak. By understanding and controlling our lives, the valleys may not be too low but the peaks may rise higher, leading to high-level wellness.

FAST FACTS

Every year, about ten million Americans suffer from severe depression, costing a total of $16 billion in therapy and days lost from work.

> ■ *PROBLEM SITUATION* A very good friend of yours gets depressed easily whenever she has any sort of negative experiences. Even reading about unhappy and threatening events in the newspaper gets her down. The depression doesn't linger too long, but it has upset her enough to talk to you about it, knowing that you're a good listener. What advice might you give, and how would you handle the problem in general? Would you recommend that she see a counselor on campus? Why or why not?

> **FAST FACTS**
>
> Hostile individuals tend to have more blockage of the coronary arteries. Also, people who are not good listeners tend to have higher blood pressure.

Anger

Emotional health, as has been pointed out, requires that a person experience a full range of emotions, not just positive ones. When the negative emotions are inaccurately perceived or inappropriately acted out, emotional pain results. Perhaps the emotion that is most difficult to deal with accurately and to express appropriately is *anger*. Society does not readily accept the direct expression of anger. For one thing, anger may imply a loss of love for many people. For another, some may fear that a show of anger may trigger a retaliatory response that is more than was bargained for. Nevertheless, when anger is recognized and freely expressed without undue fear, it leads to open communication and may bring about needed changes.

In managing your anger, it is important to direct the expression of it toward the precise cause of the anger, not toward everyone and everything. First you must pinpoint exactly what you are angry about and then clearly communicate to the person involved just what is causing you to become angry. Let the person know that you still like them, or perhaps even love them, and that you are angry only at a particular behavior or situation. Even though anger can involve aggression, it needn't be manifested in an overly violent manner, which can cause the other person to react similarly. The challenge is to learn to express anger constructively.

A problem that often occurs when the source of anger isn't accurately identified or dealt with is that it gets directed at an unrelated object. Sometimes this redirective behavior may be helpful, such as if you're physically threatened by someone, but eventually the source of anger must be directly confronted. If we do not allow our anger to be vented because of unpleasant immediate consequences, it may be replaced by prolonged fear. For example, if we are never allowed to show anger towards our parents, our attitudes toward other authority figures can be negatively influenced.

Also important is how you cope with anger when it is directed towards you. Can you accept the expression of anger by another without feeling that it equates to being unloved? Anger, after all, is not the same as withdrawal of love and acceptance.

Guilt

Another emotion, *guilt,* is the concern that we have perpetrated some sort of moral wrong through action or thought. All of us experience guilt at one time or another. Some guilt stems from things that we have done (or not done) that may have contributed to pain or prevented a goal from being met. Guilt acts as a social indicator of wrong-doing, and in this sense it can be beneficial. However, much guilt is taken on unnecessarily, as when we are accused of actions that are beyond our control or when we ourselves take responsibility for things that we cannot personally affect.

Imagine, if you will, a girl who quarreled frequently with her mother and therefore entertained thoughts of being rid of her. If her mother were to become ill and die, the daughter might think that her bad thoughts and arguments caused her mother's death, which could lead to a lifetime of unwarranted guilt feelings. Obviously this would have a detrimental effect on the girl's subsequent behavior and self-concept. Most guilt that we feel can easily be handled by becoming aware of its source and talking it out with a good listener/friend. If it is too intense, then professional counseling can be sought. The same is true for anxiety and fear.

Anxiety and Fear

Fear, an emotion aroused by impending danger, and the resultant feelings of apprehension and uneasiness called *anxiety,* have some far-reaching effects on our feelings and behavior. A certain amount of anxiety and fear is natural in some situations and may be helpful to optimal functioning. However, intense, chronic, or unidentified general anxiety and worry can inhibit normal functioning. We may feel the physical manifestations of anxiety, such as decreased appetite or increased heartbeat, but not have any idea what is causing them. Of course, if we are able to accurately identify the source of our fear and anxiety, there is a much greater chance of dealing with it directly and satisfactorily.

Fear can be such an uncomfortable emotion that it may be denied or repressed, and it may manifest itself later in a harmful way. Although directly facing up to our fears may be temporarily painful, it is more fulfilling and growth-enhancing than "sticking our heads in the sand." For example, because of the fear of possible rejection and the concomitant anxiety it may cause, you may avoid approaching another person for whom you feel affection.

Loneliness

A frequent problem of college life is the feeling of being isolated or alienated in some way from others on campus—what is labeled *loneliness.* Before examining the roots of loneliness, we need to differentiate between being alone and being lonely. It is important to be comfortable with being alone and engaging in solitary activities. It has been said that in the core of our minds, we are born alone and we die alone, although we usually live among others. In this sense, then, even in a crowd of people we are alone. Solitude, as compared to loneliness, is a self-satisfied state of contentment in which we learn about ourselves, our relation to the world we live in, and the mysteries of the universe. It is an energy-enhancing and growth-producing condition.

Feelings of loneliness take two basic forms—a personal feeling of separation or **alienation,** and the societal form of feeling apart from members of a different group, whether it is racial, sexual, religious, political, cultural, or geographical. In his classic work, *The Pursuit of Loneliness,* Philip Slater points to three human wants that are inhibited by American culture, thus leading to social loneliness. The first is the need to live in harmony and trust with all other human beings—the desire for community. This desire is frustrated by the value we place on competition at the expense of cooperation. Second is the societal tendency to avoid long-term commitments to solving social problems; because of this, change becomes superficial and the basic frustrations remain. Third is the desire for dependence or the need for shared responsibility over one's life. We are continually encouraged to be independent and not to ask others for "favors." Rugged individualism seems to be a dominant cultural value in the United States; we are often taught to make it on our own and outdo all competitors.

One way to help overcome loneliness is through the establishment of a social network (discussed in Chapter 3) consisting of people we can trust and rely on. Sometimes such networks take time to develop, especially when we're in a new and unfamiliar environment.

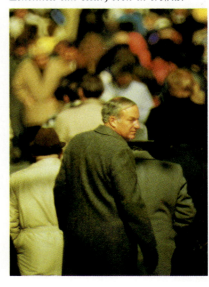

Loneliness can occur, even in crowds.

Ironically, another way to deal with loneliness is to allow for occasional periods of solitude. Being free from the judgments of other people provides the setting necessary to get to know ourselves and to discover our purposes in life. Thoreau sought solitude at Walden Pond. By getting closer to nature, it enabled him to explore his life and the world around him and to place things in their proper perspective.

> ▰ *PROBLEM SITUATION* There are times when each of us feels alienated or lonely, even in a crowd of people. You have had this feeling a lot lately and would like to do something about it. How can you overcome your loneliness and alienation? Who can you rely on to talk about it with?

Shyness

Sometimes loneliness stems from a person's anxiety over meeting new people in new situations. *Shyness* occurs when someone avoids interactions with others as a way of dealing with this fear. Most people are shy in certain situations, but when shyness prevents normal, everyday interactions, it is problematic and requires definite action to overcome.

If you feel that shyness is a problem that you should be working on, you might want to use the CARE approach to behavior change described in Chapter 1. You may also want to make a contract with yourself stating how you will go about effecting changes in your behavior. No matter what method you use, start with the realization that you are a good and lovable person. Then make short-term goals, stating specifically how you will approach, meet, and interact with people. Begin with people and situations that are most comfortable and familiar for you, and then practice talking with strangers in "safe" settings. You should also give yourself a schedule for interacting with a certain number of people each day. The more you interact, the more comfortable you'll be in social situations, and the more you'll like yourself.

▰ Suicide

Suicide, a self-intentioned act that leads to an earlier death than expected, is preceded by a period of extreme, seemingly unbearable psychological pain. In almost all cases, however, it pays to bear the suffering until it is resolved; suicide is not worth it. This may seem to be an easy statement to make; people who commit suicide don't see a way out of their predicament.

There are various levels of suicidal behavior. First, there are those people who exhibit certain characteristic predisposing signs such as depression, but who haven't really considered attempting suicide. At the second level are those who actually think about suicide as an alternative. Most of us, at one time or another, have experienced these two levels, although our thoughts of suicide were only fleeting. A more serious level is reached if one makes an overt verbal threat of committing suicide. Even though most people who threaten suicide do not carry it out, such threats should be taken very seriously as a call for help. At the fourth level is an actual suicide attempt, and at the final level is successfully committing suicide.

About three times as many women as men attempt suicide but three times as many men are successful. This is probably because men use more violent means (guns, in particular) whereas women usually attempt suicide by taking

---

FAST FACTS

Shy people tend to be in careers with minimal contact with others such as computer programming.

SELF-INVENTORY 2.2

Mental Health Assessment

Directions: In the exercises that follow, circle one response for each question. Place the score on the line next to the question. Add up your score and put the total in the box at the end. Then go to the next section.

Self-Esteem

_____ 1. Generally, would you say that you like yourself?
   9 Yes, definitely
   7 Yes, for the most part
   4 I don't know
   3 No, not too well
   0 No, not at all

_____ 2. Are you a self-confident person?
   4 Yes, all of the time
   3 Yes, most of the time
   2 Some of the time
   1 Seldom
   0 Never

_____ 3. Are you comfortable with your sexual feelings?
   4 All or most of the time
   2 Frequently
   2 Some of the time
   1 Seldom
   0 Never

_____ 4. How comfortable are you doing things alone?
   3 Very comfortable
   2 Somewhat comfortable
   1 I don't know
   1 Not very comfortable
   0 Very uncomfortable

_____ **SELF-ESTEEM TOTAL**

If you scored less than 7, your self-esteem is low. You need to consider ways to improve your confidence. A score of 15 or more indicates that you probably have high self-esteem. Keep it up.

Coping with Emotions

_____ 5. Are you in control of your anger and your temper?
   3 Most of the time
   2 Frequently
   2 Some of the time
   1 Seldom
   0 Never

_____ 6. How much of the time do you feel guilty?
   0 Most or all of the time
   1 Frequently
   2 Some of the time
   2 Seldom
   3 Never

_____ 7. Does fear keep you from doing things you like to do?
   3 No, never
   2 Seldom
   2 Some of the time
   1 A lot of the time
   0 Most or all of the time

_____ 8. If someone seeks help from a professional counselor, would you say that person is weak?
   2 Definitely not
   1 Not particularly
   1 I don't know
   0 Yes, for the most part
   0 Definitely

_____ **COPING WITH EMOTIONS TOTAL**

If you scored 8 or above, you tend to handle emotions in a healthy way. A score below 4 indicates that you could use some help coping with your emotions.

SOURCE: Adapted from *Helping Yourself* (California State Department of Mental Health, 1989).

> **FAST FACTS**
>
> The most common method of suicide for both males and females in the 15- to 24-year-old age group, is firearms. Use of guns accounts for most of the increase in suicides among young adults in the past thirty years.

drugs, often in a less-than-lethal dose. As far as race is concerned, the suicide rate for whites is higher than for nonwhites for both males and females.

Although the age group over 45 has the highest risk of dying from suicide, there has recently been a disturbing trend of suicides among children less than 15 years old. For the age group 15 to 24, suicide is the third leading cause of death behind motor-vehicle accidents and homicide. This is not an entirely accurate picture, because some motor-vehicle deaths are intentional, a fact that would raise the actual suicide rate. The most common reasons for suicide attempts among youth are the following:

1. Disturbances in a relationship, such as a breakup with one's boyfriend or girlfriend, leading to a sense of loss and alienation (It could involve one's parents, as well.)
2. School difficulties
3. Unwanted pregnancy
4. Sudden changes in one's life situation
5. A negative self-image connected with failure

Those who attempt suicide are usually in the midst of serious depression, other intolerable emotional disturbances, and an unsettled life pattern. They have a tunnel vision of the world, and they are unable to see alternative ways out of their dilemma. All options seem to be closed for these people.

The steps leading to a suicide attempt begin with an acute crisis situation. This is followed by a period of ambivalence, during which the person doesn't know whether to live or die. There also exists, in the person's mind, a vacillation between love and hate for himself/herself and others. This ambivalence eventually ceases once that person has decided to take action leading to suicide. At this point there are usually some warning signs, which are sometimes subtle and sometimes direct. These may be a direct verbal statement, "I want to kill myself"; a behavioral sign such as involvement in a one-car accident; or a syndrome of patterned depression, disorientation, or extreme dependency. Extreme stress also could signal a possible suicide attempt. As you can see, the circumstances surrounding suicide are complex.

People who are suicidal feel hopeless (they have given up), helpless (they see no way out), and hapless or abandoned. Although they may want help, they may not be able to ask for it or accept it when offered. What can you do to assist someone like this? First, you can show the person that you care so that he or she will not feel abandoned. That's part of overcoming the haplessness. Then you can physically go with the person to set up an immediate appointment with a counselor or therapist to insure that action will be taken. You should also take steps to expand and solidify the person's social support system.

If you should happen to be in a situation in which a friend, family member, or even an acquaintance is threatening suicide, there are some crisis-intervention steps that you can take.

1. First establish trust. Be calm, speak in a gentle tone of voice, and maintain constant contact.
2. Obtain information. Ask, "Are you thinking of harming yourself?" If the answer is "yes," ask the person how he or she plans to do it. Find out the *specific* means, whether these means are *available,* and how *lethal* the method is. This will help you evaluate the real suicide potential.
3. Once you have clarified for both the person at risk and yourself what the focal problem is and have evaluated the person's chances of actually attempting

> **FAST FACTS**
>
> The suicide rate for 15 to 19 year olds has more than doubled in the past twenty years.

suicide, assess his or her strengths and resources. The key question here is, "What has kept you alive until now?"

4. At this point you can formulate an immediate plan of action. The plan should involve getting the person into professional counseling NOW, committing the person to seeing you in the near future, and getting him or her into a strong social network.

> ■ *PROBLEM SITUATION* A close friend of yours tells you that he is seriously contemplating suicide. He is constantly depressed, sees no way out of his emotional pain, and lacks the energy and motivation to do anything really beneficial for himself. What kinds of questions might you ask him to evaluate the situation, and how would you then intervene in an attempt to prevent him from committing suicide?

You can do all that you can to keep someone from committing suicide, but eventually you must let the person be responsible for his or her own life. If that person, or any other person, does subsequently commit suicide, you should feel no guilt about it. After all, we are all ultimately responsible for our own living and dying.

Unfortunately, society has sometimes viewed suicide as an immoral or criminal act, even as a sickness. It is none of these. Suicide is an act of despair, an attempt to rid oneself of overwhelming pain. Usually this pain is psychological, although it can also be unbearable physical pain. In the best of all worlds, people would not commit suicide, but if death does occur by this means, it should not tarnish the memory of that person or the status of the survivors.

■ Mental Ill Health

Mental Illness Defined

The first thing to clarify when describing mental illness is whether we are referring to the brain or the mind. Mental illness encompasses both organic brain disorders and psychological problems of coping with daily living. People are labeled "mentally ill" because their character traits are so different that, in the judgment of psychologists and psychiatrists, they are unable to function adequately in society. These deviations may be psychological or organic in origin. (For a listing of types of mental disorders, see Appendix B.)

Mental illness is usually a result of conflict or disharmony within people as they try to adjust to the demands and expectations of society. When one's inner and outer worlds become too far apart, mental ill health can result. One's culture determines what is "acceptable" behavior and thereby defines, to a large extent, what constitutes mental dysfunction. Some behaviors are expected in one culture but are considered a sign of mental illness in another. In the United States, alcoholism is generally considered to be a disease; in some places in the world it is acceptable, and in other places it is a criminal offense.

■ Caring For Mental Health Problems

You don't have to be "crazy" to benefit from professional psychological help. When your body is ailing, you quickly go to a physician. When your mind is troubled, it makes sense to go to a mental health professional. People who walk

FAST FACTS

Scientists can now map the functions of the cerebrum (called brain imaging), which allows them to understand how the normal brain works. Based on this information, they can map abnormalities involved in some mental illnesses.

into counseling services on campus, or anywhere else as outpatients, are not necessarily more disturbed than others; they simply recognize that their problem exists and have taken steps to alleviate it.

Types of Psychotherapies

There are two aspects of personality that we have mentioned—the inner world of experience and the outer world of behavior. You can choose to conceal or to become aware of your inner world. With the aid of **psychotherapy,** you attempt to put experience and behavior together so that they are consistent and function to help you live your life optimally.

Whatever form of therapy you choose, all of them employ deliberate methods aimed at assisting you with the array of psychological problems that you may encounter. They can help with disorders of thinking (cognitive problems), emotions, or mood swings, and behavioral control. Table 2–1 lists just some of the more than 250 psychotherapeutic approaches in common practice today.

Psychotherapy is a learning process rather than a treatment per se. It may influence you by facilitating self-understanding, enhancing your sense of control, boosting morale, and establishing a safe setting for the emotional reaction necessary for change to take place. Because you are ultimately responsible for your own thoughts, emotions, and behavior, the "cure" lies within *you*, not within the therapist.

Psychotherapies may be *individual*, which involve a one-to-one encounter between therapist and client; *family*, in which the entire family works on solving interactional problems that they face in daily living; or *group*, in which individuals deal with their personal problems through group interaction and the insight of peers. Psychotherapeutic approaches may employ either **insight therapy, action therapy**, or a combination of both.

Insight therapy includes those approaches in which the therapist *talks* with the patient so that both can understand why the patient is the way he or she is and so that the patient's inner stress can be relieved through this understanding. As the patient talks, the therapist listens, pieces together the puzzle, and gives limited but crucial feedback for self-understanding to be achieved.

Action therapy, in contrast, aims at relieving symptoms of psychological distress rather than focusing on the motives that cause people to behave the way they do. It is based on how people learn their patterns of behavior and emotional responses. In this form of therapy, the therapist lays out a plan of action with and for the patient, usually involving modifying the environment that led to the problem so that a new behavior can be more easily implemented. Action therapy is more appropriately used to control such self-destructive practices as overeating, smoking, drug abuse, or any other specifically identified pattern.

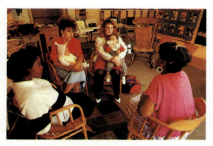

Psychotherapies may be of an individual, group or family nature.

Mental Health Practitioners

Who are these people who call themselves psychotherapists? They are generally found in one of three professions. **Psychiatrists** are medical doctors who spe-

TABLE 2–1 ■ **Characteristics of Selected Psychotherapies**

Name	Characteristics
Psychoanalysis	Developed by Sigmund Freud; examines unconscious forces, uses free association and dream analysis
Existential Psychotherapy	Focuses on human isolation and the realization that "I am"
Family Therapy	Focuses on the family as a whole and the existing relationships
Humanistic Psychology	Focuses on the person as central to all
Person-Centered Therapy	Developed by Carl Rogers; the therapist shows genuine caring, is nonjudgmental, and uses a nondirective approach
Transpersonal Psychology	Focuses on the spiritual dimension but looks at the physical, social, and psychological realms as well in a holistic manner
Cognitive Therapy	Utilizes mental and intellectual control of emotions and behavior
Behavioral Psychology	Holds that maladaptive behavior is learned and can be unlearned and changed by manipulating one's personal environment
Reality Therapy	Focuses on behavior in the present, enables the individual to see and face reality with no personal threat
Transactional Analysis	Developed by Eric Berne; used in group therapies, it is a theory of personality organization that recognizes a parent, adult, and child aspect of each person
Logotherapy	Developed by Victor Frankl; focuses on meaning and purpose in life

cialize in treating mental disorders. They can, by law, administer physically based treatment in the form of drugs, **electroconvulsive** (formerly called electroshock) **therapy,** and **neurosurgery. Clinical psychologists** are often Ph.D.s with training in human behavior who employ general and specific techniques to help patients cope with problems of living. They can also conduct psychological assessments of personality and intelligence. **Psychiatric social workers** have the credentials of Licensed Clinical Social Worker and Master of Social Work degrees. They are trained to focus on emotionally disturbed individuals and families in the community, providing special services as needed.

There are also many others who provide formal and informal psychotherapy, such as psychiatric nurses; vocational, guidance, and rehabilitation counselors; occupational therapists; art therapists; play therapists; horticultural therapists; marriage and sex therapists; and so on. Ministers, many of them specifically trained in psychotherapy, do pastoral counseling. Nevertheless, probably the greatest source of actual psychological help is provided by friends and neighbors who have a reputation for giving sage and sound practical advice when it comes to personal problems. They provide a shoulder to cry on, an ear to listen, and wise counsel to follow.

Issues In Mental Health

Who is mentally healthy and who is mentally ill? It is not as easy to determine this as it might seem. This is because mental illness rarely presents overt physical signs or **pathology,** such as brain damage. In a classic study conducted in New York City, it was concluded that 80 percent of the 1,600 residents responding to a survey suffered from one or more of the symptoms of mental illness. Among the lower socioeconomic classes, this figure rose to 95 percent. Thus, one may conclude that almost everyone exhibits one or more characteristics of mental illness. This is mainly because certain behavioral patterns are considered to be components of mental illness merely because they deviate from culturally accepted norms.

There are particular groups of people who are more vulnerable to mental illness than others, both because of their status in our culture and because they are singled out for being different. Black Americans, Hispanic Americans, and Native Americans all have above-average rates of mental illness and underserved mental health needs. When they do come in contact with the mental health "establishment," they are often misunderstood because they do not speak the same "language" as mental health workers, who usually come from different cultural backgrounds. They may, as a cultural trait, for example, speak loudly and stand close to those with whom they are communicating, conveying a false impression of belligerence.

Women face special mental health problems today because of their changing roles in society (although this can also be a potential problem for men who are threatened by changes in traditional roles). A more immediate problem exists, however, and that is the different treatment that women receive in dealing with their mental health problems. Much more psychosurgery, electroconvulsive therapy, and psychotherapeutic drugs are administered to women, predominantly by male psychiatrists.

Special problems exist for the poor and homeless, because many suffer from undiagnosed forms of disturbances in their ability to cope with psychological demands, including the cognitive knowledge necessary to manage daily affairs. Some homeless people are on the streets by choice, and some are homeless because they don't know how to get and hold a job or manage their limited resources. In many states, in which mental hospitals have been closed and mental health funding severely reduced, homelessness has increased significantly.

Does anyone ever achieve an ideal state of mental wellness? The answer is no. First, this is because none of us is perfectly healthy physically, socially, spiritually, or mentally. Secondly, the science of psychology is not precise enough to be able to establish an ideal for everyone. Therefore, be satisfied with who you are, but know that there is always room for improvement in mental well-being, as in other dimensions of personal health. Also remember that help is available when needed.

FAST FACTS

Women who have been sexually and physically abused have a significantly greater chance of developing psychiatric illness, usually of a depressive type, than those who have no history of abuse.

POSITIVE BEHAVIORS

I. *Place a check mark in front of each behavior that you now practice.*

_____ 1. I accept myself and like myself. (LIKE SELF)

_____ 2. My sources of gratification are many and varied. (GRATIFICATION)

_____ 3. I deal comfortably with my entire range of emotions. (EMOTIONS)

_____ 4. I take concrete steps aimed at becoming aware of my mental and spiritual health status and pursue changes when appropriate. (AWARE)

_____ 5. I am basically a joyful person but accept and express sadness when it occurs. (JOY/SADNESS)

_____ 6. When depressed, I usually know why, and I work on overcoming it as soon as possible. (DEPRESSION)

_____ 7. When I feel lonely, I don't dwell on it but take steps to overcome the feeling of alienation. (LONELINESS)

_____ 8. I do not tend towards self-destructive behavior, but if I were in a state of depression and emotional turmoil and had thoughts of suicide, I would immediately seek professional counseling. (SUICIDE)

_____ 9. I have identified several good listener/friends on whom I can rely. (GOOD LISTENER)

_____ 10. I am aware of the various types of psychotherapies and therapists and would be comfortable seeking them out when and if I needed their help. (THERAPY)

II. *For each behavior that you DO NOT ENGAGE IN, write the KEY WORD(S) that is in the parentheses located at the end of the statement in the column below. Then put a check mark in the appropriate column to indicate whether you are going to keep or change that behavior.*

Behaviors I Don't Engage In   **KEEP/CHANGE**

_____/_____
_____/_____
_____/_____
_____/_____
_____/_____
_____/_____
_____/_____
_____/_____
_____/_____
_____/_____

III. *For each of the preceding behaviors that you choose to KEEP, write a statement indicating why you are choosing to keep that behavior.*

I choose to keep behavior _____ because:
                          KEY WORD

For each of the preceding behaviors that you choose to CHANGE, write a statement indicating how you plan to implement that change.

I will change behavior _____ by:
                        KEY WORD

Now You Know

1. TRUE. The ability to give and receive love enables one to develop all other aspects of mental wellness.
2. TRUE. This combination of roles, qualities, and belongingness determines our selves.
3. TRUE. Everyone of us is lovable and capable and good in our own eyes simply because we are alive.
4. FALSE. Science and spirituality have very definite connections, as evidenced by the rash of scientists who are correlating their scientific discoveries with spirituality.
5. TRUE. Suffering and pleasure are both qualities of human life, and they contribute insight that helps us identify purposes in living.
6. TRUE. Most depression passes with time and may only require talking things over with a good listener/friend. If it's long-lasting or painful, a professional counselor should be seen.
7. FALSE. Although personal loneliness involves the feeling of separation from a substantial portion of the community (that is, alienation), solitude is the desirable feeling of being alone, a condition that's necessary from time to time.
8. TRUE. Women usually use less lethal means (pills as opposed to guns) when attempting suicide than men.
9. TRUE. Action therapies attempt to correct counterproductive behaviors, whereas insight therapies work on understanding a person's reasons for his or her behavior.
10. TRUE. Women are, for example, much more likely to be medicated when under a psychiatrist's care. It should be noted that the majority of psychiatrists are men.

Summary

1. Personal mental wellness consists of many characteristics, such as possessing self-acceptance, being loving, being socially responsible, having purpose in life, being active and productive, having a variety of sources of gratification, being able to deal with life's stressors, and utilizing one's full range of emotions.
2. Normal mental health is not precisely measurable but may be more accurately described as a range of emotions and behaviors that reflects societal definitions and expectations.
3. Besides helping us to find meaning in life and form a system of ethical conduct, spiritual health enables us to possess an attitude of caring for others, be a loving person, and develop a concept of the cosmos or universe.
4. To develop mental well-being requires personal awareness, determination of appropriate directions in life, and the ability to follow through on needed and desired changes.
5. Probably the most important self-care step that you can take towards maintaining high-level mental wellness is to cultivate a good listener/friend.
6. Having emotional control means that you are able to use your full range of emotions in a beneficial way rather than stifling them because you're uncomfortable displaying them.
7. Emotions of anger, sadness, depression, guilt, loneliness, and anxiety are not always pleasant to experience, but they need to be expressed directly and appropriately.
8. Loneliness, an emotion we've all experienced, can occur even when we're in the midst of a crowd. It differs from solitude, which is a condition that we all need from time to time.
9. A certain amount of anxiety is normal in some situations, but if it becomes too great, it can be paralyzing, especially if we are not aware of its source.
10. There are steps you can take to help a person who is contemplating suicide, but if you should fail to prevent the suicide, you should accept the fact that it was the other person's action that led to death, and you should not harbor any guilt about it.
11. Mental illness may be induced by organic brain damage, or it may be a functional psychological disorder.
12. Although we must give certain mental disorders labels in order to talk about them, this can lead to problems, such as people living up to expectations posed by such labeling or being thought of in terms of their labels rather than being seen as the individuals that they are.
13. The various forms of psychotherapy help people by enabling and facilitating self-understanding, a sense of control, improved morale, and emotional involvement.
14. Mental health providers may be psychiatrists, clinical psychologists, counselors, or even your best listener/friend.

References

1. Aguilera, Donna, and Janice Messick. *Crisis Intervention: Theory and Methodology*. St. Louis: C. V. Mosby, 1986.
2. Banks, Rebecca. "Health and the Spiritual Dimension: Relationships and Implications for Professional Preparation Programs." *Journal of School Health* 50(1980): 195–202.
3. Bedworth, Albert, and David A. Bedworth. *Health for Human Effectiveness*. Englewood Cliffs, N.J.: Prentice-Hall, 1982.
4. Bieliauskas, Linas A. *The Influence of Individual Differences in Health and Illness*. Boulder, Colo.: Westview Press, 1983.
5. Buscaglia, Leo. *Love*. Thorofare, N.J.: Charles B. Slack, Inc., 1972.
6. Campbell, Robert N. *The New Science: Self-Esteem Psychology*. New York: University Press of America, 1984.
7. Camus, Albert. *The Myth of Sisphyus and Other Essays*. New York: Vintage Books, 1955.
8. Chapman, Larry S. "Developing a Useful Perspective on Spiritual Health: Well-being, Spiritual Potential and the Search for Meaning." *American Journal of Health Promotion* 1(1987): 31–39.
9. *Diagnostic and Statistical Manual of Mental Disorders: DSM–III–R*. Washington, D.C.: American Psychiatric Association, 1987.
10. Frank, Jerome. *Persuasion and Healing*. Baltimore, Md.: The Johns Hopkins University Press, 1973.
11. Frankl, Viktor E. *Man's Search for Meaning*. New York: Washington Square Press, 1963.
12. Gale, Raymond F. *Who Are You*. Englewood Cliffs, N.J.: Prentice-Hall, 1974.
13. Gerald, Michael C. *Pharmacology: An Introduction to Drugs*. Englewood Cliffs, N.J.: Prentice-Hall, 1981.
14. Gordon, James S., Dennis T. Jaffe, and David E. Bresler. *Mind, Body and Health: Toward an Integral Medicine*. New York: Human Sciences Press, 1984.
15. Hunt, Morton. "Navigating the Therapy Maze." *New York Times Magazine,* August 31, 1987, 28+.
16. Jourard, Sidney. *The Transparent Self*. New York: D. Van Nostrand Co., 1971.
17. Jung, Carl G. *The Archetypes and Collective Unconscious*. Princeton, N.J.: Princeton University Press, 1969.
18. Kahn, Marvin W. *Basic Methods for Mental Health Practitioners*. Cambridge, Mass.: Winthrop Publishers, 1981.
19. Krassner, Albert. *Journey to Be*. Washington, D.C.: Veridon Editions, 1983.
20. Luft, Joseph. *Group Processes: An Introduction to Group Dynamics*. Palo Alto, Calif.: National Press Books, 1970.
21. Maslow, Abraham. *New Knowledge in Human Values*. New York: Harper and Row, 1959.
22. Matarazzo, Joseph D., et al. *Behavioral Health: A Handbook of Health Enhancement and Disease Prevention*. New York: John Wiley and Sons, 1984.
23. May, Gerald. *Will and Spirit: A Contemplative Psychology*. New York: Harper and Row, 1982.
24. May, Rollo. *Love and Will*. New York: W. W. Norton, 1969.
25. Mead, George H. *Mind, Self and Society: From the Standpoint of a Social Behaviorist*. Chicago: University of Chicago Press, 1934.
26. Morgan, Arthur. *Search for Purpose*. Yellow Springs, Ohio: Antioch Press, 1955.
27. Moustakas, Clark. *Loneliness and Love*. Englewood Cliffs, N.J.: Prentice-Hall, 1972.
28. Peck, Scott. *The Road Less Traveled*. New York: Simon and Schuster, 1978.
29. Powys, John C. *A Philosophy of Solitude*. New York: Simon and Schuster, 1933.
30. Progoff, Ira. *At a Journal Workshop*. New York: Dialogue House Library, 1975.
31. Ray, Oakley. *Drugs, Society and Human Behavior*. St. Louis: C. V. Mosby, 1982.
32. Schmolling, Paul, William Burger, and Merrill Youkeles. *Helping People: A Guide to Careers in Mental Health*. Englewood Cliffs, N.J.: Prentice-Hall, 1981.
33. Shneidman, Edwin S. "Suicide," in *Encyclopaedia Britannica*. Chicago: Encyclopaedia, Inc., 1973.
34. Silverman, Irwin. *Pure Types Are Rare*. New York: Praeger Publishers, 1983.
35. Slater, Philip. *The Pursuit of Loneliness*. Boston: Beacon Press, 1970.
36. Szasz, Thomas. *The Myth of Mental Illness*. New York: Delta Publishing Co., 1961.
37. Thackeray, Milton G., Rex A. Skidmore, and O. William Farley. *Introduction to Mental Health: Field and Practice*. Englewood Cliffs, N.J.: Prentice-Hall, 1979.
38. Tillich, Paul. *The Essential Tillich: An Anthology of the Writings of Paul Tillich*. New York: Macmillan, 1987.
39. Vaughan, Frances. *The Inward Arc*. Boston: New Science Library, 1985.

Suggested Readings

Adler, Mortimer J. *A Vision of the Future*. New York: Macmillan, 1984.

Bolen, Jean Shinoda. *Goddesses in Everywoman*. New York: Harper and Row, 1984.

Bolen, Jean Shinoda. *Gods in Everyman*. New York: Harper and Row, 1989.

Castaneda, Carlos. *The Power of Silence: Further Lessons of Don Juan*. New York: Simon and Schuster, 1987.

Dass, Ram, and Stephen Levine. *Grist for the Mill*. Berkeley, Calif.: Celestial Arts, 1987.

Jampolsky, Gerald G. *Out of Darkness, Into the Light*. New York: Bantam Books, 1989.

Peck, Scott. *The Road Less Traveled*. New York: Simon and Schuster, 1978.

Vaughan, Frances. *The Inward Arc*. Boston: New Science Library, 1985.

Zilbergeld, Bernie. *The Shrinking of America*. Boston: Little, Brown and Co., 1983.

Zimbardo, Philip. *Shyness*. New York: Jove Publications, 1987.

CHAPTER 3

Managing Stress

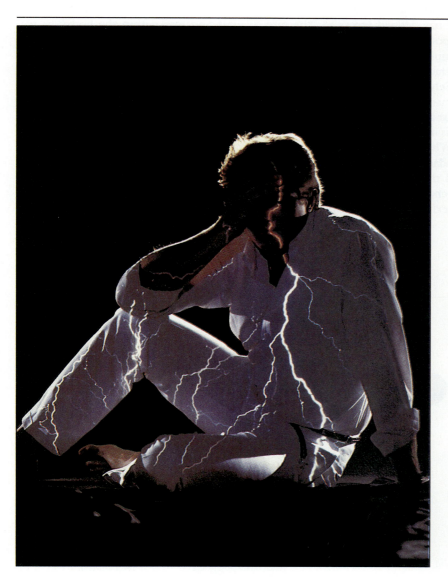

What Do You Know?

Are the following statements true or false?

1. Stress is harmful and therefore should be avoided.
2. Chronic stress can lead to organic damage such as high blood pressure, kidney disease, and cancer.
3. The biggest source of interpersonal stress is one's family.
4. Anyone who undergoes many extreme changes in his or her life, such as the death of a close family member, divorce, loss of job, or flunking out of school will experience an increase in the frequency and severity of illness within the following two to three years.
5. When crisis has occurred, resulting in disequilibrium, it is necessary to have a realistic perception of the situation, adequate support, and adequate coping skills in order to restore balance.
6. Stress management is best approached holistically by simplifying and balancing positive health practices dealing with environmental, material, spiritual, and personal actions.
7. The best relaxation technique is meditation.
8. A social-support system consists of people who sustain us emotionally, give us tangible material support, and provide us with information and advice.
9. Although we know social support to be important for high-level human wellness, this fact hasn't really been proved empirically by research.
10. Having pets at home has been demonstrated to have positive health effects on elderly and homebound people.

What Is Stress?

There's a bumper sticker that reads, "My worst day fishing is better than my best day working." We conjure up the image of someone out on a sunny day, drifting on a lake in a boat or sitting on the shore, without a care in the world. Our stereotyped image of that same person at work is of someone being hassled, trying to meet deadlines, and experiencing various other sorts of pressures.

Without a doubt, most of our waking and productive hours involve stress in one form or another; it can occur during work or play (including fishing). As we shall see, stress is not bad in and of itself, and a certain amount of it may be necessary for achieving a high quality of life. The optimal amount of stress may vary from person to person. Nevertheless, too much stress can be harmful, especially if steps are not taken to control the effects of inevitable stress.

A well-known researcher in the science of stress has been Dr. Hans Sclye. He has defined **stress** as "the rate of wear and tear within the body" as we respond to environmental stressors. The stressors may be the result of excessive stimuli or they may stem from stimulus deprivation, such as lack of physical contact.

Selye also defined stress as "the nonspecific response of the body to any demand made upon it." The key point to this definition is the fact that the body must adjust to any demand in an attempt to maintain a condition of **equilibrium.** This means that adaptation is the central purpose of the body's reaction to stress.

When stressors have a negative effect, such as causing stomach cramps or headaches, the effect is called **distress.** Not all stressors are harmful, however, and the term **eustress** has been coined to distinguish those stressors that are psychologically beneficial. An example of eustress is the elation that comes after an exhausting but satisfying performance in an athletic contest.

Stress can have an effect on all aspects of an individual.

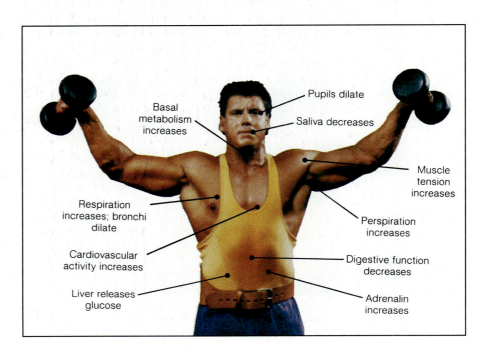

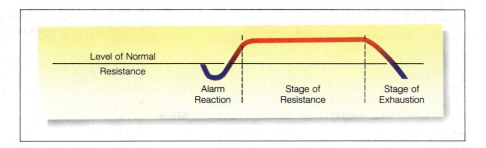

FIGURE 3–1 ■ **General Adaptation Syndrome**

SOURCE: Adapted from Hans Selye, *Stress Without Distress* (New York: S. B. Lippincott, 1974).

A person's reaction may be to coexist with the stressor or to directly combat the source of stress. One important factor is whether the person has learned to perceive stress as being personally threatening. Regardless of whether stressful events are pleasant or unpleasant, stress triggers the same general physiological reaction in the body. What may be more important is the *intensity* of its demands on the body's adaptive mechanisms.

Physiology of Stress

You are about to go on stage to perform in a play or concert. You are about to start an athletic competition—a ball game or a race. You are about to go out on a date with someone who you like but have only recently met. STRESS! Your heart starts pounding fast. Your palms and underarms become sweaty. You get a queasy feeling in the pit of your stomach. All of your body functions seem to be operating at double time. You probably recognize these symptoms as your body's response to the stressful situation.

Even though you tell yourself to keep calm, your body maintains its excited state. Why and how do these reactions occur? How does the brain and **neuroendocrine** system transform a psychological stress, such as taking an exam, into a physiological response? What is the nature of the response, and how does it effect bodily defenses and disease causation?

Selye has categorized the body's reactions to environmental stress into three phases, which he calls the *general adaptation syndrome* (GAS) (see Figure 3–1). In the first stage, there is a nonspecific, general *alarm reaction*, during which the **hypothalamus** portion of the brain is activated by the stressor. The hypothalamus, in turn, activates the **autonomic nervous system** and regulates the **pituitary gland**, which causes specific body defenses to be aroused. During this second phase of the GAS, called the *stage of resistance*, the hormone **epinephrine** is released, which helps the body either fight the stressor directly or take flight to avoid the stressor's harmful effects. If exposure to the same stressor is continued over a long period of time, the body will no longer be able to adjust or resist, and a *stage of exhaustion* will prevail. Adaptability is not infinite; we eventually succumb to the effects of the stressor, and our resistance breaks down. As you will see in the chapter dealing with AIDS, when the body's **immune system** is no longer able to cope with disease-causing organisms, death ensues.

Patterns of Stress

There are three basic patterns of stress response:

1. A stressor is present and is followed by adaptive change that returns the individual to a stress level no higher or lower than before (Figure 3–2a).

FIGURE 3–2 ■ Short- and Long-Term Stress Responses

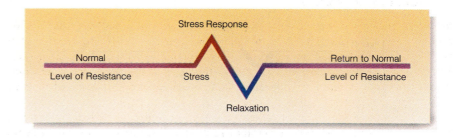

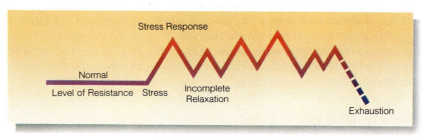

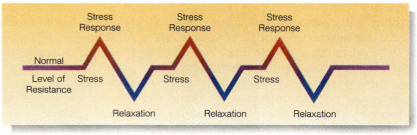

FAST FACTS

Chronic exposure to traffic jams tends to lead to higher baseline blood pressure, decreased frustration tolerance, an increase in aggressive driving behavior, and negative mood.

2. There is an increase in the level of stress but with no adaptive change strong enough to offset the stressful effects (Figure 3–2b).

3. Stress continues to escalate but it is accompanied by therapeutic actions aimed at maintaining normalcy (Figure 3–2c).

Selye discovered that chronic stress suppresses the immune system, thus diminishing the body's disease-fighting capabilities. In addition, continued chronic stress causes the body to produce excessive amounts of hormones, which, in turn, may lead to chronic diseases such as hardening of the arteries, high blood pressure, and arthritis.

■ *PROBLEM SITUATION* When it comes to making speeches in class, you always get anxious and experience thumping heartbeat and upset stomach beforehand. Although you recognize that it is beneficial to your maturing and learning process to encounter little stresses such as this, you'd like to control your body's physiological response to some degree. What steps can you take to diminish the immediate and direct effects of this stress, as well as the long-term stress reactions?

Sources Of Stress

Stressors can be found in all sorts of situations, forms, and environments. Table 3–1 identifies common sources of stress that bring tension and anxiety into your life. List a potential source of stress for yourself in each of these categories. Which areas seem to provide the most stress for you? What are your main sources of distress and eustress? How can you control the sources of distress and enhance eustress?

Stress can be either primary or secondary. A stimulus that results directly in a stress response is said to be a **primary stressor**. A **secondary stressor** occurs when, as a result of the initial stress response, further stress is created.

Assume, for example, that you and a friend have been looking forward to going to a concert, but as you get ready to leave the house, you discover that you have lost the tickets. You never do get into the concert. Instead you go to a local eatery and "pig out" on food and beer, a secondary stress response. If you create additional stress by feeling guilty for overindulging and hungover from excessive alcohol, further adaptive responses could be necessary.

Life Events and Change

A direct correlation exists between stressful life events and the occurrence of disease. Drs. Thomas Holmes and Richard Rahe, as well as others, have studied accumulated, stress-producing changes in people's lives. Their research confirms the notion that people with more stressful events in their lives have higher morbidity and mortality rates. One study by Holmes and Rahe found that 80 percent of those who had more than 300 Life Change Units (LCUs) on the Social Readjustment Rating Scale (see Self-Inventory 3.1) within the past year developed an illness within the next two years. This compared to a 37-percent chance of getting sick in the following two years for those who had less than 150 LCUs and a 51-percent risk of developing illness for those who scored between 150 and 300 LCUs. In addition, when those with over 300 LCUs did get sick, they were more likely to develop serious illnesses like cancer, heart

> **FAST FACTS**
>
> About 14 percent of all occupational disease claims in 1988 were attributed to stress, compared to 5 percent in 1980.

> **FAST FACTS**
>
> A 75-year old man who won $1,683 on a $2 bet at the racetrack was so stressed that he died of a heart attack as he stepped up to the window to cash in his winning ticket.

TABLE 3–1 ■ Common Sources of Stress

Classification	Explanation
1. *Intrapersonal conflict*	The turmoil within you that concerns which paths to take in life including goals, values, priorities, and decisions.
2. *Interpersonal relationships*	Stress resulting from interaction with others. Friends or peers are common sources of stress as you deal with the differences between you and learn to communicate and compromise.
3. *Family*	Although a major source of support, the family is also a source of stress because of the strength of the emotional ties among the people involved. Also, interaction among family members is more frequently of a judgmental nature.

(continued on page 62)

TABLE 3-1 ■ **Common Sources of Stress,** continued

Classification	Explanation
4. *Work and school settings*	Involves work satisfaction and meeting standards expected of you.
5. *Money concerns*	Always with you, especially as college students, money problems are usually not a matter of having enough to survive (although it may seem like that at times) but how to prioritize how you spend your income.
6. *Global instability*	In the United States, we are more isolated from the type of regional war that occurs in many other parts of the world, but conflict in another part of the globe can have immediate, deleterious effects here. In addition, awareness of the destructive presence of nuclear arms can produce "passive" stress.
7. *Environmental abuse*	Can come in the form of pollution, crowding, crime, overstimulation (especially by the media), and ecological damage.
8. *Technology*	Advances such as the automobile, computer, and nuclear energy are stressful because they require adaptive change and speed up the pace of life. Most technological advances are associated with increased risk, such as the toxic waste and threat of radiation that accompany nuclear plants or the more than 50,000 accidental deaths per year in the United States involving automobiles.
9. *Change*	Any sort of change is a source of stress, although certain changes are clearly more stressful than others. The more changes present in your life and the faster these changes come about, the greater the stress you will encounter.
10. *Time pressure*	Time pressures can cause stress directly or increase the stress brought on by other factors. Many people are not instinctively effective at time-management skills.
11. *Spiritual issues*	Coming to terms with discovering meaning in your life or developing a code of ethical and moral behavior can be stressful, especially if it involves rejecting previously held beliefs. If no recognition is given to the spiritual dimension, it can affect how you cope with stress because of a lack of direction in your life.
12. *Health patterns*	Illness, injury, dietary imbalances, exposure to toxic substances, and the like are fairly obvious forms of stress. The physiological stress response is often more clearly seen in these instances than in situations involving social and psychological stress.

SELF-INVENTORY 3.1

The Social Readjustment Rating Scale

Life Event	Mean Value
1. Death of spouse	100
2. Divorce	73
3. Marital separation	65
4. Jail term	63
5. Death of close family member	63
6. Personal injury or illness	53
7. Marriage	50
8. Fired at work	47
9. Marital reconciliation	45
10. Retirement	45
11. Change in health of family member	44
12. Pregnancy	40
13. Sexual difficulties	39
14. Gain of new family member	39
15. Business readjustment	39
16. Change in financial state	38
17. Death of close friend	37
18. Change to different line of work	36
19. Change in number of arguments with spouse	35
20. Mortgage over $10,000	31
21. Foreclosure of mortgage or loan	30
22. Change in responsibilities at work	29
23. Son or daughter leaving home	29
24. Trouble with in-laws	29
25. Outstanding personal achievement	28
26. Spouse begin or stop work	26
27. Begin or end school	26
28. Change in living conditions	25
29. Revision of personal habits	24
30. Trouble with boss	23
31. Change in work hours or conditions	20
32. Change in residence	20
33. Change in schools	20
34. Change in recreation	19
35. Change in church activities	19
36. Change in social activities	18
37. Mortgage or loan less than $10,000	17
38. Change in sleeping habits	16
39. Change in number of family get-togethers	15
40. Change in eating habits	15
41. Vacation	13
42. Christmas	12
43. Minor violations of the law	11

Interpretation

Refer to the score range below to classify your life change score.

Score Range	Interpretation	Susceptibility
300+	Major life change	Major illness within year
250–299	Serious life change	Lowered resistance to diseases
200–249	Moderate life change	Depression
150–199	Mild life change	Colds, flus occasional depression
149–0	Very little life change	Good health

General Observations

1. Change in one's life is followed, about a year later, by associated health changes. Is this true of your life style?
2. Life changes tend to cluster significantly around health changes. Is this true in your case?

SOURCE: T. H. Holmes and R. H. Rahe, "The Social Readjustment Rating Scale," *Journal of Psychosomatic Research* 11 (1967): 213–218. Copyright 1967, Pergamon Press, Ltd.

SELF-INVENTORY 3.2
A Social Readjustment Rating Scale for College Students

Column A		Life-Change Event	Column B	Column C
_____	(1)	Entered college	50	_____
_____	(2)	Married	77	_____
_____	(3)	Trouble with your boss	38	_____
_____	(4)	Held a job while attending school	43	_____
_____	(5)	Experienced the death of a spouse	87	_____
_____	(6)	Major change in sleeping habits	34	_____
_____	(7)	Experienced the death of a close family member	77	_____
_____	(8)	Major change in eating habits	30	_____
_____	(9)	Change in or choice of major field of study	41	_____
_____	(10)	Revision of personal habits	45	_____
_____	(11)	Experienced the death of a close friend	68	_____
_____	(12)	Found guilty of minor violations of the law	22	_____
_____	(13)	Had an outstanding personal achievement	40	_____
_____	(14)	Experienced pregnancy, or fathered a pregnancy	68	_____
_____	(15)	Major change in health or behavior of family member	56	_____
_____	(16)	Had sexual difficulties	58	_____
_____	(17)	Had trouble with in-laws	42	_____
_____	(18)	Major change in number of family get togethers	26	_____
_____	(19)	Major change in financial state	53	_____
_____	(20)	Gained a new family member	50	_____
_____	(21)	Change in residence or living conditions	42	_____
_____	(22)	Major conflict or change in values	50	_____
_____	(23)	Major change in church activities	36	_____
_____	(24)	Marital reconciliation with your mate	58	_____
_____	(25)	Fired from work	62	_____
_____	(26)	Were divorced	76	_____
_____	(27)	Changed to a different line of work	50	_____
_____	(28)	Major change in number of arguments with spouse	50	_____

disease, and extreme depression than milder illnesses like common colds. A similar scale, based on the original Holmes and Rahe scale, was developed specifically for college students (see Self-Inventory 3.2).

The scores on these scales represent only a likelihood of an illness or injury occurring. There are too many other factors associated with individual susceptibility to make accurate predictions. Still, the results of these scales should make you consider whether or not to take overt steps to control the effects of high levels of stress in your life.

In a recent study, college students in Kentucky were asked which factors they thought were most stressful for them. Table 3–2 indicates the top 21 factors

Column A		Life-Change Event	Column B	Column C
_____	(29)	Major change in responsibilities at work	47	_____
_____	(30)	Had your spouse begin or cease work outside the home	41	_____
_____	(31)	Major change in working hours or conditions	42	_____
_____	(32)	Marital separation from mate	74	_____
_____	(33)	Major change in type and/or amount of recreation	37	_____
_____	(34)	Major change in use of drugs	52	_____
_____	(35)	Took on a mortgage or loan of less than $10,000	52	_____
_____	(36)	Major personal injury or illness	65	_____
_____	(37)	Major change in use of alcohol	46	_____
_____	(38)	Major change in social activities	43	_____
_____	(39)	Major change in amount of participation in school activities	38	_____
_____	(40)	Major change in amount of independence and responsibility	49	_____
_____	(41)	Took a trip or a vacation	33	_____
_____	(42)	Engaged to be married	54	_____
_____	(43)	Changed to a new school	50	_____
_____	(44)	Changed dating habits	41	_____
_____	(45)	Trouble with school administration	44	_____
_____	(46)	Broke or had broken a marital engagement or steady relationship	60	_____
_____	(47)	Major change in self-concept or self-awareness	57	_____
			TOTAL	_____

Directions for scoring: List the number of times each event hås occurred to you within the past 12 months in Column A. Multiply that by the corresponding numerical value in Column B. Place that number in Column C. Total the scores in Column C.

Interpretation: High Risk 1450+ points
Medium Risk 890 points
Low Risk 347− points

SOURCE: Martin B. Marx, Thomas F. Garrity, and Frank R. Bowers, "The Influence of Recent Life Experiences on the Health of College Freshmen," *Journal of Psychosomatic Research* 19 (1975): 97, Copyright 1975, Pergamon Press Ltd.

for men and women. Notice that most stressors relate to academics and relationships. Which factors seem to be most stressful for you? What other factors not on this list should make the top 21, in your opinion?

> ■ **PROBLEM SITUATION** During the past year and a half, you have accumulated an abundance of Life Change Units (see Self-Inventory 3.1 or 3.2) that put you into the high-risk category for experiencing illness or injury. What actions can you take that will ameliorate the distressing effects of the major life changes that you're going through?

TABLE 3–2 ■ **Perceived Intensity of Stress Factors for College Students**

Rank	Males	Rank	Females
1.	Death of a parent	1.	Death of a parent
2.	Loss of intimate relationship	2.	Involved in pregnancy or abortion
3.	Final-exam week	3.	Final-exam week
4.	Breaking off a relationship	4.	Loss of a close friend
5.	Involved in pregnancy or abortion	5.	Breaking off a relationship
6.	Divorce or remarriage of parents	6.	Loss of intimate relationship
7.	Selecting or changing major	7.	Divorce or remarriage of parent
8.	Career opportunities after graduation	8.	Change in schools
9.	Change in schools	9.	Loss of close relative
10.	Loss of close friend	10.	Test anxiety
11.	Financial pressures	11.	Making plans for future
12.	Finding someone acceptable to date	12.	Oral presentations
13.	Putting off assignments or responsibilities	13.	Finding someone acceptable to date
14.	Making plans for future	14.	Academic workload
15.	Guilt for not doing better	15.	Financial pressure
16.	Oral presentations	16.	Deciding about or planning for marriage
17.	Loss of a close relative	17.	Putting off assignments or responsibilities
18.	Test anxiety	18.	Overweight or underweight
19.	Deciding about or planning for marriage	19.	Selecting or changing major
20.	Roommate adjustment	20.	Guilt for not doing better
21.	Concern about sexually transmitted diseases	21.	Career opportunities after graduation

SOURCE: Herman Bush, Merita Thompson, and Norman Van Tubergen, "Personal Assessment of Stress Factors for College Students," *Journal of School Health* 55(November 1985), 370–375.

FAST FACTS

Approximately 15 percent of Vietnam veterans have been found to have combat-related stress disorders.

Managing Crises

When intense emotional stress becomes too great to handle, a crisis situation can arise. A **crisis** is any risky event or crucial time in life that cannot be managed with resources and actions that have worked in the past. It can lead to further anxiety that hampers one's ability to clearly think through solutions or that stymies independent action.

Figure 3–3 shows how crisis progresses from a condition of relative balance to a state of **disequilibrium.** The first step in dealing with this crisis, then, is to feel the need to restore the balance that has been disturbed. The satisfactory restoration of balance will depend on a number of factors, the first of which is our perception of the unbalancing event. If we are not aware of the source of the tension, it will be harder to handle. Can you see in Figure 3–4 the results of Mary having incorrectly perceived the reason for failing an exam as personal failure rather than insufficient studying?

A second factor in overcoming a crisis is the availability of and access to an adequate support system consisting of friends, family members, and others involved in your life. It can include, for example, your good listener/friend or an empathetic counselor on campus.

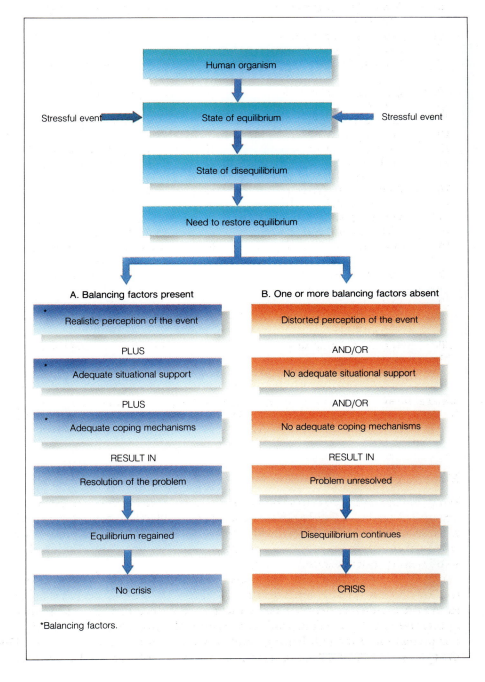

FIGURE 3–3 ■ **Paradigm: The Effect of Balancing Factors in a Stressful Event.**

SOURCE: Reproduced by permission from: Donna Aguilera and Janice Messick, *Crisis Intervention: Theory and Methodology* (St. Louis: C. V. Mosby, 1986).

The final factor in rebalancing emotional equilibrium is the adequacy of the set of personal coping mechanisms that you have developed. If your coping skills are not well developed, disequilibrium will continue. Once again, this is where a professionally trained counselor or therapist can help you. Thus, if you have a realistic perception of the stressful event or object, strong social support, and adequate coping skills, the problem can be resolved and balance restored.

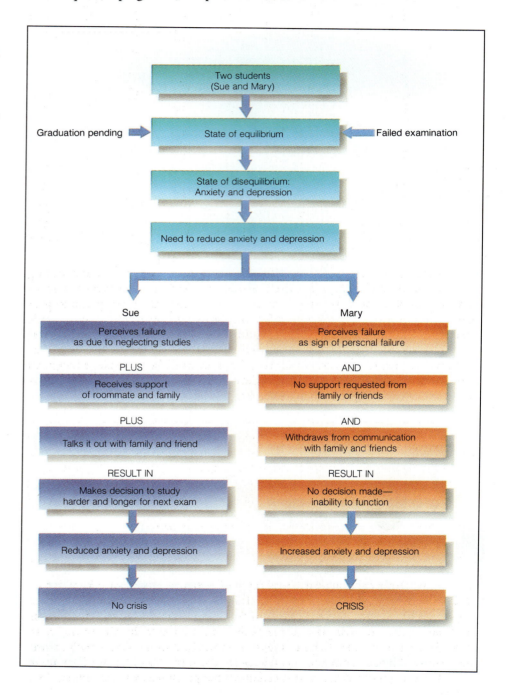

FIGURE 3–4 ■ Paradigm Applied to Case Study

SOURCE: Reproduced by permission from: Donna Aguilera and Janice Messick, *Crisis Intervention: Theory and Methodology* (St. Louis: C. V. Mosby, 1986).

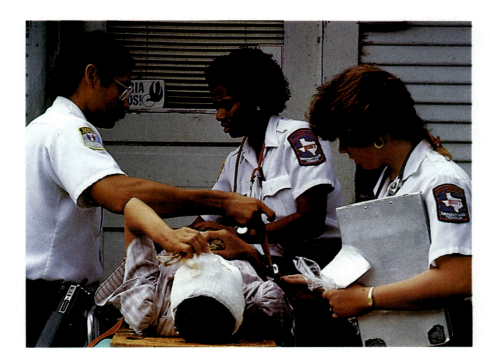

When crisis occurs we should be prepared to handle it properly.

Anticipatory crisis may occur before many events and can be just as disabling as crisis produced by the event itself. Stress perceived as being great before an event takes place, such as prior to exams, can be beneficial, forcing you to gear up for the event, or can be harmful, mushrooming into a full-blown panic reaction. A certain amount of anticipation is good, but when stress interferes with the achievement of your goals, concrete action needs to be taken. For example, academic counselors and workshops are available on college campuses for students who suffer from math anxiety and who have formed mental blocks when it comes to understanding mathematical concepts.

> ■ *PROBLEM SITUATION*   A good friend of yours is doing well in school academically but has encountered a critical financial situation because this person's parents have lost their family business and have declared bankruptcy. How could this potential crisis be dealt with satisfactorily? Using Figure 3–3, what are some factors that might prevent this from developing into a crisis for your friend, and what might cause it to escalate?

■ Manifestations Of Stress

Do you remember the ancient Greek myth of Achilles? His mother learned that if she dipped him in the River Styx when he was a baby, the water would make him invulnerable to injury or harm in battle. However, she held him by his heel, and therefore that part of his body wasn't covered by the water. Sure enough, later in his life, Achilles was shot in the heel in combat, which caused his demise. Hence, from this legend comes the term "Achilles heel," or weak spot. What is yours? When you succumb to the pressures of stress, where does it hit?

Why is it that when people are exposed to the same or similar psychological and pathological stressors, some remain healthy while others become sick? One approach to answering this question is to study the development of good health, called **salutogenesis,** an area that has been investigated extensively by the sociologist Aaron Antonovsky. Salutogenesis is an individual's ability to successfully cope with life's problems and the stressors encountered along the way.

Antonovsky found that people with a strong **sense of coherence** (knowing who they are in their environment and having a sense that they "fit") are less likely to succumb to stressors and therefore enjoy good health. He defines sense of coherence as:

> . . . a global orientation that expresses the extent to which one has a pervasive, enduring though dynamic feeling of confidence that one's internal and external environments are predictable and that there is a high probability that things will work out as well as can reasonably be expected.

This definition emphasizes that a reasonable outcome is both *predictable* and *expected* for a person with a strong sense of coherence. The three core elements of one's sense of coherence are (1) making sense of the whole array of stimuli (stressors) that one is faced with, (2) having a realistic perception that the resources to manage daily problems are at one's command, and (3) seeing one's situation in the world as having meaning and purpose.

Managing Your Stress

We have seen what stress is and is not, and where stress usually comes from. We have also investigated how stress becomes manifest in the body and why people may differ in their reactions to it. Assuming that you have taken in all of this information, let's look at some things that you can do to promote eustress and diminish distress in your own life.

Coping Strategies

The basic, overriding principles of avoiding distress and promoting a long and healthful life can be traced at least as far back as the year 2697 B.C., which was when *The Yellow Emperor's Classic of Internal Medicine* (called the *Nei Ching* in Chinese) was put in written form. The *Nei Ching* says that to enjoy a full life, free from the harmful effects of stress, one should live in harmony with the natural way of things. It calls for moderation in drinking and eating plus a regular schedule of rising, working, playing, sleeping, and resting. The ancient Chinese gave excellent advice when they said that simplicity in living is the key to reducing stress and getting the most out of life.

This approach to stress management is very holistic in nature, because it fosters such positive practices as appropriate consumption of material goods, environmental awareness, concern for humanity in living and working, personal growth, and self-determinism. In practical everyday terms, it boils down to managing stress by engaging in good habits of exercise, rest, nutrition, social networking, and spiritual awareness and by experiencing positive stimulation and the achievement of aesthetic satisfaction.

Another key factor in stress management involves managing the limited amount of time that each of us has. There are only 60 minutes in an hour and 24 hours in a day. As a student, the chores you have to fit into that limited time frame include going to classes, studying and preparing for class, working, participating

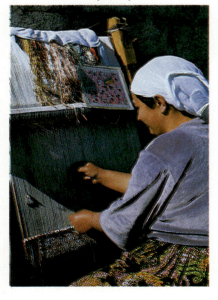

Each of us has our own way of managing stress. What do you do to help control the stresses in your life?

in extramural activities, family responsibilities, personal time for your hobbies, exercising, social affairs, and so on. Somehow you must either simplify your life when there is not enough time to do all that you must do or closely monitor and organize your time.

The first thing to understand about time management is that you really must manage yourself, because you are flexible and time is not—it just keeps moving along. If you've ever run a race and tried to "beat the clock," you're aware that the second hand never stops. Here are some suggestions that may help you manage your time, if that's a problem for you.

1. *Prioritize* what's truly important in your life. Don't overplan. If you are overscheduled, perhaps you can, for example, graduate from college a semester later without sacrificing anything really important.

2. You can't add more hours or minutes to your day, but you can *increase usable time*. Organize your schedule to make the most of what time you have. Identify and reduce "wasted" time, delegating certain activities to others in your social network instead of taking on too much by yourself. Schedule enough time for your high-priority activities. A problem that most of us have to some degree is procrastination—putting off today what may or may not wait until tomorrow. As far as academic procrastination is concerned, focus on avoiding or controlling distractions. For example, study in the library, where distractions are minimal.

3. You may want to *reduce the urgency* of time. Perhaps that task does not really have to be completed in the arbitrarily self-assigned time.

4. Another problem that affects optimal use of time is striving for perfection in the task that you're doing, thereby delaying its completion. It's okay to *give yourself permission to be imperfect*. You certainly don't want to do sloppy work, but recognize that most projects could be improved if only you began working on them sooner in order to spend more time on them.

5. Finally, be aware of procrastination that is caused by the fear of not being able to accomplish a task. If it seems overwhelming, *break the task down into smaller sub-tasks* to be done a piece at a time. If, however, the fear of failure stems from a lack of self-confidence in your ability to perform, you must *develop a positive attitude*. After all, you can't learn unless you try, and just because you fail at a task does not mean that you are not a good and capable person. With

GUIDELINES TO YOUR GOOD HEALTH

Positive thinking can be nurtured by taking these steps:

1. Psych yourself up for important events. Think over the upcoming situation and visualize it as being a successful experience.
2. Talk to yourself in a positive manner. It's like when Dorothy in the *Wizard of Oz* keeps telling herself, "I can. I can."
3. Be prepared. Develop a plan of action as well as contingency or alternate plans to use just in case circumstances change.
4. Label an upcoming event that might possibly cause undue tension a "positive learning experience." Look at exams, for example, as an opportunity to tell what you know, not as a test of what you don't know. What a feeling of power this can give you, if you're prepared.

this attitude, it's easier to undertake a task with the anticipation that it will be a life-enhancing experience. As important as it may be to develop relaxation and stress-reducing techniques, having a positive mental attitude is equally vital.

On the negative side of the ledger, many people try to cope with stress through artificial, chemical means, which is rarely a satisfactory method in the long run. Unfortunately, the most widely prescribed drug in the United States is Valium (diazepam), a tranquilizer. Other popular, over-the-counter substances, usually contain nothing more than multiple vitamins. They have no proven stress-reducing properties.

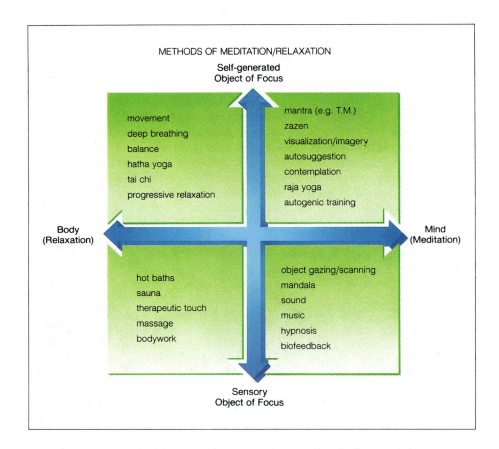

FIGURE 3–5 ■ **Methods Of Meditation/Relaxation**

SOURCE: Courtesy of Arnold Shapiro, M.D., Student Health Services, San Francisco State University.

■ *PROBLEM SITUATION* Whenever you go through a stressful event, you seem to develop a headache, back ache, or a stiff neck. Knowing this pattern, what steps can you take that will help prevent or alleviate these bothersome, stress-related pains?

Relaxation Techniques

In Figure 3–2, we saw a graph of a long-term stress response showing elevated body activity that stayed at a high level without resolution. To alleviate this

GUIDELINES TO YOUR GOOD HEALTH

The following are basic conditions for eliciting a relaxation response using a meditative technique:

1. Find a *quiet place* where you will be free from extraneous noise, interruptions, or other distractions.
2. Get into a *comfortable position* (yet not so comfortable that you fall asleep). Sit or lie down, removing or loosening restrictive clothing and shoes.
3. A *passive attitude* is the next requirement for an optimal relaxation response. To help clear your mind, do some deep breathing, inhaling deeply and then emptying your mind as you slowly exhale. If you did nothing more than a few deep breathing exercises every hour or two during the day, you would be well ahead of the game of stress reduction.
4. Have a *mental focus* to dwell on. Closing your eyes will help you concentrate on this relaxing thought, image, or other mental device.
5. Allow for 15 to 30 minutes of *uninterrupted time*.

continued state of physiological readiness, we can perform various exercises aimed at activating the **parasympathetic nervous system,** which is that part of the nervous system responsible for taking in energy and initiating a relaxation response.

In Figure 3–5, the methods of relaxation are categorized as primarily involving the body (called relaxation activities) or the mind (called meditation exercises) and as having either a self-generated object of focus or a sensory focus. Which ones you choose to use depends on your personal preferences; there is no scientific evidence that one is better than the others.

Meditative skills consist of being quiet and paying attention. Some techniques encourage a free flow of ideas entering and leaving the mind, whereas others rely on either totally emptying the mind or concentrating on a single object.

The focus in a meditative exercise may be the body itself (as in concentrated deep rhythmic breathing), a repetitive sound (a word, phrase, or simple musical tune), or an imagined peaceful scenario. The focus may be a **mantra,** which is a word or phrase, often sanskrit, that is repeated over again in a melodic rhythm. The purpose of having an object of focus is to prevent the undisciplined "monkey mind" from flitting from subject to subject as various thoughts and stimuli enter the consciousness. As you become more experienced at meditating, it is easier for you to prolong and sustain concentration.

Besides concentrative meditation, there is a meditative form that involves "letting go" or "going with the flow" in such a way as to become more sensitive to your environment. To do this, first get into a comfortable, meditative position, sway back and forth as you "settle in," take some deep breaths, and let go a little each time you exhale. Sometimes intentionally relaxing a given part of the body for a while is helpful prior to "free" thinking. Thoughts are allowed to flow from one to the other without making an attempt to manipulate them. Distractions are allowed to be played out until attention can be gently brought back to the peaceful present. The aim of this sort of meditation is to lose self-consciousness and not to think in the perspective of "I." The self is forgotten, and the world of NOW opens up. It is crucial to be in a quiet, serene place such as the shore, the woods, or a quiet place at home for this type of meditation.

Positive, creative imagery can have a suggestive effect that starts the mind moving toward a goal and weakens or overcomes negative images. By imagining where you want to be and visualizing how you will achieve that goal, you have gone a long way toward facilitating success. If you imagine failure, you are bound to fail; if you imagine success, you are more likely to succeed.

As with other relaxation techniques, visualization takes practice to work best. To practice creative imagery, first become "centered," or self-focused in the here and now, by getting relaxed as described previously. When you are fully relaxed, with your eyes closed and your breathing slow and steady, "breathe in energy and breathe out fatigue." Now begin to conjure up images in your mind, either of purely sensory sensations (for example, seeing blue skies, touching cottony clouds, smelling lemony fragrances, or hearing soft music) or of a desired scenario (for example, going out on the perfect date or spending 24 perfect hours). You can place yourself in an energy-enhancing environment and just allow good, peaceful thoughts to flow through your mind, imagining fantasies that are fulfilling and totally relaxing to you.

Physical exercise, preferably of the aerobic type (see Chapter 6), can also be a relaxation-evoking activity. A slow long-distance run, walk, swim, or bike ride can relieve stress and provide the added benefit of increasing physical fitness.

Keeping a Journal

Journaling is an excellent and powerful tool that can help you to understand and manage your stress, although it has the potential to be used in many areas of mental health. A personal journal is different from a diary in that the journal is more directive or tied to a theme or goal. It is kept in order to help you develop the self-directing and self-healing capacities in your life. The aim is to focus inward, encouraging spontaneity of thought and action by writing freely, followed by objective analysis. There is as much to gain from reading over and analyzing the journal as there is from actually keeping the journal. The following questions and answers will help you create a personal journal from which you can learn.

1. *What shall I write in?* Whatever you choose to write in, it will be a sort of companion of yours, so it should be easy to carry around and expandable.
2. *Where is the best place to write?* There is no single best place, but it is a good idea to write at a regularly scheduled time and in a place with minimum distractions, such as in your bedroom, the library, or even a quiet setting outdoors.
3. *How should I write?* It is important to write quickly and spontaneously with complete honesty and openness. This is your own personal journal; because you may not want to share it with another person, take some precautions to insure privacy. When you do make entries, they should focus primarily on the *positive*, although you'll want to examine all aspects of yourself.
4. *How often should I write in it?* This depends on what purpose your journal serves for you, but it should be on a regular basis. An intensive journal is done every day or so, whereas an occasional journal is written in on particular occasions.
5. *How shall I structure the journal and what shall I write about?* Journals have some degree of organization; they aren't merely free writing exercises. How you organize your journal is a highly individual and creative undertaking. First

decide what you want to learn from your journal, and then you will be able to choose the approach you'll take.

6. *What should I be looking for when I read it over?* In order to help examine your journal analytically, you might look for certain key-word indicators, such as labels used for people, where and how often the word "I" is used, or judgmentally laden words such as "never," "always," or "should." When reading over your journal, you may ask, "Do I still feel the same, or have I changed some of my views?" You might also write a summary statement of the journal as a means of becoming aware of your feelings, intuitions, senses, and intellect.

> ■ *PROBLEM SITUATION* Your health education professor has assigned you to keep a personal journal of your total health status and health behaviors. It is an open-ended assignment, allowing you to create the journal to meet your own desires and inclinations. How would you structure the journal and what would you write about? What would your journal look like? When would you write in it and where? Would you share it with anyone else?

■ Social Well-Being And Stress

So far we considered what the individual alone can do to help control the effects of stress. Of equal importance in handling stress are the social aspects of wellness.

There isn't a person reading this book who hasn't been depressed by some event or bad news and needed to talk to someone about it. Perhaps you have needed to talk things over with someone because a difficult decision had to be made, such as what to major in at school or whether to drop a class or drop out of school altogether. Think back to a recent time when you felt particularly down in the dumps. Who did you call on for assistance or solace? When was the last time a friend, classmate, co-worker or relative needed some sort of help or support, and you were the one who provided it?

GUIDELINES TO YOUR GOOD HEALTH

Here are some suggested themes for personal journal entries:

■ Create *guided imageries* or fantasies centered on specific people, environments, or situations.
■ Write *unsent letters* to different people.
■ Create *dialogues* with various people, including public figures, personal acquaintances, or fictitious characters. You can even create dialogues with objects, events, or society in general.
■ Write *period logs* discussing particular times in your life, such as during high school or when you participated in a special activity or group.
■ Make *lists* of "things I love to do," "traits I like in friends," "people I'd like to spend time on a deserted island with," and so on.
■ Compose *portraits* of your ideal teacher, friend, doctor, parent, lover, clergyman, and so on.
■ Make *topical entries,* such as ones covered in this book, about mental health, spirituality, families, drugs, AIDS, parenting, physical fitness, and so on.

Social support systems help meet basic human needs.

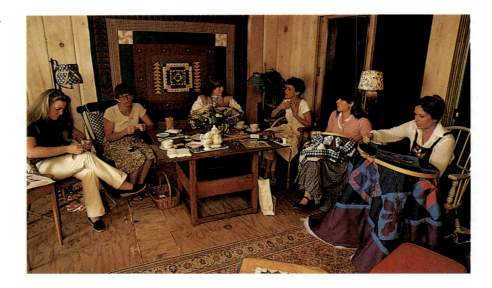

FAST FACTS

Individuals who repress their feelings and who may be called "loners" are 16 times more likely to develop cancer than those who act out their emotions in an overt manner.

This give and take of assistance and support forms the very heart of what is considered to be social well-being. We depend on others to meet our physical-survival and mental health needs as well as for human and spiritual fulfillment. The need for love, in particular, is based on the human desire for connectedness with others. The ability to interact with people in a satisfactory way and to establish close interpersonal relationships is a sign of social wellness.

Two basic terms that will come up frequently are *social support* and *social network*. A **social support** is any person or persons who provide some sort of assistance in helping us meet basic needs. A social-support system may give *emotional support* by helping us maintain self-esteem and a positive self-concept; *feedback* about ourselves and our perceptions of others; *information and advice;* and *tangible support* in the form of money, time, or skills.

Social networks refer to specific relationships among people in a group that can be analyzed according to various properties of existing relationships. The questions that are usually examined are: how do the people in the network connect with one another as a whole, what is the nature of the relationships within the network, and what function does the network serve? Social networks may exist in a natural form and meet general needs, such as those involving family and friends, or they may be formal groups created intentionally to help meet the specific needs of their members, such as a support groups for cancer patients or for people who abuse alcohol or drugs.

Social Support and Health

It has been only within the last two decades or so that research has been conducted that points directly to social support as a factor in preventing disease, lessening its severity and improving rehabilitation. General susceptibility to disease increases as social ties lessen or disintegrate. Of course, there are other factors that may lower general resistance, but lack of a substantial social network is an important influence with many ramifications.

A landmark study linking disease to social networks was conducted in Alameda County, California, between 1965 and 1974. More than 7,000 people were included in the study, which found that both morbidity and mortality increased significantly among those who had few social ties as compared to those with strong social-support systems. This finding was consistent in all ethnic groups, sexes, and socioeconomic levels.

Another interesting study looked at two groups of nursing-home residents, each of whom was given a plant. The experimental group's members were told that the plant was theirs and that they had the responsibility to care for it, whereas the control group's members were told that the staff would take care of the plant just as the staff took care of the patients. Not only did people in the experimental group, who had the responsibility of caring for the plants, display better mental and physical health, but after a period of 18 months, they had a death rate that was half that of the control group's. Having a responsibility for the well-being of any organism provides a reason for living and maintaining good health. Similar studies have shown that elderly people who have pets such as dogs or cats are healthier, live longer, and recover from illnesses more quickly than senior citizens who are isolated and live alone.

How Social Supports Help

Exactly why social support promotes good health is not known at the present time, but two general explanations have been suggested. The first of these, called the *buffering* effect of social support, explains that when people are exposed to environmental stressors that can cause or contribute to illness, having strong social ties helps control the adverse effects of these stressors. The buffering effect of social support helps people to cope by allowing them to control their mood (for example, to avoid depression) and by enhancing normal functioning. The buffering effect also helps them to maintain feelings of self-esteem and a sense of mastery when exposed to adversity.

The second explanation of the positive effects of strong social ties on health and well-being is called the *direct* effect. The reasoning here is that an extensive support system may provide people with unconditional approval, which leads to general well-being that enables them to better cope with stress. The direct effect of social support may also prevent people from being exposed to certain environmentally harmful stressors, because they may follow good health practices recommended by members of their social groups. In a study done in Oregon that looked at the medical records of 2,600 adults during a period of seven years, it was found that having social ties, being trustful of others, and perceiving more control were all related to better health status. An interesting part of these findings was that people's belief that they have control over their lives is as important as whether they actually do have such self-control.

The following are some of the specific functions that social networks serve.

Esteem. Self-esteem is a basic need that all humans attempt to fulfill. When threats to our self-esteem arise, it becomes important to have someone around to talk to and to gain reassurance that we are accepted and valued.

Status. It is essential to have a strong sense of who we are in relation to our society, and our social network clarifies and strengthens our roles among family members and friends. Besides fulfilling the roles of parent, child, spouse, or boyfriend or girlfriend, we also belong to other community groups that provide a degree of status, showing us that we are valued within the larger community.

FAST FACTS

A study of 110 men who were forcibly unemployed because of plant closures concluded that those men whose families and friends were highly supportive had fewer mental and physical health problems than those with fewer opportunities for social interactions.

Social Companionship. We live in a culture in which the majority of things we do outside our home and work are done with other people. On certain occasions we go to public events alone—and it is good to feel comfortable about being alone in public—but most people enjoy going to movies, sporting events, parties, and other forms of entertainment with someone else. Unfortunately, some people (such as elderly people who live alone and aren't very mobile) don't have natural companions with whom they can share these events. Companionship is desirable for its own sake, but it also leads to other forms of tangible and emotional support. Perhaps you can volunteer some of your time to provide temporary companionship to a person who is without a network of friends. Not only will it help that other person, but it will also make you feel good.

Information. Much of the information that we rely on to help us solve problems and make decisions comes in the form of advice and guidance. This information may not always be accurate, but because it comes from a source that we cherish as part of our social network, it is usually highly credible to us. Others within our social network often have insights into our problems and can be far more objective than we can be about ourselves.

Material Support. Let's face it, a great deal of our time during our waking moments is spent in the pursuit of material goods, because they are necessary for survival and they help satisfy other basic needs. If it weren't for social networking, it would be more difficult for us to acquire these goods and services. Tangible support may come in the form of money that is either given or loaned, time that is given to assist in a project, transportation, help in times of illness or distress, tutoring when we find it difficult to understand something, or any of a number of other offerings that lessen our burdens.

> ■ **PROBLEM SITUATION** As a new student on campus with no established social-support system in town, you realize the need for friends and other sources of support to help you deal with the stresses associated with academic life, financial needs, and independent living. What are some of the steps you can take to *assess* your social-support needs concerning emotional support, tangible resources, companionship, information, or simply having someone to bounce ideas off? How can you go about meeting these needs?

In spite of the helpful aspects of social networks, there are some potentially negative aspects about them. For one thing, the group to which one belongs imposes demands on its members, and these may not always be in their best interests and might create conflict. Some groups may blame problems on scapegoats, thus reinforcing prejudices, or they may put down their own members from time to time. We know that abuse does occur within families and that it may be physical or psychological, including sexual abuse.

Even when those on whom we depend for social support mean well, they may do more harm than good. For example, they may simply pass along information to us that is incorrect. More insidious is the pressure put on us when group members give advice (such as parents give to children) and expect us to follow it without question. Resentment often occurs when we believe that others are trying to control us. By and large, however, social networks operate in a positive manner to help us meet our needs.

POSITIVE BEHAVIORS

I. *Place a check mark in front of each behavior that you now practice.*

_____ 1. I keep my life as simple as is practical. (SIMPLIFY)

_____ 2. When I get nervous before an event, I take the time to practice a relaxation response. (NERVOUS)

_____ 3. When stress starts building up, I always take overt steps to reduce the sources of stress or alleviate their detrimental effects. (STRESS REDUCTION)

_____ 4. When my life gets too hectic, I set up a daily time-management calendar for myself that isn't too ambitious but that allows me to accomplish all of my most important tasks. (TIME MANAGEMENT)

_____ 5. When I encounter an overwhelming primary stressor, I always take direct positive action rather than allowing it to cause secondary stress. (PRIMARY STRESS)

_____ 6. I am aware of the amount and seriousness of personal life changes I am undergoing, and I take steps whenever possible to prevent too many changes from occurring in a short time span. (LIFE CHANGES)

_____ 7. I have a wide array of activities that I rely on to help me cope with life's stressors. (COPING)

_____ 8. I supply emotional and material support for my friends, relatives, and others within my social network whenever I am able. (SUPPORT OTHERS)

_____ 9. I maintain a social network that is strong enough to meet my needs for health and happiness. (NETWORK)

II. *For each behavior that you DO NOT ENGAGE IN, write the KEY WORD(S) that is in the parentheses located at the end of the statement in the column below. Then put a check mark in the appropriate column to indicate whether you are going to keep or change that behavior.*

Behaviors I Don't Engage In   **KEEP/CHANGE**

_____ / _____
_____ / _____
_____ / _____
_____ / _____
_____ / _____
_____ / _____
_____ / _____
_____ / _____
_____ / _____

III. *For each of the preceding behaviors that you choose to KEEP, write a statement indicating why you are choosing to keep that behavior.*

I choose to keep behavior _____ because:
                              KEY WORD

For each of the preceding behaviors that you choose to CHANGE, write a statement indicating how you plan to implement that change.

I will change behavior _____ by:
                          KEY WORD

Now You Know

1. FALSE. Stress is always present and can be beneficial as well as harmful.
2. TRUE. Excessive stress causes a weakening of the immune system and lowering of general resistance.
3. TRUE. Because we spend so much time growing up with our families and because emotional attachment is great, our families influence us in all ways, including being a source of stress.
4. FALSE. It is true that there is a correlation between life changes, stress, and illness, but not everyone is adversely effected.
5. TRUE. All three factors are necessary for resolution of the problem and restoration of equilibrium.
6. TRUE. Keeping our lives simple and harmonious is the best overall approach to stress control. This includes time management, positive self-perception, and regular relaxation exercises.
7. FALSE. There is no one best relaxation technique that suits everyone. For some it's meditation, but for others it may be jogging, swimming, painting, playing the piano or guitar, reading poetry, or listening to music.
8. TRUE. Social-support systems do these things and more, including giving us feedback about our ideas and actions, helping us maintain high self-esteem, and providing companionship.
9. FALSE. Many studies have shown a direct correlation between social support and health status.
10. TRUE. Not only are dogs, cats, fish, birds, and other pets beneficial to serving social needs, but even plants are valuable in giving people who live alone "someone to care for."

Summary

1. Stress has been defined by Dr. Hans Selye as "the rate of wear and tear within the body" as well as "the nonspecific response of the body to any demand made upon it."
2. Beneficial environmental stimuli lead to a state of *eustress,* whereas those stimuli that are damaging cause *distress.*
3. The body reacts to stressors in three stages—a general reaction stage, followed by a specific stage of resistance and, ultimately, exhaustion if the stress is too great. Selye calls this physiological pattern the General Adaptation Syndrome (GAS).
4. Stress my be short term or it may continue chronically over a period of time, in which case there are likely to be harmful effects on the body caused by excessive hormonal activity and imbalances.
5. Stress may occur directly from a primary stressor or as a result of a maladaptive response to the primary stressor, called secondary stress.
6. When too much change occurs in a person's life over too short a period of time, that individual has a significantly greater chance of becoming sick and also becomes less able to overcome illness.
7. It is important to recognize when situations have reached crisis proportions in our lives and to know how to go about reversing the imbalances created by these crises.
8. Exposure to the same forms and intensity of stress have different effects on different people. One possible explanation is that people have varying strengths of the sense of coherence (or the feeling of fitting into their environments). Those with a strong sense of coherence feel that they have better control of themselves.
9. Perhaps the best general approach to stress management is still to live simply and in harmony with the nature of things, maintaining balance and moderation, a philosophy that was advocated as long as 5,000 years ago in China.
10. Besides simplifying our lives, we can manage stress by better managing our time, doing regular relaxation exercises, and developing strong social supports.
11. One's social-support system consists of all people who provide help in meeting one's needs. A social network consists of our specific relationships among people in groups.
12. Having a substantial social network is an important factor in resistance to illness and recovery from disease.
13. A social-support system promotes good health by acting as a buffer against the harmful effects of stress and by increasing one's general resistance.
14. Social supports increase our bodies' general resistance by providing support for self-esteem, status, information gathering, companionship needs, and acquisition of material goods and services.
15. Although social networks are generally supportive and positive, they can also possess certain potentially negative qualities, such as when group members make demands that are too rigid or inappropriate.
16. How beneficial one's social network is depends on such factors as emotional closeness between members, the size and complexity of the network, the similarities of group members, and the frequency of interactions among members.

References

1. *A Guide to Managing Stress*. Daly City, Calif.: Krames Communications, 1985.
2. Antonovsky, Aaron. *Health, Stress, and Coping*. San Francisco: Jossey-Bass, 1979.
3. Barrera, Manuel Jr., Irwin N. Sandler, and Thomas B. Ramsay. "Preliminary Development of a Scale of Social Support: Studies of College Students." *American Journal of Community Psychology* 6(1981): 435–447.
4. Benson, Herbert. *The Mind/Body Effect*. New York: Simon and Schuster, 1979.
5. Berkman, Lisa, and Leonard Syme. "Social Networks, Host, Resistance and Mortality: A Nine-Year Follow-up Study of Alameda County Residents." *American Journal of Epidemiology* 109(1979): 186–204.
6. Bush, Herman S., Merita Thompson, and Norman Van Tubergen. "Personal Assessment of Stress Factors for College Students." *Journal of School Health* 55(1985): 370–375.
7. Curtis, John D., and Richard A. Detert. *How to Relax: A Holistic Approach to Stress Management*. Palo Alto, Calif.: Mayfield Publishing Company, 1981.
8. Dohrenwend, Barbara S., and Bruce Dohrenwend (eds.). *Stressful Life Events and Their Contexts*. New York: John Wiley and Sons, 1984.
9. Flynn, Patricia Anne Randolph. *Holistic Health*. Bowie, Md.: Robert J. Brady Company, 1980.
10. Friedman, Meyer, and Diane Ulmer. *Treating Type A Behavior—and Your Heart*. New York: Alfred A. Knopf, 1984.
11. Gordon, James S., Dennis T. Jaffee, and David E. Bresler. *Mind, Body and Health*. New York: Human Sciences Press, 1984.
12. Gottlieb, Benjamin H. (ed.) *Social Networks and Social Support*. Beverly Hills, Calif.: Sage Publications, 1981.
13. Gottlieb, Benjamin H. *Social Support Strategies*. Beverly Hills, Calif.: Sage Publications, 1983.
14. Greenberg, Jerrold S. *Comprehensive Stress Management*. Dubuque, Ia.: Wm. C. Brown, 1983.
15. Holmes, Thomas H., and Richard H. Rahe. "The Social Readjustment Rating Scale." *Journal of Psychosomatic Research* 11 (1967): 213–218.
16. Maguire, Lambert. *Understanding Social Networks*. Beverly Hills, Calif.: Sage Publications, 1983.
17. Minkler, Meredith. "The Social Component of Health." *Journal of Health Promotion* 1(1986): 33.
18. Milsum, John H. *Health, Stress and Illness*. New York: Praeger Publishers, 1984.
19. Pelletier, Kenneth R. *Mind as Healer, Mind as Slayer*. New York: Dell Books, 1977.
20. Schneiderman, Neil, and Jack T. Tapp. *Behavioral Medicine: A Biopsychosocial Approach*. Hillsdale, N.J.: Lawrence Erlbaum Associates, 1985.
21. Selye, Hans. *Stress Without Distress*. New York: J. B. Lippincott, 1974.
22. Selye, Hans. *The Stress of Life*. New York: McGraw-Hill, 1976.
23. Vieth, Ilza. *Huang Ti Nei Ching Su Wen: The Yellow Emperor's Classic of Internal Medicine*. Berkeley: University of California Press, 1966.

Suggested Readings

Cohen, Sheldon, and S. Leonard Syme (eds.). *Social Support and Health*. Orlando, Fla.: Academic Press, 1985.

Curtis, John D., and Richard A. Detert. *How to Relax: A Holistic Approach to Stress Management*. Palo Alto, Calif.: Mayfield Publishing Company, 1981.

Dohrenwend, Barbara S., and Bruce Dohrenwend (eds.). *Stressful Life Events and Their Contexts*. New York: John Wiley and Sons, 1984.

Gillespie, Peggy Roggenbuck, and Lynn Bechtel. *Less Stress in 30 Days: An Integrated Program for Relaxation*. New York: New American Library, 1986.

Girdano, Daniel A., and George S. Everly. *Controlling Stress and Tension: A Holistic Approach*. Englewood Cliffs, N.J.: Prentice-Hall, 1986.

Greenberg, Jerrold S. *Stress and Sexuality*. New York: AMS Press, 1987.

Rosch, Paul J., and Kenneth Pelletier. *Occupational Stress*. New York: AMS Press, 1988.

The Women's World: A Holistic Approach to Dealing with Stress. New York: AMS Press, 1987.

SECTION II

Body Dynamics

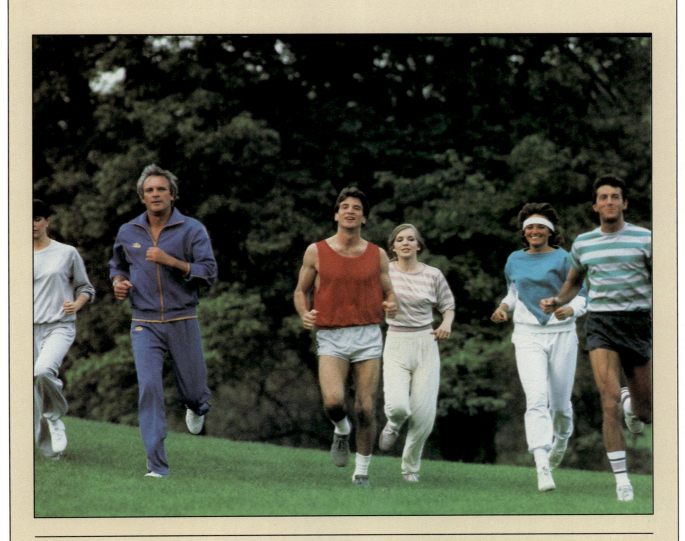

Chapter 4: Food Facts
Dietary Guidelines for Americans
What Are Nutrients?
Calorie Awareness
Carbohydrates: The Total Picture
Protein
Fats
Vitamins
Minerals
Vitamin and Mineral Supplements

Water
Health Foods
An Anti-cancer Diet

Chapter 5: Eating Behaviors
Body Weight
Body Composition
The Decision to Lose Weight
The Decision to Gain Weight
Theories of Weight Control

Weight Reduction
Eating Disorders

Chapter 6: Getting Physical
Definition of Physical Fitness
Benefits of Exercise
Principles of a Fitness Program
Developing Your Exercise Program
Athletic Training

CHAPTER 4

Food Facts

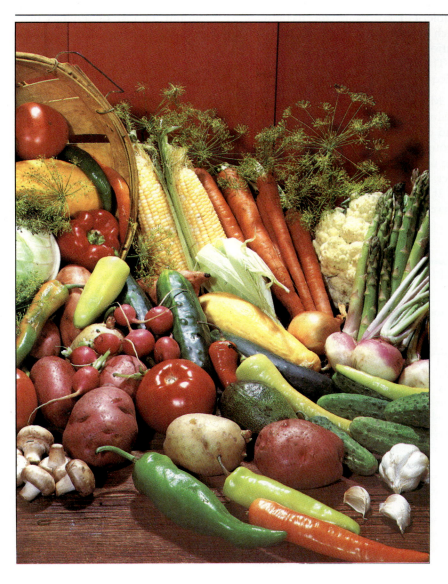

What Do You Know?

Are the following statements true or false?

1. Meats, butter, eggs, and milk are the primary sources of dietary cholesterol.
2. The more protein an individual eats, the healthier he or she becomes.
3. A totally vegetarian diet cannot provide all the essential amino acids needed to synthesize protein.
4. Vitamins supply the body with energy.
5. The biggest single component of the body is bone tissue.
6. The greatest percentage of daily calories should come from eating protein.
7. A sudden, large increase in dietary fiber may cause abdominal cramping and distention.
8. Vitamin and mineral tablets are needed to supplement a well-balanced diet.
9. Oils from vegetable sources, such as corn, sunflower, and safflower oils, are high in saturated fats.
10. Perspiration and thirst are the body's signals that more water is needed in order to replace what has been lost.

Good nutrition is an essential component of good health. By eating a well-balanced, nutritious diet, you can help keep your body healthy. Eating for good health requires a balanced intake of carbohydrates, protein, fat, vitamins, minerals, fiber, and water. Too much or too little of any of these nutrients can affect the optimal functioning of your body. Good eating habits entail knowing how to select foods and knowing how many servings of each to eat daily. A commonly used system in the United States is the Four Basic Food Groups Plan. Foods of similar nutrient value are placed in one of the four following food groups:

- Meat and high-protein foods
- Milk and milk products
- Fruits and vegetables
- Breads and cereals (whole-grain or enriched)

This plan specifies that a certain amount of food must be eaten from each group. Table 4–1 represents the recommended minimum number of servings from each food group that should provide a balanced intake of essential nutrients for various members of the population.

The Four Basic Food Groups Plan provides a basis for assuring nutritional adequacy; however, be aware of the following potential built-in problems:

- Many of the foods we eat do not fit into any of the four food groups—for example, butter, sour cream, gravies, salad dressing, relishes, soft drinks, cakes, and candy, just to mention a few. Foods that do not fit into any of the food groups are called "extra" foods. These foods are usually high in fat or sugar or are used for flavoring. They usually do not provide anything nutritious to the diet.
- It is possible to choose the least nutritious foods from among the four groups, thereby leading to some nutrient deficiency. For example, daily servings from

TABLE 4–1 ■ Recommended Minimum Number of Servings from the Four Basic Food Groups

Food Group	Recommended Minimum Number of Servings*					
	Child	*Teenager*	*Adult*	*Pregnant Woman*	*Lactating Woman*
Meat	2	2	2	3	2
Milk	3	4	2	4	4
Fruit-Vegetable	4	4	4	4	4
Bread-Cereal	4	4	4	4	4

*Serving size varies according to the specific type of food. Usually, however, a serving of meat is 2 to 3 ounces of cooked, lean, boneless meat, fish, poultry, or protein equivalent or 1 egg.

A serving of milk is 1 cup milk, yogurt, or calcium equivalent or ½ to 1 ounce of cheese. (A serving of cheese can be used for either the milk *or* meat group, but not both.)

A serving of fruit or vegetable is ½ to 1 cup or 1 medium-size fruit or potato.

A serving of bread or cereal is 1 slice of bread, ½ to ¾ cup of cooked cereal, rice, or pasta, or 1 ounce of ready-to-eat cereal.

the fruits and vegetables group should always include a food rich in vitamin C and one rich in vitamin A. Failure to make these choices could result in deficiency.

■ It might be possible to overload on one type of nutrient. For example, high-fat foods may be selected from three of the groups, thus contributing an excessive amount of fat to the overall diet.

■ Individuals have different metabolic rates and physical activity levels. What might be an adequate intake of calories and nutrients for one person might be too little or too excessive for another.

■ The terminology used may be inappropriate for the vegetarian who may desire to avoid the meat and milk groups altogether. However, knowledge that a combination of dried peas and beans may be an alternate food in the meat group helps to alleviate this problem.

■ An individual may follow this plan and still be deficient in vitamin B_6, vitamin E, iron, magnesium, and zinc.

With proper understanding of the Four Basic Food Groups, these problems can be avoided by selecting a wide variety of foods.

The United States Departments of Agriculture and Health and Human Services have established dietary guidelines to help individuals achieve and maintain sound eating patterns for good health. These guidelines recommend calorie control, increased consumption of starches and fiber, and reduced consumption of fat, sugar, and sodium. Which of the following guidelines have you already incorporated into your diet, and which are you neglecting?

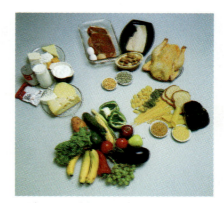

Eating a variety of foods from the Four Basic Food Groups will provide individuals with a balanced intake of essential nutrients.

■ Dietary Guidelines for Americans

1. *Eat a variety of foods.* Restricting a diet to only a few foods, or emphasizing one particular nutrient, can result in a nutritionally deficient, or even dangerous, diet.

2. *Maintain ideal body weight.* The key to weight control is calories. Your weight marks the balance between what you eat and your level of activity. It is easier to achieve and maintain your desired weight through a program including both proper diet and exercise.

3. *Avoid too much fat, saturated fat, and cholesterol.* Dietary fat is an essential nutrient, but too much saturated fat and cholesterol in the diet has been linked to the development of heart disease. Limit your intake of fats on and in foods by choosing low-fat protein and dairy sources.

4. *Eat foods with adequate starches and fiber.* To add starches and fiber to your diet, eat whole-grain breads and cereals, fresh fruits and vegetables, and legumes.

5. *Avoid too much sugar.* Foods with sugar as a major ingredient generally have few vitamins, minerals, and fiber. Satisfy your desire for sweets with small amounts of fresh fruits and juices, which have sugar but also provide additional nutrients.

6. *Avoid too much sodium.* Diets high in sodium have been linked to serious health problems. The major source of sodium is salt. Cut down or eliminate adding salt to your foods. You can enhance the natural flavors of food by minimal cooking and a few carefully selected herbs and spices.

7. *If you drink alcohol, do so in moderation.* Alcohol contains few nutrients other than calories. Excessive amounts of alcohol can lead to health problems. Even small amounts of alcohol during pregnancy can have adverse effects on the developing fetus.

What Are Nutrients

Nutrients are substances found in food that meet the body's needs for energy, growth, and good health. Humans have an essential requirement for a variety of nutrients. There are six nutrients considered necessary in human nutrition. They are carbohydrates, fats, protein, vitamins, minerals, and water. Vitamins is the name given to a group of organic compounds, other than protein, carbohydrate, and fat, that are present in foods and are essential to maintaining good health. The nutrient, minerals, consists of many mineral elements such as calcium, phosphorus, and iron that are present in foods and essential to the functioning of the body. Each nutrient is needed in a certain amount in order to adequately perform its function. Do you know how much of each nutrient is needed by your body?

In the United States, the amounts of certain of these nutrients have been established by the Food and Nutrition Board of the National Academy of

TABLE 4–2 ■ Recommended Dietary Allowances (RDA), 1989

		Weight[b]		Height[b]			Fat-Soluble Vitamins			
Category	Age (years) or Condition	(kg)	(lb)	(cm)	(in)	Protein (g)	Vitamin A (µg RE)[c]	Vitamin D (µg)[d]	Vitamin E (mg α-TE)[e]	Vitamin K (µg)
Infants	0.0–0.5	6	13	60	24	13	375	7.5	3	5
	0.5–1.0	9	20	71	28	14	375	10	4	10
Children	1–3	13	29	90	35	16	400	10	6	15
	4–6	20	44	112	44	24	500	10	7	20
	7–10	28	62	132	52	28	700	10	7	30
Males	11–14	45	99	157	62	45	1,000	10	10	45
	15–18	66	145	176	69	59	1,000	10	10	65
	19–24	72	160	177	70	58	1,000	10	10	70
	25–50	79	174	176	70	63	1,000	5	10	80
	51+	77	170	173	68	63	1,000	5	10	80
Females	11–14	46	101	157	62	46	800	10	8	45
	15–18	55	120	163	64	44	800	10	8	55
	19–24	58	128	164	65	46	800	10	8	60
	25–50	63	138	163	64	50	800	5	8	65
	51+	65	143	160	63	50	800	5	8	65
Pregnant						60	800	10	10	65
Lactating	1st 6 months					65	1,300	10	12	65
	2nd 6 months					62	1,200	10	11	65

[a] The allowances, expressed as average daily intakes over time, are intended to provide for individual variations among most normal persons as they live in the United States under usual environmental stresses. Diets should be based on a variety of common foods in order to provide other nutrients for which human requirements have been less well defined.
[b] Weights and heights of Reference Adults are actual medians for the U.S. population of the designated age, as reported by NHANES II. The median weights and heights of those under 19 years of age were taken from Hamill et al. (1979). The use of these figures does not imply that the height-to-weight ratios are ideal.

(continued on page 89)

Sciences/National Research Council. The Recommended Dietary Allowances (RDA) represent the levels of intake of essential nutrients considered to be adequate to meet the nutritional needs of practically all healthy persons in the United States. The current RDA are listed in Table 4–2, the tenth revision since they were initiated in 1943.

An individual must interpret the RDA with care. They have been established for the average-sized male or female at a given age. They have also been designed for healthy persons and do not take into account persons such as alcoholics, the chronically ill, crash dieters, junk-food addicts, the very poor, or the elderly. So use the RDA as a guide to nutritional needs, but remember that they have their limitations. The best way to assure getting all the essential nutrients in your diet is to eat a variety of foods, because no one food contains all the nutrients a human body needs.

FAST FACTS

RDAs for vitamin K and selenium are established for the first time in the tenth edition printed below.

TABLE 4–2 ■ Recommended Dietary Allowances (RDA), 1989, continued

	Water-Soluble Vitamins						Minerals						
Vitamin C (mg)	Thiamin (mg)	Ribo-flavin (mg)	Niacin (mg NE)ƒ	Vitamin B₆ (mg)	Folate (µg)	Vitamin B₁₂ (µg)	Calcium (mg)	Phos-phorus (mg)	Mag-nesium (mg)	Iron (mg)	Zinc (mg)	Iodine (µg)	Sele-nium (µg)
30	0.3	0.4	5	0.3	25	0.3	400	300	40	6	5	40	10
35	0.4	0.5	6	0.6	35	0.5	600	500	60	10	5	50	15
40	0.7	0.8	9	1.0	50	0.7	800	800	80	10	10	70	20
45	0.9	1.1	12	1.1	75	1.0	800	800	120	10	10	90	20
45	1.0	1.2	13	1.4	100	1.4	800	800	170	10	10	120	30
50	1.3	1.5	17	1.7	150	2.0	1,200	1,200	270	12	15	150	40
60	1.5	1.8	20	2.0	200	2.0	1,200	1,200	400	12	15	150	50
60	1.5	1.7	19	2.0	200	2.0	1,200	1,200	350	10	15	150	70
60	1.5	1.7	19	2.0	200	2.0	800	800	350	10	15	150	70
60	1.2	1.4	15	2.0	200	2.0	800	800	350	10	15	150	70
50	1.1	1.3	15	1.4	150	2.0	1,200	1,200	280	15	12	150	45
60	1.1	1.3	15	1.5	180	2.0	1,200	1,200	300	15	12	150	50
60	1.1	1.3	15	1.6	180	2.0	1,200	1,200	280	15	12	150	55
60	1.1	1.3	15	1.6	180	2.0	800	800	280	15	12	150	55
60	1.0	1.2	13	1.6	180	2.0	800	800	280	10	12	150	55
70	1.5	1.6	17	2.2	400	2.2	1,200	1,200	320	30	15	175	65
95	1.6	1.8	20	2.1	280	2.6	1,200	1,200	355	15	19	200	75
90	1.6	1.7	20	2.1	260	2.6	1,200	1,200	340	15	16	200	75

ᶜRetinol equivalents. 1 retinol equivalent = 1 µg retinol or 6 µg β-carotene. See text for calculation of vitamin A activity of diets as retinol equivalents.
ᵈAs cholecalciferol. 10 µg cholecalciferol = 400 IU of vitamin D.
ᵉα-Tocopherol equivalents. 1mg d-α tocopherol = 1 α-TE.
ƒ1 NE (niacin equivalent) is equal to 1 mg of niacin or 60 mg of dietary tryptophan.
SOURCE: Reproduced from Recommended Dietary Allowances, 10th ed. (1989), with permission of The National Academy of Sciences, Washington, D.C.

> **FAST FACTS**
>
> A twelve-ounce soft drink contains from eight to ten teaspoons of sugar.

Calorie Awareness

Most people are familiar with the term "calorie." **Calories** in food represent a form of potential energy to be used by the body to produce heat and perform work. In nutrition, the calorie or **kilocalorie** (kcal.), is the main expression of a food's energy-producing value. A glass of whole milk, for example, has about 160 kcal. of energy.

Consumption of calories is a necessity if the body is to function at all. Because a calorie is a unit of energy, and because energy can neither be created nor destroyed, those calories that we eat must either be expended or conserved in the body. Simply put, if you take in more calories than you expend, you will gain weight; if you expend more than you take in, you will lose weight. To maintain your body weight, caloric intake and output must be equal. One pound of body fat equals 3,500 calories. Therefore, for every decrease in food intake or increase in physical activity to total 3,500 calories, you will lose one pound. The opposite is true if you want to gain one pound of body weight. Now that you know a little more about the caloric concept of weight control, how can you figure out how many calories you are consuming?

You first need to know that calories can only come from carbohydrates, proteins, and fats. They are the only nutrients that can be oxidized in the body to yield energy. They are, therefore, referred to as the *energy nutrients*. Even though alcohol can serve as an energy source, it is not considered to be a nutrient because it cannot be used by the body to promote growth, maintenance, or repair. Of the total calories consumed daily, the following proportion of calories should be derived from each of the energy nutrients: protein, 12 percent; fat, 30 percent; and carbohydrates, 58 percent.

The energy value of foods depends primarily on the relative amounts of carbohydrate, protein, fat, and alcohol that they contain. The following values can be used to determine the caloric content of the foods we eat.

> 1 gram of carbohydrate = 4 kcal.
> 1 gram of protein = 4 kcal.
> 1 gram of fat = 9 kcal.
> 1 gram of alcohol = 7 kcal.

A food's energy value may be computed by multiplying the number of grams of each energy nutrient in a given serving of the food by the caloric values per gram of carbohydrate, protein, and fat. Using this formula, let's determine what the energy value of an eight-ounce glass of whole milk would be. Milk contains 12.0 grams of carbohydrate, 9.0 grams of protein, and 8.0 grams of fat in an eight-ounce serving. The caloric value is calculated as follows:

Nutrient	Total Grams		kcal./g.		Total kcal.
Carbohydrate	12.0	×	4	=	48.0
Protein	9.0	×	4	=	36.0
Fat	8.0	×	9	=	72.0
			Total	=	156.0 kcal.

Therefore, an eight-ounce glass of whole milk has 156.0 kcal.

The number of calories an individual needs daily depends on a variety of factors, such as age, sex, current health status, body weight, **basal metabolic rate (BMR),** and level of physical activity. How many calories are you consuming daily? Are you consuming too many or too few for your body's needs?

CHAPTER 4 ■ FOOD FACTS   91

> ■ *PROBLEM SITUATION* You have been feeling very tired and listless lately. As the saying goes, "your get-up-and-go just got up and went." What in your diet might be affecting this condition? What changes can you make in your diet to improve the way you feel?

■ Carbohydrates: The Total Picture

A large group of substances in our food is called **carbohydrates.** Carbohydrates provide most of the energy in the average diet. Chemically, carbohydrates are made up of the elements carbon, hydrogen, and oxygen. These three elements are combined in many different ways to make the different types of carbohydrates found in foods.

In general terms, carbohydrates may be categorized as either simple or complex. The **simple carbohydrates** are the **disaccharides** and **monosaccharides,** commonly known as sugars. The **complex carbohydrates** are the **polysaccharides,** commonly known as starches. Carbohydrates are usually ingested in the forms of polysaccharides (starches) and disaccharides (sugars), although some monosaccharides (**glucose, fructose,** and **galactose**) can be found in the diet.

Without going into the complexity of the digestive process, what essentially occurs is a breakdown of the polysaccharides and disaccharides to the monosaccharides. All carbohydrates must be broken down into monosaccharides before they can be absorbed and used by the body. The fructose and galactose that are absorbed into the blood are eventually transported to the liver, where they are converted to glucose. It is the glucose that circulates in the bloodstream and is used for energy. That is why glucose is known as "blood sugar." After assimilation into the blood, glucose may be used as an immediate energy source or stored as glycogen in the liver and muscles. When the cells' immediate energy needs are met and the glycogen stores are full, the liver will break the extra energy compounds into the more permanent energy-storage compounds—fat. Unlike the liver cells, which can only store about half a day's worth of glycogen, the fat cells can store unlimited quantities of fat. Body fat can never regenerate glucose to feed the brain.

Without glucose, the body is forced to use protein and fat differently. When body protein is used as an energy source, the body breaks down its own muscles and other protein tissues to make glucose. Without sufficient carbohydrate, fats cannot be used efficiently. The body converts fat into ketones (unusual products of fat breakdown), incurring **ketosis.** Ketosis during pregnancy can cause brain damage and irreversible mental retardation to the fetus. Still other problems occur when the diet lacks carbohydrates: fatigue, dehydration, nausea, vomiting, loss of appetite, and a temporary drop in blood pressure when getting up from a reclining position.

Although it is true that carbohydrates are a major source of energy, they can and should provide more than just calories. The problem arises when we eat too many of the empty calories and too few of the nutritious ones. Americans have replaced many of the nutritious carbohydrates with highly refined flour and sugars. Increased consumption of these refined products has already been linked to several major health problems, such as obesity, heart disease, tooth decay, diabetes, and colon cancer. There are three types of carbohydrates that

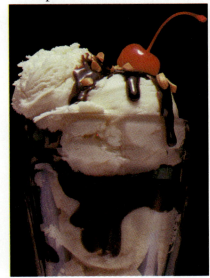

Blood sugar level would soar after eating this temptation.

have significant effects on an individual's health when included in the diet. These types are the simple carbohydrates, or sugars; the complex carbohydrates, or starches; and fiber.

Simple Carbohydrates or Sugars

Simple carbohydrates are found naturally as part of fruits and vegetables or as a refined product in foods such as table sugar, syrups, sodas, cakes, and candy. The natural sources of sugar are healthy. Eating a peach, for example, provides the body with vitamin A, vitamin C, fiber, potassium, and small amounts of niacin and iron in addition to the sugar. Most of the simple sugar we consume, however, is in the form of table sugar, soft drinks, candy, and desserts. Simple sugar contains about thirteen calories per teaspoon, but nothing else. Sugared foods are stripped of natural fiber, vitamins, and minerals and are mostly just a source of calories. Remember that one gram of carbohydrate is equal to 4 kcal.

If you believe that substituting honey for white sugar is better for your health because honey is "natural," think again. After digestion, honey and white sugar are identical. Spoonful for spoonful, however, white sugar contains fewer calories than honey, because the crystals of sugar take up more space. Remember, sweeteners such as honey or brown sugar are still primarily a concentrated form of calories.

A word about alcohol is in order here. Although not a true carbohydrate, alcohol is derived from carbohydrate foods either by natural fermentation, as in beer and wines, or from a distillation process to produce hard liquor such as whisky. Alcoholic beverages are generally a source of empty calories, and if you combine a sweet mixer with the alcohol, you are just adding additional sugar and calories.

It is all right to occasionally indulge yourself by eating a rich pastry, but since it is mostly just a source of calories, limit the quantity while enjoying the quality.

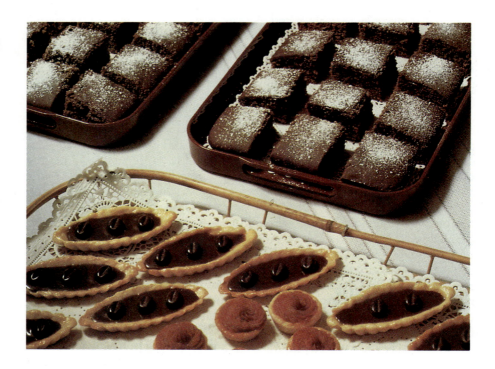

GUIDELINES TO YOUR GOOD HEALTH

Consider the following guidelines for minimizing sugar in your diet:

1. Drink beverages that contain little or no sugar. Many people drink sugared beverages without realizing the amount of sugar and extra calories they contain. Did you know that a 12-ounce can of soda contains approximately 150 calories?
2. Reduce your intake of processed foods. Much of the sugar we consume is hidden in these foods.
3. Eat plain yogurt. Many commercial yogurts are high in sugar. Buy plain yogurt and add fresh fruit, if desired.
4. In recipes calling for sugar, reduce the amount you add by a third to a half.
5. Become a label reader. Try to select foods with the lowest amount of sugar. Because ingredients are listed in the order of their amount by weight, there is at least some basis for comparison.
6. Be on the lookout for various forms of sugar or sweeteners found in foods. Corn syrup, corn sweeteners, honey, molasses, and maple syrup are all caloric sweeteners. All ingredients ending in "ose," such as sucrose, fructose, lactose, maltose, and glucose, are forms of sugar.
7. Eat breakfast cereals low in sugar or, better still, without added sugar. Sweeten cereal with fresh fruit instead of table sugar.
8. Avoid or cut down on sweet desserts. Substitute fresh fruit or milk deserts for cakes and pies.
9. Eat fresh fruits. Before eating canned fruits, drain them and rinse the syrup from them. The syrup has the unnecessary sugar you want to avoid.
10. Avoid or limit candy. Many candies are made up almost entirely of sugar. Chocolate candy is not only high in sugar but also high in fat.
11. Do not keep sweets (candy, cookies, soda, etc.) around the house if you cannot resist the snacking temptation.

Complex Carbohydrates or Starches

Complex carbohydrates are found as starches in whole grains, fruits, vegetables, and **legumes** (dried peas and beans). They are composed of long chains of sugar molecules. Because these chains must be broken down to simple sugars before being absorbed by the body, complex carbohydrates release their energy into the body over a longer period of time than do the simple carbohydrates. As a result, starchy foods satisfy your hunger better than sugars do. Even though one gram of complex carbohydrate is equal to 4 kcal., complex carbohydrates are in their whole or unrefined form, thus providing the body with vitamins, minerals, and fiber as well as calories. Fiber has recently been shown to be beneficial in the prevention and treatment of many health problems. The increased consumption of complex carbohydrates is highly recommended under the **Dietary Goals for the United States** published in 1977 (see Table 4–3).

TABLE 4–3 ■ **The Current Diet and the Recommended Dietary Goals for Americans**

Current Diet (percentage of kcal/day)	Dietary Goals (percentage of kcal/day)
Fat = 42%	Fat = 30%
Protein = 12%	Protein = 12%
Complex Carbohydrates = 22%	Complex Carbohydrates = 48%
Simple Carbohydrates = 24%	Simple Carbohydrates = 10%

The average American is presently getting 22 percent of his or her daily calories from complex carbohydrates. It has been recommended in the Dietary Goals that 48 percent of one's daily calories be derived from complex carbohydrates and that the daily consumption of fat and sugar be greatly reduced.

Fiber

Fiber is a general term that describes the indigestible portions of plant foods. It is often referred to as "bulk" or "roughage." These indigestible substances help make up the structure and the outer coverings of plants. Examples of fiber are the stringy parts of celery, the bran from grains, and the skins on fruits and vegetables. Fiber is unlike sugars or starches in its chemical structure. This structure causes the fiber to be indigestible for humans. It is this characteristic that makes fiber so important in the diet, because it provides roughness to help move food wastes through the body. Even though there is no Recommended Dietary Allowance for fiber, nutritionists recommend eating between 25 and 50 grams of dietary fiber daily. Presently, the average American consumes about 10 to 20 grams daily.

Starchy foods are the major sources of fiber in the diet. Unfortunately, much of the fiber is taken out of the foods we eat today. This is especially true of breads. Bread is made from a particular grain, such as wheat, oats, corn, rice, and rye. A grain consists of three parts: the **endosperm, germ,** and **bran.** (see Figure 4–1) To make refined flour, which is used in white bread, only the endosperm is used. The endosperm is the soft, inside portion of the grain containing starch and proteins. To make unrefined flour, which is used in whole-wheat bread, the entire grain is used, including the germ and bran. The germ is rich in vitamins and minerals, and the bran is an excellent source of fiber. We often hear the argument that white flour is as nutritious as whole-grain flour because it is enriched with vitamins and minerals. **Enrichment** is the addition of vitamins and minerals—specifically thiamine, riboflavin, niacin, and iron—to processed cereal and grain products to restore the amount lost in processing. Unfortunately, enrichment does nothing to replace the fiber and trace minerals that have also been lost during the processing.

Not only is fiber important for proper body functioning, but the *type* of fiber eaten is equally as important in the protection against certain diseases. Two types of dietary fiber, **insoluble** and **soluble,** have been identified as having positive health effects on the body. The best sources of insoluble fiber are whole-grain breads and cereals, especially whole-wheat products, and most fruits and

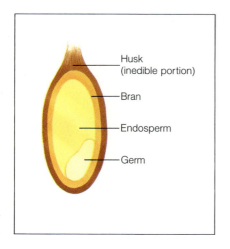

FIGURE 4–1 ■ The Three Parts of a Grain

CHAPTER 4 ■ FOOD FACTS

vegetables. Insoluble fiber speeds up the movement of food through the intestines and promotes regularity, thereby contributing to an *anti-cancer diet*. The best sources of soluble fiber are oat bran and dried beans, such as kidney, garbanzo, pinto, and navy beans. This type of fiber appears to lower blood-cholesterol levels, thereby contributing to a *healthy-heart diet*. Soluble fiber has also been found to help stabilize blood-sugar levels in people with diabetes.

The best way to increase dietary fiber is to increase consumption of complex carbohydrates (whole grains, fruits, and vegetables), legumes (dried peas and beans), nuts, and seeds. A sudden, large increase in fiber may cause uncomfortable flatulence, cramping, and distention. Add fiber gradually to your diet. Drink plenty of liquids, especially with more fiber in your diet. Liquids help you to avoid gas, constipation, and intestinal blockage. Whole-grain products spoil and turn rancid more quickly than refined grains; therefore, remember to store them in tightly sealed containers and keep them in a cool place.

FAST FACTS

Psyllium-containing breakfast cereals are being marketed as a source of high-soluble fiber that can help lower blood cholesterol, making psyllium the latest natural "wonder fiber."

GUIDELINES TO YOUR GOOD HEALTH

Consider the following guidelines for increasing fiber in your diet:

1. Eat whole-grain breads and cereals daily.
2. Include whole fruits in your diet more often than fruit juice. If you eat half a grapefruit instead of drinking grapefruit juice, you will be getting more fiber and more satiety value for your calories.
3. Eat more raw vegetables. They provide fiber and are richer in nutrients than cooked ones. If you do cook your vegetables, steam them. Steaming preserves nutrients and some fiber.
4. Eat legumes (dried peas and beans) more frequently.
5. Read food labels carefully. Don't be fooled by a product that proclaims itself to be a "one-hundred percent grain product." That is not the same as a "one-hundred percent WHOLE grain product."
6. Don't be fooled by a bread or cereal that looks brown. Food manufacturers frequently add caramel coloring to white grain to make it look brown. The only way to be sure is to READ THE LABEL.

FAST FACTS

Dried figs have 41 percent more dietary fiber than dried apricots and nearly 150 percent more than seedless raisins.

■ Protein

Contrary to popular belief, protein's key value is not in supplying energy but in furnishing the building material for bodily structures. **Protein** compromises the hard and insoluble coverings of the body, such as hair, skin, and nails. It also contributes to the formation of three important body chemicals: (1) enzymes, which aid digestion and other body processes; (2) antibodies, which fight off diseases and infection; and (3) hormones, which regulate the body's chemistry. Most of the protein in our body is found in the muscle tissue, but it is also distributed in soft tissues, bones, teeth, blood, and other body fluids.

Protein is made up of chains of **amino acids** and, like fats and carbohydrates, contains carbon, hydrogen, and oxygen. Protein, however, also contains nitrogen. It is only through protein foods that we obtain this important element.

Our bodies can produce many of the amino acids that make up proteins. However, eight, or possibly nine, of these amino acids are called **essential amino acids** because they can be supplied to the body only through foods and it is essential that the diet provides them. The rest of the amino acids are called **nonessential amino acids.** This does not mean they are not needed; it simply means that the body can produce them from other substances present in the body if they are not provided by the food that is eaten. All of the essential amino acids must be present at the same time if protein is to be synthesized. An absence of any one can limit protein synthesis, and the food will be used as calories instead. Remember, one gram of protein is equal to 4 kcal. Protein production depends on whether or not the foods consumed provide a balance of essential amino acids.

Most Americans eat more protein than they actually need. Many people think that the more protein they eat, the healthier they will become. What really happens is that once the body's protein requirement is met, excess protein is stored as body fat. When it comes to eating protein foods, you must estimate your protein requirement and choose foods that are low in saturated fats and cholesterol. Protein-rich animal foods such as meat, milk, eggs, and dairy products are excellent sources of protein, but the saturated fat, cholesterol, and calories that come with them have contributed to the high incidence of obesity, heart disease, and certain types of cancer. Americans need to get more of their proteins from plant sources. Foods such as grains, legumes, nuts, and seeds provide protein without the saturated fat and cholesterol. Plant foods are also higher in fiber and richer in certain vitamins and minerals.

Animal proteins are generally of higher quality than those from plant sources. Because animal proteins contain sufficient amounts of all of the essential amino acids, they are called **complete proteins.** Most plant proteins are deficient in

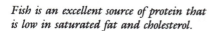

Fish is an excellent source of protein that is low in saturated fat and cholesterol.

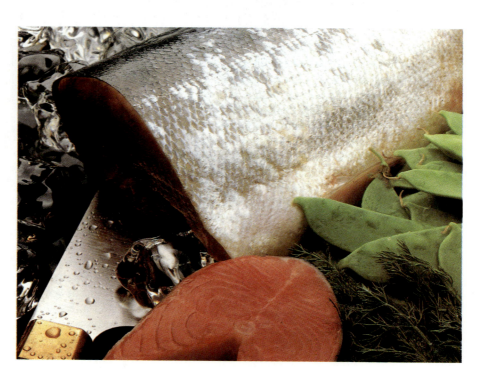

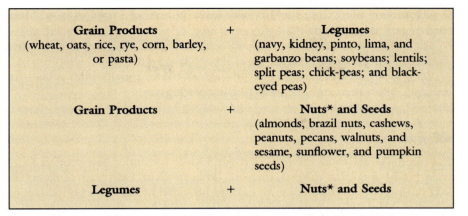

FIGURE 4–2 ■ Complementary Protein Combination

one or more of the essential amino acids and are therefore called **incomplete proteins.** Although it is true that plant proteins are not as well-balanced with respect to essential amino acids as animal proteins, a balance can be attained by eating a combination of plant proteins. By doing so, the amino acids deficient in one plant source are supplied by another. For example, rice and beans eaten together supply a good balance of amino acids, even though each alone is low in certain amino acids. This process of combining incomplete proteins is known as **complementary protein combination.** Knowing how to combine different protein sources is the key to replacing animal protein in the diet. Figure 4–2 shows food combinations for adequately balanced protein intake.

If you want to include quality protein in your diet without high amounts of calories, saturated fats, and cholesterol, remember the following guidelines:

■ Limit the amount of red meats, whole milk, eggs, and dairy products.
■ Substitute low-fat protein sources for high-fat sources. For example, use low-fat milk, yogurt, and cheeses or products made from nonfat milk.
■ Include more fish and poultry in your diet.
■ Include combinations of grain products, legumes, nuts, and seeds in your diet.

Protein for the Vegetarian

The **vegetarian** faces a special problem in diet planning—obtaining adequate amounts of protein from fewer food sources. There are two major classes of vegetarians (with many variations):

1. Lacto-ovo vegetarian: A vegetarian who excludes animal flesh from the diet but eats such animal products as milk and eggs.
2. Vegan: A strict vegetarian; one who excludes all animal flesh and animal products from the diet, eating only plant foods.

You can be a vegetarian and still obtain sufficient amounts of protein in the diet. Consider the following points when planning your meals:

■ As a lacto-ovo vegetarian, you can get high-quality sources of protein from eggs, cheese, milk, and milk products.

- Eliminating meat from the diet may result in a lower intake of iron. Make sure to eat iron-rich foods.
- The vegan, who excludes meat and dairy products, should find alternative sources of calcium and vitamin D and should take a vitamin B_{12} supplement.
- Eat foods in combinations that provide all the essential amino acids—for example, black bean and rice soup (legume with grain).

Fats

Fat is a misunderstood, essential nutrient. Ounce for ounce, fats provide more energy, and thus more calories, then any other nutrient. One gram of fat equals 9 kcal. That's twice the amount of calories provided by either carbohydrates or proteins. Many individuals believe that fat should be omitted from the diet, since fatty foods are calorie-loaded, nonnutritious, and associated with serious health problems. Although there is truth to these accusations, fat is still an important part of the diet. To judge both the positive and negative aspects of fat, you first need to understand about the different kinds of dietary fats and how each contributes to the functioning of the body.

Fats, whether in the body or in foods, are chemical compounds made up of carbon, hydrogen, and oxygen. The more scientific name for fat is **lipid.** Lipid simply means "fat-like." The basic building blocks of fats are fatty acids. Fats provide energy, enable vitamins A, D, E, and K to be absorbed by the body, form a protective cushion around bones and vital organs, insulate the body against heat loss, and make up part of the structure of individual cells.

When we speak about fat, we need to differentiate between dietary fat (the fat found in foods) and body fat (the fat your body produces and stores). The information presented in this section will focus on dietary fat. Body fat will be discussed at a later time when the topic of weight control is addressed.

The average American consumes as much as 40 to 45 percent of his or her calories as fat. This percentage is too high. Experts recommend that fat should provide about 30 percent of calories consumed daily. The chief sources of fat in the American diet are meats, milk, butter, eggs, and cheese. Most people are conscious of ingesting fat when they eat butter or meat gravies, but what about those invisible fats? It is estimated that about 60 percent of the fat we eat is hidden in foods, such as dairy products, egg yolks, baked goods, and nuts. Did you know that one medium egg has 64 percent of its calories from fat, one ounce of American cheese has 75 percent, a plain donut has 41 percent, and one ounce of walnuts has 85 percent. That's quite a lot of invisible fat being consumed! Table 4–4 lists the calorie, fat and cholesterol content of hamburgers from popular fast food restaurants.

High-fat diets have been correlated with such serious health problems as obesity, heart disease, and cancer of the breast, colon, and prostate. Altering dietary habits could greatly reduce the risk of developing these health problems. To understand what dietary changes are needed, let's look at two important components of dietary fat: triglycerides and cholesterol.

Triglycerides

Dietary fats are found mostly in the form of **triglycerides.** There are three distinct types of triglycerides: **saturated, monounsaturated,** and **polyunsat-**

TABLE 4–4 ■ **Calorie, Fat and Cholesterol Content of Hamburgers from Popular Fast Food Restaurants**

Restaurant and Type of Burger	Calories	Fat (gm.)	% Calories from Fat	Cholesterol (mg.)
Burger King				
Hamburger	275	12	39	37
Whopper Jr.	322	17	48	41
Whopper	626	38	55	94
Carl's Jr.				
Happy Star Hamburger	330	13	35	40
Famous Star Hamburger	530	32	54	70
Super Star Hamburger	780	50	58	155
Hardee's				
Hamburger	276	15	50	*
Big Deluxe Hamburger Sandwich	503	29	52	*
Jack in the Box				
Hamburger	276	12	38	29
Jumbo Jack	485	26	48	64
McDonald's				
Hamburger	263	11	39	29
Quarter Pounder	427	24	50	81
Big Mac	570	35	55	83
Roy Rogers				
Hamburger Sandwich	456	28	56	73
RR Bar Burger	611	39	58	115
Wendy's				
Hamburger	350	18	46	65

*Data not available.
SOURCE: Jacobson et al., 1986, pp. 136–214.

urated. Saturated fats are full of hydrogen, so they are solid at room temperature. In excessive amounts, saturated fats have a tendency to raise the blood-cholesterol level, thus increasing the risk of heart disease. Foods from animal sources, such as meat, eggs, milk, cheese, and butter, are high in saturated fats. In addition, some vegetable oils, such as palm oil and coconut oil, contain large amounts of saturated fat.

Polyunsaturated fats are liquid at room temperature and remain liquid even when refrigerated. They have a tendency to lower the blood-cholesterol level, thus decreasing the risk of heart disease. They are found most abundantly in plants. Examples of polyunsaturated fats include corn, sunflower, safflower, cottonseed, sesame seed, and soybean oils. If an oil has a high polyunsaturated content, it contains a considerable amount of linoleic acid. **Linoleic acid** is an essential fatty acid that can be obtained only through food sources.

Monounsaturated fats are liquid at room temperature but become solid when refrigerated. Once believed to have little or no effect on the blood-cholesterol level, evidence continues to accumulate that diets high in monounsaturated fatty

FAST FACTS

A cup of coconut milk has about twice as much fat as the amount found in an entire quart of whole milk.

TABLE 4–5 ■ Fatty Acid Composition Of Oils And Fats

Oil/Fat	Percentage of Total Fatty Acids		
	Saturated	Monounsaturated	Polyunsaturated
Canola (rapeseed oil)	6	62	32
Safflower oil	9	13	78
Sunflower oil	11	20	69
Corn oil	13	25	62
Olive oil	14	77	9
Soybean oil	15	24	61
Peanut oil	18	48	34
Sockeye salmon oil	20	55	25
Cottonseed oil	27	19	54
Lard	41	47	12
Palm oil	51	39	10
Beef tallow	52	44	4
Butterfat	66	30	4
Palm kernel oil	86	12	2
Coconut oil	92	6	2

acids may be effective agents for the prevention of coronary heart disease. Examples of monounsaturated fats include olive, canola, avocado, and peanut oils. If an oil has a high monounsaturated content, it contains a considerable portion of **oleic acid.**

Table 4–5 lists the fatty-acid composition of oils and fats found in the foods we eat. The list is structured in order of increasing saturation, thus making canola the oil with the least-saturated fatty acids and coconut oil the most saturated.

Your body needs a variety of natural fats daily, but use the three types of dietary fat sparingly in an effort to reduce total fat consumption. Even though polyunsaturated fats tend to lower the blood-cholesterol level and are, therefore, encouraged as a substitute for saturated fats, they still contribute to total fat and have just as many calories as other types of fat. When making food choices regarding dietary fat, remember that your overall goals are to reduce total fat consumption and to balance the types of fat in the diet by eating less saturated fat. To reduce the amount of saturated fat, decrease overall intake of the following:

- Saturated fats such as butter, lard, and hydrogenated shortenings
- Fat-rich meats
- High-fat dairy products such as whole milk, cream, sour cream, and cheeses
- Fat-rich pastries and desserts

Cholesterol

Cholesterol is a fat-like substance. It is found in all body tissue, especially the brain, nerves, adrenal cortex, and liver. Cholesterol is a component of bile, serves as a precursor for vitamin D, and is involved in the synthesis of some hormones. Even though cholesterol is vital to normal body functioning, an elevated blood-cholesterol level is associated with an increased risk of heart disease. Cholesterol will not mix with water. In order for cholesterol to be transported in the blood, it must be wrapped within protein molecules. The combination of cholesterol and protein is called a lipoprotein. When an individual's blood cholesterol is measured, the ratio of the types of lipoproteins present in the blood is an important indicator of the individual's risk of developing coronary heart disease. (Detailed information about the relationship of lipoproteins to heart disease is discussed in Chapter 16). Cholesterol comes from two sources: it can be supplied in the diet or produced by the body. Dietary cholesterol can come only from foods of animal origin. The amount produced by the body is somewhat dependent on the amount provided by the diet; if you eat more, the body produces less. According to a 1989 report published by the National Research Council, the average American male is currently consuming 435 milligrams of cholesterol daily and the average female is consuming 304 milligrams daily. The American Heart Association maintains that 300 milligrams of cholesterol a day is the most a person should eat. People should limit themselves to 100 milligrams of cholesterol for every 1,000 calories consumed.

There are several dietary factors that affect the blood-cholesterol level. They are excess cholesterol; excess fat, particularly saturated fat; excess sugar; and inadequate fiber. Large amounts of cholesterol, saturated fat, and sugar in the diet increases the blood-cholesterol level. Dietary fiber decreases the absorption of cholesterol and increases its excretion from the body. So, to help keep blood cholesterol at a safe level, remember the following dietary guidelines:

- Reduce dietary cholesterol.
- Reduce saturated fats.
- Decrease sugar consumption.
- Increase dietary fiber.

Vitamins

Vitamins are organic compounds that are found in small amounts in most foods. Although vitamins are often said to provide energy, they actually cannot. They do not have any caloric value. They act with enzyme systems in initiating and giving impetus to many body functions, such as freeing energy from carbohydrates, proteins, and fat, enabling blood to clot, and maintaining healthy teeth and bones. Vitamins are an essential part of the diet because they cannot be synthesized by the body at a sufficient rate to satisfy its needs. Their absence will result in specific vitamin-deficiency diseases.

There are two general classes of vitamins: those that are soluble in fat and those that are soluble in water. Thirteen vitamins exist in all. The **fat-soluble vitamins**—A, D, E, and K—are stored in body fat and in the liver until needed. The **water-soluble vitamins**—Vitamin C and eight different B vitamins—dissolve in water and cannot be stored in the body. An excess of these vitamins is excreted in the urine. You should include foods with these vitamins in your diet every day.

Table 4–6 lists the thirteen vitamins along with their importance to the body, the results of deficiency, and quality food sources.

FAST FACTS

The kiwifruit, a fruit about the size of a large egg, contains more than 100 percent of the RDA for vitamin C.

TABLE 4–6 ■ **Thirteen Essential Vitamins**

Vitamin	Importance to the Body	Results of Deficiency	Quality Sources
FAT-SOLUBLE			
Vitamin A	For healthy skin and mucous membranes within the digestive, respiratory, and urinary tracts; Prevents night blindness	Dry and scaly skin; Night and glare blindness; Intestinal infection	Beef liver; Dark-green leafy and yellow vegetables; Whole milk; Cheese; Butter; Egg yolks; Fish liver oils
Vitamin D	Helps calcium and phosphorus absorption; Utilized in the formation of bones and teeth	Inadequate calcium metabolism; Bone deformities; Retarded growth; Muscle weakness	Fortified milk; Fish liver oils; Tuna; Salmon; Dairy products; Produced in the body by exposing the skin to sunlight
Vitamin E	Serves as an antioxidant; Protects cells from destruction by strengthening their cellular membranes	Deficiency states are rare in adults; Possible anemia in premature babies	Vegetable oils; Wheat germ; Seeds; Legumes; Nuts
Vitamin K	Vital to the blood-clotting process	Slow blood clotting; body bruises easily	Green, leafy vegetables; Pork; Corn; Tomatoes; Vegetable oils; Main supply appears to be formed in the intestines by bacterial action
WATER-SOLUBLE			
Vitamin C	Maintenance of cartilage, bone, and tendon, as well as healthy gums and teeth; Involved in the healing of wounds; Helps body absorb iron	Swollen and bleeding gums; Pain in joints; Impaired healing; Weakness; Fatigue	Citrus fruits; Strawberries; Melons; Tomatoes; Green pepper; Broccoli; Cabbage
Vitamin B_1 (Thiamine)	Essential for growth, normal appetite, digestion, and healthy nerves	Retarded growth; Poor appetite; Mental confusion; Irritability; Insomnia; Abnormal fatigue	Pork; Lean meat; Poultry; Whole-grain and enriched breads and cereals; Milk; Legumes

TABLE 4–6 ■ Thirteen Essential Vitamins, continued

Vitamin	Importance to the Body	Results of Deficiency	Quality Sources
Vitamin B₂ (*Riboflavin*)	For cellular enzyme systems that help release energy from food; Essential for normal growth	Impaired growth; Feelings of weakness; Cracks in the corners of mouth; Red, scaly areas around the nose	Meats Liver Eggs Milk Green, leafy vegetables Whole-grain and enriched breads and cereals
Niacin	Helps release energy from food; Involved in cellular respiration; For normal functioning of the gastrointestinal (G.I.) tract and the nervous system	Swollen, beefy, red tongue; Weakness; Loss of appetite; G.I. disturbances; Mental disturbances; Irritability	Lean meats Poultry Fish Whole-grain and enriched breads and cereals Legumes
Vitamin B₆	For the metabolism and synethesis of amino acids; Aids hemoglobin synthesis	Greasy dermatitis located on the face; Depression; Nausea; Vomiting	Meat Poultry Fish Vegetables Seeds Whole-grain cereals
Vitamin B₁₂	Formation of healthy red blood cells; Maintenance of the sheath surrounding and protecting nerve fibers; Promotion of normal growth	Pernicious anemia; Swollen tongue; Weakness; Loss of weight; Nervous system disorders	Meats Poultry Fish Milk Cheese Eggs (Not found in plant foods)
Folacin (*B-complex*)	Formation and maturation of blood cells; Helps body form protein tissues	Anemia; Smooth, red tongue; Fatigue; Diarrhea; Loss of appetite; Weight loss	Green, leafy vegetables Organ meats Whole-wheat products Legumes Milk Oranges Cantaloupe
Pantothenic Acid (*B-complex*)	Aids in the metabolism of carbohydrates, fats, and proteins	Rarely experienced	Meats Poultry Fish Milk Legumes Whole-grain products (Distributed widely in foods)
Biotin (*B-complex*)	Coenzyme necessary for the synthesis of fat and glycogen; Involved in amino-acid metabolism	Dermatitis; Muscle pain; Nausea; Loss of appetite; Depression; Fatigue; Sleeplessness	Meats Vegetables Legumes Nuts

■ Minerals

Minerals are inorganic elements found in nature. Unlike the other nutrients, minerals are not organic, because they do not contain carbon. Neither do they contain hydrogen or oxygen. In nutrition, the term *mineral* is used to list those elements essential to life processes.

Minerals are generally divided into two groups: the major, or macrominerals, and the trace minerals. **Macrominerals** are defined as those needed in amounts greater than 100 milligrams a day. They include calcium, phosphorus, sodium, potassium, chlorine, sulfur, and magnesium. **Trace minerals** are those needed in amounts less than 100 milligrams a day. They include iron, iodine, zinc, copper, and fluorine, just to mention a few. Table 4–7 lists the macrominerals and some of the trace minerals along with their importance to the body and quality food sources.

Most of the functions that minerals perform in the body may be divided into three categories: structural, functional, and regulatory. As structural components, minerals make up the bony structures of the body. As functional components, minerals occur in soft tissues and fluids throughout the body, enabling cells to perform many functions. For example, minerals make possible normal

> **FAST FACTS**
>
> A cup of brewed tea can have up to three times more fluoride than a cup of fluoridated water.

TABLE 4–7 ■ Minerals

Mineral	Importance to the Body	Quality Sources
MACROMINERALS		
Calcium	Maintains strong bones and healthy teeth Essential for proper muscle action Aids the nervous system in impulse transmission	Milk and all milk products Green vegetables Sardines Salmon
Phosphorus	Gives strength to bones and teeth Aids in energy transfer occurring during cellular metabolism Helps transport lipids in the blood	Meat Fish Eggs Poultry Whole grains Nuts Seeds
Sodium	Regulates muscle contraction and nerve stimulation Regulates the balance of water in the body Aids in keeping calcium and other minerals soluble in the blood	Salt Processed foods Kelp
Potassium	Regulates heart beat Maintains the fluid volume and the acid-base balance inside body cells	Fruits Green leafy vegetables

TABLE 4–7 ■ Minerals, continued

Mineral	Importance to the Body	Quality Sources
Chlorine	Works with sodium and potassium to regulate the acid-base blood balance	Salt
Sulfur	Essential component of proteins	Meat Fish Eggs Dried beans Nuts
Magnesium	Aids in proper nerve and muscle functioning Necessary for the conversion of blood sugar into energy	Dark green vegetables Legumes Seeds
TRACE MINERALS		
Iron	Major component of hemoglobin Vital to cellular respiration	Liver Red Meats Fish Poultry Egg Yolks Spinach Legumes
Iodine	Component of the thyroid hormones Promotes proper growth Regulates metabolic rate	Iodized salt Seafood
Zinc	Aids in enzyme reactions Essential for protein synthesis Component of the hormone, insulin Promotes healing of wounds Aids in healthy reproductive functioning	Red meats Shellfish Milk Eggs Whole grain products
Copper	Necessary for the conversion of iron into hemoglobin Aids in the manufacturing of collagen Helps maintain the sheath around nerve fibers	Legumes Whole grain products Organ meats Nuts
Fluorine	Strengthens bones and teeth	Fluoridated drinking water Seafood Brewed Tea

rhythm of the heart beat and contractability of all muscles. As regulatory components, minerals occur as essential parts of many of the enzymes and hormones that regulate most of the body's reactions. Even though we identify each mineral separately, it should be understood that they act together and in various combinations. Certain minerals serve specific purposes in the body, but they seldom act alone in accomplishing these purposes.

In meeting the body's needs for minerals, a general rule is to consume a variety of foods from each of the Four Basic Food Groups. Minerals not present in one food will probably be found in another. Do you know which mineral is most likely to be excessive in the diet? Do you know which one is most likely to be deficient? Well, read on!

GUIDELINES TO YOUR GOOD HEALTH

To get the maximum amount of vitamins and minerals present in foods, remember the following points:

1. Minimize the amount of processed foods you eat. Over-processing often results in the loss of important vitamins and minerals.
2. Eat whole fruits and vegetables. They are usually higher in vitamin and mineral content. When selecting vegetables, choose those that are bright and natural in color and free of decay. When selecting fruits, choose those that are firm, plump, and free from bruises.
3. Refrigerate vitamin-rich foods to help slow down the enzyme activity that causes oxidation. The longer fruits and vegetables are stored, the more vitamins are destroyed through oxidation.
4. Avoid soaking and cooking fruits and vegetables in water, because vitamins and minerals can be dissolved.
5. Avoid exposing vitamin-rich foods to light and extreme heat, because these factors can destroy vitamins.

Electrolytes

Sodium, chlorine, and potassium are present in the body in relatively large amounts as compared to other minerals. They are unique among minerals because they become electrically charged when in the body fluids. Because of their electrical charges, sodium, chlorine, and potassium are called **electrolytes.** The electrical charges help these minerals to perform their roles in the body.

In the body fluids, sodium takes on a positive electrical charge. Sodium is normally found in extracellular fluids and in the blood. Chlorine, in the form of chloride, takes on a negative electrical charge in body fluids. It, too, is found in extracellular fluids; however, it can pass through the cell walls if the body needs it within the cells. Potassium takes on a positive electrical charge in body fluids, and it is found mainly in intracellular fluids. The electrolytes help to regulate the acid–base balance and the overall water balance in the body. Sodium and potassium are involved in muscle contraction and proper activity of the nervous system.

When the amount of electrolytes is much greater or much less than needed, problems can result from the imbalance. Since sodium is a major part of the American diet, let's look at how it affects our health. Most Americans consume much more sodium than they need. The National Academy of Sciences says that the safe and adequate daily intake of sodium for healthy adults is 1,100 to 3,000 milligrams. For adolescents, the level is 900 to 2,700 milligrams. A general rule to follow is 1,000 milligrams of sodium for every 1,000 calories consumed. The most common form of sodium in the diet is table salt, or sodium chloride, which is 40 percent sodium. Many people believe that the saltier a food tastes, the higher its sodium content. This is not necessarily true. Sodium is found in a wide range of non–salty tasting foods. It occurs naturally in foods from animal sources, and high amounts can be found in processed, canned, dried, and frozen foods. In general, fresh fruits and vegetables and grains are naturally low in sodium.

Too much sodium in the diet has been found to have detrimental effects on an individual's health. A certain amount of excess sodium will be excreted in the urine and lost through perspiration during physical activity. In many instances, however, too much sodium can cause edema (swelling of body tissues) and contribute to the development of high blood pressure. Although the problems of an excessive intake of sodium are rather well-known, the other side of the coin cannot be ignored. There are instances in which the sodium level in the body is inadequate. This is created by excessive losses of sodium without adequate replacement. Sodium depletion can occur as a result of excessive vomiting, diarrhea, burns, or sweating. When sodium and water losses are great, potassium shifts outside the cells to replace the lost sodium and draws out the fluid from the cells with it. This leads to **dehydration,** a potentially dangerous situation. A clue to the development of dehydration is thirst. At this point, water and sodium may need to be replaced immediately.

The use of diuretics can cause a significant loss of water from the body and may result in an imbalance of electrolytes. A **diuretic** is a chemical that increases water excretion from the body. With the loss of water, however, also comes the loss of potassium. In severe cases of potassium loss, there will be abnormalities in the functioning of the heart, kidney, and lungs. More about diuretics and potassium loss will be mentioned when dieting and weight control is addressed.

FAST FACTS

Some types of TV dinners contain as much as 2,200 milligrams of sodium.

The Trace Mineral Iron

The amount of iron needed by the body is small in comparison to other minerals. Why, then, is iron deficiency one of the most common nutritional deficiencies in the world? Who is at greatest risk of experiencing such a deficiency? Let's learn more about iron.

The major function of iron in the body is the formation of compounds essential to the transportation of oxygen. The vast majority of iron is used to form **hemoglobin,** a protein–iron compound that transports oxygen from the lungs to the body tissues. Iron has to be absorbed through the intestinal wall before it is available to form hemoglobin and other iron-containing compounds. Only a small amount of iron from foods is absorbed. The actual amount your body absorbs depends on the body's needs for iron, what the food is, and which other nutrients are present. If there is an adequate level of iron in your body, the absorption rate from food may be less than 10 percent. If the iron level is

Even though this delicious piece of roast beef is a high-level source of iron, it is also a high-level source of saturated fat and cholesterol. The choice is yours.

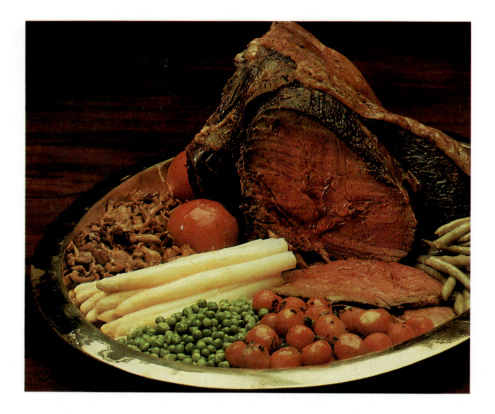

low, the absorption rate may be as high as 30 percent. Unabsorbed iron is excreted in the feces. About 1 mg. of iron a day is lost through urine, sweat, and sloughed-off skin. Bleeding is the principal way of losing iron.

The body conserves iron very efficiently. When red blood cells are broken down, the iron is reused to form new cells. Even with the continual recycling of iron, there is need for replacement from foods being eaten. Excellent sources of dietary iron include liver, heart, red meats, dried fruits, dark-green leafy vegetables, whole-grain breads and cereals, and blackstrap molasses. The iron found in animal products is more effectively absorbed than that found in plants.

The RDA for iron is 10 mg. for men and 18 mg. for women and teenagers of both sexes. Low levels of iron are most common in infants, young children, teenage girls, women of childbearing age, and the elderly. Part of the reason for low levels of iron in infants and young children is the fact that milk is not a good source of iron. The diets of teenage girls and the elderly are often inadequate in foods that are rich sources of iron. Women need greater amounts of iron during menstruation, pregnancy, and lactation.

How can you determine if you are iron deficient? All that is needed is a blood test. A low level of iron indicates a condition called iron-deficiency anemia. One very noticeable sign is a constant, overall feeling of fatigue. Frequently, this condition can be corrected by including iron in the diet. Severe cases may require medical attention.

Although remote, there may be dangers associated with excess iron in the body. Chronic iron toxicity occurs when large amounts of iron are taken over an extended period of time. Normally this only happens if a person is taking an iron supplement, because iron levels in food are usually not high enough to cause excessive build-up. The iron salts of the type usually present in iron pills are acutely toxic at high doses. Some children have died from swallowing their parents' pills.

Now that you know the implications associated with an iron deficiency, here's how you can help your body absorb adequate amounts of iron.

- Eat iron-rich foods.
- Eat a good source of vitamin C in combination with an iron-rich food.
- Make sure that the protein content of your diet is adequate.
- Include food sources of copper and the B vitamins in your diet.
- Substances such as antacids, calcium, phosphate salts, and tannic acid in tea may interfere with iron absorption. Avoid these substances if they affect your iron level.

Vitamin And Mineral Supplements

Vitamins and minerals continue to be among the most widely used and abused nutrient supplements in the United States today. According to the National Research Council, 40 to 60 percent of Americans routinely swallow nutrient supplements. Annual sales are approaching the $3 billion mark.

Vitamin/mineral-pill manufacturers and advertisers have attempted to convince members of the American public that they are not receiving an ample supply of vitamins and minerals in the foods they eat. There is no solid evidence to indicate that the average healthy American, eating a well-balanced diet, is suffering from vitamin or mineral deficiencies and related diseases. A well-balanced diet contains all the necessary vitamins and minerals needed by the average healthy individual; however, there may be certain situations in which supplements are recommended.

FAST FACTS

Vitamin C supplements are often manufactured using the simple sugar glucose.

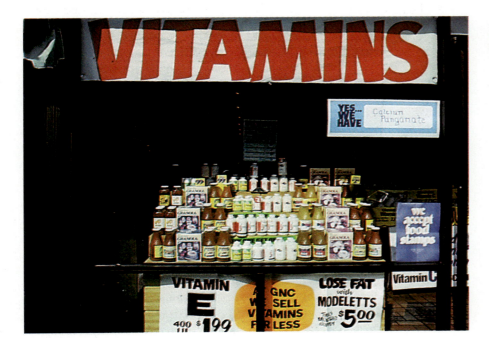

The marketplace is filled with gimmicks intended to entice individuals into buying all types of dietary supplements.

> **FAST FACTS**
>
> A new form of vitamin C, under the trademark Ester C, contains much less acidity than regular vitamin C and is being promoted as a supplement for those who cannot tolerate the more common forms of vitamin C.

Vitamin/mineral supplements may be needed during certain stages of development or to make up for losses caused by certain medications or environmental conditions. For example, oral contraceptives may increase the need for vitamins B_6, B_{12}, C, and folacin; smoking may increase vitamin C needs; and a strict vegetarian will need a B_{12} supplement. Other factors, such as illness, surgery, pregnancy, stress, high fever, and extensive burns, will increase vitamin and mineral requirements.

The American Dietetic Association has stated that it sees no harm in individuals taking daily multivitamin/mineral preparations containing 100 percent of the Recommended Dietary Allowances; however, they have documented serious side effects from higher doses of certain nutrients. For example, vitamin A may cause permanent liver damage after seven to ten years of use. Also, large amounts of zinc appear to upset the body's balance of minerals (such as copper) as well as reduce the number of high-density lipoproteins in the blood. In 1985, there was a 50 percent increase in calcium-supplement sales. This rise was due to the publicity about calcium's role in preventing osteoporosis. The long-term effects of consuming calcium supplements are not yet known.

Taking excess amounts of vitamin/mineral supplements will not serve any useful purpose. In fact, the effects may be harmful, even toxic, to the body. If you think supplements are needed, consult a qualified physician, especially because you may not be suffering from a dietary deficiency but from some other health problem. Deficiency conditions can be diagnosed by a doctor through the use of medically sound tests. Physicians are now being asked to report adverse reactions to vitamin/mineral supplements to the Food and Drug Administration. It is hoped that this action will serve as a warning to the public that taking high doses of vitamins and minerals can be a dangerous health practice.

Water

Do you think of water as a nutrient? Well, it is! It is of critical importance for proper functioning of the body. An individual can get along for days, even weeks, without food, but death will result in a matter of days without water. Water is essential if the other nutrients are to function properly within the body.

Water is the main transportation mechanism in the body. It transports oxygen, nutrients, hormones, and other compounds to the cells for their use, and it carries waste products to various organs for excretion from the body. Water is of primary importance in the regulation of body temperature. When the body becomes too hot, an individual will perspire. The evaporation of water from the skin's surface can help to dissipate excess body heat.

In addition, water is part of the material that makes up each body cell. In fact, the biggest single component of the body is water. Water composes about 60 percent of the body's weight. It is stored in various body compartments, although there is a constant movement of water between these compartments. The vast majority of the body's water is stored inside the body cells (intracellular water), and the remainder is outside the cells (extracellular water). Proper water and electrolyte balance within these compartments is of vital importance. The electrolytes are dissolved and ionized in water, and any major changes in their concentration may adversely affect cellular function. Water in close association with the major electrolytes also helps to regulate the acid–base balance in the body.

Nutritionists recommend that people drink about four to eight glasses of water daily. Not all the water you drink needs to come from the water faucet, however. Fruit and vegetable juices, milk, and soups are also good sources of water. Another way to include water in the diet is to eat fruits and vegetables. These foods have a high water content. The general recommendation of four to eight glasses of water daily will meet the body's needs for water under normal conditions. Sometimes illness, hot weather, or physical activity may increase the body's need for water. When you feel thirsty or start to perspire, recognize these as signals from your body. Drink up!

Health Foods

Have you ever eaten an organic- or natural-food product? To answer this question, you would have to know what the words *organic* and *natural* mean in reference to food. Although chemists define organic substances as those that contain carbon, health-food proponents consider **organic foods** to be those foods grown without chemical fertilizers and pesticides. Although there is no legal definition for "natural," **natural foods** usually refer to those foods that have undergone minimal processing and do not contain artificial ingredients.

Advocates of these so-called health foods believe that organically grown and natural foods are more nutritious and safer than conventionally grown foods. But are they? Many Americans believe that if a food is promoted as a "health" food, it must be good for you. What should be realized is that all foods can contribute to health or detract from health, depending on how they are used.

There is no evidence that organic and natural foods are nutritionally superior to foods produced by conventional means. The nutritional quality of a plant is largely determined by genetics, climate, and stage of maturity when harvested, not by whether a natural or synthetic fertilizer was used. Plants can absorb nutrients from the soil only in inorganic form, and they don't care if these nutrients have been supplied by manure or by chemical fertilizers. Even worn-out soil affects only the amount, not the nutritional value, of what manages to grow in it.

Let's look at two examples of foods that gained their popularity by being labeled "natural." Are the ingredients found in these foods really more nutritious? Quaker 100% Natural Cereal is sweetened with brown sugar and honey instead of with processed white sugar (sucrose). Are these "natural" sources of sweetener healthier for your body? Virtually all sugars eaten are changed into glucose once they are absorbed; therefore, the end product turns out to be the same. Brown sugar and honey, although they do have very small amounts of certain nutrients, are still concentrated sources of energy that should be limited in the diet. (see Figure 4–3) Another "natural" food that many people enjoy as a snack is banana chips. Individuals buy them by the pound at health-food stores and supermarkets. Banana chips are made by thinly slicing bananas, mixing the slices with sugar and honey, and then frying them in coconut oil. Sounds delicious, but are they nutritious? A once-nutritious banana has now become loaded with calories and soaked in a highly saturated fat. In other words, banana chips are to bananas what potato chips are to potatoes. If you are really health-conscious, stick to eating the banana in its original form. From these examples, it is obvious that "natural" is not necessarily healthier. When buying these types of foods, read what ingredients are found in them so you become aware of their nutritional value.

FIGURE 4–3
A "Natural" Food Label

What about the argument that organic foods are safer to eat because they were grown without the use of chemicals. Nature, as well as humans, adds toxic compounds to food. Hundreds of toxicants are known to occur naturally in foods. For example, aflatoxin, a mold product that grows naturally under some conditions on corn, peanuts, and other grains, is a powerful carcinogen. The Food and Drug Administration monitors foods for **aflatoxin** and has established safe minimum levels in some foods. Foods containing aflatoxin above these safe levels cannot be marketed. There is no way, however, that the FDA can assure that all foods are entirely free of such naturally occurring toxins. In most cases, the toxin is present at low-enough levels and the food is not consumed in large-enough quantities to cause problems. In other instances, the food can be prepared in a way that reduces or eliminates the toxin. Don't become neurotic thinking that every food you eat has the potential of poisoning you; simply exercise common sense by eating a balanced diet from a wide variety of foods.

Now that you know more about organic and natural foods, don't be misled into believing that they are any healthier or safer to eat. These foods often cost more than conventional foods, yet there are no more tangible benefits to be gained by eating them than by eating other foods. As always, the final decision is yours, but at least now you have more factual information on which to base your decision.

An Anti-cancer Diet

Although there are several contributing factors to the causes of certain cancers, most nutritionists and physicians agree that the incidence of cancer could be substantially reduced if people would make some dietary changes. Table 4–8 lists the effect that food has in the prevention of specific types of cancer. The American Cancer Society also advocates dietary modifications in order for individuals to increase the chances of a healthier life and to reduce the risk of developing cancer. There is no guarantee that eating a specific food or following a certain diet will prevent cancer; however, based on research findings, an individual *may* lessen the chances of getting cancer by following these dietary guidelines.

1. Maintain ideal body weight. Obesity increases an individual's risk of developing cancers of the uterus, breast, gallbladder, kidney, stomach, and colon. By eating properly (more about diet will be discussed in Chapter 5) and by exercising regularly (more about exercise will be discussed in Chapter 6), ideal body weight can be maintained.
2. Reduce the amount of fat in the diet. As previously stated, an individual's total fat consumption for the day should not exceed 30 percent of the total calories. A high-fat diet increases an individual's risk of developing cancers of the prostate, colon, and breast.
3. Increase dietary fiber. Fiber helps to reduce the amount of time **carcinogens** might stay in the intestines. A high-fiber diet, especially consisting of wheat bran and whole grains and vegetables, may offer protection against the development of colon cancer.
4. Include **cruciferous** vegetables in the diet. Consumption of cruciferous vegetables, such as broccoli, brussel sprouts, cauliflower, cabbage, kale, and kohlrabi, may reduce the risk of colorectal, stomach, and respiratory cancers.
5. Include foods rich in vitamins A and C in the diet. Dark green, deep yellow, and orange-colored vegetables are rich in beta-carotene, a form of vitamin A

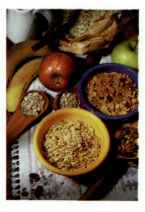

There are many sources of food available that can provide the body with sufficient amounts of complex carbohydrates and fiber.

TABLE 4–8 ■ The Effect that Food has in the Prevention of Specific Types of Cancer

Foods that Decrease the Risk	Types of Cancer	Foods that Increase the Risk
Fresh fruits and vegetables Wheat bran Whole grain breads and cereals	Colon	Refined breads and cereals High-fat content (such as red meats, whole milk, eggs, and high-fat cheese)
Foods rich in Vitamin A (such as dark green and deep yellow vegetables, sweet potato, carrots, peaches, apricots, and tomatoes)	Larynx Lung	
Foods rich in Vitamin A Foods rich in Vitamin C (such as citrus fruits, green and red peppers, cantaloupe, and strawberries)	Esophagus	Salt-cured, smoked and nitrite-cured foods (such as hot dogs, sausage, bacon, luncheon meats, and smoked fishes) Heavy alcohol consumption
Foods rich in Vitamin C	Stomach	Salt-cured, smoked and nitrite-cured foods
Cruciferous vegetables (cabbage, broccoli, kohlrabi, brussel sprouts, kale, and cauliflower)	Gastro-intestinal Respiratory	
Low-fat content (such as complex carbohydrates)	Breast Colon Prostate	High-fat content (such as red meats and high-fat dairy products)
	Mouth Throat Liver	Heavy alcohol consumption

that may lower the risk of cancers of the larynx, lungs, and esophagus. Oranges, grapefruit, strawberries, red and green peppers, and tomatoes are examples of foods rich in vitamin C. Vitamin C may offer protection against cancers of the esophagus and stomach. A good food source of vitamins A and C should be included in the diet daily.

6. Limit consumption of smoked, salt-cured, and nitrite-cured foods, such as bacon, hot dogs, certain hams and sausages, and smoked fishes. Eating large quantities of these foods over a long period of time may increase the risk of developing cancers of the esophagus and stomach. These foods do not need to be completely eliminated from the diet. If you do choose to eat them, however, do so only occasionally and in moderation.

Research continues to be directed at determining what roles diet and nutrition play in relation to the cause and prevention of cancer.

SELF-INVENTORY 4.1

Are You A Healthy Eater?

Read the following statements and place a check mark in the appropriate column. Be as honest as possible in order to obtain a true analysis.

	Yes	Some-Times	No
1. I eat nonfat or low-fat milk products.	___	___	___
2. I eat meats such as cold cuts, bacon, bologna, and hot dogs.	___	___	___
3. I eat salads that contain a variety of vegetables.	___	___	___
4. I use sugar, honey, jellies, and syrups sparingly or not at all.	___	___	___
5. I use generous amounts of butter, margarine, mayonnaise, or salad dressing.	___	___	___
6. I include deep green or yellow vegetables in my daily diet.	___	___	___
7. I eat white breads, refined cereals, and white rice.	___	___	___
8. I eat large portions of red meat.	___	___	___
9. I eat fresh or water-packed fruits.	___	___	___
10. I use whole milk or cream.	___	___	___
11. I limit my egg consumption to no more than 3 to 4 eggs a week.	___	___	___
12. I salt foods after they have been prepared.	___	___	___
13. I drink soda and other sweetened fruit-flavored drinks.	___	___	___
14. I eat whole-grain breads and cereals.	___	___	___
15. I eat rich desserts and snacks.	___	___	___
16. I use unsweetened fruits, cereals, and juices.	___	___	___
17. I eat convenience foods such as TV dinners and fast foods.	___	___	___

Scoring

If you answered YES to questions 1, 3, 4, 6, 9, 11, 14, and 16 and NO to questions 2, 5, 7, 8, 10, 12, 13, 15, and 17, you are an *extremely healthy eater*.

If you answered YES to the majority of these questions (1, 3, 4, 6, 9, 11, 14, and 16) and NO to the majority of these questions (2, 5, 7, 8, 10, 12, 13, 15, and 17), you are *on the right track toward being a healthy eater*.

If you answered SOMETIMES to all of the questions or to the majority of them, you have the potential for being either a healthy or an unhealthy eater. Be aware of the factors and situations that may lead you *away* from healthy eating and those that may lead you *toward* unhealthy eating.

If you answered YES to the majority of these questions (2, 5, 7, 8, 10, 12, 13, 15, and 17) and NO to the majority of these questions (1, 3, 4, 6, 9, 11, 14, and 16), you are *going astray and heading toward being an unhealthy eater*.

If you answered YES to questions 2, 5, 7, 8, 10, 12, 13, 15, and 17 and NO to questions 1, 3, 4, 6, 9, 11, 14, and 16, you are an *extremely unhealthy eater*.

POSITIVE BEHAVIORS

I. *Place a check mark in front of each behavior that you now practice.*

_____ 1. I find ways to deal with my emotions other than by eating. (EMOTIONS)
_____ 2. I limit the amount of sugar I eat. (SUGAR)
_____ 3. I eat a variety of foods. (VARIETY)
_____ 4. I eat at least one dark green or deep yellow vegetable daily. (VEGETABLE)
_____ 5. I limit the size of my food portions. (PORTIONS)
_____ 6. I drink four to eight glasses of water daily. (WATER)
_____ 7. I avoid stocking up on "problem" foods. (PROBLEM FOODS)
_____ 8. I avoid or limit high-calorie snacks. (SNACKS)
_____ 9. I eat whole-grain breads and cereals. (WHOLE-GRAIN)
_____ 10. I eat fish and poultry more frequently than red meats. (RED MEATS)

II. *For each behavior that you DO NOT ENGAGE IN, write the KEY WORD(S) that is in the parentheses located at the end of the statement in the column below. Then put a check mark in the appropriate column to indicate whether you are going to keep or change that behavior.*

Behaviors I Don't Engage In   KEEP/CHANGE

_____ / _____
_____ / _____
_____ / _____
_____ / _____
_____ / _____
_____ / _____
_____ / _____
_____ / _____
_____ / _____
_____ / _____

III. *For each of the preceding behaviors that you choose to KEEP, write a statement indicating why you are choosing to keep that behavior.*

I choose to keep behavior _____ because:
                                                  KEY WORD

For each of the preceding behaviors that you choose to CHANGE, write a statement indicating how you plan to implement that change.

I will change behavior _____ by:
                                    KEY WORD

Now You Know

1. TRUE. Dietary cholesterol can come only from foods of animal origin.
2. FALSE. Once the body's protein requirement is met, excess protein is stored as body fat.
3. FALSE. You can be a vegetarian and still obtain sufficient amounts of protein in the diet. Although it is true that plant proteins are not as well-balanced with respect to essential amino acids as animal proteins, a balance can be attained by eating a combination of plant proteins.
4. FALSE. Although vitamins are often said to provide energy, they actually cannot. They do not have any caloric value.
5. FALSE. The biggest single component of the body is water. Water composes about 60 percent of the body's weight.
6. FALSE. Of the total calories consumed daily, 12 percent should be derived from protein. The greatest percentage of calories consumed (48 percent) should come from eating complex carbohydrates.
7. TRUE. Add fiber gradually to your diet. Drink plenty of liquids, especially with more fiber in your diet. Liquids help you to avoid gas, constipation, and intestinal blockage.
8. FALSE. A well-balanced diet contains all the necessary vitamins and minerals needed by the average healthy individual.
9. FALSE. Most oils from vegetable sources are high in polyunsaturated fats. Palm oil and coconut oil, however, are exceptions to the rule. They are vegetable oils that are high in saturated fats.
10. TRUE. Water is of primary importance in the regulation of body temperature. When the body becomes too hot, an individual will perspire. Also, thirst is a clue to the possible development of dehydration.

Summary

1. Nutrients are substances found in food that meet your body's needs for energy, growth, and good health. There are six nutrients considered to be necessary in human nutrition. They are carbohydrates, fats, proteins, vitamins, minerals, and water.
2. The Recommended Dietary Allowances (RDA) represent the levels of intake of essential nutrients considered adequate to meet the nutritional needs of practically all healthy persons in the United States.
3. Calories represent a form of potential energy to be used by the body to produce heat and work. Carbohydrates, fats, and proteins are referred to as the "energy" nutrients.
4. To compute the energy value of food, it is necessary to know that 1 gram of carbohydrate equals 4 kcal., 1 gram of protein equals 4 kcal., and 1 gram of fat equals 9 kcal.
5. Specific daily caloric needs depend on such factors as age, sex, current health status, body weight, basal metabolic rate, and level of physical activity.
6. Carbohydrates are the major energy source for the body. Simple carbohydrates, commonly known as sugars, are mainly a source of nothing more than calories. Complex carbohydrates, or starches, also provide calories; however, they also contribute vitamins, minerals, and fiber to the diet.
7. Fiber is an indigestible form of carbohydrate. The bran from grains and skins on fruits and vegetables are examples of fiber. Fiber is extremely important in the diet, because it provides roughness to help move food wastes through the body.
8. Protein helps to build and repair body tissues. Amino acids are the building blocks of protein. Those amino acids that must be supplied through the foods we eat are called "essential" amino acids. Those amino acids that our bodies can produce are called "nonessential" amino acids.
9. Complete proteins are foods that contain sufficient amounts of all the essential amino acids. Animal proteins are examples of complete proteins. Incomplete proteins are foods that are deficient in one or more essential amino acid. Most plant proteins are incomplete, but a balance can be attained by combining plant proteins. The process of combining incomplete proteins is known as "complementary protein combination."
10. Fat is a calorie-laden nutrient. Dietary fats are found mostly in the form of triglycerides. The three types of triglycerides are saturated, monounsaturated, and polyunsaturated. Eating foods high in saturated fats increases the risk of heart disease. Eating foods high in polyunsaturated fats decreases the risk.
11. Vitamins are organic compounds that are an essential part of the diet. The fat-soluble vitamins—A, D, E, and K—are stored in body fat and in the liver until needed. The water-soluble vitamins—vitamin C and eight different B vitamins—cannot be stored in the body and should be included in the diet daily.
12. Minerals are inorganic elements essential to life processes. The macrominerals, such as calcium and phosphorus, are those minerals needed in amounts greater than 100 mg. a day. The trace minerals, such as iron and iodine, are those minerals needed in amounts less than 100 mg. a day.

13. The average healthy American eating a well-balanced diet normally does not need to take vitamin and mineral supplements. There may be certain situations, however, in which supplements are recommended. Factors such as pregnancy, taking certain medications, illness, surgery, stress, high fever, and extensive burns increase vitamin and mineral requirements.

References

1. *A Guide to Food, Exercise and Nutrition.* Rosemont, IL: National Dairy Council, 1985.
2. *An Eating Plan for Healthy Americans.* Dallas, TX: American Heart Association, 1987
3. Bailey, Covert. *The Fit-or-Fat Target Diet.* Boston: Houghton Mifflin, 1984
4. "Beware of Snacks Made with 'Pure Vegetable Oil'." *Tufts University Diet and Nutrition Letter* 5:3 (May 1987): 1–2.
5. Blume, Elaine. "Trouble from the Tropics." *Nutrition Action Healthletter* 13:7 (July/August 1986): 7–8.
6. Blumenthal, Dale. "A Simple Guide to Complex Carbohydrates." *FDA Consumer* 23 (April 1989): 13–17.
7. Hamilton, Eva May Nunnelley, Eleanor Noss Whitney, and Frances Sienkiewicz Sizer. *Nutrition: Concepts and Controversies,* 4th ed. St. Paul: West Publishing Co., 1988.
8. Jacobson, Michael F. and Sarah Fritschner. *The Fast-Food Guide.* New York: Workman Publishing Co., 1986.
9. Kowalski, Robert E. *The 8-Week Cholesterol Cure.* New York: Harper and Row, 1987.
10. Lappé, Frances Moore. *Diet for a Small Planet.* New York: Ballantine Books, 1982.
11. *Nutrition and Cancer: Cause and Prevention.* San Diego: American Cancer Society.
12. *Nutrition, Common Sense and Cancer.* San Diego: American Cancer Society, 1984.
13. *Nutrition Myth-Information.* Rosemont, IL: National Dairy Council, 1988.
14. Roth, Eli M., and Sandra Streicher. *Good Cholesterol, Bad Cholesterol.* Rocklin, CA: Prima Publishing and Communications, 1989.
15. *Taking Control: 10 Steps to a Healthier Life and Reduced Cancer Risk.* San Diego: American Cancer Society, 1985.
16. Williams, Sue Rodwell. *Nutrition and Diet Therapy,* 6th ed. St. Louis: Times Mirror/Mosby College Publishing, 1989.
17. Wilson, Josleen. *The Oat Bran Way.* New York: Berkley Books, 1989.

Suggested Readings

Cholesterol: Your Guide for a Healthy Heart. Lincolnwood, IL: Publications International, Ltd. 1989.
Jacobson, Michael F., and Sarah Fritschner. *The Fast-Food Guide.* New York: Workman Publishing Co., 1986.
Lappé, Frances Moore. *Diet for a Small Planet.* New York: Ballantine Books, 1982.
Nutrition Action Healthletter. Washington, D.C.: Center for Science in the Public Interest, current issues.
Roth, Eli M., and Sandra Streicher. *Good Cholesterol, Bad Cholesterol.* Rocklin, CA: Prima Publishing and Communications, 1989.
Tufts University Diet and Nutrition Letter. New York: William H. White, current issues.
U.S. Department of Health and Human Services. *The Surgeon General's Report on Nutrition and Health.* New York: Warner Books, 1989.

CHAPTER 5

Eating Behaviors

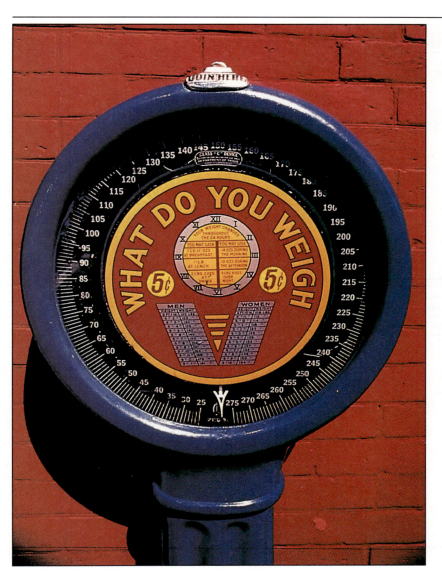

What Do You Know?

Are the following statements true or false?

1. To lose one pound, an individual must experience a deficit of 3,500 calories.
2. Dieting decreases the number of fat cells.
3. Protein consumed in excess of what the body needs is converted to energy or stored as fat.
4. Obesity is a bodily condition characterized by excessive storage of fat.
5. Physical activity accounts for the largest component of the average person's daily energy expenditure.
6. Anywhere from 15 to 25 percent of people who lose weight regain it within a year.
7. It has been found that obese individuals absorb more food than lean individuals.
8. The body has two types of fat tissue: white fat and brown fat.
9. Sometimes sugar-free products have the same number of calories as their sugared counterparts.
10. Bulimia is an eating disorder characterized by self-imposed starvation.

Body Weight

We have all heard at one time or another that there is an ideal body weight for our particular height. But ideal in terms of what? Health? Appearance? Physical performance? Standard tables of weight and height have been developed to enable people to determine if they are overweight. Ideal body weight has been traditionally defined by reference to the tables compiled by the Metropolitan Life Insurance Company. (Table 5–1 represents the most recently revised version.) To correctly determine your desirable body weight, you need to know your height (in shoes with one-inch heels) and your body-frame size. You know how to measure your height, but how do you measure the size of your body frame? The Metropolitan Life Insurance Company gives the following guidelines:

TABLE 5–1 ■ Height and Weight Tables*

Men

Height (Feet)	Height (Inches)	Small Frame	Medium Frame	Large Frame
5	2	128–134	131–141	138–150
5	3	130–136	133–143	140–153
5	4	132–138	135–145	142–156
5	5	134–140	137–148	144–160
5	6	136–142	139–151	146–164
5	7	138–145	142–154	149–168
5	8	140–148	145–157	152–172
5	9	142–151	148–160	155–176
5	10	144–154	151–163	158–180
5	11	146–157	154–166	161–184
6	0	149–160	157–170	164–188
6	1	152–164	160–174	168–192
6	2	155–168	164–178	172–197
6	3	158–172	167–182	176–202
6	4	162–176	171–187	181–207

Women

Height (Feet)	Height (Inches)	Small Frame	Medium Frame	Large Frame
4	10	102–111	109–121	118–131
4	11	103–113	111–123	120–134
5	0	104–115	113–126	122–137
5	1	106–118	115–129	125–140
5	2	108–121	118–132	128–143
5	3	111–124	121–135	131–147
5	4	114–127	124–138	134–151
5	5	117–130	127–141	137–155
5	6	120–133	130–144	140–159
5	7	123–136	133–147	143–163
5	8	126–139	136–150	146–167
5	9	129–142	139–153	149–170
5	10	132–145	142–156	152–173
5	11	135–148	145–159	155–176
6	0	138–151	148–162	158–179

*In shoes with one-inch heels and indoor clothing weighing five pounds for men and three pounds for women.
SOURCE: Metropolitan Life Insurance Company, 1983 version.

TABLE 5-2 ■ **Measuring your Frame Size**

Men	
Height in 1-Inch Heels	*Elbow Breadth**
5 ft 2 inches to 5 ft 3 inches	2½ to 2⅞ inches
5 ft 4 inches to 5 ft 7 inches	2⅝ to 2⅞ inches
5 ft 8 inches to 5 ft 11 inches	2¾ to 3 inches
6 ft 0 inches to 6 ft 3 inches	2¾ to 3⅛ inches
6 ft 4 inches and over	2⅞ to 3¼ inches

Women	
Height in 1-Inch Heels	*Elbow Breadth**
4 ft 10 inches to 4 ft 11 inches	2¼ to 2½ inches
5 ft 0 inches to 5 ft 3 inches	2¼ to 2½ inches
5 ft 4 inches to 5 ft 7 inches	2⅜ to 2⅝ inches
5 ft 8 inches to 5 ft 11 inches	2⅜ to 2⅝ inches
6 ft to 0 inches and over	2½ to 2¾ inches

*Approximations for medium-frame individuals.
SOURCE: Metropolitan Life Insurance Company.

Extend one arm and bend the forearm upward at a 90 degree angle. Keep fingers straight and turn the inside of your wrist toward your body. Place the thumb and index finger of your other hand on the two prominent bones on either side of your bent elbow. Pull your fingers away, maintaining the space between them. Measure the space between your fingers and compare it with those in the table (see Table 5–2), which are for medium-frame people. Measurements lower than these indicate a small frame and higher measurements, a large frame.

The reason that these weight ranges are generally considered "desirable" is because it has been found that people within this range of weight are at the lowest risk of dying prematurely. These tables do have shortcomings, however. For example, the sample of people used was not representative of the entire population. Minority groups were underreported, and people who were not covered by life insurance were not considered in deriving the tables. Also, age was not taken into account. Given these shortcomings, the tables should serve as a general guideline for determining body weight. Perhaps an individual's best determinant of ideal body weight should be what weight makes that person look and feel good and causes no major health problems.

■ Body Composition

Body composition refers to the component parts of the body. For our discussion, the body may be regarded as being composed of two components: (1) **body fat** and (2) **lean body mass**. For the average adult male and female, the following values represent approximate percentages of the body weight that a specific tissue composes:

	Adult Male	Adult Female
Muscle	43	36
Bone	15	12
Total fat	15	26
Essential fat	3	15
Storage fat	12	11
Other Tissues	27	26
Total	100%	100%

Total body fat consists of both **essential fat** and **storage fat.** Essential fat is necessary in the structure of various types of cells and also for protection of some internal organs. Storage fat is the accumulation of excess fat, most of which is found under the skin in the subcutaneous tissue. There is a need for the essential body fat; however, an individual can function efficiently with relatively low levels of storage fat. The average percentage of body fat for college men is about 12 to 15 percent, and for college women it is about 22 to 26 percent. Those men and women involved in athletic competition report lower percentages of body fat. Body composition is influenced by such factors as sex, age, diet, and exercise.

The Body Fat Component

The amount of body fat (**adipose tissue**) that is stored is determined by two factors: (1) the number of fat-storing cells (adipocytes) and (2) the size or capacity of the fat-storing cells. The number of fat cells cannot be decreased by exercise or dietary restrictions once adulthood is reached. During weight reduction involving fat loss in adults, it is the size, not the number, of fat cells that decreases.

Research on fat cells had suggested that there were three critical periods in life when the number of fat cells could be increased: during the fetus's development in the third trimester of pregnancy, during infancy and early childhood (up to about two years of age), and during preadolescence and throughout adolescence in girls. Recent studies now show that when fat cells reach a critical size, they divide to form new fat cells. What this means is that the number of fat cells can increase at any time throughout an individual's lifetime, and once formed, they take up permanent residence.

The Lean Body Mass Component

When the weight of body fat is subtracted from the total body weight, the remaining weight is referred to as lean body mass. Lean body mass reflects mainly the skeletal-muscle mass, but it also includes the weight of other tissues and organs such as bone, skin, liver, and heart. The less body fat, the more lean body mass. The average lean body mass of college-age men is about 85 percent of their total body weight, and that of college-age women is about 75 percent of their total body weight.

■ The Decision to Lose Weight

If you are having difficulty deciding whether or not you need to lose weight, there are many ways to determine degree of fatness. One simple test is to pinch

---

FAST FACTS

In general, beginning during puberty, females deposit more fat and males develop more muscle tissue.

the fat away from the underlying muscle at the back of the upper arm about midway between the shoulder and elbow. Hold this fat between your thumb and forefinger and measure the width of it with a ruler. Normal values are between one-half and one inch. Percentage of body fat is most accurately measured by underwater weighing. It is more frequently estimated, however, from skinfold or fat-fold measurements because of the method's simplicity. Using special calipers, skinfold measurements are made at specific sites of the body to estimate percentage of body fat. Skinfold measurements also give information about the distribution of body fat. As far as heart disease is concerned, the distribution of body fat may be a better indicator of potential health problems than total body weight.

Losing weight is not impossible, but it does require a commitment. If you want to lose weight, it involves not just knowing *what* you eat but also becoming aware of *how, why, when,* and *where* you eat. As is the case with anything worth doing, careful planning and some hard work are necessary. This is why the "quick and easy" weight-loss programs are so appealing, yet so fraudulent. It should be obvious that when several new diets are published daily, each one claiming to be the best, something is questionable. There is no diet now, and there never will be a diet, that cures obesity. The reason for this is that diets do not attack the fundamental problem of the overweight person. Sure, diets help people to lose weight; but losing weight is not the basic problem. The problem is keeping the lost weight off. It is an unfortunate statistic, but anywhere from 75 to 95 percent of people who lose weight regain it within a year.

For the normal, healthy individual attempting to lose weight, the principles of dieting are rather basic. If you consume more calories than you expend, body weight will increase. If you expend more calories than you consume, body weight will decrease. The ultimate control of body weight appears to involve a balance of energy. Energy input and output, in the form of calories, is responsible for the control of body weight on a long-term basis. An excess expenditure of 3,500 calories is required in order to lose one pound.

Calorie awareness is very important if you are trying to lose weight. To know the number of calories you should consume daily in order to lose weight, you must first know how many are needed to maintain your present weight. That depends on two things. One is your basal metabolic rate (BMR), which refers to the number of calories required to maintain all the cellular activities that are necessary to sustain life. Basal metabolism accounts for the largest component of the average person's daily energy expenditure. A simple way to estimate your BMR is to multiply your current weight by ten. For example, if a woman weighs 120 pounds, her BMR calorie needs are 1,200 calories. The second thing you need to figure out is how many calories you use for daily activities. The amount of energy needed depends on the involvement of the muscles, the amount of weight being moved (a heavier person needs more calories because it takes extra effort to move the additional body weight), and the duration of the activity. How would you classify your activity level? If you lead a sedentary lifestyle (mostly sitting), you can figure about 30 percent of BMR for activity calories; for light activity, about 40 percent; for moderate activity, about 50%; and for strenuous activity, about 60 percent. So, if our 120-pound female leads a sedentary lifestyle, we would estimate the energy she needs for physical activities by multiplying her BMR calories per day by 30 percent. She would therefore need 360 calories daily (1,200 calories per day × 0.30) for her physical activities. Her total daily energy needs would be 1,560 calories [1,200 calories (BMR)

FAST FACTS

Skipping or skimping on breakfast and lunch and then having a large dinner is likely to result in the intake of more calories in a 24-hour period than having three or more smaller meals throughout the day.

+ 360 calories (activities)] if she wanted to maintain her current weight. Because this figure is based on estimates, it would be best to express her needs as falling within a range of plus or minus 50 calories.

> ■ *PROBLEM SITUATION* You have decided that you want to lose some weight. You know that to do so, you must take in fewer calories than you use up. How many calories do you need to maintain your present weight? Without altering your activity level, how many calories a day should you consume if you want to lose one pound by the end of the week?

Balanced, low-calorie diets that provide 1,000 to 1,200 calories a day for women and several hundred more for men are the most healthful and effective diets for losing weight and keeping it off. The best feature of a balanced diet is that you can choose from a variety of foods that provide adequate amounts of all the necessary nutrients. By eating a variety of foods in limited quantity, you avoid the cravings for those "missed" foods. Also, you can stay with this type of diet even after you have reached your desired weight; and by continuing to make wise food choices, you will maintain the weight loss. Stay away from diets that advise you to eat "none of this and all of that." These diets are unbalanced because they concentrate on one food group and restrict others.

FAST FACTS

The American Medical Association says a person leading a moderately active life needs 15 calories per pound per day to maintain his or her weight.

Assessment of Eating Habits

Becoming aware of the circumstances under which you tend to overeat may help you to change your eating behaviors. How do these factors affect your eating?

■ *Type of food and amount.* Steer clear of "red light" foods. If ice cream is something you just can't get enough of, make another selection. Choose a food that you feel confident you can control but that still has the qualities you desire.

■ *Meal or snack.* You may find yourself snacking several times a day as well as eating your three basic meals. Beware of raids on the refrigerator.

■ *Time of day.* Do you eat at regular hours, or do your day's activities revolve around eating?

■ *Degree of hunger.* How hungry are you when you eat? Are you eating from habit rather than from hunger?

■ *Activity.* What are you doing while eating? Watch out for automatic eating—at the movies, in front of the television, while reading a book, and so on.

■ *Location.* Where do you eat? Have a designated eating place at the kitchen table. Avoid bringing food into other rooms to eat.

■ *Persons involved.* Do you eat more when alone or with others? Do certain people trigger a tendency to overeat? Don't be pressured into eating just to be sociable. At parties, choose low-calorie foods. Don't stand next to the food table and be a "glutton" for punishment.

■ *Emotional feelings.* How do you feel when eating? Do certain emotions trigger overeating?

■ *Purchasing of food.* Do your food shopping when you are not hungry. Prepare a shopping list and do not deviate from it. Avoid filling your refrigerator and cabinets with tempting foods.

■ *Visibility of foods.* Keep food out of sight. A bowl of candy or nuts sitting on a table is hard to walk by without taking a handful. Don't test your willpower by seeing if you can pass it up. Why put yourself through such frustration?

Understanding the Labels

When you buy a food product, do you take time to read the label? All packaged foods have labels. They must provide at least the following information: the name of the product; the name and location of the manufacturer, packer, or distributor; and the net contents or net weight.

Regulations adopted by the Food and Drug Administration (FDA) in 1973 require manufacturers to provide nutrition information on their product label only if one or more nutrients are added to the food or if a nutritional claim is made about the product. The nutrition information must include the number of calories and the amount of protein, fat, carbohydrate, and sodium in a specified serving. In addition, the label must show the percentage of the Recommended Dietary Allowances (RDAs) for seven essential vitamins and minerals (vitamin A, vitamin C, thiamine, riboflavin, niacin, calcium, and iron) in each serving. There may be an optional listing that includes the fat content by degree of saturation and the amount of cholesterol. Slightly more than half of all packaged foods today carry nutrition information.

Reading a food label can be difficult if you don't understand the terms being used. To help the health-conscious consumer interpret some confusing terms, the following list was compiled by the staff of *Tufts University Diet and Nutrition Letter*.

FAST FACTS

Since July 1986, the FDA has required sodium content in nutrition labeling.

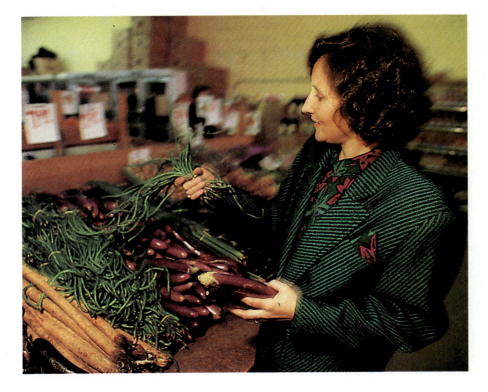

It is not only important to examine the quality of fresh produce, but shoppers also need to read the label posted above each item to determine cost as well as nutritive value.

FAST FACTS

If a food product label says "substitute," what you are buying is nutritionally equivalent to the food it resembles.

- *Low calorie*—These foods cannot contain more than 40 calories per serving or no more than 0.4 calories per gram.
- *Reduced calorie*—These foods must be at least one-third lower in calorie content than similar foods that contain the usual amount of calories.
- *Imitation*—This means that the product is not "the real thing" and that it is usually nutritionally inferior.
- *Light or lite*—This can mean anything from a lighter color or texture to less sodium, calories, or fat. The label doesn't always provide the answer. The FDA has no legal definition for "light."
- *Low-fat*—Referring to dairy products, it means that they must contain between 0.5 and 2 percent milk fat. Referring to meat, it means no more than 10 percent fat by weight.
- *Sugar-free or sugarless*—Although these foods cannot contain sucrose (table sugar), they can have other sweeteners, including honey, corn syrup, fructose, sorbitol, and mannitol. Sometimes sugar-free products have the same number of calories as their sugared counterparts.
- *Naturally sweetened*—The FDA does not have a regulation regarding this term. Many manufacturers use it when they sweeten with a fruit or juice instead of with sugar.
- *Sodium-free*—Indicates that the food has less than 5 milligrams of sodium per serving.
- *Reduced sodium*—Indicates that the sodium levels have been reduced by at least 75 percent. The label must show before and after sodium levels.
- *Natural*—This means that there are no additives or artificial ingredients of any kind and that the food was produced and marketed with a minimum of processing.
- *Organic*—This term has no legal meaning, so a manufacturer may use it without any guidelines.

Remember, manufacturers are out to sell their products. So the next time you read a food label that seems ambiguous or misleading, realize that it just may be intentional. Perhaps knowing some of the preceding terms will help to make you a wiser shopper.

■ The Decision to Gain Weight

Although most individuals in our society have a desire to lose excess weight, there are some individuals who want to gain weight, either to improve their physical appearance or to have greater body mass. No matter what the reason for wanting to gain weight, an individual should be concerned about where the extra pounds will be stored. Excess body fat will not improve physical appearance or physical performance. It may detract from both. To put on body weight, an individual has to concentrate on means to increase lean body mass, particularly muscle tissue, with little or no increase in body-fat stores.

There may be a variety of reasons for an individual to be **underweight.** The most obvious cause is inadequate consumption of food. Other factors may include a genetic predisposition, a metabolic disorder, medical problems, social pressures, or a psychological disturbance. It is important to determine the cause of being underweight before beginning a weight-gain regimen. If being underweight is not symptomatic of any medical problem, measures can be taken to gain body weight. For the underweight individual who simply is expending more calories than are being consumed, weight gain will consist of increasing caloric consumption and decreasing energy expenditure.

When you initiate a program to gain body weight, the following guidelines may help you to maximize your gains in muscle mass and keep body fat increases relatively low:

1. Increase your caloric intake. Eat greater quantities from the Four Basic Food Groups in three balanced meals plus several high-calorie, high-nutrient snacks. The weight gain should be primarily muscle tissue and not body fat.
2. Decrease the intake of bulky foods that are filling yet contain few calories.
3. Although the amount of saturated fat and simple sugars will normally increase in this type of diet, try to keep the intake of these types of food to a minimum. Use vegetable fats and oils rather than animal fats.
4. Muscle-building exercises should be included in your exercise regimen in order to increase muscle mass.

Adequate rest, increased caloric intake, and a proper weight-training program may be effective as a means to gain the right kind of body weight. Remember to consult your physician before initiating such a program to determine whether such a regimen could be detrimental to your health.

Theories of Weight Control

Is dietary fat the culprit responsible for body fat? If you answered "yes" to this question, you may see fat as an unnecessary evil in your diet. After all, if you get rid of fatty foods, you get rid of a fat body. Right? Wrong! Excess body fat is produced when there is an overconsumption of any of the three energy nutrients. The human body can make fat from whatever it is fed—carbohydrates, proteins, or fats. Overeating itself, not any one nutrient, leads to storage of body fat.

Being overweight is an extremely complicated physiological, psychological, and social issue. It has different meanings in different segments of the population. For example, in less affluent societies, fatness is valued as a sign of success and wealth. In some societies, female beauty is judged by sheer bulk, and young females are sent to fattening houses before marriage. In American society, the majority of young females will tell you that "thin is in and flab is drab." Striving to attain a great physique or a beautiful body has been turned into an issue of aesthetics. Wanting to "look good" has become the main reason for losing weight, and most people will go to almost any lengths to achieve this goal. Now, there is certainly nothing wrong with wanting to look good, but there are also important health reasons for maintaining desirable body weight. Health conditions such as diabetes, **hyperlipidemia,** and high blood pressure are known to be related to or caused by obesity, whereas other conditions such as respiratory illnesses, cirrhosis of the liver, and coronary heart disease may be aggravated by the body's extra weight load.

Americans have become *so* weight conscious that an extra pound or two on the scale puts them into a tail spin. The assumption that being overweight is a "condition to be gotten rid of" should be questioned. Understanding the difference between being **overweight** and being **obese** is very important.

Being overweight implies a quantity of heaviness. It actually means greater-than-normal weight for a certain height and body-frame size. *How much* greater can vary. A person can be one pound or ten pounds overweight. Approximately

FAST FACTS

Nearly 90 percent of Americans think they weigh too much, and more than 35 percent want to lose at least fifteen pounds.

FAST FACTS

Obesity is the most prevalent nutritional disorder in the United States.

34 million Americans are considered to be overweight. Being obese, however, refers to an excessive amount of body fat. A person with a fat percentage of more than 20 percent of the recommended weight for men or more than 25 percent of the recommended weight for women is usually classified as obese. Studies indicate that 25 to 45 percent of adult American men and women suffer from being obese, and approximately 25 percent of all American children are obese. Whereas obesity has potentially negative consequences in all realms of an individual's life, being overweight may pose little or no problem. Many people find it easier to deal with being some degree overweight than to cope with the constant bouts of frustration each time a dieting attempt fails.

It is not uncommon for a person to learn to cope with an emotional problem by overeating. Food can be a welcomed friend when you are feeling depressed, bored, lonely, angry, or stressed. It temporarily gets you through the rough time—but when the eating is done, the problem is still there, along with the new-found emotion of guilt for having "pigged out." Do your ways of dealing with emotional upset involve eating?

> **PROBLEM SITUATION** You walk into a restaurant to have dinner with your family. Once seated, you see your sweetheart walking out of the restaurant, behaving extremely intimately with someone you do not know. What emotion(s) would you be feeling? In what way would these feelings affect your food selection and eating behavior?

When trying to determine *why* some people become fat and gain weight faster than others, the following information was discovered:

- Obese individuals do not have an increased absorption of food.
- There is no increase in thyroid deficiency among obese individuals.
- Obese individuals do not seem to have a greater desire for sweet foods than do thin people.
- There is no conclusive evidence that obese individuals are less active than thin people.

If these are *not* factors contributing to obesity, what are some of the factors? The following section will examine four physiological theories of obesity. They include genetic predisposition theory, fat-cell theory, white fat versus brown fat activity theory, and the setpoint theory.

Genetic Predisposition Theory

One theory states that the tendency for obesity is inherited. Children inherit their body type from their parents. The skeletal frame of a child will be similar to that of one of his or her parent's. The terms **ectomorph, endomorph,** and **mesomorph** have been established to define the different body types. The ectomorph has a slender, wiry body frame and has a lesser capacity for storing fat. The endomorph has a soft, rounded appearance and has a greater capacity for storing fat. The mesomorph has a muscular body frame and tends to be less likely to have a weight problem. (See Figure 5–1.)

It is usually evident when you see parent and child together that "the apple doesn't fall far from the tree." Studies indicate that if one parent is obese, the child has a 40 percent chance of being overweight. If both parents are obese, the percentage rises to 80. If the genetic predisposition theory is correct, this means that the *tendency* is inherited. The word "tendency" is very important,

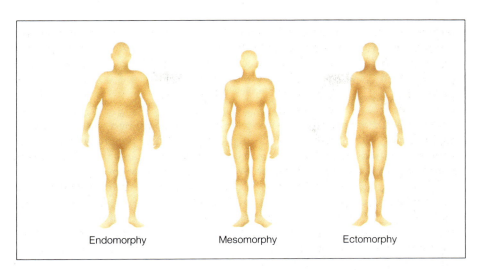

FIGURE 5–1 ■ **The Three Basic Body Types**

because it still allows an individual to be in control of his or her fate. By establishing wise eating habits and incorporating regular exercise into one's lifestyle, obesity *can* be avoided!

Fat-Cell Theory

Another theory states that the number of fat cells in the body predisposes an individual to obesity. As previously mentioned in this chapter when we were discussing the body-fat component, an individual is born with a certain number of fat cells, and this number is genetically determined. However, a pregnant woman can alter this number in her last trimester of pregnancy. If during this time, the woman overeats and consumes a high-fat, high-sugar, diet, the number of fat cells in the fetus will increase. Also, overfeeding a child during infancy and up to about two years of age will increase the number of fat cells. Thus, what you have, by the age of two, is a child who has a much greater number of fat cells than was genetically predetermined.

There is a saying that "A fat baby is a healthy baby." Nothing could be farther from the truth. It is a myth that plump babies will "outgrow" their baby fat. It is estimated that 80 percent of today's extremely overweight children will be tomorrow's fat adults. Everybody has fat cells, but the greater the number, the greater the capacity to store more energy in the form of fat.

White Fat versus Brown Fat Activity Theory

It has been proposed that people who have weight problems have little brown-fat activity. The human body has two types of fat tissue: white fat and brown fat. Most of the fat that is stored in cells is called white fat. In the living body, it is actually pink in color because of the blood flowing through it. White fat accumulates mainly in the subcutaneous tissue, the abdominal cavity (around the internal organs), and the intramuscular tissue. The other type of fat tissue is called brown fat. Brown fat is less abundant in the body and accounts for about 1 percent of body weight. It is found in the back and shoulder region and in the back of the neck. At birth, our bodies have relatively large amounts of brown fat, but we lose it as we get older. Brown fat has a high metabolic activity potential. It has the ability to burn part of the food we eat and expend the excess energy as heat. It is speculated that obese individuals may have inefficient brown-fat tissue. Research is being conducted to learn more about brown fat, but to date, there is no known way to stimulate brown fat to work at a faster pace.

The Setpoint Theory

The setpoint theory proposes that body weight is controlled by a weight-regulating mechanism (WRM) located in the hypothalamus. The weight level that this mechanism chooses to maintain is called the setpoint, and the WRM works continuously to maintain this level. When the stability of the setpoint weight is threatened, the WRM functions in two ways. First, it increases or decreases the individual's appetite as needed to maintain the setpoint weight. This may account for why an individual becomes hungrier and more obsessed with food when he or she is dieting. Second, this mechanism triggers body systems to expend energy if the individual overeats or to conserve energy if the individual eats too little. What this means is that the WRM will conserve energy to maintain the setpoint even if an individual is trying to lose weight by eating less. This most likely explains why some people can eat very little and still remain overweight whereas others eat a lot and never gain a pound.

The setpoint theory sheds light on why people usually gain back the weight that has been lost on extremely low-calorie diets. If an individual restricts daily caloric intake to below 1,000 calories, the body automatically slows down its metabolism to conserve energy. This can lead to as much as a 15 to 30 percent decrease in basal metabolic rate. Lack of energy expenditure leaves the individual feeling listless and fatigued, which in turn decreases his or her desire and ability to maintain normal activity levels. Decreased activity levels raise the setpoint, and because not enough food is being consumed to maintain this higher setpoint, the WRM takes action in an effort to restore stability. How is this done? Well, if you have ever experienced food cravings and hunger pangs, or the uncontrollable urge to eat, just thank the WRM.

Why bother trying to lose weight if the WRM undermines your efforts? It seems like a losing battle, with the bulge winning out—right? Not necessarily! There are ways to lower your setpoint level so that the WRM is satisfied with less food. On the other hand, there are also ways to raise your setpoint. It is important to be aware of the factors that affect the setpoint level so that you can work toward lowering it rather than raising it.

Factors That Affect the Setpoint. The following factors have been found to lower an individual's setpoint level:

1. *Aerobic exercise, performed regularly, at moderate intensity*—(Chapter 6 will discuss aerobic exercise and the guidelines to follow to achieve optimal results.) Not only is exercise essential in lowering the setpoint, but it also increases the metabolic rate, maintains muscle mass, and increases the enzymes that burn fat.
2. *Reduced consumption of high-fat foods*—As mentioned in Chapter 4, an individual's fat consumption should not exceed 30 percent of the daily caloric intake.
3. *Reduced consumption of simple carbohydrates*—High levels of sugar in the bloodstream cause an overproduction of insulin, and excess insulin can cause increased fat storage. Also, because simple carbohydrates are rapidly absorbed, there is usually a strong desire to eat again within a short period of time.

FAST FACTS

Women who are between 18 and 25 percent body fat seem to be healthiest both physically and emotionally.

4. *Reduced consumption of artificial sweeteners*—Artificial sweeteners seem to increase the desire for sweets, and they also may raise the setpoint.
5. *Reduced consumption of caffeine*—Caffeine stimulates the production of insulin.
6. *Increased consumption of complex carbohydrates*—Because complex carbohydrates are absorbed more slowly than simple carbohydrates, they do not stimulate an overproduction of insulin.

The following factors have been found to raise an individual's setpoint level:

1. *Eating irregularly or skipping meals*—Your body interprets this deprivation of food as a threat to your survival and therefore takes the necessary actions to conserve energy.
2. *Stress*—Stress-related hormones, such as epinephrine (Adrenaline), trigger excess insulin production.
3. *Certain mineral deficiencies*—Mineral deficiencies can interfere with the proper metabolic processing of sugars; therefore, it is extremely important to eat well-balanced meals in order to obtain adequate amounts of these needed minerals.

Even though these suggestions can help to lower your setpoint, it is important to realize that it takes time to reprogram the setpoint. It may take several months before you notice any change. Also, it is not known how far down your setpoint will go. You may follow the preceding suggestions to a tee but may still never reach your fantasized weight. Remember, what your setpoint will accept as your ideal weight as compared to what you have dreamed about weighing can be two very different things. You can achieve success only if you are realistic about the end results.

Weight Reduction

Most people judge how successful a diet is by the amount of weight they have lost. Weight loss, however, is a poor indicator of success. Total body weight consists of fat, muscle, bone, and water. When you lose weight, it is important to know where that loss is coming from. Is most of your loss water weight? Is it a loss of lean muscle tissue? Is it a loss of body fat? The *type* of weight lost is more important to the success of a diet than the number of pounds shed.

Because numbers seldom give a realistic picture, how can you determine if any progress is being made when you are dieting? One thing you can do is to periodically take your body measurements. As you lose fat, your waist, hip, and thigh measurements will decrease even if total body weight doesn't change. Another way to indicate success is to try on clothing that was previously tight on you. Does it feel any looser? Also, do you notice an improvement in your energy level or in your overall health status? Do you feel mentally and physically better in comparison to how you felt before you started the diet? If a diet is working for you, the signs of success will be there. You just need to know where to look!

FAST FACTS

About 70 percent of the weight loss during the first few days of a reduced calorie diet is due to body water losses.

> **PROBLEM SITUATION** After procrastinating for months about losing weight, you finally accept the fact that you need to lose fifteen to twenty pounds to be in good health. How might you motivate yourself to begin losing this weight? What obstacles might interfere with your intended weight loss, and how can you avoid them? What approach will you pursue to reach your desirable weight?

GUIDELINES TO YOUR GOOD HEALTH

Before selecting a particular weight-reduction diet, ask yourself the following questions:

1. Does the diet work? Does it have a proven track record?
2. Does the diet show long-term maintenance of weight loss?
3. Is the diet easy to follow?
4. Does the diet instill principles of sound nutrition and wise eating habits? Does it include low-calorie/high nutrient foods from the Four Basic Food Groups?
5. Can following the diet impair my health or well-being?
6. Is the diet flexible, and does it allow me to eat the foods I like?
7. Can I incorporate the diet comfortably into my life-style, whether I eat most of my meals at home or away?
8. Is the diet a life-long diet, one that I can continue even after my desired weight is attained?

Combining a diet program with an exercise program is the most effective way to lose weight. Together they promote fat loss while preserving lean body mass. If you want to lose weight and maximize the chances of keeping it off, you should not lose more than two pounds per week.

FAST FACTS

Over 2,500 books now in print recommend unproven and unscientific nutrition practices.

Popular Diets

There are thousands of weight-reduction diets available to try, and each one claims to be better and more effective than all of the others. No matter how ridiculous the claims or the logic behind them, if a diet promises instant weight loss without much effort or deprivation of favorite foods, people are extremely anxious to try it. But what do you really know about the various diets being advertised? Let's look at some of the more popular diets to see if any are really the "best and most effective."

Complete Fasting Diet. A fasting diet is the most drastic way to reduce caloric intake. **Fasting** is equivalent to starvation. The main difference is that when a person fasts, he or she voluntarily deprives the body of food; when a person is starving, it is usually not out of choice. The body does not differentiate between fasting and starving. When there is food deprivation, the body switches to a **wasting metabolism,** drawing on its stored food reserves. As fasting begins, the body calls up its glycogen reserves (stored glucose) in the liver and converts them back to glucose. The brain cells can use only glucose for their source of fuel. When the glycogen reserves are used up, the body calls on protein. Glucose can be obtained from proteins, but not as easily as from carbohydrates. Because no proteins are available from food sources, the body breaks down muscle and lean tissue to supply protein for conversion to glucose.

The body also breaks down fat into fatty acids to obtain fuel. Sufficient amounts of carbohydrates are not available to completely metabolize the fatty acids, so the fatty acids break down into ketone bodies. The accumulation of ketones in the body produces a condition known as ketosis. Ketosis can lead to an acid condition of the body (**acidosis**) and cause a rise in the level of uric acid in the blood. Ketosis in a pregnant woman can cause brain damage and irreversible mental retardation in the developing fetus. Also, the accumulation of ketones causes a person to feel nauseated, which in itself can suppress the desire to eat. As ketosis begins, substantial weight loss occurs.

Prolonged fasting causes the body to drastically reduce its energy output in order to conserve both its lean and fat tissue. As the muscles waste, they do less work, thus reducing energy needs. Because of the decreased metabolic rate, the loss of fat falls to a bare minimum—less, in fact, than the amount that would be lost on a sensible, reduced-calorie weight-reduction diet.

There is no doubt that fasting produces weight loss; however, most of the loss is due to water rather than fat. Once eating is resumed, the lost water is regained and so is the weight! Prolonged fasting leads to metabolic imbalances, dangerously low blood pressure, mineral imbalances, and possible liver impairment and kidney damage. One-day fasts usually have no lasting negative health consequences. Because of the potential hazards of fasting and the need for continuous medical supervision, fasting as a means of weight reduction is not recommended.

> **FAST FACTS**
>
> Fasting has been shown to lower the rate of metabolism by as much as 20 percent within a few days, but lowered metabolism usually means less weight loss too.

Low-Carbohydrate Diets. The amount of carbohydrates that can be eaten are limited in low-carbohydrate diets and protein consumption is encouraged. Diets high in protein are usually high in fats and cholesterol. We should all know by now the negative health problems associated with fats and cholesterol. A diet low in carbohydrates will also produce ketosis. (You should remember the effects caused by ketosis, having just read about fasting.) As a general rule, a minimum of 100 grams of carbohydrate should be eaten each day in order to avoid the breakdown of protein tissue and prevent ketosis. Diets advocating lower levels of carbohydrate intake are not recommended.

Protein-Supplemented Modified Fast Diet. This type of diet conserves lean tissue while maximizing fat loss. High-quality protein food or drink containing 300 to 500 calories is consumed daily. A multivitamin and mineral supplement along with a potassium and calcium supplement is taken daily. This diet regimen should not be followed by preadolescent individuals, pregnant women, or individuals with heart, liver, or kidney disease. Any individual attempting this diet should be under the constant care and monitoring of a physician.

The Cambridge Diet. The Cambridge diet is a protein powder sold in cans. Water is added, and the mixture is drunk three times a day in place of meals. Various diets are available, ranging from 330 to 800 calories, although the 330-calorie diet seems to be the most popular. The protein powder is not sold in stores and can only be bought through a "counselor." Criteria for the selection of counselors are unclear; however, a nutrition background is not a prerequisite. Because this diet is dangerously low in calories, it should not be used as the sole source of nutrition. Even if this diet is to be supplemented with small meals, I would strongly recommend consulting your physician before trying it.

Fit for Life Diet. This specific diet is worthy of mention because it was the bestselling diet book in 1986. *Fit for Life* made publishing history by selling one million hardcover books in a six-week period. The diet emphasizes a high-carbohydrate, high-fiber, low-fat eating regimen. This part of the diet has merit, especially since the American Heart Association recommends such a diet. In addition to this regimen, however, the authors suggest limiting animal proteins in the diet and totally eliminating dairy products. This diet is probably not dangerous if followed for only a few weeks, but since it is deficient in calcium, vitamin D, vitamin B_{12}, zinc, and possibly protein, continued practice could predispose an individual to negative health problems.

The Beverly Hills Diet. Another unique diet plan needs to be mentioned. *The Beverly Hills Diet* was a top-selling book in 1981. The author, Judy Mazel, recommends that for the first ten days, the dieter eat nothing but fruit. Essentially no protein is eaten until the eleventh day, and an adequate amount of protein is not eaten until the nineteenth day of this diet. Ms. Mazel claims that in order for food to be properly digested, only one type (carbohydrate, protein, or fat) should be eaten each day. Besides the fact that this diet is possibly monotonous to follow, it does not adhere to the principles of healthy nutrition, which recommend that a person eat a variety of foods from the Four Basic Food Groups each day.

The Rice Diet. This diet needs to be mentioned because it is potentially life threatening. This diet recommends "going for as long as possible" eating one and one-half cups of rice a day in addition to five servings of fruit and selected beverages. The total caloric daily intake is 700 calories. Consumption of animal proteins are not allowed until later stages of the diet. Milk products are discouraged, sodium is severely restricted, and herbs and spices are eliminated. The diet must be followed "exactly as it is written." This diet is deficient in several vitamins and minerals, and the protein deficiency can be very dangerous.

Prescription Diet Pills

Amphetamine, a central-nervous-system stimulant, was once widely used to suppress appetite, but it was found that its adverse effects outweighed any usefulness as a diet aid. Although amphetamine temporarily suppresses appetite, tolerance quickly develops, and the individual must take higher doses to maintain the drug's effects. Prescription diet pills produce nervousness, irritability, insomnia, and fatigue. High doses can cause abnormal heart rhythms and produce psychosis. For the few pounds that are lost during the first few months of use, the negative health consequences far outweigh any benefit. A responsible physician will not prescribe amphetamine as a diet aid.

Over-the-Counter Diet Preparations

The following over-the-counter (OTC) diet preparations are sold to help control one's desire to eat. How safe and effective are they?

■ **Phenylpropanolamine** is a nasal decongestant and the active ingredient found in many OTC diet pills. Doses high enough to suppress appetite may cause headaches, blurred vision, dizziness, rapid pulse, nervousness, insomnia, and elevations in blood pressure.

FAST FACTS

The National Council Against Health Fraud warns individuals to be wary of any weight-control program that encourages use of special products rather than teaching how to make wise food choices from the conventional food supply.

- **Benzocaine** is a local anesthetic used in chewing gum and lozenges. By dulling nerve endings in the mouth, benzocaine is supposed to decrease a person's sense of taste, thereby decreasing interest in eating. It has been found not only to dull nerve endings but also to create a feeling of numbness in the mouth. As for decreasing a person's sense of taste, it removes most of the taste in *all* food.
- **Bulk producers** are indigestible, noncaloric substances that absorb water during digestion and supposedly trick the stomach into thinking that it is full. There has been no substantial proof that bulk producers reduce hunger or appetite. They do, however, produce flatulence and diarrhea.

That people purchase all of these products is just another indication of how far they will go to lose weight. At least if these diet plans and aids were harmless (although ineffective), people would only be wasting their time, money, and energy (which is bad enough). Unfortunately, many of them are *both* harmful and ineffective. And too many people don't realize this until it is too late!

> **FAST FACTS**
>
> Americans spend $200 million a year on over-the-counter appetite suppressants that, for the most part, do not effect permanent weight loss.

Surgical Procedures

Surgery for weight-loss purposes is considered a radical approach. Complication rates can be quite high, so these procedures should be used mainly by individuals who are 100 pounds or more above their desirable weight. The following procedures are available.

- *Intestinal bypass surgery*—This surgery involves removal of a portion of the small intestine. People who have bypass surgery lose large amounts of weight because they cannot absorb as much food as they could before. The disadvantages of this surgery are that it can cause severe diarrhea and lead to possible malnutrition because of nutrient losses that result from the impaired absorption. It can also lead to liver disease and kidney stones.
- *Stomach reduction*—This surgery closes off part of the stomach by means of stitches, staples, or the implanting of a balloon. People lose large amounts of weight because they feel full on smaller amounts of food. This type of surgery causes fewer complications than bypass surgery; however, there is no guarantee that the lost weight will be kept off.
- *Jaw wiring*—Wiring the jaw allows the individual to feed only on beverages and liquified foods. It leads to rapid loss of weight, but most people regain their losses once the wiring is removed. The disadvantages of jaw wiring are that it can cause considerable pain, lead to dental decay, and possibly weaken and cause atrophy of the jaw muscles.
- *Liposuction*—This surgery involves the suctioning of fat deposits from under the skin. This procedure is used for people who have unsightly pockets of fat that won't go away with dieting and exercise. It is performed more often on overweight people than on the obese. Liposuction is not intended as a replacement for proper dieting and exercise. This procedure should be done by a qualified plastic surgeon, and no more than five pounds of fat should be removed at one time. When too much fat is removed, large quantities of fluids are also lost. If these fluids are not replaced, the individual can go into shock. The disadvantages of this surgery are that postoperative bruising, swelling, tenderness, and a numbing or burning sensation in the suctioned area can last for several weeks to months following the surgery. To locate a qualified physician, contact the American Society of Plastic and Reconstructive Surgeons.

136 SECTION II ■ BODY DYNAMICS

Having the support of other people when trying to lose weight is extremely important. The 100-pound weight loss experienced by this man is a shared victory.

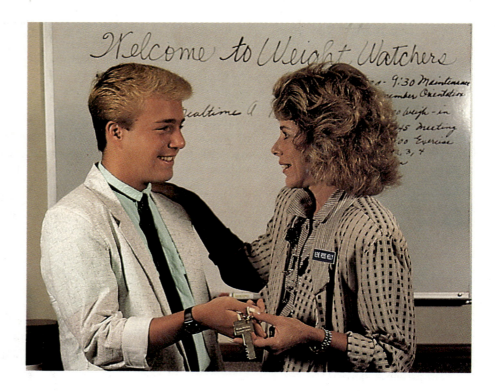

Self-Help Groups

Many people need to be motivated in order to stay on a weight-reduction diet. The support from other people who are also trying to lose weight can be very helpful. Support must extend not only during the period of weight loss but also after the loss is achieved so that the weight is not regained. Organizations such as Weight Watchers, TOPS (Take Off Pounds Sensibly), and OA (Overeaters Anonymous) provide great help to many individuals wanting to lose weight. According to Abraham and Llewellyn-Jones, self-help groups have the following advantages:

1. The leaders of the group have been able to alter their own eating habits and have achieved and maintained their weight goal; therefore, they are able to serve as good role models.
2. It is easy to join and to leave the group (there is no obligation to stay).
3. The group exerts a positive effect, which may help the person counter the psychological and social pressures that encourage relapse.
4. This method helps the person to feel that he or she has achieved the eating-behavior changes by his or her own efforts.
5. The person is not converted into a "patient" with a "disease."
6. Usually the courses provided by these groups are less expensive than those provided by professional therapists.
7. Most of these groups are accessible at all times to help a person who perceives himself or herself to be in "crisis."

Self-help groups may not be appropriate for helping individuals whose overweight problems are caused by physical or psychological conditions. These individuals need to consult with a qualified health professional.

SELF-INVENTORY 5.1

Are You in Control of Your Weight?

Read the following statements and place a check mark in the appropriate column. Base your responses on your current eating behaviors.

	Fre-quently	Some-times	Rarely
1. I eat slowly and chew my food thoroughly.	___	___	___
2. I tend to overeat.	___	___	___
3. I maintain my weight in an ideal range for my height and body frame.	___	___	___
4. I eat while doing other activities, such as watching television or reading.	___	___	___
5. I make a list and stick to it when I go food shopping.	___	___	___
6. I eat even when I am not hungry.	___	___	___
7. I carefully plan what my daily meals and snacks will be.	___	___	___
8. I make raids on the refrigerator.	___	___	___
9. I take time to sit down and enjoy my meals.	___	___	___
10. I position myself near the food table at social functions.	___	___	___
11. I eat small portions of food and take only one serving.	___	___	___
12. I eat when other people around me are eating.	___	___	___
13. I am able to eat one piece of candy or one cookie and feel satisfied.	___	___	___
14. I go for long periods at a time without eating.	___	___	___
15. I limit alcohol consumption to an average of not more than one drink per day.	___	___	___
16. I reward myself for "a job well done" by eating a treat.	___	___	___

Scoring:

Total Control—Checked "Frequently" for all the odd numbered questions and checked "Rarely" for all the even numbered questions.

Fair to Good Control—Checked "Frequently" for more than 50 percent of the odd numbered questions and checked "Rarely" for more than 50 percent of the even numbered questions.

Marginal Control—Checked "Sometimes" for the majority of questions. You are at the threshold of being able to either gain control or lose control. Be aware of any changes in your eating behaviors to determine in which direction you are heading.

Losing Control—Checked "Rarely" for more than 50 percent of the odd numbered questions and checked "Frequently" for more than 50 percent of the even numbered questions.

No Control at All—Checked "Rarely" for all the odd numbered questions and checked "Frequently" for all the even numbered questions.

What does your score tell you?

What changes do you need to make in your eating behaviors in order to have more control?

Eating Disorders

Eating disorders occur because a person loves food and either seeks to control this love (as is the case with anorexia nervosa and bulimia) or give into it (as is the case with obesity). An eating disorder, in itself, is not an illness. It becomes an illness, however, when it interferes with the person's mental or physical comfort, disorganizes the person's life to a marked degree, or produces severe medical problems. The following sections will discuss the eating disorders of anorexia nervosa and bulimia.

Anorexia Nervosa

Being underweight has a variety of effects on the body, depending on its severity and duration. Being slightly underweight may actually reduce the risk of certain diseases and prolong life. In its severe forms, however, being underweight impairs growth and mental development in children, decreases resistance to infection, reduces neuromuscular performance, inhibits sexual functioning, and interferes with the normal activity of the heart.

The obsession for thinness reaches its most extreme form in a condition called **anorexia nervosa.** This is a severe, self-imposed starvation that results from an intense fear of gaining weight. Anorexia affects females fifteen times more commonly than males and usually begins during adolescence or in early adulthood. It is estimated to occur in one out of every 200 females aged twelve to eighteen. The incidence in eight- to eleven-year-olds is said to be increasing. Because male victims are few, anorexia is viewed primarily as a female disorder. Anorectics are described as having low self-esteem and feeling that others are controlling their lives. The anorectic becomes obsessed with a fear of fat and with losing weight. In her mind, she sees normal folds of flesh as fat that must be eliminated. The preoccupation with food usually prompts strange food-related patterns, such as crumbling food, moving it about on the plate, and cutting it into very tiny pieces to prolong meals. An anorectic individual may feel hungry but suppresses her hunger and refuses to eat normally because of her obsession to be thin.

Anorexia may be a sudden, limited episode, or the illness may gradually work itself into the victim's life and go on for years. Many of the anorectic's behaviors and bodily changes are typical of any starvation victim. The starving body tries to protect itself by slowing down or stopping less vital body processes. Menstruation ceases, blood pressure and respiratory rate slow down, and thyroid function diminishes. With depletion of fat, the body temperature is lowered. Soft hair called **lanugo** forms over the skin. Electrolyte imbalance can become so severe that irregular heart rhythm and heart failure occur.

According to the American Psychiatric Association, the following criteria must be met for a case to be recognized as an occurrence of anorexia:

1. Intense fear of becoming obese, even when underweight.
2. Disturbance in the way in which one's body weight, size, or shape is experienced—for example, claiming to "feel fat" even when emaciated.
3. Refusal to maintain body weight over a minimal normal weight for age and height.
4. In females, absence of at least three consecutive menstrual cycles when otherwise expected to occur.

CHAPTER 5 ■ EATING BEHAVIORS   139

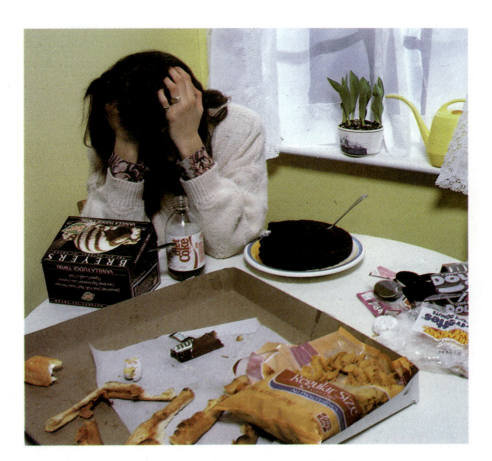

The bulimic's desire to eat is uncontrollable during a binge period.

Bulimia

Bulimia, an eating disorder characterized by compulsive **bingeing** and **purging,** is found in 40 to 50 percent of persons suffering from anorexia. Bulimia was considered to be a part of anorexia nervosa until recently, but it is now accepted as a separate illness. This disorder affects between 3 and 7 percent of women between the ages of fifteen and thirty-five. The true prevalence may be higher, because these statistics only reflect those women seeking medical treatment. People with bulimia rapidly eat tremendous amounts of food and then get rid of the food by vomiting or other means. Actual diagnosis of this disorder may not be made until a person is in her thirties or forties. In the January 1985 issue of *Cosmopolitan,* for example, actress Jane Fonda revealed that she had been a secret bulimic from age twelve until her recovery at age thirty-five—bingeing and purging as many as twenty times a day.

Most binge eaters are secretive about their behavior. The binge may start at any time of the day, but many binge eaters have specific times, such as weekends. Factors such as tension, unhappiness, loneliness, and boredom may trigger a binge. Hunger is seldom the triggering factor. Bingeing episodes may occur as frequently as two to three times a week or as infrequently as twice a month. The food eaten is usually considered by the individual to be junk food, fattening food, or "bad" food. The amount of food eaten during a binge varies from

FAST FACTS

A bulimic's fear of fatness is as great as her love of food.

TABLE 5–3 ■ **Food Eaten During a "Bad" Binge Lasting Eight Hours (as Reported by a Patient)**

3 loaves bread, 5 lb. potatoes (chips), 1 jar honey, 1 jar anchovies (on bread), 1 lb. rolled oats, 2 lb. flour (as pancakes), 1 lb. macaroni, 2 instant puddings, 4 oz. nuts, 2 lb. sugar, 1 large package Rice Bubbles, 1½ lb. margarine, 1 pint oil (for cooking), 4 pints milk powder, 1 tin condensed milk (in porridge, on bread, or in a drink), 4 lb. ice cream, 1 lb. sausages (or meat rissoles), 1½ lb. onions, 12 eggs (in milk shake, scrambled eggs), 1 lb. liquorice (liquorice allsorts), 2 family-size blocks chocolate, 1 lb. dried figs, 2 packages sweets, 6 'health bars,' assorted cream cakes (up to 12) eaten while shopping, 1 lb. sultanas (on bread or in porridge), left-overs found in fridge, 1 bottle orange cordial.

This amount of food gives a total of:

Energy	54,000 kcal.
Protein	1,071 g.
Fat	1,964 g.
Carbohydrate	14,834 g.

three to thirty times the amount usually eaten in one day. (Table 5–3 shows an example of food eaten during an eight-hour binge.)

To lose the gained weight, the bulimic begins purging, which may include using laxatives, diuretics, or self-induced vomiting. Between binges, the bulimic may fast or exercise excessively. Most bulimics show frequent swings in body weight. The binge-purge cycle can be devastating to health in a number of ways. It can upset the body's balance of electrolytes, which can cause fatigue, seizures, muscle cramps, irregular heartbeat, and decreased bone density. Repeated vomiting can damage the esophagus and stomach, cause the salivary glands to swell, make the gums recede, and erode tooth enamel. Some bulimics use the **emetic** syrup of ipecac to induce vomiting after a binge. Recording artist Karen Carpenter was an anorectic who died of syrup of ipecac abuse. Building up over time, the alkaloid emetine in the ipecac irreversibly damaged her heart muscle, which eventually led to her death by cardiac arrest.

According to the American Psychiatric Association, the following criteria must be met for a case to be recognized as an occurrence of bulimia:

1. The individual has recurrent episodes of binge eating (rapid consumption of a large amount of food in a discrete period of time).
2. During the eating binges, there is a feeling of lack of control over the eating behavior.
3. The individual regularly engages in either self-induced vomiting, use of laxatives, or rigorous dieting or fasting to counteract the effects of binge eating.
4. There must be a minimum average of two binge-eating episodes per week for at least three months.

More research is needed to determine the incidence and causes of anorexia and bulimia. One theory about these two eating disorders is that many females feel excessive pressure to be as thin as some ideal perceived in the media. Other theories suggest that certain biological factors may predispose individuals to the onset of these eating disorders. These disorders may even be triggered by an inability to cope with a situation in life.

FAST FACTS

Bulimia was first defined as a medical disorder in 1980.

Early treatment is important to recovery. As either disorder progresses, damage to the body becomes less reversible. For treatment to be effective, the individual must first perceive that she has an eating problem. Secondly, she must believe that if the disorder continues, it will produce serious health complications. Finally, she must make a commitment to change her eating behavior.

> ■ *PROBLEM SITUATION* A female friend shows all the signs of being anorectic. You are worried about her because she refuses to eat but also refuses to admit that she has a problem. How can you get her to realistically see herself as she is and seek appropriate treatment?

POSITIVE BEHAVIORS

I. *Place a check mark in front of each behavior that you now practice.*

____ 1. I maintain my weight within a normal range for my height. (WEIGHT)
____ 2. I am aware of approximately how many calories I consume daily. (CALORIES)
____ 3. I eat when I am hungry and not out of habit. (HUNGRY)
____ 4. I avoid raids on the refrigerator. (RAIDS)
____ 5. I know my danger periods when I am most likely to overeat. (DANGER PERIODS)
____ 6. I go food shopping when I am not hungry. (FOOD SHOPPING)
____ 7. I avoid diet crazes. (DIET CRAZES)
____ 8. I read food labels to obtain nutritional information about the food. (LABELS)
____ 9. I do not stand next to the food table at social functions. (FOOD TABLE)
____ 10. My daily food intake includes foods from each of the Four Basic Food Groups. (FOOD GROUPS)

II. *For each behavior that you DO NOT ENGAGE IN, write the KEY WORD(S) located in the parentheses at the end of the statement in the column below. Then put a check mark in the appropriate column to indicate whether you are going to keep or change that behavior.*

Behaviors I Don't Engage In   KEEP/CHANGE

_____   _____/_____
_____   _____/_____
_____   _____/_____
_____   _____/_____
_____   _____/_____
_____   _____/_____
_____   _____/_____
_____   _____/_____
_____   _____/_____
_____   _____/_____

III. *For each of the preceding behaviors that you choose to KEEP, write a statement indicating why you are choosing to keep that behavior.*

I choose to keep behavior _____ because:
                              KEY WORD

For each of the preceding behaviors that you choose to CHANGE, write a statement indicating how you plan to implement that change.

I will change behavior _____ by:
                          KEY WORD

Now You Know

1. TRUE. One pound of body fat equals 3,500 calories. Therefore, for every decrease in food intake or increase in physical activity that totals 3,500 calories, an individual will lose one pound.

2. FALSE. The number of fat cells cannot be decreased by dietary restriction. During weight reduction involving fat loss in adults, it is the size, not the number, of fat cells that decreases.

3. TRUE. Energy or body fat is produced when there is an overconsumption of protein.

4. TRUE. Obesity refers to an excessive amount of body fat. Persons who have a fat percentage of above 25 percent of the recommended body weight are usually classified as obese.

5. FALSE. Basal metabolism accounts for the largest component.

6. FALSE. Anywhere from 75 to 95 percent of people who lose weight regain it within a year.

7. FALSE. Obese individuals do not have an increased absorption of food.

8. TRUE. White fat is primarily a storage place for excess energy. Brown fat has the ability to burn part of the food we eat and expend the excess energy as heat.

9. TRUE. Although sugar-free products cannot contain sucrose, they can contain other sweeteners, such as honey or corn syrup.

10. FALSE. Bulimia is an eating disorder characterized by binge eating followed by a period of purging.

Summary

1. An individual's body is composed of body fat and lean body mass. Body fat consists of essential and storage fat. Lean body mass reflects mainly the skeletal-muscle mass. Body composition is influenced by such factors as sex, age, diet, and exercise.

2. The amount of body fat that is stored is determined by the number and size of fat-storing cells present in the body. The number of fat cells cannot be decreased by exercise or dietary restrictions. During weight reduction involving fat loss, it is the size, not the number, of fat cells that decreases.

3. Energy input and output in the form of calories is responsible for the control of body weight. Losing one pound requires an excess expenditure of 3,500 calories. Balanced, low-calorie diets that provide 1,000 to 1,200 calories a day for women and several hundred more for men are the most effective and healthful diets for losing weight and keeping it off.

4. An individual wanting to gain weight should be concerned about where the extra pounds will be stored. Healthful weight gain involves increasing muscle mass while keeping body-fat increases relatively low.

5. Being overweight involves physiological, psychological, and social factors. Being overweight means having greater-than-normal weight for a certain height and body-frame size. Being obese refers to an excessive amount of body fat. Persons having a fat percentage of above 25 percent of the recommended body weight are usually classified as obese.

6. There are four physiological theories of obesity. The genetic predisposition theory states that the tendency for obesity is inherited. The fat-cell theory states that the number of fat cells in the body predisposes an individual to obesity. The white fat versus brown fat activity theory states that people who have weight problems have little brown fat activity. The setpoint theory states that body weight is controlled by a weight-regulating mechanism located in the hypothalamus.

7. Total body weight consists of fat, muscle, bone, and water. The type of weight lost is more important to the success of a diet than the number of pounds lost. Combining a diet program with an exercise program is the most effective way to lose weight. Together they promote fat loss while preserving lean body mass.

8. There are hundreds of weight-reduction diets, and each one claims to be the quickest, easiest, and most effective way to lose weight. A healthy reducing diet allows an individual to choose from a variety of foods that provide adequate amounts of all the necessary nutrients.

9. Other methods used to lose weight include prescription diet pills, over-the-counter diet preparations, surgical procedures, and self-help groups.

10. Anorexia nervosa and bulimia are two types of eating disorders. Anorexia is a self-imposed starvation that results from an intense fear of gaining weight. Bulimia is characterized by compulsive binge eating followed by a period of purging. Both disorders can be extremely harmful to the body. As either disorder progresses, damage to the body becomes less reversible. Early treatment is important to recovery.

References

1. Abraham, Suzanne, and Derek Llewellyn-Jones. *Eating Disorders*. New York: Oxford University Press, 1987.
2. *A Guide to Losing Weight*. Dallas, TX: American Heart Association, 1987.
3. Berland, Theodore. *Rating the Diets*. New York: Beekman House, 1983.
4. Burtis, Grace, Judi Davis, and Sandra Martin. *Applied Nutrition and Diet Therapy*. Philadelphia: W. B. Saunders Co., 1988.
5. Collipp, Platon J. *Childhood Obesity*. New York: Warner Books, 1986.
6. Dove, Jody. *Facts about Anorexia Nervosa*. Washington D.C.: National Institute of Child Health and Human Development.
7. Dusek, Dorothy E. *Weight Management: The Fitness Way*. Boston: Jones and Bartlett, 1989.
8. Katch, Frank I., and William D. McArdle. *Nutrition, Weight Control, and Exercise*, 3rd ed. Philadelphia: Lea and Febiger, 1988.
9. Krause, Marie V., and L. Kathleen Mahan. *Food, Nutrition, and Diet Therapy*, 7th ed. Philadelphia: W. B. Saunders, 1984.
10. Lamb, Lawrence E. *The Weighting Game: The Truth about Weight Control*. Secaucus, NJ: Lyle Stuart, Inc., 1988.
11. Remington, Dennis W., A. Garth Fisher, and Edward A. Parent. *How to Lower Your Fat Thermostat*. Provo, UT: Vitality House International, 1988.
12. "Test Your Food Label Knowledge." *FDA Consumer* 22 (March 1988): 16–21.
13. "Things are not Always What They Appear to Be," *Tufts University Diet and Nutrition Letter* Vol. 4 (September 1986): 3–6.
14. *Weight Loss and Nutrition*. San Diego: Health Media of America, 1986.
15. Williams, Sue Rodwell. *Nutrition and Diet Therapy*, 6th ed. St. Louis: Times Mirror/Mosby College Publishing, 1989.
16. Yetiv, Jack Z. *Popular Nutritional Practices: Sense and Nonsense*. New York: Dell Publishing, 1988.

Suggested Readings

Bailey, Covert, and Lea Bishop. *The Fit-or-Fat Woman*. Boston: Houghton Mifflin, 1989.

Lamb, Lawrence E. *The Weighting Game: The Truth about Weight Control*. Secaucus, New Jersey: Lyle Stuart, Inc., 1988.

Siegel, Michele, Judith Brisman, and Margot Weinshel. *Surviving an Eating Disorder*. New York: Harper and Row, 1988.

Tribole, Evelyn. *Eating on the Run*. Champaign, Ill.: Life Enhancement Publications, 1987.

Yetiv, Jack Z. *Popular Nutritional Practices: Sense and Nonsense*. New York: Dell Publishing, 1988.

CHAPTER 6

Getting Physical

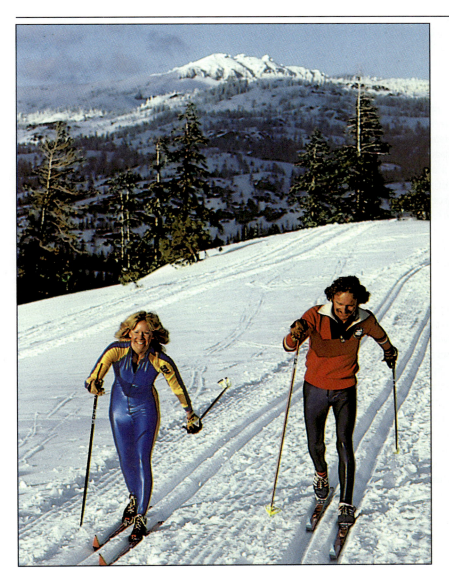

What Do You Know?

Are the following statements true or false?

1. Americans are exercising less.
2. Cardiovascular fitness is a health-related fitness component.
3. Flexibility is the improvement and maintenance of one's ability to exert force through progressive and gradual resistance activities that overload a muscle group.
4. Regular aerobic exercise will reduce one's risk of heart disease.
5. Improved collateral circulation through exercising can increase your longevity.
6. Frequency, intensity, and duration are the principles of a fitness program.
7. We all should "go for the burn" when exercising.
8. The term *aerobic* means "with oxygen."
9. Isokinetic weight training involves lifting a constant weight through a full range of motion.
10. Ballistic stretching is an excellent way to improve flexibility.
11. Steroids are dangerous drugs.
12. We all should warm up before we stretch to prevent injuries.

■ Definition of Physical Fitness

The music begins and we start dancing. The starter's gun goes off and we begin the race. We've done our stretching and other warm ups, we're attired in the "right" outfit for physical exercise, and we move into strenuous exertion of some form or other, be it aerobic dance, jogging, biking, or swimming. But wait a minute . . .

Why are we bothering to spend an hour or more every other day on such activity? Will it reduce the saddlebags on our thighs or the roll of fat around our middles? What level of physical fitness are we trying to attain? How did we decide to engage in our particular form of sport? Are we doing it correctly? What is physical fitness?

The President's Council on Physical Fitness defined *physical fitness* as "the ability to carry out daily tasks with vigor and alertness, without undue fatigue, and with ample energy to enjoy leisure time pursuits and to meet unforeseen emergencies." A major outcome of physical activity is fitness. For some of us, fitness means having a lean, muscular body. For others, fitness means "being in top shape," having the capacity to participate in strenuous exercise, such as hiking, swimming, running, or skiing. But a thin, strong body or exceptional physical abilities represent the extreme of the concept of fitness. Most people do not have the time, physiological capacity, or desire to become models of fitness. Some of us are lucky not to get out of breath racing across campus to our next class. Fortunately, nearly everyone can reach a level of fitness that is synonymous with good health, with their life goals, and with their individual capacities.

Each year more and more Americans engage in regular exercise. Regular exercise is defined by the Surgeon General of the United States as exercising three times weekly at one's target heart rate for at least twenty minutes. A 1979 national survey revealed that 35 percent of people eighteen to thirty-five exercised regularly; a 1980 study identified nearly 70 million people, or more than one-half the adult population, who were practicing exercise for self-improvement. And in 1989, the number of adults exercising was approximately 60 percent. It is clear that among the adult population in the United States, the exercise boom is here to stay. Aerobic exercise, jogging, swimming, yoga, and sports continue to attract more people each year. Exercise and diet books continue to be best sellers as Americans crave information on exercise, nutrition, and healthy lifestyles. Millions of Americans have realized exercise's positive benefits to their energy level, appearance, and overall health.

Approximately two thousand years ago, Hippocrates claimed that all parts of the body that have a function become healthy, well developed, and slow to age if exercised; if they are not exercised, they become liable to disease, defective in growth, and quick to age. This claim is universally regarded as the basis for the prescription of exercise for physical fitness. There are so many fitness recipes; a few are useful, many are not, and, unfortunately, some can prove to be injurious to the participant. Millions of people believe that spot reduction of subcutaneous fat in specific areas of the body is possible, and exercises, pills, belts, and gadgets that perpetuate this fallacy are still merchandised. For some people, exercise means taking the dog for a walk around the block, pushing the cart around in the grocery store, or vacuuming the house. Some people sit in steam baths, lose a small amount of their body water through sweating, and then believe that they have permanently burned up fat in the heat. Weight is lost, but it only

---

FAST FACTS

Exercise will increase one's energy level and decrease fatigue.

lasts for a few hours—enough time to get into a tight pair of jeans for a special date. This chapter provides the tools and information you will need to guide your exercise decisions so that you can meet your personal physical fitness goals.

Components of Physical Fitness

To go beyond the simple definition of physical fitness, it is important to understand the dual elements that make up the criteria by which to judge your current physical fitness level and develop your personal goals. Physical fitness can be categorized into *health-related* and *performance-related* components. To maintain or improve health, the emphasis should be on health-related components; to learn, maintain, or improve athletic ability, the emphasis should be on performance-related components. The two components complement one another, and both need to be taken into consideration when planning an exercise program.

Health-Related Fitness Components. The physiological physical fitness components that are believed to offer some protection against degenerative diseases such as obesity, coronary heart disease, and various musculoskeletal disorders are termed the **health-related fitness components.**

To attain cardiovascular fitness, we must improve and maintain cardiorespiratory efficiency through regular aerobic activities of sufficient duration and intensity to achieve a training effect. Activities that involve the large muscle groups in continuous repetitious movements meet the requirements for cardiovascular fitness. These activities will strengthen the heart and the lungs by boosting the body's ability to use oxygen.

Muscular fitness includes two aspects—muscular endurance and muscular strength. **Muscular strength** involves improving and maintaining our ability to exert force through progressive and gradual resistance activities that overload a muscle group. Strength in muscle groups helps prevent injuries. **Muscular endurance** involves improving and maintaining the ability of muscle groups to persist in physical activity by working against resistance for increasing periods of time. Good muscular endurance leads to better posture, fewer backaches, and resistance to fatigue.

Flexibility entails improving and maintaining the functional capacity of specific muscles and joints by increasing their full range of motion through static stretching techniques. Stretching is especially important for injury prevention.

Another aspect of health-related fitness components include body fat composition. To achieve optimal body-fat composition, we must improve and maintain the relative percentage of lean body mass to fat mass through regulating caloric consumption and expenditure. We should strive for 75 to 80 percent lean tissue weight (muscle and bone) and less than 20 to 25 percent body fat. Those of us who are leaner are usually healthier and live longer.

Performance-Related Fitness Components. Goals such as agility, balance, coordination, power, reaction time, and speed are **performance-related** goals. Proficient athletes have honed these skills to a fine degree. These components are not necessary for health but are essential for sports and exercise performance. Many of us participate in tennis, basketball, racquetball, and other games that

FAST FACTS

To rid yourself of cramps while exercising, slow your pace and take slow, rhythmic breaths.

SECTION II ■ BODY DYNAMICS

Volleyball includes both health-related and performance-related components of physical fitness.

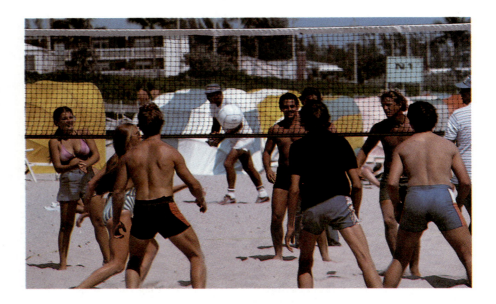

combine both types of fitness. For example, your physical fitness goal might be to improve your tennis skills, which would involve both performance-related and health-related components of physical fitness. You might be in training for your college football team or the Olympic volleyball team, which would also involve both performance- and health-related components.

FAST FACTS

Mild exercise, such as walking or swimming, reduces anxiety, tension, and blood pressure on the first day of exercise.

■ Benefits of Exercise

Research findings indicate that aerobic exercise benefits the body both physiologically and psychologically, including the cardiovascular and respiratory systems. Muscle function, strength, and stamina are all improved through exercise. Risk factors can be reduced and disease can be prevented.

Seven out of the ten leading causes of death have been strongly linked to behavior such as lack of exercise, drinking in excess, smoking, drug abuse, distress, poor nutrition, and obesity. As we can observe from this list, lifestyle behaviors are the leading influences on mortality in our country. As discussed in Chapter 1, there are four major factors that influence our health, lifestyle being the most influential. The prescription for the prevention of the major causes of death in our country, as well as the reduction of risk factors such as hypertension, is a formula that includes the lifestyle choice of exercise over and over again. Regular aerobic exercise reduces tension, high blood pressure, cholesterol, fat, causes weight reduction, and increases cardiovascular function and high-density lipoprotein/low-density lipoprotein (HDL/LDL) ratios.

Positive contributions of regular aerobic exercise to overall health and wellness have been well documented. A study in *Runners' World* reviewed the corporate fitness programs of the Fortune 500 group of companies. At one office of Prudential, employees participating in fitness programs had 45.7 percent fewer major medical expenses than nonparticipants. They also had 42.6 percent fewer days of disability. Not only did the individuals participating in the fitness programs benefit from them, but the corporations benefited as well through fewer days lost from work by employees and lower health-care costs for employees.

Disease Prevention

The major cause of mortality in our country today is heart disease, which is associated with a number of risk factors, among them obesity, stress, high blood pressure, and a history of heart disease. There is much evidence that habitual vigorous exercise is associated with a reduced risk of heart disease. In the last two decades, there has been a 28 percent decline in heart-attack deaths in the United States. Aerobic exercise is one of the positive lifestyle habits (in addition to improved nutrition, a reduction in cigarette smoking, blood pressure screening and control, and better medical diagnosis and treatment) that most authorities agree have contributed to the decline.

Several research studies have indicated that physical activity may be related to the prevention and control of atherosclerosis, diabetes, and osteoporosis. Hypertension, which can begin as early as twenty years of age, can be prevented to a great degree by exercise, along with other positive lifestyle habits. Recent research with Harvard alumni indicated that regular exercise significantly reduced the lifetime risk of breast cancer, colon cancer, and cancers of the reproductive system. Exercise is a very important ingredient in our recipe for a healthy life.

> **FAST FACTS**
>
> Moderate exercise can enhance one's immune response, helping to fight off infection.

Physiological Benefits

The cardiovascular benefits of exercise include effects on both the heart itself and the blood vessels. The stroke volume—the amount of blood pumped through the body with each contraction of the heart—is increased. As a consequence, the heart rate slows down. This increase in blood volume results from strong heart-muscle tissue, which in turn results in stronger muscle contractions and more complete filling and emptying of the left ventricle with each heartbeat. These benefits all result in a stronger, more efficient cardiovascular system.

Individuals who exercise vigorously have resting heart rates as low as 40 to 50 beats per minute (normal range is around 70 beats per minute) as well as much lower heart rates during physical exercise than their less fit counterparts. For example, a physically fit runner may have a heart rate of 140 beats per minute while running a marathon. A less fit person running the marathon might have a heart rate as high as 180 or more. In addition, after exercise, the heart rate of a fit individual will return to normal more quickly than that of someone not in good physical condition.

Blood pressure is also reduced by regular exercise. By following a regular program of aerobic exercise, you can lower your blood pressure as much as twenty points. If your normal blood pressure is 120/80 before starting your exercise program, it may be as low as 100/60 or so just a few months later. If your blood pressure is too high at the beginning of your program, you could possibly lower it into the normal range through exercise. As with heart rate, blood pressure also returns to normal more quickly after exercise in the fit individual. In urban western cultures, blood pressure tends to rise gradually with age. This process seems to be slowed in physically fit individuals.

The blood's capacity to carry oxygen to all body tissues is increased through regular exercise. The total volume of blood, the total number of red blood cells, and the amount of hemoglobin (which carries the oxygen in the circulating blood) are all increased. These effects combine to improve the body's overall

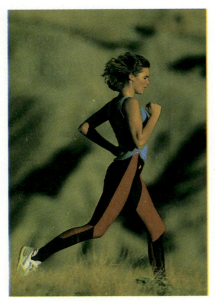

Running, one form of aerobic exercise, is beneficial for the respiratory and the circulatory systems of the body.

ability to deliver oxygen to muscles during physical activity, which leads to increased stamina and endurance—just what you need for a fun evening of dancing!

Collateral circulation (alternative pathways of blood flow) tends to develop in areas of skeletal-muscle activity. This increases the body's ability to deliver oxygen to those muscles. This process is well documented. Some evidence suggests that regular aerobic exercise may also increase collateral circulation to the heart muscle, but this theory is still controversial. If such is the case, the increased blood flow to the heart muscle would make the heart a more efficient pump and would likely extend its life. Improved collateral circulation through exercising can increase longevity. Research studies with laboratory animals have shown development of such collateral circulation with exercise, but evidence in human research is not conclusive.

Aerobic exercise helps to reduce levels of circulating cholesterol and lipids and also causes an increase in high-density lipoprotein/low-density lipoprotein (HDL/LDL) ratios. High-density lipoproteins (the good cholesterol) are responsible for transporting excess fats to the liver, where they are metabolized and eliminated from the body. Low-density lipoproteins (the bad cholesterol) transport fat to storage locations in the body. (You know where they are!) For further discussion of HDLs/LDLs, see Chapter 16. It is interesting to note that during exercise itself, blood cholesterol levels tend to be higher than normal. This might demonstrate the effect of exercise in removing excess fat from fat stores, which plays an important role in preventing atherosclerosis.

The muscles of the respiratory system increase in both strength and endurance with aerobic exercise. This leads to an increase in the amount of air you can inhale with each breath while working out. The amount of air exhaled per breath also increases, and the amount of air left in the lungs after a breath decreases. Blood circulation to lung tissue is improved, leading to more effective oxygenation of respiratory muscles. Blood flow to the alveoli also is augmented, and the amount of oxygen entering the blood rises. All these factors combine to prevent shortness of breath during physical exertion and to increase the overall efficiency of the respiratory system. After you've been exercising regularly for a while, you won't run out of breath next time you go hiking or dancing or engage in other strenuous exercise.

An important change that occurs when you exercise aerobically on a regular basis is that you burn calories, which contributes significantly to weight loss. After all, don't most of us exercise because of vanity? Dieting alone can lead to weight reduction; however, research has indicated that within seven to twenty-one days after this weight loss occurs, 95 percent of the dieters will regain this weight plus five pounds extra. To lose weight, you should reduce your caloric intake by eating less and increase your energy expenditure by exercising. When you diet without exercising, the resulting loss is about 70 percent fatty tissue and 30 percent lean muscle. Add regular aerobic exercise to the formula and you will increase your fatty-tissue loss to 95 percent. Both human and animal research indicates that physical activity decreases appetite. See Figure 6–1 for caloric expenditure during different forms of exercise.

Aerobic exercise also appears to play a role in the setpoint theory. This theory indicates that the body automatically alters its metabolism to expend more or fewer calories, thus keeping the body weight at a particular point. This explains why people who lose weight on reducing diets quickly return to their original weight, as if their bodies "wanted" to weigh a certain amount. This theory is supported by animal research, but there is insufficient evidence in human research to validate the theory at this time. Researchers are currently studying the preliminary findings that exercise can lower one's setpoint by increasing energy expenditure through an increase in metabolism or by decreased energy intake through a decrease in appetite. For further discussion of the setpoint theory, see Chapter 5.

Psychological Benefits

The idea that mental and physical fitness are linked is not new, but in our past thinking about the mind-body connection, we put the mind over the body in the equation. Now psychologists, counselors, and psychiatrists are asking the question in reverse: Can exercising the body soothe the mind? Many studies conclude that aerobic exercise is a practical way to treat the emotional problems of daily living. Harvard psychiatrist Dr. Thomas Hackett says that for recovering coronary patients, exercise is "the single most effective way to lift a patient's spirits and to restore feelings of potency about all aspects of life." Exercise can help reduce anxiety, relieve depression, improve self-esteem, and increase one's zest for life. After considering individual patient needs, mental health professionals are recommending exercise programs that include an activity's duration, intensity, and frequency. Refer to Table 6–1 to determine the type of exercise to improve your peace of mind. When your goal is to exercise to cope with stress or anxiety, it is important to exercise for its intrinsic benefits rather than for competitive reasons. Competing to win increases stress.

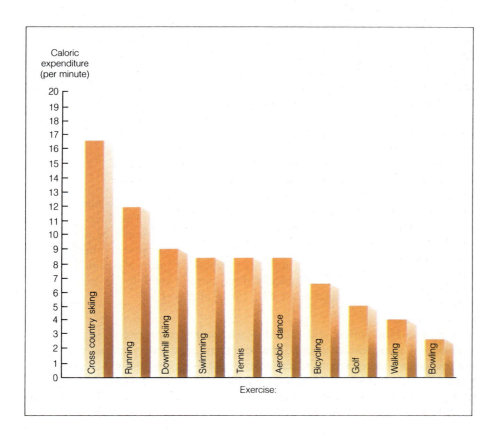

FIGURE 6–1 ■ **Caloric Expenditure during Various Exercises**

SOURCE: President's Council on Physical Fitness

TABLE 6-1 ■ **Exercise to Improve Your Peace of Mind**

Goal	Intensity	Frequency	Duration	For Maximum Benefits
To reduce tension	Average pace	3–5 days a week	20–30 minutes	For any of these problems, add meditation and progressive-relaxation exercises to reduce tension, stress, and anxiety.
To reduce depression	Fast pace	5 days a week	40–60 minutes	For serious psychological problems, schedule counseling with a licensed professional.
To improve your psychological well-being	Average to fast pace	3–5 days a week	20–60 minutes	

SOURCE: Adapted from Dianne Hales and Robert Hales, "Using the Body to Mend the Mind," *American Health* Vol. 4, No. 5 (June 1985): 26–31.

■ Principles of a Fitness Program

When you begin an exercise program or develop new goals, you need to plan your activities based on the principles of a fitness program. The three principles are frequency, duration, and intensity. These principles should be planned in this progression for the best training benefits and to prevent injuries. The standard recommendation of the American College of Sports Medicine (ACSM) is that you should exercise aerobically three times a week for at least twenty minutes at 70 percent target heart rate. (See Table 6–1.)

Frequency. How often you exercise each week determines your program's *frequency*. Researchers have found that exercising moderately at least three days a week for twenty to sixty minutes will produce a training effect that will result in cardiovascular benefits. When you exercise two days a week or less, detraining occurs; you begin to lose the good effects of earlier sessions. When you exercise five days a week or more, there is no added cardiovascular value, but body fat will decrease.

Duration. The amount of time you exercise each session is called *duration*. Twenty- to sixty-minute sessions of continuous aerobic activity are recommended by the ACSM. The duration will depend on the intensity. With higher-intensity activities like jumping rope or jogging, you can achieve a training effect in as short a time as twenty or thirty minutes. With activities like walking or bicycling, longer sessions are needed. To reduce body fat, thirty minutes or longer is necessary.

Intensity. The rate at which you exercise is the *intensity*. According to the ACSM, healthy adults should exercise at a rate known as the target heart rate (THR) which is the percent of aerobic activity that meets your fitness goals. Your pulse rate should not exceed your THR during your exercise session. Research data support the notion that an intensity level equivalent to 70 percent of the aerobic capacity represents the threshold above which a cardiovascular training effect occurs for young and middle-aged people. At the same time, 85 percent of the aerobic capacity is recognized as the upper limit of exercise for the development of physical fitness.

Controversy over Activity Level

A controversy has arisen over these recommendations concerning activity level. Recently, many research studies have indicated that at high intensity levels physical activity can be dangerous to our health. Another group of studies has shown that moderate to low levels of activity can have significant health benefits. We do know that those of us who don't exercise at all don't receive any health benefits and are in danger of becoming couch potatoes!

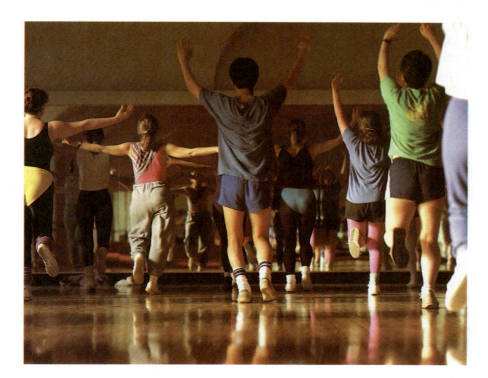

Physical activity must involve the large muscle groups in continuous, repetitious movements to be considered cardiovascular exercise.

High Activity. In the belief that more is better, many people are exercising at between 80 to 90 percent THR. As a result, many people are overtraining. This occurs when exercisers do too much too often, resulting in injuries, fatigue, sudden loss of weight, or an increase in the resting pulse rate. Of the twenty-seven million people who began doing aerobic dancing when it first became popular, 60 percent sustained minor injuries, mostly stress fractures and other orthopedic injuries.

A lifetime of regular exercise strengthens bones in women and helps prevent osteoporosis. But with high levels of exercise, hormonal changes occur. Up to 50 percent of female endurance athletes (marathon runners) fail to have regular menstrual cycles or stop having menses altogether. As a result, some women experience temporary infertility and spinal bone loss associated with lower estrogen, calcium, and fat levels. These problems can be reversed by reducing the intensity of exercise. Menstruation can begin again after the woman either stops training for a period of time or drastically reduces the amount and intensity of exercise. Increasing calcium and caloric intake can also assist in getting the body into its natural rhythms again. Overdoing exercise is definitely out of vogue.

Moderate Activity. First came "lite" beer, then "lite" wine, then you could have an entire "lite" meal. Now that Americans have seen the light, it should come as no surprise that next up is "lite" exercise. Many researchers have come to the conclusion that the public has been oversold in the value of "go for the burn" exercise. There has been a major shift in philosophy among physical-fitness experts. Dr. Kenneth Cooper, the physician who popularized aerobic exercise with his book *Aerobics* in 1968, has been running less after suffering from bone fractures and heel problems. Jane Fonda, the actress and exercise entrepreneur who popularized the term "go for the burn," has sold more than $4 million worth of exercise books and videotapes. Her latest videotape features moderate rather than high-intensity exercises.

Dr. Henry S. Miller, considered to be the father of cardiac rehabilitation and medical director of Bowman Grey School of Medicine in North Carolina, presented a research paper at the 1987 ACSM meeting reporting findings that showed no difference in the recovery of heart-attack patients who were on low-intensity or high-intensity exercise regimes. A twenty-year Harvard study by Dr. Ralph Paffenberger found that if you want to live longer, it's not important how you burn your calories just as long as you burn them. Those who engaged in moderate exercise such as walking and climbing stairs lived up to two years longer than their sedentary peers. Most important, the people who participated in vigorous exercise did not gain any significant health advantage over those who enjoyed moderate activity. Paffenberger's study also suggests that the heavy exerciser pays a price for the excess activity with a high injury rate and extreme fatigue.

Low Activity. Many experts state that there has been far too much emphasis on the intensity of exercise and not enough on the exercise itself. A 1980 study reported in *Lancet* tracked 18,000 English civil servants and found that those who engaged in low levels of activity gained health advantages comparable to those achieved by people engaged in vigorous sports. Both groups in the study had less than half the incidence of heart disease of their more sedentary colleagues. Energetic gardening for more than half an hour and at least five minutes of brisk walking every two days were positively linked to heart-disease prevention.

No Activity. The "go for the burn" philosophy has scared many people into never exercising. In this country, an idealized image of fit young people doing highly vigorous activity is perpetuated, which dissuades many overweight or out-of-shape people from beginning any kind of exercise program. If you're one of these people, the information in this chapter should convince you that even low levels of activity can increase your fitness. So, instead of just pushing the grocery cart around the store or driving your car instead of walking, let's exercise!

Despite the preceding evidence, the theory that the moderate approach to exercise is the best formula is still controversial. Cardiologist Dr. Harvey Simon of Harvard Medical School says that although some exercise is better than none, vigorous exercise is best of all. There are five major studies that show that high levels of exercise significantly reduce heart disease. Even experts that advocate the moderate approach concede that a person who participates in vigorous exercise will have more energy. The ACSM still recommends that healthy Americans should exercise at least twenty minutes three times a week at around 70 percent target heart rate. But Dr. Paffenberger says that the increase in heart rate during exercise can be as low as 50 percent of the heart's maximum capacity and still be associated with notable health benefits. And Dr. Steven Van Camp, medical director of the Adult Fitness Program at San Diego State University, states that physical activities directed at "health goals require less intense exercise than exercising to achieve a high fitness level." The traditional ACSM recommendations should be considered optimal goals and not the bare minimum necessary for health.

We can conclude from this controversy that you will receive health benefits from exercising at any level. The old belief that exercising below a vigorous

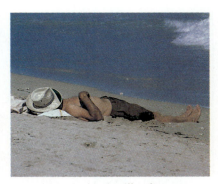

Resting on the beach will reduce stress but will not aid in improving cardiovascular fitness or reducing weight!

GUIDELINES TO YOUR GOOD HEALTH

The following guidelines will help you to plan an exercise program.

1. Evaluate your current physical fitness level. Use Self Inventory 6.1.
2. Define your goals. Make them realistic.
3. Choose your activities. Select activities that you think are fun.
4. Review your resources. Evaluate how much time you have, your equipment needs, and where you plan to exercise.
5. Make a plan. Organize the plan so that you will want to continue.
6. Determine positive and negative reinforcers. *Positive:* Give yourself a reward—do something special or buy a small gift for yourself each time you reach a goal. *Negative:* Take away a pleasure when you don't reach a goal; for example, don't watch your favorite television program, or do fifty sit-ups.
7. Re-evaluate your plan and readjust it as necessary. Each day is a new beginning. Change your plan as often as you need to make it work for you.

SELF-INVENTORY 6.1

How Physically Fit Are You?

Test	Purpose	Procedure
1. Pinch test	Identify body fat 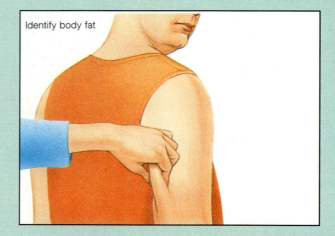	Use the thumb and index finger to pinch a deep fold of skin in the back of the upper arm, the thigh, the back of the upper leg, and the abdomen. Rating: When the fold is greater than one inch, you need to reduce overall body fat. When the fold is less than one inch, you're in great shape.
2. Ruler test	Identify abdominal fat 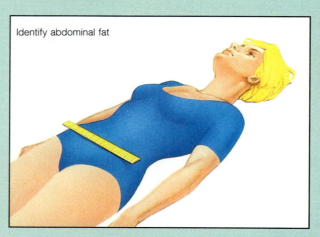	Place a ruler on your abdomen, attempting to touch the pelvic area on both sides. An individual with normal body fat should have no trouble because this area is normally flat or concave. Rating: If the ruler does not touch the pelvic area on both sides, overall body fat should be reduced. If the ruler touches both sides, you're looking good.
3. Twelve minute run test	To determine aerobic endurance 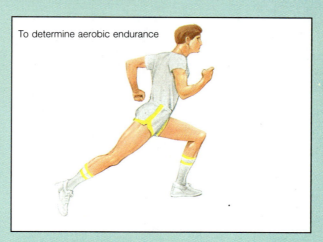	Measure the distance you can run in fractions of a mile in twelve minutes:

Rating	Men (miles)	Women (miles)
Excellent	1.9	1.5
Very good	1.8-1.89	1.4-1.49
Fair	1.6-1.79	1.1-1.39
Poor	1.5-1.59	1.0-1.09
Very poor	1.4-1.49	Below 0.9

Test	Purpose	Procedure
4. Sitting toe touch	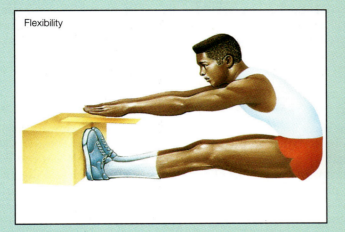 Flexibility	Sit on the floor with your legs fully extended and the bottoms of your feet against a box projecting from the wall. Reach your arms forward as far as you can, attempting to touch your toes or past your toes. Use a ruler that extends nine inches from the edge of the box. Measure the distance that you can reach. **Flexibility scoring** Rating / Men (inches) / Women (inches) Excellent — 17 — 18 Good — 14-16 — 15-17 Average — 10-13 — 10-14 Poor — 7-9 — 7-9 Very poor — 6 or less — 6 or less
5. Pushups	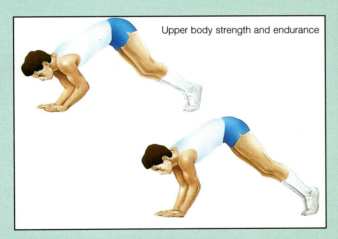 Upper body strength and endurance	With feet 2 - 4 inches apart, knees relaxed, buttocks up above the rest of the body, hands under the ears, push up slowly. <u>Rating:</u> Ten is the minimum number for women to pass. Twenty is the minimum for men. Less than three - you need to begin an upper body strength building program.
6. Curl-downs	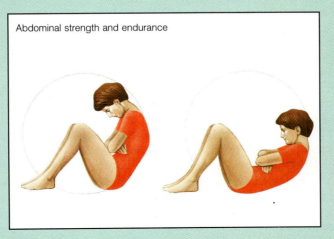 Abdominal strength and endurance	Sit with your knees very bent and your chin tucked in. Uncurl the spine slowly almost down to the floor and then slowly curl up. <u>Rating:</u> 20 is the minimum for women to pass and 30 for men. Fewer curl-downs suggests that your abdominal endurance needs building up.

level would not result in cardiovascular benefits doesn't hold anymore. Those of you who exercise moderately now have research to prove that you are preventing heart disease. Even those of you who exercise at a low activity level live two years longer than your sedentary friends. Regardless of the many research studies with varying results, the level of exercise you choose to meet your personal exercise goals will greatly enhance your life and health in many ways. Dr. Paffenberger puts it this way: "As a whole, the population is likely to benefit more if the least active begin to do a little more than if the most active do even more (exercise)."

■ Developing Your Exercise Program

The most important element of any exercise program is a viable plan. Many of us have started an exercise program only to stop because we found that our goals were set too high or our muscles felt sore. When you start exercising or when you increase one of your fitness goals, you should use the following steps to plan a program that meets your needs: (1) evaluate your current level of physical fitness, (2) define your goals, (3) choose your exercise activities, (4) review your resources, (5) develop a personal contract, and (6) start exercising. Readjust your plan as necessary.

Evaluation of Current Physical Fitness Level

Every commercial on television advertising an exercise program includes a disclaimer stating that each individual should have a medical examination before beginning any exercise regimen. It's always a good idea to check with a doctor before beginning an exercise program, particularly if you have been physically inactive or have health problems. The next step is to complete a self-assessment test of your flexibility, strength, and cardiovascular fitness levels. See Self-Inventory 6.1, "How Physically Fit Are You," for assistance in identifying your strengths and weaknesses.

Did Jim Fixx have a medical examination before he started his exercise program or on a regular basis during his training program? James Fixx was the person most responsible for encouraging Americans to run. He published a best-selling book, *The Complete Book of Running,* made many guest appearances on radio and television, wrote articles and books, and was considered the spokesperson for amateur running in the United States. At the age of fifty-three, Jim Fixx died of a sudden heart attack while running. If running is supposed to be so good for you, why did Jim Fixx, considered the runner's runner, die at such an early age of a heart attack?

We can come to no conclusions, but we do have some facts. Before Fixx reached the age of forty, he had many of the risk factors associated with heart disease. He smoked, was overweight, had extreme stress at work, and his family had a history of heart disease. Another possible contributing factor is that he had complained of tightness in the chest and throat in the weeks preceding his death. These symptoms are suggestive of heart trouble, but Fixx did not see a doctor during this time because he and his family thought that he was healthy and fit. Sports physicians state that Jim Fixx's death does not mean that running or any other form of aerobic exercise will lead to an early death. Considerable research points out that the opposite is more likely. Yet no one can expect to live forever because of superior physical fitness. Every body has its limits, and the wise individual learns to pay attention to the body's signals.

Defining Your Goals

Because exercise is multifaceted and can be organized in many ways, it can meet different objectives. For example, the appropriate selection of types of physical exercise can help the overweight to lose weight or the underweight to gain it. First you must determine what you want to accomplish through your exercise program. The more specific your goals are, the easier it will be to plan an individualized program to meet your goals. Do you want to lose weight or participate competitively in cycling, running, diving, or tennis? Do you want to increase your energy level, improve your appearance, or overcome depression? Are you interested in restructuring your body, having fun, or meeting new people by exercising? Some individuals want to reduce their risk of heart disease by exercising to lower their blood pressure and blood cholesterol or want to improve the strength of their bones.

Goals aimed at maintaining wellness should be your first priority, with those directed at achieving specific fitness and training goals to follow. If you have several goals, rank them in order of importance. Often, more than one goal may be pursued concurrently. Set attainable goals, and don't expect too much too soon. Consistency is the key; you must exercise regularly to achieve your objectives.

Choosing Your Exercise Activities

After you have listed your goals, you can choose the different activities to meet your objectives. There are three components of exercise: cardiovascular fitness, flexibility, and muscular fitness (which includes muscular strength and muscular endurance). Each of these components is important, but a well-balanced fitness-for-life program will include all three aspects. You'll want to stretch for flexibility, build up your cardiovascular system, and develop your strength. The list of exercise activities to achieve your goals should be varied. You can attend a yoga class for your stretching, race walk for cardiovascular fitness, and work out at a gym for your strength-building activities. All of these choices will give you opportunities to socialize and have fun in addition to improving your physical fitness.

> ■ **PROBLEM SITUATION** You really enjoy bicycle riding, but the demands of studying and working part-time leave you little time left over for exercising. How can you incorporate bicycle riding into your daily routine?

Cardiovascular Fitness. The ability of the heart, lungs, and blood vessels to mobilize the body's energy represents **cardiovascular fitness.** Exercise that meets this need involves the use of the large muscle groups in repetitious movements.

Aerobic Exercise. Dr. Kenneth H. Cooper was a pioneer in the field of **aerobic exercise.** He published his book *Aerobics* in 1968 after completing many years of fitness research with the United States Air Force. The term *aerobic* means

FAST FACTS

A varied exercise program of running, swimming, bicycling, etc. will crosstrain all major and minor muscle groups.

SECTION II ■ BODY DYNAMICS

> **FAST FACTS**
>
> Physical fitness teachers should be certified by the American College of Sports Medicine (ACSM).

"with oxygen." As you exercise at a level between approximately 60 to 85 percent target heart rate, you will be able to meet your oxygen needs continually during sustained exercise. There are many activities you can choose to increase your heart rate besides cozying up to your loved one. Activities that involve the large muscle groups in continuous repetitious movements such as jogging, fast walking, jumping rope, roller skating, cross-country skiing, swimming, and bicycling are examples of aerobic exercise.

There are two tests to determine whether you are pacing yourself at an appropriate aerobic level. One simple test is that you should be able to talk out loud comfortably (not huff and puff) while doing any aerobic exercise. The second test is that you are exercising at your target heart rate (see Table 6–2). As you improve your physical condition, you will have to work harder to get to your target heart rate. You need to take your pulse during exercise to determine if the intensity of your workout is too heavy, just right, or too light. A ten-second pulse count multiplied by six is recommended to arrive at your heart rate per minute.

Whichever aerobic exercise you choose, your workout should follow the same time pattern (see Figure 6–2). You should warm up to elevate your body temperature and prepare your body for more vigorous exercise. Jogging in place is ideal. Then you should stretch to loosen your muscles and prevent injuries. Exercise at your target heart rate. Cool down by moving more slowly. If you've been jogging, fast walking and then slower walking will cool you down. Finish by stretching to prevent injury and soreness the day after.

High-Impact Aerobics. Jogging and aerobic dancing are both high-impact aerobic activities. High-impact aerobics involve jumping, hopping, and leaping movements. Each time you do a jumping jack, you jump up in the air and land

FIGURE 6–2 ■ Time Pattern for Ideal Fitness Program Exercise

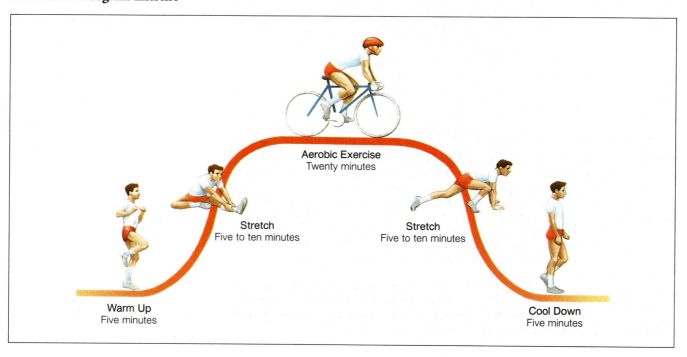

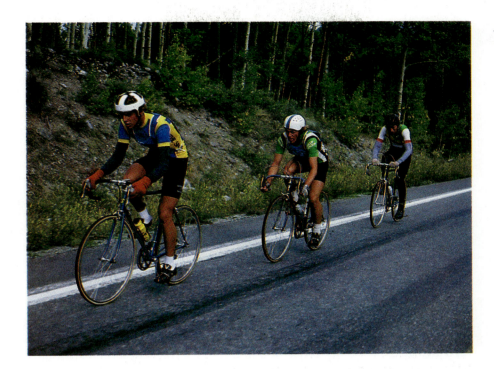

Bicycling with friends is a fun aerobic activity.

with a vertical force considerably exceeding the weight of the body. This may often result in shin splints or joint and feet problems.

As aerobic dancing became the favorite exercise regimen for more than 24 million people, many injuries occurred. A study conducted by the National Injury Prevention Foundation and San Diego State University showed that nearly 45 percent of the students and 75 percent of their instructors were being sidelined with injuries. All of the bouncing, hopping, and jumping movements were creating continued stress on the lower body that was beyond what the musculoskeletal system is designed to absorb.

TABLE 6-2 ■ Determining Your Target Heart Rate

To calculate your target heart rate, do the following:

1. Measure your resting heart rate by finding your radial pulse. Place the first two fingers (pointer and middle fingers) of your right hand on the underside of your left hand near the base of the palm (on the thumb side). Or find your carotid pulse with your right two fingers on the right side of the lower part of your neck just above your collar bone. You will feel pulsations of blood passing under your fingers. Count these pulsations for a full sixty seconds to determine your resting heart rate per minute.
2. Find your maximum heart rate by subtracting your age from 220. This is an estimate of the highest beat per minute possible during intense exercise for your age. Don't exercise at this pace.
3. Locate your target heart rate. Choose your target from 60 to 85 percent, according to your fitness goals. Subtract your resting heart rate from your maximum heart rate. Multiply this figure by 60 through 85 percent. Add that figure to your resting heart rate. Figure 6-3 illustrates how to take your radial and carotid pulses.

FIGURE 6-3 ■ Taking Your Radial or Carotid Pulse

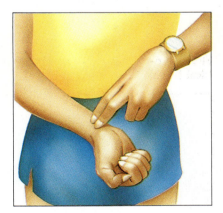

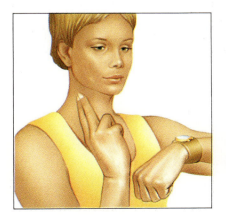

GUIDELINES TO YOUR GOOD HEALTH

Selection of the proper exercise shoe will help minimize muscle and joint injuries. Match the shoe structure with your foot structure and your specific footwear needs using the following guidelines:

1. Purchase the shoe late in the day to allow for true measurement of your foot's width. Feet tend to swell as the day goes on.
2. Bring your running socks with you to better evaluate shoes.
3. Make sure that there is a thumbs width between the big toe and the end of the shoe on each foot. Be sure to measure this standing up.
4. Examine your shoes by placing them on a level surface. Observe from the front and back. Alignment of the heel should be perpendicular to the sole, and the soles should be level with the surface.

Long-distance runners are also vulnerable. Up to 20 percent of joggers each year have to stop running because of running-related injuries. The main problems involve the knees, legs, hips, and feet. Two factors are responsible for most of their injuries: (1) failure to progress slowly, and (2) not giving the musculoskeletal system enough time to adapt to intensity. Dr. Kenneth Cooper states that if you're running more than twenty miles per week, you're running for reasons other than cardiovascular health.

Low-Impact Aerobics. With the evolution of modern fitness programs has come the knowledge that less is more. By reducing exercise intensity, greater gains in fitness can be achieved. An increasing number of physical-fitness instructors are teaching the "be-kind-to-your-body" low-impact aerobics. This means that you keep one foot on the floor at all times, substituting side steps for jumping jacks, marching for jogging, and gliding for leaping, which lessens stress on joints, shins, feet, and lower back. Accentuating the use of the upper body by motions such as bicep curls and arm presses increases the heart rate enough to receive cardiovascular benefits. One problem with this is that many low-impact exercisers overwork the shoulders; this can lead to tendonitis. Another problem with low-impact exercise is that during the lateral movements on carpet, exercisers sometimes sustain ankle injuries. It is safer to do low-impact exercise on wood floors, as long as the wood floor is not layered on concrete.

High-Impact versus Low-Impact Aerobic Exercise. A common misconception is that the greater the exercise intensity, the more fat that is burned. In reality, fat can only be burned when oxygen is being used—that is, during aerobic exercise. When the body is working at high intensities (anaerobically, at a heart rate above 85 percent), it naturally uses its most efficiently burning fuel—carbohydrate. When working at lower intensities (aerobically), the body can afford to fall back on its less efficiently burned calorie source—fat. For the first thirty minutes of aerobic exercise, stored glycogen is used almost exclusively. Then free fatty acids begin to be used more and more, resulting in more direct use of fat in exercise at over 30 percent of heart rate. As many of us exercise to lose weight, we can exercise at least five times per week at a lower intensity and longer duration that will use fat stores as the primary fuel source—more weight loss for less effort.

Many people believe that exercising at high intensities burns significantly more calories. This is not true. Katch and McCardle, in their book *Nutrition, Weight Control, and Exercise,* say that a 150-pound person expends about 110 calories while jogging a mile in 12 minutes. If the same person runs one mile at a faster pace of 5½ minutes per mile (over twice as fast), only about 130 calories are expended. Exercise twice as hard and only 20 additional calories are burned. Is all that extra work worth the small benefit? Longer duration of exercise is the critical factor for burning more calories, and longer duration is achieved by adding more exercise time.

Another motive for engaging in low-impact exercise is that there are many injuries sustained with high-intensity exercise such as jogging or aerobic dancing. These activities result in injuries because in the moment between strides, both feet are off the ground at the same time. For example, the jogger achieves a moderate amount of elevation, and while the arms are moving, the primary action occurs in the legs. Each time the foot hits the ground, the vertical force considerably exceeds the weight of the body, resulting in injuries to the hip joints, knees, and shins. As you lower the impact, the injury rate is also lowered.

There are many benefits to both high-impact and low-impact aerobic exercising. It is recommended that you alternate between high- and low-impact workouts and plan *cross-training* workouts, which involve a combination of flexibility, strength-training, and aerobic activities, including both low- and high-impact exercising. Some video exercise programs are reviewed in Table 6–3.

> ■ **PROBLEM SITUATION**   You are overweight and would like to lose about thirty pounds. How can you use exercise to help you achieve your goal? What type of exercise will you use?

TABLE 6–3 ■ Comparison of Video Exercise Programs

Aerobics

Jane Fonda's Low-Impact Aerobic Workout

This video is an excellent beginning workout. It has six minutes of warm-up, thirty-five minutes of low-impact aerobics, and ten minutes of a cool-down. If you want a low-key workout or you haven't exercised before, this is the tape for you. This video was designed with Dr. James G. Garrick, director of the Center for Sports Medicine, Saint Francis Memorial Hospital, San Francisco.

Martina Navratilova Fitness and Conditioning Workout Program

This is a program for those who want to challenge themselves. Martina demonstrates the program she has used to become one of the best tennis athletes in the world. She's strong and very agile, and her aerobics routine is rough. An excellent video for those who are ready to match their strength and stamina to Martina's.

TABLE 6–3 ■ **Comparison of Video Exercise Programs, continued**

Running

Running Great with Grete Waitz

Grete is one of the fastest female runners in the world; she won a silver medal in the 1984 Olympics. This is a tape to watch, as Grete demonstrates and instructs her viewers on her four-point training program. Grete says that if you are currently running twelve miles a week, you can increase to twenty-five to thirty miles a week in just two months. This progression is good for advanced runners; beginners should use this video to integrate Grete's tips into their personal training program.

Biking

Cyclevision Tours

As you pedal away on your stationary bicycle, you watch these videos, which take you on a tour of the Grand Tetons, through Vermont, to San Francisco, or, if you wish a challenge, to join a "race." The program includes a warm-up, a workout at your training rate, and a cool-down.

Rowing

Rowing Machine Companion

This video is a lot of fun. The thrill begins after the warm-up and instructions on how to use a stationary rowing machine. The race starts in a racing shell in the water, continues with the sound of the oars cutting the water, and finishes with the end of the race. In the second phase, Seth Baller, a bronze medalist, leads the training for the Olympic event.

Swimming

Swimming for Fitness

Don't even consider using this video near a pool, as you could electrocute yourself. The program doesn't pretend to teach you how to swim, but it does give you a detailed training program for beginning, intermediate, and advanced swimming workouts. Donna de Varona, an Olympic gold medalist, provides drills and techniques and a stretching segment for before and after swimming. This is also an instructional video; it is well done, and every swimmer will pick up some pointers.

Anaerobic Exercise. During **anaerobic exercise,** the body's demand for oxygen exceeds the supply, producing "oxygen debt"; this occurs during high-intensity, short-term exercise. Sprinting a short distance or running up three flights of stairs as fast as possible are examples of anaerobic exercise. The runner goes so fast that he or she can replace only part of the oxygen the body uses during the sprint itself and has to make up for the oxygen debt afterward by labored breathing. When you are exercising at an intensity above 85 percent target heart rate, anaerobic exercise is taking place. Sports such as racquetball, handball, squash, football, track, and baseball require all-out efforts in the form of sprints for several seconds. To be able to make these repetitive but intense efforts, you must improve your anaerobic conditioning level by practicing short sprints, which form the foundation of an anaerobic training program.

Muscular Fitness. In the past decade, more and more Americans have been exercising and shaping up—from the waist down. The most popular exercises that we participate in are bicycling, jogging, and aerobic dancing. All of these activities primarily use our legs. Our upper-body muscles are underdeveloped, flabby, and weak. Although aerobic workouts condition your heart and lungs, they don't exercise many of the muscles that shape your body and provide strength when you need it to lift a heavy box or hold a child in your arms.

Muscular fitness can be increased by working on muscular strength and muscular endurance. These two abilities are closely related, and the terms are often used interchangeably to refer to skeletal-muscle function. Both functions are important in exercise. **Muscular endurance** is the capacity of the same muscle or a group of muscles to sustain a series of repetitive contractions. Chin-ups and sit-ups are examples of muscular endurance. **Muscular strength** refers to the amount of force (weight) that a muscle or a group of muscles can exert for one repetition. Lifting or moving a desk essentially depends on muscular strength. Your muscular fitness programs should involve both muscular strength and endurance.

To gain muscular fitness, you can begin with calisthenics. This will involve doing sit-ups, leg lifts, and push-ups, among others. It is important for you to do calisthenics safely. For example, do not do complete sit-ups fast or straight-legged or with your feet hooked under something or with your arms behind your head. Another way to develop muscular fitness is through weight training. You must choose one of three methods: isokinetic, isotonic, or isometric programs.

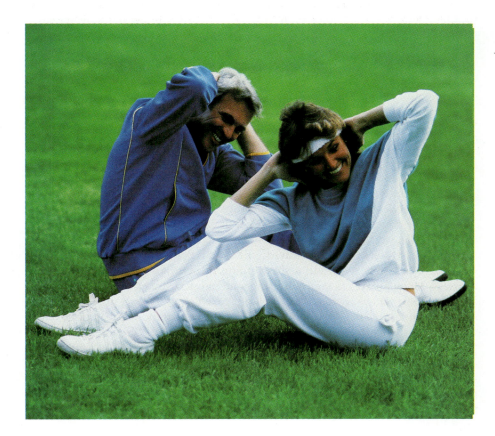

Calisthenics will aid in warming up before exercise, as well as in improving muscle tone.

Isokinetic Programs. Weight training programs that are **isokinetic** enable muscles to contract against the same level of resistance (on Nautilus or Cybex or some other specialized equipment) throughout a full range of motion. Many experts believe that isokinetic programs are the best for developing both muscular strength and endurance. One of the disadvantages of an isokinetic program is that it requires specialized equipment, such as Nautilus and Cybex, which is expensive. This equipment can be found not only in spas and health clubs but also on college campuses in the physical education department.

Isotonic Programs. Exercise that is **isotonic** involves lifting a constant weight through a full range of motion. Isotonics entail the use of free weights (such as barbells and dumbbells) or machines, and they can help you to develop both muscular strength and endurance. You should use free weights which have equal weight for right and left sides. This will allow for equal distribution in both arms and legs.

Isometric Programs. Weight training that is **isometric** involves the individual pushing or pulling against a fixed resistance or an immovable object. This requires a steady muscle contraction against an immovable resistance object, like a wall or a door jamb. The range of motion is restricted, which results in the muscle becoming strong at a particular angle only.

Flexibility. The ability to use the joints fully, to move them easily through the range of motion available, is called **flexibility**. A person may be flexible in some joints and not in others. It depends on many factors: your age, your sex, posture, whether you have bone spurs, and how fat or muscular you are. Women tend to be more flexible than men because of differences in their muscle mass, skeletons, and body composition. Prevention of low back pain and injury are the main contributions of practicing flexibility movements.

Flexibility can be improved through exercises that promote the elasticity of the soft tissues of the joints. There are two major types of flexibility stretches—static (or passive) and ballistic (or dynamic). Bob Anderson, the author of *Stretching*, states that static stretching is the safest way to stretch. **Static stretching** is a relaxed, gradual stretch that you hold for fifteen to thirty seconds. Static stretching is less likely to cause injuries, produces no muscle soreness, and consumes less energy. **Ballistic stretching** is characterized by rapid bouncing or jerking movements, such as a series of up-and-down-bobs as you reach again and again to touch your toes with your hands. These bounces can stretch muscle fibers too far, and the muscle reacts by contracting rather than stretching.

For safe stretching, follow these guidelines. Before you begin stretching, increase your body temperature by running in place for a few minutes. Cold muscles are vulnerable to injury. Raising your temperature increases the pliability of connective tissue (such as tendons, joint capsules, and skin), provides greater potential for increased flexibility, and lessens the likelihood of injury. When you stretch, reach to the point of discomfort, then back off slightly, relaxing and allowing the muscle to adjust for fifteen to thirty seconds. You should hold the stretch until the tension diminishes. Continue breathing rhythmically throughout your stretch routines. Practice stretching on a regular basis; the more you stretch, the more flexible you will become. The "use it or lose it" motto applies to stretching; when you don't stretch, you lose your flexibility and become prone to injury.

> ■ *PROBLEM SITUATION* You have a friend who is in a wheelchair. Suggest an exercise program for your friend that will improve her physical fitness.

Injury Prevention. One of the best ways to prevent injuries is to maintain good muscle tone and flexibility in the legs, abdomen, and back. Injuries can occur from overuse. These are usually caused by pushing the body too hard, too fast, and often without proper training or equipment. The most common overuse injuries are tendinitis and stress fractures. Common acute injuries include fractures, sprains, strains, and tendon tears. To protect knees, it's important to improve support by strengthening the quadriceps muscles and keeping hamstrings stretched. To keep feet flexible, stretch your Achilles tendons. Some exercises should be avoided (see Figure 6–4).

Any time you exercise, you should start out by increasing your body temperature for at least one minute and then do five to ten minutes of warm-up stretches. This will help you to avoid cramps, sprains, and other injuries. Exercise should always begin at a slow pace—don't do too much too soon. To allow your muscles to recover from exercise, you should exercise hard on one day and less strenuously the next. Remember to take days off for rest and relaxation. If you do injure yourself and can't get to a doctor immediately, you should apply first aid. See Appendix A for further discussion of first aid. Many of us are so impatient to start exercising that we conveniently forget to stretch. Of the three components of physical fitness, stretching is the least popular and the most important for injury prevention.

Sports. Competitive sports are a wonderful way to meet your fitness goals. You can join teams to play volleyball, tennis, football, and many other sports. Performance-related components of physical fitness will be met by your participation in sports. They are also an excellent method of maintaining and improving physical fitness. Most sports will not improve your conditioning level, as many of these activities are not aerobic in nature. You will need to supplement your sports involvement with aerobics and strength-building activities.

Reviewing Your Resources

Now that you've evaluated your current physical fitness level, defined your goals, and chosen your exercise activities, it is time to review your resources. One aspect of your plan is to improve your strength. How much money, time, and equipment do you need to reach your goal? Can you afford the fees at a gym, can you buy the equipment for home, or should you plan to take a weight-training course on campus? If you plan to join a gym, is it on your way home or to work or school? If it's not convenient, you won't continue working out. Statistics show that most people stop attending a gym approximately three months after they join, even after they've paid their fees for a year. Carefully review your resources before you complete your physical fitness contract.

Designing Your Plan

Completing a physical fitness contract provides a good motivation to exercise on a regular basis. It will help you achieve your physical fitness goals. Complete the physical fitness contract in Table 6–4.

FAST FACTS

Drink five to eight ounces of fluid (any beverage with less than 10 percent sugar) every fifteen minutes before, during, and after exercise.

168   SECTION II ■ BODY DYNAMICS

FIGURE 6-4 ■ **Stretching for Exercise**

Safe stretches	Correct	Incorrect	Unsafe stretches
Raised leg crunches	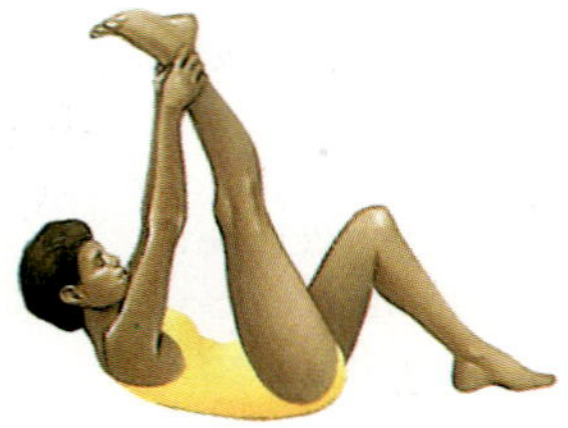	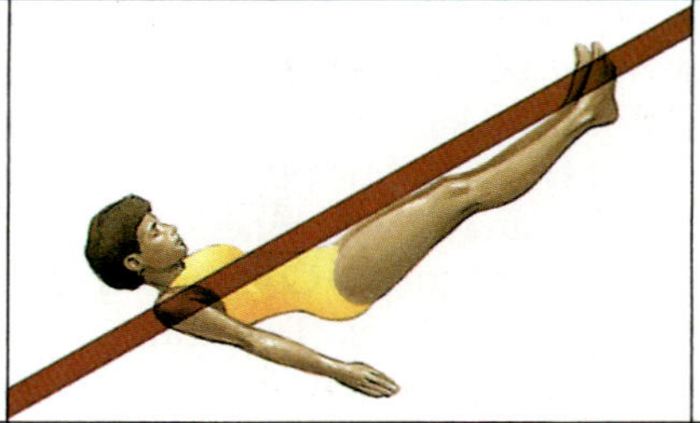	Double leg lifts
Side neck stretches	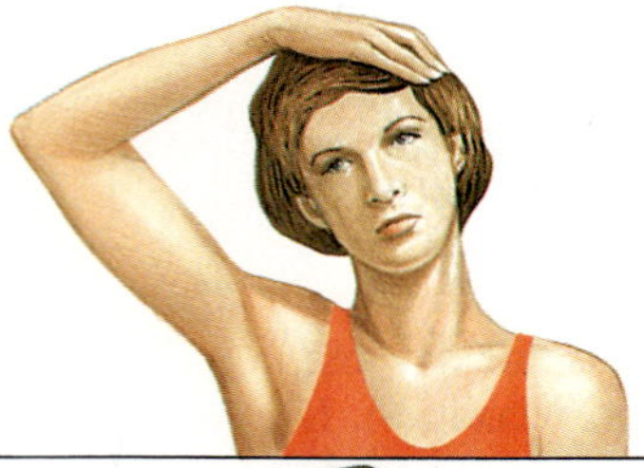	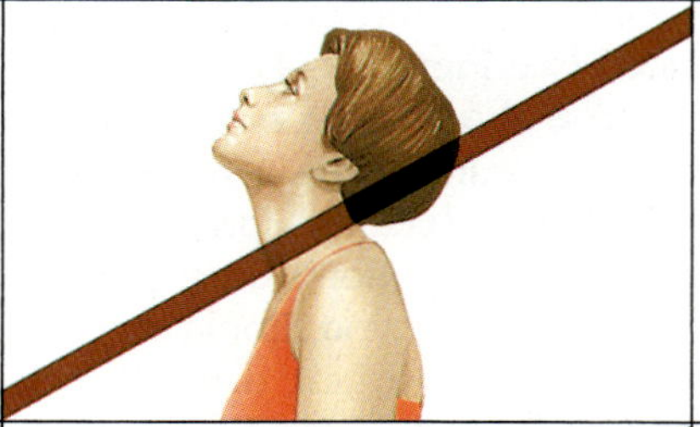	360 head rolls
Partial squats	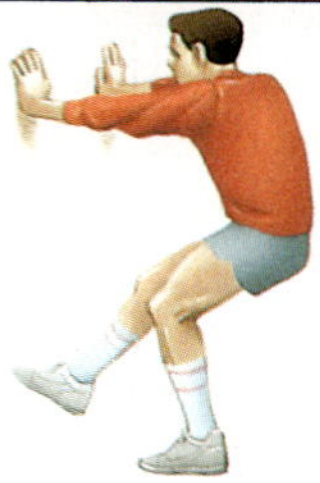	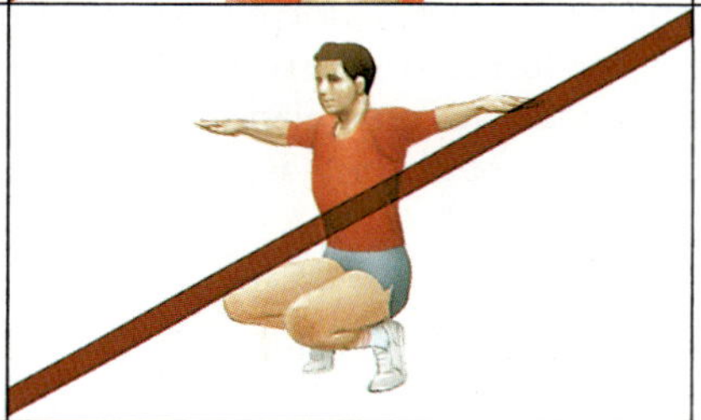	Full squats
Knee rolls	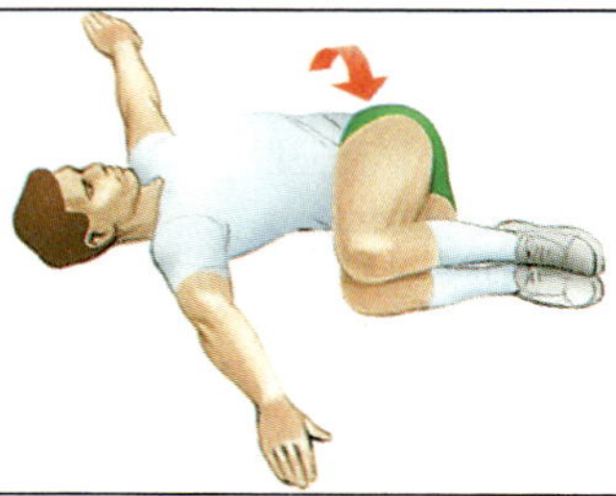	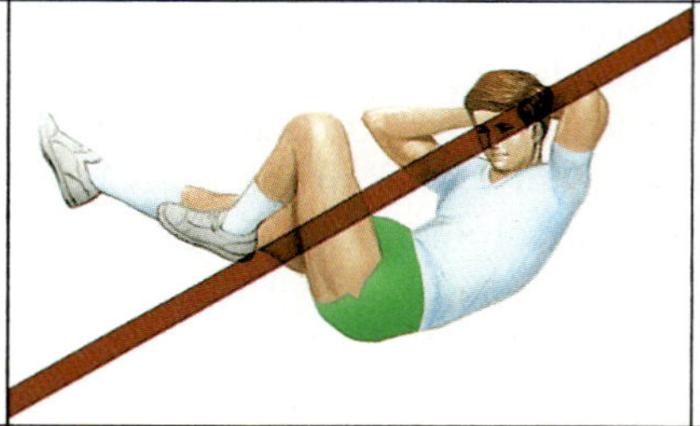	Alternating bent-leg sit-ups
Fold-up stretch	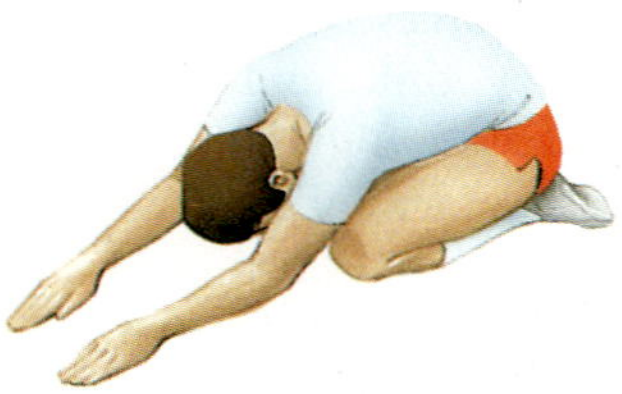	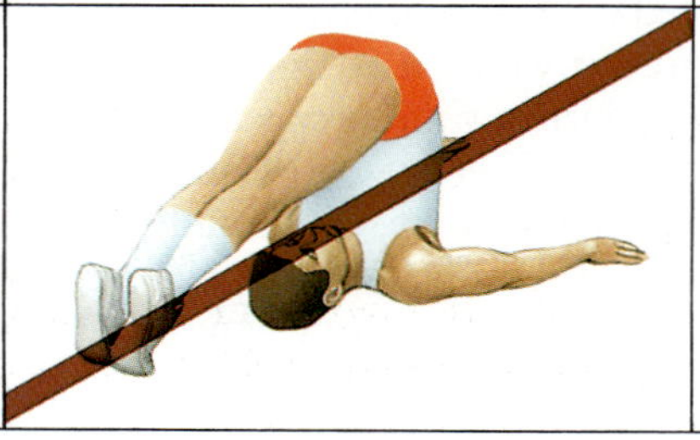	Yoga plow

TABLE 6–4 ■ Physical Fitness Contract

I, _____ agree to the following:

a. I will stretch _____ times a week to increase my flexibility.
   I will stretch before and after my strength-building or aerobic activity. I will stretch using these activities: _____

b. I will spend _____ minutes at least three times a week doing strength-building activities.
   I will increase my muscular strength by these activities: _____
   I will increase my muscular endurance by these activities: _____

c. I will spend _____ minutes at least three times a week doing aerobic activities.
   I will improve my cardiovascular fitness by doing these activities: _____

I plan to complete my physical fitness program at _____
_____ (name the place) at
_____ (name the time).
I plan to discuss my progress at least biweekly with: _____

   I plan to change the following attitudes and beliefs I now hold to the positive belief of: _____
   I plan to reward myself with one of the following pleasures when I achieve my daily goals in increased activity:
   1.
   2.
   3.
When I do not meet my daily exercise goals, I will agree to do the following:
   1.
   2.
   3.
I agree to the preceding conditions and I will follow this contract until I meet my physical fitness goals. I will then make new goals with a new contract.

Signed _____ Date _____ Witness _____

FAST FACTS

As little as twelve minutes of stationary bicycling three times a week can produce a significant improvement in maximum oxygen consumption.

■ Athletic Training

Concepts of Training

Whether you are planning a fitness program or an athletic training program, certain concepts need to be taken into account. One of these elements is *specificity*, which is choosing a particular aspect of fitness to be specific to your goal. If your primary goal in your physical fitness program is to increase your cardiovascular endurance, you will choose an aerobic activity such as swimming or jogging. But if you want to improve your muscular strength, you will develop a weight training program.

Fitness experts also suggest that you use the concept of *overload*, subjecting muscles to a greater-than-normal load to increase their size and strength. You

> **FAST FACTS**
>
> Fasting and fluid restriction when reducing body weight can cause kidney malfunction and reduction in muscle strength.

can systematically overload until you reach your goal. Once you reach your goal, you will need an additional increase in the load or weight used in order to reach the next goal. *Progressive resistance* refers to gradually increasing the resistance, adding extra weight to maintain overload. Many athletes training for tennis, swimming, and other competitive sports will use specificity, overload, and progressive resistance in their training programs.

Progression is planning the frequency, duration, and intensity of your fitness program, in this order. You must gradually work up to your fitness goals. If you are capable of running for only fifteen minutes twice a week, you will find it difficult to run at 85 percent intensity. Frequency, duration, and intensity must be planned as a whole to reduce injuries and maximize fitness.

Carbohydrate Loading

There is one dietary practice that will be of value in building endurance. *Carbohydrate loading* can lengthen the time the athlete can exercise before "running out of steam." It involves packing the muscles with extra glycogen by eating large amounts of carbohydrate for several days before an event. The athlete will eat approximately 70 percent of total calories from complex carbohydrates, consisting of whole grain breads and cereals, fresh fruits, and vegetables. This will be helpful only in events in which the individual will be competing or exercising continuously for ninety minutes or more or engaging in multiple competitions.

Carbohydrate loading should be done only by healthy adults no more than three or four times a year. Carbohydrate loading has relevance only to endurance trainers exercising for more than two hours; it will not assist in strength-building or help you move faster if you exercise for less than two hours at a time.

Steroids

Despite many dangerous side effects, anabolic steroids are primarily used by athletes who want to gain additional muscle mass as an extra edge on their competition. Anabolic steroids can promote body-tissue building processes and slow down the breakdown of tissue. Like the natural hormone testosterone, anabolic steroids aid in the storage of nitrogen, resulting in the syntheses of protein, which enhances muscle size, stamina, and tissue repair. The use of steroids is against the rules in competition sports; this has led to many athletes being disqualified in international sports events. New ultrasensitive drug detectors can detect even one-billionth of a gram of an illegal drug.

Both amateur and professional athletes use steroids in the belief that the drugs will increase their athletic prowess and success. According to the latest research, only half of the studies have found strength improvements from the steroids commonly used (androgenic anabolic steroids, human growth hormone, and human chorionic gonadotropin). The other half found improvements to be attributable to the placebo effect.

> ■ **PROBLEM SITUATION** Your roommate comes home one day with a bottle of steroids given to him by his friend. He intends to take them to improve his athletic ability. What advice should you give him and why?

Athletes frequently take dangerously large doses of steroids, which can lead to many serious side effects. Because the drugs raise the level of testosterone in the blood, steroids can cause the pituitary gland to stop stimulating the natural production of testosterone in the testicles, resulting in atrophy of the testicles as well as a diminished sperm count. Other side effects include impotence, bladder irritability, a deepening of the voice, permanent hair loss, and liver damage. Adolescents who use steroids can end up with shorter stature, which is the reverse of what the drugs are being taken for. Clearly, the negative aspects of steroids far outweigh the potential gains.

POSITIVE BEHAVIORS

I. *Place a check mark in front of each behavior that you now practice.*

_____ 1. I stretch three times a week. (STRETCH)
_____ 2. I warm-up and cool-down each time I exercise. (WARM, COOL)
_____ 3. I participate in aerobic exercise three times a week. (AEROBIC)
_____ 4. When I stretch, I do static stretches. (STATIC)
_____ 5. I do not take steroids or other drugs to increase my athletic powers. (STEROIDS)
_____ 6. I do weight training three times a week. (WEIGHT)
_____ 7. When I do aerobic exercise, I workout at 70 percent of my target heart rate. (70 PERCENT)
_____ 8. Each time I do aerobic exercise, I work out for at least twenty minutes. (TWENTY MINUTES)

II. *For each behavior that you DO NOT ENGAGE IN, write the KEY WORD(S) located in the parentheses at the end of the statement in the column below. Then put a check mark in the appropriate column to indicate whether you intend to keep or change that behavior.*

Behaviors I Don't Engage In   KEEP/CHANGE

_____   _____/_____
_____   _____/_____
_____   _____/_____
_____   _____/_____
_____   _____/_____
_____   _____/_____
_____   _____/_____
_____   _____/_____

III. *For each of the preceding behaviors that you choose to KEEP, write a statement indicating why you are choosing to keep that behavior.*

I choose to keep behavior _____ because:
                              KEY WORD

For each of the preceding behaviors that you choose to CHANGE, write a statement indicating how you plan to implement that change.

I will change behavior _____ by:
                          KEY WORD

Now You Know

1. FALSE. Each year Americans exercise more. Currently, 60 percent of the population exercises regularly.

2. TRUE. Cardiovascular fitness is a health-related fitness component that strengthens the heart and the lungs by boosting the body's ability to use oxygen.

3. FALSE. Flexibility is the improvement and maintenance of the functional capacity of specific muscles and joints by increasing their full range of motion through static stretching techniques.

4. TRUE. Regular aerobic exercise will not only reduce one's risk of heart disease but can also prevent heart disease and cancer.

5. TRUE. Improved collateral circulation through exercising can increase your longevity. It increases the body's ability to deliver oxygen to muscles.

6. TRUE. The principles of a fitness program are frequency, intensity, and duration.

7. FALSE. "Going for the burn" when exercising can cause injuries.

8. TRUE. *Aerobic* means "with oxygen." Your body will be able to meet its oxygen needs during sustained exercise.

9. FALSE. Isokinetic weight training programs enable muscles to contract against the same level of resistance throughout a full range of motion.

10. FALSE. Ballistic stretching is characterized by rapid bouncing and jerking movements, which result in injuries; static stretching is a relaxed, gradual stretch that is excellent for improving flexibility.

11. TRUE. Steroid use can result in atrophy of testicles, diminished sperm count, bladder irritability, hair loss, liver damage, and shortness of stature.

12. TRUE. We should warm up before we stretch to prevent injuries.

Summary

1. According to the *Random House College Dictionary*, fitness is defined as being "in good physical condition or health." A major outcome of physical activity is fitness.

2. There are three health-related components of physical fitness: cardiovascular fitness, muscular fitness, and flexibility. The performance-related goals include agility, balance, coordination, power, reaction time, and speed.

3. There are many research studies providing evidence that regular vigorous exercise is associated with a reduction of heart disease, the leading cause of mortality in the United States. In the past two decades, there has been a 28 percent decline in heart-disease deaths, partly because Americans are exercising.

4. Regular aerobic exercise reduces risk factors associated with heart disease and cancer. Exercise reduces tension, high blood pressure, cholesterol, fat, brings about weight reduction, and improves cardiovascular function and HDL/LDL ratios.

5. Aerobic exercise decreases depression, mental tension, and anxiety and improves self-esteem and one's zest for life.

6. The three principles of a fitness program involve frequency, duration, and intensity.

7. You can exercise at low, moderate, or high activity levels to receive health benefits. Low activity levels will increase your longevity by two years, moderate activity levels will prevent heart disease, and high activity levels will significantly reduce heart disease.

8. To develop your exercise plan, you should evaluate your current level of physical fitness, define your goals, choose your exercise activities, review your resources, develop a personal contract, and then start exercising, re-evaluating your plan as necessary.

9. The term *aerobic* means "with oxygen." During aerobic exercise, your body is able to meet its oxygen needs continually during a sustained period. Anaerobic exercise produces "oxygen debt." Your body's demand for oxygen will exceed the supply.

10. High-impact aerobic activities like aerobic dancing and jogging make the exerciser vulnerable to more injuries. Low-impact aerobics, in which you keep one foot on the ground at all times, lower your risk of injuries.

11. Muscular fitness is made up of muscular endurance and muscular strength. You can achieve your muscular fitness goals with isokinetic, isometric, or isotonic weight training programs.

12. Flexibility is important in the prevention of injuries. You should stretch before and after every exercise session.

13. Fifty percent of research studies concerning anabolic steroids indicate strength improvements from the drug, but the other 50 percent attribute the results to the placebo effect. Steroid use results in many serious side effects.

14. One of the best methods to prevent injuries is to maintain good muscle tone and flexibility in legs, abdomen, and back.

References

1. American College of Sports Medicine. *Guidelines for Graded Exercise Testing and Exercise Prescription*. Philadelphia: Lea and Febiger, 1980.
2. Alter, Judy. *Surviving Exercise: Judy Alter's Safe and Sane Exercise Program*. Boston: Houghton Mifflin, 1983.
3. Anderson, Bob. *Stretching*. Shelter Publications, 1980.
4. Ardell, Donald B., and Mark J. Tager. *Planning for Wellness: A Guidebook for Achieving Optimal Health*. Wellness Media, 1981.
5. Bailey, Covert. *Fit or Fat: A New Way to Health and Fitness through Nutrition and Aerobic Exercise*. Boston: Houghton Mifflin, 1979.
6. Physical Education Handbook Committee. *Handbook for Physical Education: Framework for Developing a Curriculum for California Public Schools*. Sacramento: California State Department of Education, 1986.
7. Hales, Dianne, and Robert Hales. "Using the Body to Mend the Mind." *American Health* Vol. 4, No. 5 (June 1985), 26–31.
8. Fox, Edward L. *Lifetime Fitness*. Saunders College Publishing, 1983.
9. Greenberg, Jerrod S., and David Pargman. *Physical Fitness: A Wellness Approach*. Prentice-Hall, 1986.
10. Kastrup, Erwin K., ed. *Drug Facts and Comparisons*. J. B. Lippincott Co., 1985, 278–280.
11. Reid, J. Gavin, and John M. Thomson. *Exercise Prescription for Fitness*. Prentice-Hall, 1985.
12. Rosato, Frank D. *Fitness and Wellness*. St. Paul: West Publishing Co., 1986.

This chapter written by Christina S. Kinney, Lecturer, California State University Dominguez Hills, Carson, California

Suggested Readings

Allsen, Philip C. *Fitness for Life*. William C. Brown, 1984.
Alter, Judy. *Surviving Exercise: Judy Alter's Safe and Sane Exercise Program*. Boston: Houghton Mifflin, 1983.
Anderson, Bob. *Stretching*. Random House, 1980.
Bailey, Covert. *Fit or Fat: A New Way to Health and Fitness through Nutrition and Aerobic Exercise*. Boston: Houghton Mifflin, 1978.
Cooper, Kenneth. *The Aerobics Program for Total Well-Being*. Leisure Press, 1985.
Dintiman, George B., and Robert Ward. *Train American: Achieving Peak Performance and Fitness for Sports Competition*. Hunt Publishing Co., 1988.
U.S. Department of Health and Human Services. *Healthy People: The Surgeon General's Report on Health Promotion*. Pub. No. 79-55-071. Washington, D.C.: Government Printing Office, 1979.

SECTION III

Understanding Your Sexuality

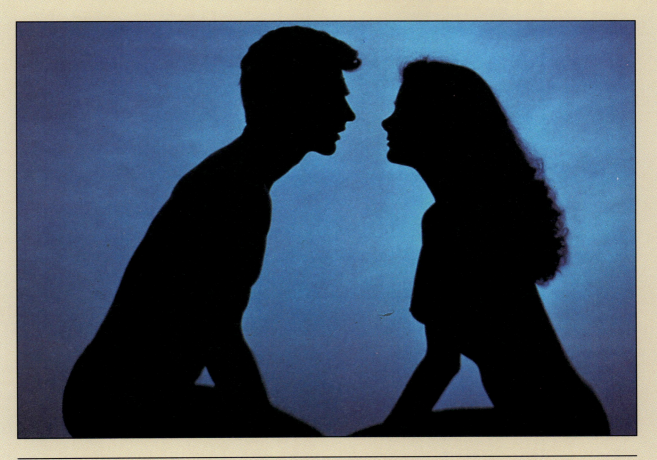

Chapter 7: Relationships
Foundations for a Healthy Relationship
Healthy versus Unhealthy Love in Adult Relationships
Exploitive Behaviors
Love and Physical Intimacy
The Romantic Love Cycle
Communication Skills
Effective Communication in a Relationship
When Love Blooms: Getting Married
When Love Fades: Getting Divorced
Picking Up the Pieces

Chapter 8: Sexual Bodyworks
Sexual Anatomy and Physiology: Male
Sexual Anatomy and Physiology: Female
Hormones and Sexual Functioning
The Major Sex Hormones
Sexual Preferences and Behaviors
The Sexual Response Cycle
The Menstrual Cycle
Menstrual Myths
Toxic Shock Syndrome
Premenstrual Syndrome

Chapter 9: Family Planning
Responsible Sexual Behavior
Birth Control versus Contraception
Birth-Control Options
Abortive Procedures
Future Trends

Chapter 10: Conception Through Birth
The Sexual Beginning
Sperm Production
Egg Production
The Process of Fertilization and Implantation
Gender Differentiation: Prenatal Variables
Determining Your Child's Sex
The Question of Parenthood
Pregnancy
Fetal Development
Childbirth
Gender Differentiation: Postnatal Variables

CHAPTER 7

Relationships

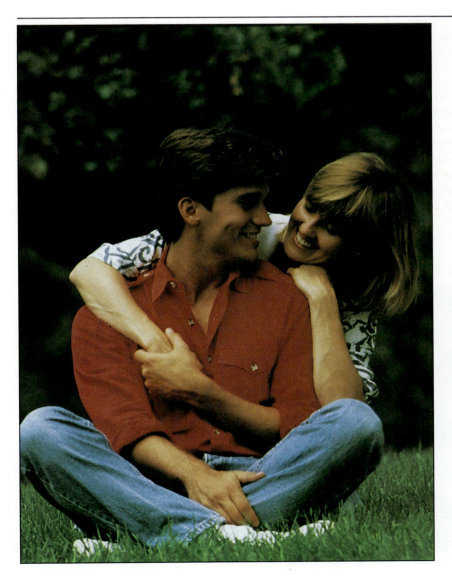

What Do You Know?

Are the following statements true or false?

1. A relationship is a positive bond between two or more people.
2. In a healthy relationship, each person maintains a sense of autonomy.
3. The difference between healthy and unhealthy love is the substance behind the love.
4. Abnormal sexual behavior seeks to give and receive pleasure.
5. Erotic love differs from other types of love in that it includes the element of sexual desire.
6. A person in a state of love readiness usually falls in love quickly.
7. About 50 percent of love relationships end by mutual consent.
8. When a relationship ends, grief is a normal reaction.
9. Staying in a relationship that should be over only prolongs the pain and guilt.
10. The best way to get over an ended relationship is to postpone or deny the pain.

A **relationship** is a bond between two or more people that exists to satisfy their needs. A relationship can exist only as long as the needs of all parties involved are met. Needs can be physical, mental, emotional, social, and economic. A person's needs can change as a result of either internal or external factors.

A relationship can be positive or negative. No relationship is perfect; problems and conflicts arise in all relationships. The way in which a person perceives and handles these difficulties is what often determines if the relationship will be positive and rewarding or negative and damaging. A person's personality and background affect the role that he or she plays in a relationship. Although there are many types of relationships (such as parent/child, sibling, peer group, and business), this chapter will focus on love relationships between consenting adults.

Foundations for a Healthy Relationship

To have a healthy and meaningful relationship, there has to be a certain initial chemistry. This involves physical attraction as well as a sense of well-being and ease. Just as one cannot put a square peg into a round hole, two people must be compatible for a relationship to work. Each person must accept the other unconditionally. When one person tries to change the other, or when one feels the need to change in order to please or accommodate the other, the relationship is no longer healthy. A person not only needs to accept his or her own strengths and weaknesses but also the strengths and weaknesses of the other person. If an individual is forced to change or compromise a part of himself or herself to please another person, it will eventually lead to anger and resentment.

In the beginning of a new relationship, the people involved are usually quite anxious to make a good impression. Have you ever done something that you disliked doing or that compromised your standards just so another person would like or accept you? Did it work? After it was over, were you still able to like and accept yourself? Maybe what you did wasn't very important, so you're saying, "Sure, I still liked myself." Or maybe it wasn't worth the stress or guilt

FAST FACTS

Physical appearance is the major factor in dating choices among college students.

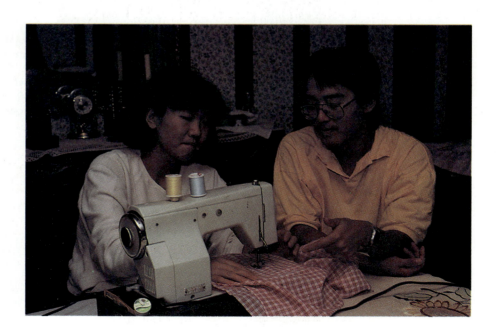

Taking an interest in activities your partner enjoys contributes to the development of a healthy relationship.

that you experienced afterwards, so you're saying, "Never again!" The point is the you have to be YOU. Relationships will come and go in your life, but YOU are a constant. YOU must face the consequences of your actions. If you are constantly doing what another person wants or being what another person expects, there is no YOU. The relationship may be real enough, but YOU are not. A relationship based on fantasy is doomed to fail. Is that the kind of relationship you want to be involved in?

> ■ *PROBLEM SITUATION* You are invited out by someone whom you really like. Both of you have a great time. The next day, however, you find out that the person asked you out only to make someone else jealous. Were you "being used"? Do you regret having gone out with that person?

How can you create and maintain a healthy relationship? The first step is to look no farther than yourself. Again, it begins with YOU. It is important for you to have a positive self-concept. Ask yourself, "Would I want to be in a relationship with a person like me?" The answer may surprise you. If you like who and what you are and think positive thoughts about yourself, others will respond to you in a similar manner.

An essential part of any good relationship is being considerate of the other person's needs and feelings. This is all well and good; however, you must not forget that you have needs and feelings, too. If you always consider the other person's needs first, you may not be meeting your own needs. Eventually you may feel cheated. Of course, you shouldn't be oblivious to or ignore your partner's feelings, because he or she may feel hurt or rejected. Either extreme will lead to conflict in the relationship. The solution is to try to strike a balance between meeting your own needs and those of the other person. Being a martyr does not strengthen a relationship. Unfortunately, the more you sacrifice, the more that is expected of you. It's great when both partners occasionally make sacrifices for each other. Yet if one person is always doing the sacrificing, it doesn't make that person more endeared; it means that the person is "being used."

The following questions should be considered when determining if a relationship is healthy and has growth potential:

1. Does each person have a secure belief in his or her own value?
2. Is each person improved by the relationship? By some measure outside of the relationship is he or she a better, stronger, more attractive, more accomplished, or more sensitive individual? Does each person value the relationship for this very reason?
3. Does each person maintain interests outside the relationship, including other meaningful personal relationships?
4. Is the relationship integrated into, rather than set off from, the totality of each person's life?
5. Does each person maintain a sense of autonomy within the relationship?
6. Are both persons beyond being possessive or jealous of the other's growth and expansion of interests?
7. Is the relationship growth-producing?
8. Can each person communicate freely with the other?
9. Are each person's needs satisfied within the relationship?
10. Is the relationship unconditional?

Most people involved in a relationship probably cannot answer "yes" to all of these questions. Obviously, the more "yes" answers, the greater the chance that you are involved in a healthy relationship with growth potential. If you answered "no" to most of these questions, maybe it's time to reevaluate the relationship.

Healthy versus Unhealthy Love in Adult Relationships

Often a relationship is started because of physical attraction; the need for love, security, and acceptance; the fear of loneliness; or convenience. Although these may be basic aspects of coupling, unless there is a true acceptance of the individuality and uniqueness of each person and the ability to allow each to grow and develop, a healthy and lasting relationship is not likely to be achieved. In order to have a loving and lasting relationship, it is important to understand what makes one person's love for another person healthy and enriching instead of unhealthy and destructive. A healthy love has the following characteristics:

- It strengthens the bond between two people in a relationship.
- It has lasting qualities that can withstand the test of time.
- It takes time to grow and develop.
- It adds fullness to life.
- It is relatively steady and secure.
- It is a realistic love; it doesn't expect perfection.
- It involves exclusivity (loving no other person in such an emotional and intimate way).
- It involves the elements of give and take.

For a person to love another person in a healthy way, he or she must be able to do the following:

1. Work to make the relationship the best it can be.
2. Share what he or she has and is with the other person.
3. Strive toward shared feelings, attitudes, ambitions, hopes, and interests.
4. Accept the other person's faults and weaknesses.
5. Openly and honestly express his or her feelings without fear of losing the love and respect of the other person.
6. Think and plan in terms of "we."
7. Work with the other person to achieve goals and ideals.
8. Help the other person grow, develop, and reach his or her potential.

An unhealthy love has some or all of the following characteristics:

- It undermines a relationship.
- It is a possessive and smothering type of love.
- It is based on idealism and fantasy rather than on reality.
- It is based mainly on erotic feelings.
- It can have negative long-term effects on the recipient of such love.
- It is an immature and insecure type of love.
- It stems out of selfish motives with little or no concern for the other person.
- It is usually centered around the ego needs of one person.

Both healthy and unhealthy love may be passionate and all-consuming. It may be difficult to distinguish between the two types. The difference, however, is based on the substance behind the love.

> **FAST FACTS**
>
> Too much self-disclosure, or self-disclosure offered too soon, can sometimes scare a person away from a relationship.

■ Exploitive Behavior

Sexual intimacy involves the consent of both individuals. Giving in to sexual activity because of a fear of angering or rejecting the other person is not consent. If an individual uses emotional blackmail to make you feel guilty or won't take "no" for an answer, that person obviously does not care much about you or your feelings. Remember, you don't have to have sex to get or keep a relationship. Sexual activity should never be used as a test of love. It is your right to have a nonexploitive, mutually consenting relationship—when you are ready for one. Sexual intercourse that occurs without consent under actual or threatened force, whether it be with a stranger, acquaintance, or even a date, is **rape.**

The incidence of **date rape** is highly underreported. Date rape, also known as acquaintance rape, is rape committed against a female by someone she knows, either well or by sight. Date rape can occur anywhere, but most incidents occur either in the victim's home or in the attacker's home. A female may not perceive the incident as being rape because she knows the attacker and because violence probably was not involved. Also, it might be very difficult for her to believe that someone she knows would want to victimize her. A female who is the victim of date rape may experience such feelings as anger, depression, guilt, shame, embarrassment, and fear. She may lose her ability to trust people as well as her ability to relate to a sexual partner. She may believe that the rape was basically her fault and agonize over how she was responsible. When a female continues to blame herself following a rape, the male who raped her is still indirectly maintaining some control over her life. A female who has been raped is often doubly victimized—first by the attacker and again by the attitudes of society. Many times the female is accused of provoking the rape because of her physical appearance or seductive behavior. Studies have shown, however, that few rapes are triggered by the victim's looks or behaviors.

Date rape *can* be prevented. First, a female must make it clear, before getting involved in a sexual situation, what her limits are. When her voice says no, her body language must also be saying no. Second, she must not get into compromising situations. This means avoiding intoxication with alcohol and other drugs so that her judgment will not be impaired, and keeping away from isolated places with someone she has just met. A female should not let a male pressure her into having sexual relations with him, even if she has had sex with him in the past. It is imperative for a female to trust her instincts and act on them. If she feels uncomfortable or uneasy in the presence of a male, she should leave immediately.

Date rape does not involve love or romance. It does not happen in the heat of passion. It is an aggressive act committed against a woman's will. It is an issue of power and control, *not* one of caring and concern. If you are a victim of date rape, you should not feel ashamed or guilty, but the incident needs to be reported to the proper authorities to lessen the chances of it happening to other women. Always remember that no one has the right to touch your body unless you allow it. A person who genuinely cares about you will not sexually exploit you and will respect your right to say No.

■ Love and Physical Intimacy

The type of love that usually exists in male-female relationships is called **erotic love.** Erotic love differs from other types of love because it includes the element

FAST FACTS

Conservative estimates indicate that a woman is raped every seven minutes and that a half million rapes occur each year in the U.S.

■ *PROBLEM SITUATION FOR MALES* You have just spent an evening wining and dining your date. When you take her home, she can barely find the lock to open the door. She invites you in for a nightcap. Once inside, she rubs up against your body and starts kissing your neck. Just when you are getting turned on, she says, "You'd better leave now." What would you do?

■ *PROBLEM SITUATION FOR FEMALES* You are on a date with a guy for the second time and you think you like him but you aren't sure. You invite him into your apartment, and before long, both of you are sitting on the couch hugging and kissing. He starts taking off your skirt, but you ask him to stop. He ignores your request and continues. How would you handle this situation?

GUIDELINES TO YOUR GOOD HEALTH

If a friend comes to you and tells you that she has just been raped, you can help her by doing the following:

1. Encourage her to call the police immediately. If she resists, try to convince her to call a physician or crisis counselor.
2. Be supportive and understanding. Give her the same type of support that you would give if she were the victim of any other kind of crisis or trauma.
3. Avoid tactless remarks such as, "I warned you about that guy," or "I told you not to wear that dress." These words offer little comfort and may just stir up guilt feelings.
4. Don't try to cheer her up. There is nothing to be cheerful about. Avoid saying, "Things could have been worse." To a female who has just been raped, *nothing* could be worse.
5. Do not force her to talk when she doesn't want to.
6. Do not, however, try to make her forget what has happened. Let her know that whenever she wants to talk, you are there to listen.
7. Don't let her be alone. See that she has a safe place to stay and someone she trusts to stay with.
8. If you are a male friend, she may act cool, distant, and even hostile toward you. Do not personalize these feelings. Try to realize that she is going through an inner struggle and that it may take time for her to recover. The best thing you can do is just let her know that you care and that you are there if she needs your friendship.

of sexual desire. It involves emotional and physical intimacy between two people. It is one of the most intense types of love that a human being can experience.

When sexual intimacy enters into a relationship, it is extremely important that there is honest communication and agreement about each person's expectations. For one partner, engaging in sexual activity may be an end in itself, an experience valued for its own returns. Nothing more may be expected from the relationship. For the other partner, sexual intimacy may be a means to the goal of a lasting relationship. If the reasons behind the intimacy are not openly shared, one partner may feel hurt, angry, guilty, or exploited. Sex may be an important component of erotic love, but by itself, it is not enough on which to build a loving relationship. In combination with such feelings as caring, respect, trust, and commitment, sex can be extremely fulfilling in a loving relationship. With little else, however, sex seldom endures the test of time.

> ■ *PROBLEM SITUATION* You are sexually attracted to someone, and you know that the feeling is mutual. Each time you're together, the physical attraction is stronger. There is a feeling of friendship between you, but no love. Would you become sexually intimate with this person if asked? Would you initiate the love-making? What factors might influence your decision?

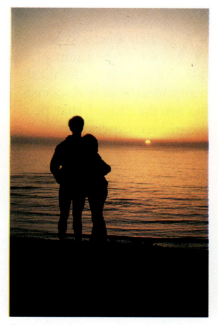

Love means being together and sharing some quiet moments

Sometimes, with a little wishful thinking and some convincing from your partner, you believe that you are in love. You very well might be. At this point, the desire for a sexual relationship may be strong. You may struggle with the question of whether or not to become sexually intimate. Factors such as upbringing, personal values and morals, previous experiences, and religious beliefs will influence your sexual decision making. Whatever you choose to do, there are no guarantees about what the outcome will be. You may feel happy and satisfied with your decision, or you may feel sorry and disappointed. If you and your partner discuss your feelings and expectations before making any decisions, there is a greater chance that neither of you will regret the outcome later on. It's ironic to learn of how many couples are intimate enough to have sexual intercourse but not open enough to share any questions, doubts, or fears they may be having. Communicate with your partner.

To help in your decision making, consider the criteria that *Marmor* has identified when deciding if sexual behavior is normal and healthy or abnormal and pathological. The following are characteristics of normal and healthy sexual behavior:

1. It is motivated primarily by feelings of affection and tenderness.
2. It seeks to give and receive pleasure.
3. It tends to be discriminating as to partner choice.
4. It is motivated by recurring erotic feelings in the context of physical attraction and affection.

In contrast, abnormal or pathological sexual behavior has the following characteristics:

1. It is used as a means of discharging anxiety, hostility, and guilt.
2. It primarily seeks to receive sexual pleasure.
3. It tends to be nondiscriminating as to partner choice.
4. It is triggered by nonerotic feelings that are often compulsive.

■ The Romantic Love Cycle

What comes to mind when you think of romantic love? Passion? Excitement? Being head-over-heels in love? Hearing bells ring and birds sing? Romance is a desirable state that most people hope to experience; however, it is only one

FAST FACTS

Romantic love is found only in cultures that idealize the concept.

> **FAST FACTS**
>
> When a person is in love, the brain produces a stimulant chemical compound that is responsible for the "high" that people in love experience.

phase in a love relationship. Masters and Johnson have proposed a theoretical model that depicts how romantic love develops called the Romantic Love Cycle. This model does not apply to all cases of romantic love; its intent is to organize one's thinking about romantic love.

> ■ **PROBLEM SITUATION** You have invited someone whom you care about to spend the evening with you. You tell that person that you will be responsible for making all of the arrangements. Now that you have the opportunity to plan your ideal romantic evening, what will it be? How will you want the other person to look and behave?

Love Readiness. The first stage of the Romantic Love Cycle is *love readiness*. This is not a physiological state but, rather, a state of mind. At this point, an individual sees love as being desirable and rewarding. There is a longing to have emotional and physical intimacy with another person. This state reflects the hope that people have about being loved. People who view falling in love as a sign of weakness or as a distraction are unlikely to experience love readiness. Some people are always in a state of love readiness but never get any farther.

Falling in Love. Most people are hopeful that love readiness will lead to *falling in love*. Falling in love happens differently for different people. Some people claim to experience "love at first sight," whereas others find themselves being attracted to another person gradually.

The newness of your love makes this an exciting stage. At this time you may feel that you're "on cloud nine" and that all's right with the world. This may be also a time of tension and insecurity, however, as you wonder if your love is going to last. Falling in love distorts objectivity. You may see the object of your affection as the ideal person who can fulfill all your wants and needs. This is the time when you are most likely to overlook weaknesses and magnify strengths. If the relationship continues, you may enter the next stage, "being in love."

> ■ **PROBLEM SITUATION** You and your teenage sister are watching a love story on television. As is often portrayed in the media, love solves all the problems in the story and the hero and the heroine live happily ever after. After the story is over, your sister tells you that she can't wait to fall in love. Would you say anything in response to your sister's statement?

Being in Love. Synonymous with the idea of romantic love is *being in love*. The person who is in love is willing to accept even the flimsiest signs of reciprocation. For some people, being in love brings with it an emotional roller coaster of ups and downs. With the excitement and the pleasure may also come an inability to concentrate, eat, or sleep, as well as, the possible deterioration of other meaningful relationships. Psychologist Dorothy Tennov coined the term **limerence** to describe a type of romantic love that is marked by obsession and preoccupation with the loved one. This intense form of love lasts an average of two years and then changes into another form of love (companionate love) or gradually terminates.

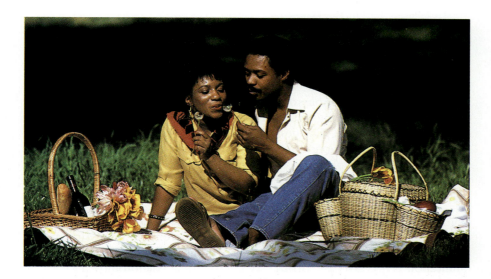

Enjoying the pleasures of nature, and one another, is a characteristic of companionate love.

Companionate Love. Once the high of romantic love begins to fade, it is replaced by a more realistic and stable love called *companionate love*. Companionate love is a steadier type of love based on affection, sharing, loyalty, trust, and togetherness. Because it is less possessive and consuming than romantic love, it allows two people to carry on their lives with a minimum of interference and a maximum of satisfaction. It can deteriorate into drabness if not sustained by continued affection and respect.

Love in Transition. Many times the feeling of being in love ceases to exist. A person may enter a stage called *love in transition*. Usually one person initiates this stage, but it is possible for both partners to experience it at the same time. During love in transition, the person feels that the initial excitement of being in love is diminishing or is gone altogether. The person may become bored or impatient with the relationship. One or both partners begins to notice imperfections in the other that were previously unobserved. The partners start to test one another and the presumed strength of their love. If the relationship does not measure up to their expectations, the conflict may lead to "falling out of love." If both people are willing to work at improving the relationship, however, measures may be taken to push the relationship into a temporary state of truce. With motivation and cooperation, the couple may resolve their difficulties, and the relationship may return to the "being in love" stage. If this occurs, the new version of the relationship may be stronger and better.

Falling Out of Love. If the difficulties cannot be resolved, eventually one or both partners will *fall out of love*. When a person is falling out of love, he or she becomes less interested in the other person. Communication is virtually nonexistent, and whatever problems occur hardly seem worth the effort to overcome. Because the majority of love relationships do not end by mutual consent, this stage is usually a painful experience for the person who may still be in love. That person may experience sorrow and heartache and grieve the loss of the relationship, or he or she may be angry and want to strike out at the other person.

FAST FACTS

When a person falls out of love, the brain stops producing the stimulant chemical, which may account for the depression that many people experience.

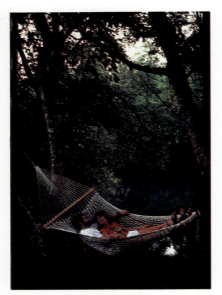

Words are not always necessary when you are trying to convey a message to someone.

Being Out of Love. Once falling out of love occurs, the person is in the stage of *being out of love*. Usually one of three things happens at this point: (1) The person goes back to a state of love readiness, perhaps wiser from the experience; (2) the person is "on the rebound" and is vulnerable to a new relationship in order to get over the previous one; or (3) the person enters a **refractory period,** finding that it is not possible to fall in love again during this time.

As long as human beings want to have intimate relationships, there will be a Romantic Love Cycle. The desire to be loved gives people the resiliency to overcome a painful relationship and the strength and courage to pursue a new one. Isn't life wonderful?

Communication Skills

Communication requires the ability to express yourself so that another person can understand what you are thinking or feeling. We communicate using spoken or written words, pictures, facial expressions, and body gestures. Effective communication is necessary for satisfactory interpersonal relationships.

Have you ever thought that there was a "failure to communicate," that even though words were spoken, communication had not occurred? Maybe communication failed because the message wasn't clearly sent or was improperly received. Listening is also a crucial part of effective communication. It is important to give feedback and to let the communicator know that his or her message has gotten across clearly. To communicate effectively, you must do the following:

1. Use words that will be understood by the person receiving the message.
2. Use words that can convey the true meaning of the message.
3. Consider the tone of voice that you will use to communicate the message.
4. Make sure that your body language is consistent with your verbal language. If you say one thing, but your facial expression or body gestures say another, you may be sending a mixed message.
5. Make sure that your timing is right. Select a time when the other person is receptive to listening.
6. Say what is on your mind. Do not give hints or make a guessing game out of what you want to communicate. This can be very frustrating for the listener.

Have you ever evaluated your listening skills? What type of listener are you? Ask yourself the following questions, and maybe you'll gain some insight.

1. Do you encourage someone to talk by showing interest in what he or she is saying?
2. Do you hear only bits and pieces of what is being said?
3. Do you become easily distracted when someone is talking to you?
4. Do you take words and meanings out of context?
5. Do you hear only what you want to hear?
6. Do you ask clarifying questions when you don't understand what is being said?
7. Do you respond with meaningful questions and comments?
8. Do you maintain eye contact with the person who is speaking?
9. Do you listen with an open mind?
10. Do you hear what is being said as well as observe the actions being communicated?

11. Do you interrupt the person who is speaking in order to change the topic of conversation?

12. Do you criticize what the person is saying or make fun of his or her remarks?

Are you a better listener than you thought, or is there much room for improvement? Just because a person is speaking to you doesn't necessarily mean that you are listening. Next time someone tries to communicate with you, ask yourself if you not only heard, but also listened, to what was said. (See Figure 7–1.)

FIGURE 7–1 ■ **Factors Needed for Effective Communication**

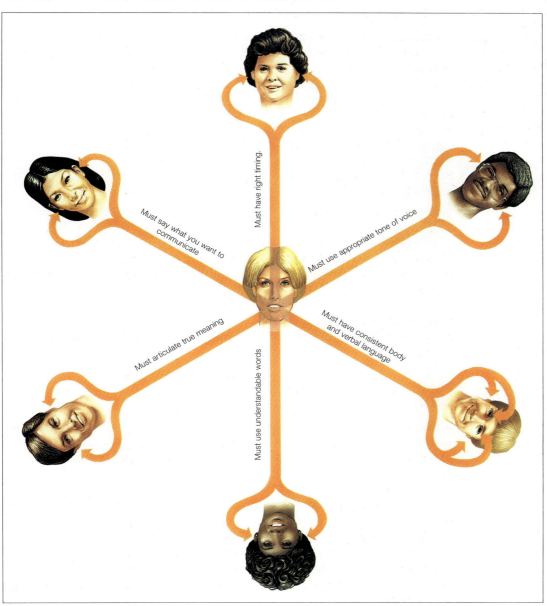

GUIDELINES TO YOUR GOOD HEALTH

Contact involves the way you meet and relate to people during the initial phase of interaction. At the core of a good contact situation, in which two or more people are really tuned in to each other, the four "C"s are always present.

Confidence

- You must convey a certain degree of self-confidence as a foundation for any successful encounter.
- Most people do not respond favorably to someone who is self-demeaning, overly apologetic, or overly boastful.

Creativity

- Being creative in making contacts means finding ways to tune in to the feelings of others.

Caring

- Showing another person that you are listening with total attention and are interested is a major indication that you care.

Consideration

- A believable concern radiating from yourself that makes other people feel a little better about themselves, even in a brief meeting, is the essence of consideration.
- It includes a combination of the other "C"s.
- It means being sensitive and aware of another person's feelings and interests.
- Being a good listener and responding with meaningful questions and comments, eye contact, and appropriate smiles shows your consideration.

Do your contact techniques include some or all of the four "C"s?

FAST FACTS

Communication is essential to the development and maintenance of intimacy.

■ Effective Communication in a Relationship

Problems arise even in the best of relationships. In fact, having problems is not always a sign of trouble. How a couple confronts and handles these problems is very important in their building of a stronger relationship. When two people openly and honestly discuss a problem, they usually can either resolve it or prevent more serious conflict from occurring. A problem situation becomes harmful when it is ignored and allowed to grow in proportion.

When a problem occurs, one person may mentally withdraw from the situation by saying nothing. A person may use silence as a way of handling conflict. If silence is used as a means of gathering one's thoughts and feelings before confronting the problem, it is healthy and acceptable. If, however, silence is used to avoid unpleasant confrontations or to hurt the other person, it is unhealthy because it stands in the way of effective communication with one's partner.

If you are dealing with a problem, it is important to stay relevant. Discuss only things that pertain to that particular problem. When you are angry or upset, it is easy to bring up other unpleasant issues. This only complicates the problem and can possibly serve to alienate your partner even further. Focus on the facts and avoid stooping to the level of "I'm right and you're wrong." This will only add fuel to the fire. Direct your energies toward resolving the problem instead of attacking the other person. Remember, those belittling or hurtful remarks may linger long after the problem is resolved. And it may be those remarks, not the initial problem, that proves to be harmful to your relationship.

■ When Love Blooms: Getting Married

At one time it was automatically assumed that once a female reached the age of eighteen, she would get married and start a family as soon as possible. As times changed, so did expectations. It was no longer assumed that *all* females would marry once they reached eighteen. Many would go to college, get a degree, and upon graduation . . . *then* get married and start a family.

As we enter into the 1990s, today's women are marrying later than at any time since 1890, when the Census Bureau began keeping marriage statistical data. The median age of American women marrying for the first time is now 23.6 years, as compared to the record low of 20.1 years in 1956. This trend has developed as women have opted for higher education and career over early marriage and children. The median age of American men marrying for the first time is 25.8 years. Since 1900, the median age of men marrying for the first time has never been less than 22.8 years. Thus, with the median age at first

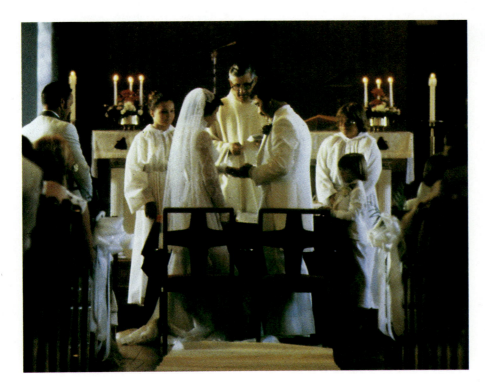

The institution of marriage will continue to thrive as long as there are people who believe in love.

marriage gradually rising, more and more individuals are choosing to remain single during part of their young adulthood.

Yet marriage still remains the most popular life-style for couples wishing to share emotional and sexual intimacy. The United States has one of the highest marriage rates. More than 90 percent of Americans marry. Such factors as love, companionship, emotional and financial security, sexual monogamy, and the desire for children are among the reasons that people marry. Marriage is also the life-style most accepted within our society and among religious affiliations.

An individual's age at marriage and his or her educational level are important factors contributing to the longevity of the relationship. The most stable first marriages occur among women who marry after the age of thirty. Teenage marriages are the least stable and the least likely to withstand the test of time. Marital satisfaction is generally higher when the partners have similar educational backgrounds. Traditionally it has been acceptable, as well as desirable, for women to marry men who are better educated than they are. The reverse, however, has not been true. A woman was said to be "marrying down" if she had more education than the man. This social norm has been changing because of the increasing number of women who have been receiving higher educational or career training. Even though marriage remains the life-style of choice for most, many young men and women are first experiencing alternatives before making the commitment to marriage and children.

When Love Fades: Getting Divorced

No one gets married with the intention of someday getting divorced; people enter into marriage believing that it will last forever. Unfortunately, things change and people change, and divorce may become inevitable. Table 7–1 lists the number and rate of marriages and divorces occurring in the U.S. since 1900. Such factors as communication difficulties, incompatibility, unhappiness, drug or alcohol problems, emotional or physical abuse, or a spouse's infidelity are some of the many reasons that individuals seek divorce.

It is often difficult to end a marriage, even when it is obvious that the problems or differences are too great to resolve. What motivates some people to stay in bad relationships? A person may stay in a bad relationship because of economic factors, convenience, children, lack of confidence about being able to find someone else, fear of loneliness, a feeling of pity for the other person, or simply not knowing how to end it. Sometimes an individual hasn't the courage to initiate the breakup. One person may deliberately start a fight in hopes that the other person will end the relationship, or one spouse may try to make the other person's life so miserable that the only choice he or she has is to leave. One thing is certain, however; staying in a marriage that should be over only prolongs the pain and guilt and prevents both people from finding happiness in another relationship.

Unfortunately, many marriages do not end in a kind way. There may be anger and bitterness, and if a person feels betrayed, he or she may say hateful things, or even spread vicious lies, about the other person, especially to the children. It is often difficult for people who are divorcing to remain friends under such circumstances, and children are usually the ones who suffer the most. Whether an individual seeks a divorce or resists it, when a marriage ends, both people experience emotional upheaval.

> **FAST FACTS**
>
> Among those who marry, about 40 percent return to single status through divorce.

TABLE 7-1 ■ The Number and Rate of Marriages and Divorces Occurring in the U.S. since 1900

	Marriage		Divorce[1]	
Year	Number	Rate[2]	Number	Rate[2]
1900	709,000	9.3	55,751	.7
1910	948,166	10.3	83,045	.9
1920	1,274,476	12.0	170,505	1.6
1930	1,126,856	9.2	195,961	1.6
1940	1,595,879	12.1	264,000	2.0
1950	1,667,231	11.1	385,144	2.6
1960	1,523,000	8.5	393,000	2.2
1970	2,158,802	10.6	708,000	3.5
1973	2,284,108	10.9	915,000	4.4
1975	2,152,662	10.1	1,036,000	4.9
1977	2,178,367	10.1	1,091,000	5.0
1980	2,406,708	10.6	1,182,000	5.2
1983	2,444,000	10.5	1,179,000	5.0
1985	2,425,000	10.2	1,187,000	5.0
1987	2,421,000	9.9	1,157,000	4.8

[1]Includes annulments.
[2]Per 1,000 population.
NOTE: Figures for most years include some estimated data. Alaska is included beginning 1959, Hawaii beginning 1960.
SOURCE: Department of Health and Human Services, National Center for Health Statistics.

■ Picking Up the Pieces

When a relationship ends, whether it results from death, divorce, or break-up of the relationship, a loss is experienced that must be acknowledged and accepted so that the person can go on with his or her life. Grief is the normal reaction to loss. When a loss occurs, the person may experience such feelings as sadness, depression, emptiness, loneliness, and even anger or guilt. There may be changes in appetite and sleep patterns. There is also a tendency to be listless, less motivated, more fatigued, and possibly accident prone. Any or all of these symptoms are to be expected during and after a loss. They are part of the body's natural healing process. The body goes through this process no matter how tragic or how seemingly trivial the loss might be. Dealing with any loss involves surviving, healing, and growing.

If you are trying to survive the loss of a relationship, the first step is to recognize that it has ended. You may struggle to believe (and wish to disbelieve) that this could have happened to you. You may feel emotionally numb. It is normal to feel pain or numbness after a loss, and it is important to the healing process that you allow yourself to experience the pain or hurt that you are feeling. The healing process takes time; the greater the loss, the more time it will take. Keep in mind, at the beginning, that there is an end. This will pass, and you will heal.

Don't blame yourself for the relationship being over. Don't dwell on negative thoughts. Disregard any thought that begins with "if only." Surround yourself with understanding and supportive family members and friends. An emotional

FAST FACTS

About 70 percent of divorced individuals eventually remarry.

SELF-INVENTORY 7.1

How Confident Are You in Social Situations?

Place a check mark in the column that most appropriately describes your feelings or behaviors in social situations.

		True	False	Some-times
1.	I like meeting new people.	___	___	___
2.	I don't mind going to parties by myself, even when I do not know anyone else.	___	___	___
3.	I can easily start a conversation with a person whom I have just met.	___	___	___
4.	I can make and keep eye contact when talking to someone.	___	___	___
5.	I get easily hurt if I think other people do not like me.	___	___	___
6.	I have difficulty finding things to talk about after the initial "hello."	___	___	___
7.	I like being noticed when I walk into a room filled with people.	___	___	___
8.	I feel uneasy when the talking stops and there is silence.	___	___	___
9.	I am a friendly, outgoing person.	___	___	___
10.	I don't feel discouraged when someone doesn't want to talk to me.	___	___	___
11.	I usually end up talking to only one person because I don't know how to end the conversation.	___	___	___
12.	I feel nervous and uneasy when I don't know anyone at a party.	___	___	___
13.	I like being the "life of the party."	___	___	___

wound is real, painful, and disabling. It is all right to need comforting. The most efficient healing takes place when enough rest and activity are alternated. Rest as much as you need, but don't become lethargic. Productive work often helps rest the emotions. Although your internal world may be chaotic, give your external world a sense of order by keeping busy.

An emotional wound requires the same attention as a physical wound. The sooner you allow yourself to be with your pain, the sooner it will pass. If you

14. I talk to many people at social functions rather than spend my time with only one person. _____ _____ _____
15. I get easily hurt if I think other people do not like me. _____ _____ _____
16. I feel embarrassed when I walk into a room filled with people and they look at me. _____ _____ _____
17. I stay off to the side and hope that someone will start talking to me when I go to a party. _____ _____ _____
18. I feel bad when another person seems disinterested in what I am saying. _____ _____ _____

Scoring:

If you answered "True" to questions 1, 2, 3, 4, 7, 9, 10, 13, and 14, you possess the confidence and skills that are necessary to meet people.

If the majority of your answers to questions 1, 2, 3, 4, 7, 9, 10, 13, and 14 is "True" or "Sometimes," you most likely feel confident in social situations but there is room for improvement. You need to assess your feelings and behaviors and determine whether you are satisfied with your present level of confidence or whether improvements need to be made.

If you answered "True" to questions 5, 6, 8, 11, 12, 15, 16, 17, and 18, you DO NOT possess the confidence and skills that are necessary to meet people.

If the majority of your answers to questions 5, 6, 8, 11, 12, 15, 16, 17, and 18 is "True" or "Sometimes," you most likely feel uncomfortable in social situations but you have the potential for gaining social confidence if you choose to work on your feelings and behaviors. You also have the potential, however, for losing what confidence you do possess. The choice is yours.

What things can you do to improve your level of confidence?

Choose one of the preceding statements that poses a problem for you and work on trying to change the feeling or behavior. How might you go about doing this?

postpone the healing process, unresolved grief can return months or even years later to haunt you. Don't try to rekindle the relationship. Futile attempts at reconciliation are painful and anti-healing. To give up this final hope may be the most difficult part of all. After recovering from this loss, however, you may find that you were able not only to survive and heal but also to grow and become stronger.

POSITIVE BEHAVIORS

I. *Place a check mark in front of each behavior that you now practice.*

___ 1. I don't pretend to be someone I'm not in order to impress a person I like. (PRETEND)
___ 2. I accept my own strengths and weaknesses. (ACCEPT)
___ 3. I am not a jealous or possessive person. (JEALOUS)
___ 4. In a relationship, I communicate openly and honestly with my partner. (COMMUNICATE)
___ 5. I am a good listener. (LISTENER)
___ 6. I maintain eye contact with the person who is speaking. (EYE CONTACT)
___ 7. I don't make belittling or hurtful remarks when I am angry. (REMARKS)
___ 8. I don't have difficulty ending relationships. (ENDING)
___ 9. I don't dwell on negative thoughts after a relationship ends. (NEGATIVE THOUGHTS)
___ 10. If I feel hurt or rejected, I don't try to get revenge. (REVENGE)

II. *For each behavior that you DO NOT ENGAGE IN, write the KEY WORD(S) located in the parentheses at the end of the statement in the column below. Then put a check mark in the appropriate column to indicate whether you are going to keep or change that behavior.*

Behaviors I Don't Engage In   KEEP/CHANGE

_____   _____/_____
_____   _____/_____
_____   _____/_____
_____   _____/_____
_____   _____/_____
_____   _____/_____
_____   _____/_____
_____   _____/_____
_____   _____/_____
_____   _____/_____

III. *For each of the preceding behaviors that you choose to KEEP, write a statement indicating why you are choosing to keep that behavior.*

I choose to keep behavior _____ because:
                          KEY WORD

For each of the preceding behaviors that you choose to CHANGE, write a statement indicating how you plan to implement that change.

I will change behavior _____ by:
                        KEY WORD

Now You Know

1. FALSE. Relationships can be positive or negative.
2. TRUE. Each person should maintain his or her own individuality and independence.
3. TRUE. Both types may be passionate and all-consuming; the difference, however, is based on the substance behind the love.
4. FALSE. Abnormal sexual behavior primarily seeks to receive sexual pleasure.
5. TRUE. It involves emotional and physical intimacy between two people.
6. FALSE. Some people are always in a state of love readiness but never succeed in getting any farther.
7. FALSE. Only about 15 percent of love relationships end by mutual consent.
8. TRUE. When a relationship ends, a person experiences a loss. Grief is the normal reaction to loss.
9. TRUE. Futile attempts at trying to rekindle the relationship are anti-healing.
10. FALSE. The sooner you allow yourself to be with your pain, the sooner it will pass.

Summary

1. A relationship is a bond between two or more people. People enter into relationships for physical, mental, emotional, social, and economic reasons.
2. A healthy and meaningful relationship requires compatibility, unconditional acceptance of the other person, and a sense of well-being and ease when with the other person.
3. When entering into a relationship, you may be overly anxious to make a good impression. It is important to be yourself and to let the other person see you as you really are. If a relationship is based on false pretenses or fantasy, it is doomed to fail.
4. The first step in creating and maintaining a healthy relationship begins with you. If you have a positive self-concept, others will respond to you positively. For a relationship to be satisfying, you must meet your own needs as well as the needs of the other person.
5. A healthy love has several characteristics, some of which include its ability to withstand the test of time, its ability to add fullness to life, and its steady and secure nature.
6. For one person to love another person in a healthy way, he or she must be open, honest, accepting, caring, and giving.
7. An unhealthy love undermines a relationship, may be based on idealism and fantasy rather than on reality, or is an immature or insecure type of love.
8. Both healthy and unhealthy love may be passionate and all-consuming. The difference, however, is based on the substance behind the love.
9. The type of love that usually exists in male-female relationships is called erotic love. It involves emotional and physical intimacy and is one of the most intense types of love a person can experience.
10. Your decisions about sexual intimacy depend on such factors as upbringing, personal values and morals, previous experiences, and religious beliefs. You and your partner should discuss the feelings and expectations you both have before making any decisions regarding a sexual relationship.
11. To help in sexual decision making, the individual should consider the criteria that make sexual behavior normal and healthy as compared with those that make it abnormal and pathological.
12. The Romantic Love Cycle is a theoretical model that depicts how romantic love develops. It involves the stages of love readiness, falling in love, being in love, companionate love, love in transition, falling out of love, and being out of love.
13. Communication requires the ability to express oneself so that another person can understand what you are thinking or feeling. Effective communication is necessary for satisfactory interpersonal relationships.
14. To effectively communicate, an individual must use words that will be understood by the person receiving the message, must make sure that body language is consistent with verbal language, and must select the right time for the communication.
15. Listening is a crucial part of effective communication. It is also important to let the communicator know that his or her message has gotten across.
16. Problems arise even in the best of relationships. Being willing to openly and honestly confront and handle problems helps to build a stronger relationship. Problems become harmful when they are ignored and allowed to grow out of proportion.
17. When a relationship ends, a person experiences a loss. Grief is the normal reaction to loss. The person may feel sad, depressed, empty, lonely, and even angry or guilty. These symptoms are part of the body's natural healing process. Dealing with an ended relationship involves surviving, healing, and growing.

References

1. Allgeier, Albert Richard, and Elizabeth Rice Allgeier. *Sexual Interactions.* Lexington, Massachusetts: D.C. Heath and Co., 1988.
2. Adams, Caren, and Jennifer Fay. *Nobody Told Me It Was Rape.* Santa Cruz, California: Network Publications, 1984.
3. Denney, Nancy W., and David Quadagno. *Human Sexuality.* St. Louis: Times Mirror/Mosby College Publishing, 1988.
4. Greenberg, Jerrold S., Clint E. Bruess, Kathleen D. Mullen, and Doris W. Sands. *Sexuality: Insights and Issues,* 2d ed. Dubuque, Iowa: William C. Brown, 1989.
5. Knox, David. *Choices in Relationships.* St. Paul: West Publishing Co., 1985.
6. Ledray, Linda E. *Recovering from Rape.* New York: Henry Holt and Co., 1986.
7. Marmor, Judd, et al. "What Distinguishes 'Healthy' from 'Sick' Sexual Behavior." *Medical Aspects of Human Sexuality.* 10(1977): 67–77.
8. Masters, William H., Virginia E. Johnson, and Robert C. Kolodny. *Human Sexuality,* 3d ed. Glenview, Illinois: Scott, Foresman and Co., 1988.
9. Strong, Bryan, and Christine DeVault. *The Marriage and Family Experience,* 4th ed. St. Paul: West Publishing Co., 1989.
10. Tennov, Dorothy. *Love and Limerence.* New York: First Scarborough Books, 1981.
11. *The 1989 Information Please Almanac.* 42nd ed. New York: Houghton Mifflin Co., 1988.
12. *What Every Woman Should Know About Rape.* South Deerfield, Massachusetts: Channing L. Bete Co., 1986.

Suggested Readings

Gordon, Sol. *Why Love Is Not Enough.* Boston: Bob Adams, Inc., 1988.

Kingma, Daphne Rose. *Coming Apart: Why Relationships End and How to Live Through the Ending of Yours.* New York: Fawcett Crest, 1987.

Ledray, Linda E. *Recovering from Rape.* New York: Henry Holt and Co., 1986.

Warshaw, Robin. *I Never Called It Rape.* New York: Harper and Row, 1988.

CHAPTER 8

Sexual Bodyworks

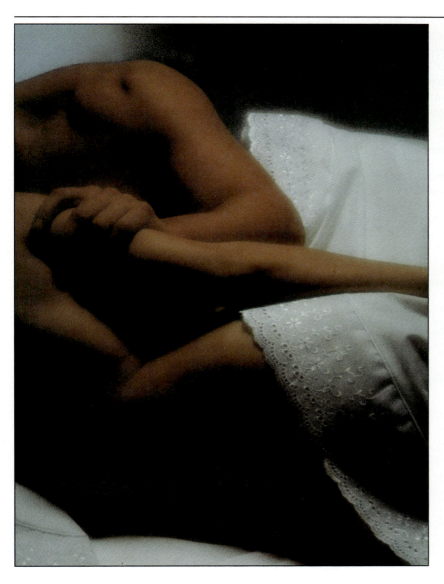

What Do You Know?

Are the following statements true or false?

1. The size of the penis determines a male's ability to give and receive sexual pleasure.
2. The testicles' only function is to produce sperm cells.
3. The collective name for the female's external genitals is the labia.
4. The inner two-thirds of the vagina is relatively insensitive to touch or pain.
5. Estrogen is a general name for feminizing sex hormones, which are present in both sexes.
6. Testosterone is responsible for sexual desire in both males and females.
7. Ovulation occurs exactly in the middle of a female's menstrual cycle.
8. The pituitary gland is the primary controlling mechanism that triggers the production and secretion of sex hormones.
9. Tampons can cause toxic shock syndrome.
10. PMS refers to the intense feelings of physical and mental discomfort that some women experience prior to menstruation.

All you need to do is take one look at a naked individual to determine if that person is biologically male or female. Males and females have anatomical features so distinct that we could not possibly confuse which sex is which. Right? As different as they appear, however, the internal and external anatomy of both sexes has similar embryological beginnings. At conception, sexual development can go in either the male or female direction, depending on the proportions of androgens and estrogens secreted. It is not until the end of the twelfth week of development that the fetus is clearly male or female in its sexual anatomy. Because knowledge of sexual anatomy and physiology provides an important foundation for understanding one's sexual self, this chapter will focus on the sexual anatomy and physiology of males and females.

Sexual Anatomy and Physiology: Male

The male reproductive system consists of both internal and external organs. Although the external genitals are visible when a male is naked, many individuals (including males) are unaware of the organs and ducts that the internal system comprises. Do you know where sperm are produced? What Cowper's glands are? What prevents a male from urinating and ejaculating at the same time? The following section will discuss the anatomy and physiology of the male reproductive system. (Figures 8–1 and 8–2 illustrate the position and relation of the organs and structures in the male reproductive system.)

External Genitals

Penis. The **penis** is the male organ through which both urine and semen are passed. It consists of a shaft and an enlarged head called the **glans.** Covering

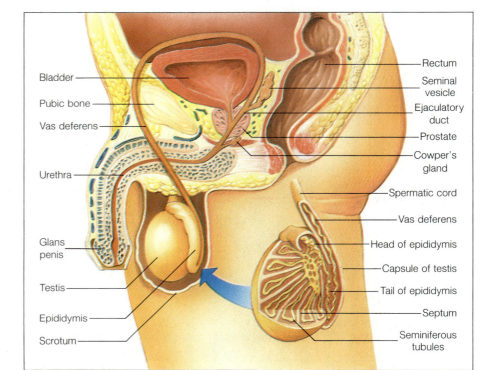

FIGURE 8–1 ■ Side View of the Male Reproductive Organs

CHAPTER 8 ■ SEXUAL BODYWORKS 199

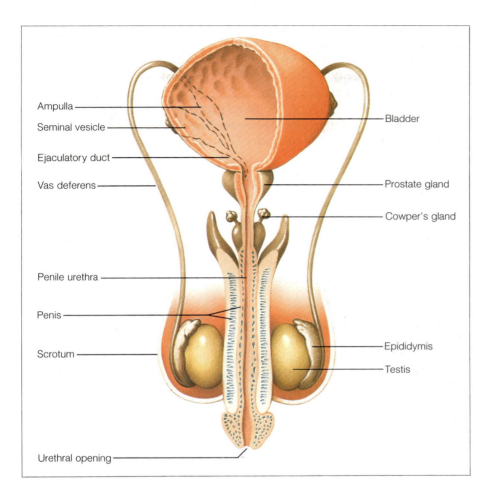

FIGURE 8–2 ■ **Front view of the Male Reproductive Organs**

the glans is a loosely fitting fold of skin called the prepuce, or **foreskin.** Surgical removal of this foreskin is called **circumcision.** It was believed that circumcision helped to prevent the spread of infection during sexual intercourse, because bacteria could not accumulate under the foreskin around the glans. Lack of circumcision, however, will not create a health problem as long as the male rolls back the foreskin and keeps the glans area clean.

The penis consists of three parallel cylinders of spongy tissue that become temporarily engorged with blood during sexual excitement. There is no muscle tissue or bone in the human penis. It is the engorgement of blood that provides the rigidity of erection. Many concerns, as well as jokes, are frequently voiced regarding penis size and sexual performance. Statements such as the following are commonly heard:

"The size and shape of the penis determines a male's ability to give and receive sexual pleasure."

"A male needs to have sexual intercourse frequently in order to prevent the penis from decreasing in size."

Do you believe that these statements are true? I hope not! Physiologically, there is no correlation between penis size and sexual satisfaction. The length of the penis mainly determines the depth of vaginal penetration, which is relatively unimportant because the majority of vaginal nerve endings are located in the

FAST FACTS

The glans is the most erotically sensitive part of the male anatomy.

outer third of the vagina. Unfortunately, many males base their feelings about their masculinity on penis size. Instead of worrying about penis size, males should focus their energy on becoming warm, caring, and sensitive partners. This will have a far greater effect on sexually pleasing their partners.

> ■ *PROBLEM SITUATION* Suppose that a male friend confides in you and says that he feels sexually inadequate because of the size of his penis. What reassurances can one male give to another? What reassurances can a female give to a male?

Scrotum. The **scrotum** is a pouch of skin located under the penis. The testes are contained within the scrotum, and for this reason, the scrotum is well-endowed with pain-sensing nerves. This is one of nature's ways of protecting exposed organs. The scrotum also serves as a temperature regulator by controlling the proximity of the testes to the body. The temperature of the testes must be a few degrees below normal body temperature in order for sperm to be produced.

Internal Organs

Testes. The **testes** or **testicles** are the male **gonads,** or sex organs. They are two small, oval-shaped organs that are housed in the scrotum. The testes have the dual function of producing sperm and the male sex hormone, testosterone.

Epididymis. The **epididymis** is a tightly coiled tube located at the top of each testis. Sperm can be stored and nourished in the epididymis until they are released for ejaculation or reabsorbed by the body.

Genital Ducts

Vas Deferens. The **vas deferens** are two slender ducts through which sperm are transported from the epididymis to the ejaculatory ducts.

Ejaculatory Ducts. The **ejaculatory ducts** are two ducts that enter the prostate gland and lead to the urethra. These ducts transport sperm along with other fluids that have been contributed by the seminal vesicles and the prostate gland.

Urethra. The **urethra** is a tube that extends through the penis. It begins at the bladder and ends at the **meatus** (the opening into the penis). Its function is to transport urine and semen out of the body.

Fluid-Producing Glands

The fluid-producing glands produce secretions that combine with the sperm to form **semen.** Semen is a grayish-white, alkaline fluid. The average ejaculate of semen is equivalent to about one teaspoon in volume, and there may be approximately 200 to 400 million sperm in one ejaculation.

FAST FACTS

Sperm account for only about 1 percent of the total volume of semen.

Seminal Vesicles. The **seminal vesicles** are saclike glands located on each side of the bladder. At the base of each seminal vesicle, there is a narrow duct that leads into the ejaculatory duct. The seminal vesicles secrete fluid directly into the ejaculatory ducts. This fluid is rich in sugar and provides an energy source for the sperm. This fluid also contains **prostaglandins,** which may help the movement of sperm by promoting subtle uterine contractions. Seminal fluid makes up about 60 percent of the total volume of semen.

Prostate Gland. The **prostate gland** surrounds the urethra and is located directly beneath the bladder. It is about the size of a walnut. The fluid from the prostate gland helps to nourish the sperm and aids in their motility. Prostatic fluid makes up about 30 percent of the total volume of semen. The prostate gland also plays an important role by preventing urine and semen from mixing. During ejaculation, the internal sphincter contracts, thereby preventing the passage of urine from the bladder into the urethra. The external sphincter opens, thereby allowing semen to be ejaculated out of the urethra.

Cowper's Glands. **Cowper's glands** (also called the bulbourethral glands) are two pea-sized glands located on each side of the urethra just beneath the prostate gland. The alkaline fluid secreted by these glands helps to neutralize the normal acidity of the urethra, making it more hospitable for the passage of sperm. During sexual arousal, Cowper's glands are responsible for the pre-ejaculatory fluid that appears on the tip of the penis. This fluid contains live sperm cells, which probably accounts for many of the unplanned pregnancies that have occurred when withdrawal was used as the method of birth control.

■ Sexual Anatomy and Physiology: Female

The female reproductive system also consists of both internal and external organs. Unlike the male's, however, the female's external genitals are not readily visible. The female's external genitals, as well as the openings into the reproductive and urinary tracts, are enclosed and protected by folds of skin. The following section will discuss the anatomy and physiology of the female reproductive system.

External Genitals

Vulva. The collective name for the female's external genitals is the **vulva.** The vulva consists of the mons veneris, the labia majora, the labia minora, the vestibule, and the clitoris (illustrated in Figure 8–3).

Mons Veneris. The **mons veneris** (also called the mons pubis) is the area over the pubic bone consisting of a cushion of fatty tissue covered by skin and pubic hair. This area may be a source of sexual stimulation.

Labia Majora. The **labia majora** ("major lips") are two large folds of skin that enclose and protect the other external genitals. The outer surfaces of the labia majora are covered with pubic hair, sweat glands, and many nerve endings.

FIGURE 8–3 ■ External Structures of the Vulva

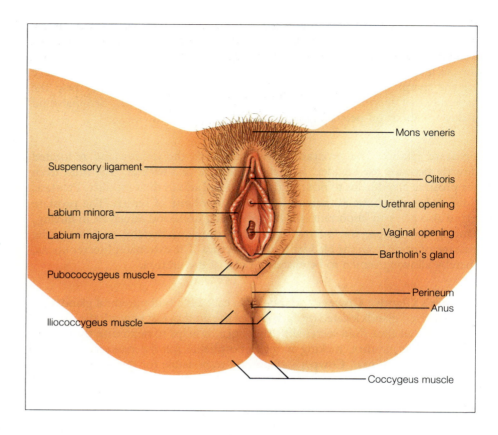

Labia Minora. The **labia minora** ("minor lips") are thin, hairless folds of skin lying within the labia majora. They enclose and protect the vaginal and urethral openings.

Vestibule. The **vestibule** consists of the area between the labia minora. Within this area are Skene's glands and Bartholin's glands (illustrated in Figure 8–3). Skene's glands are located on each side of the urethral opening. They secrete mucus to keep the vestibule moist. Bartholin's glands, which are located on each side of the vaginal opening, produce minimal amounts of alkaline lubrication.

Clitoris. The **clitoris** is a small organ composed of highly sensitive erectile tissue that is located just below the point where the labia minora converge at the top of the vulva. It is the most erotically sensitive part of the female anatomy.

Internal Organs

Vagina. The **vagina** is a hollow, muscular organ about three to four inches in length. In its normal state, its appearance is similar to a collapsed tube of toothpaste, but during sexual arousal or childbirth, its walls expand greatly. The vagina has three reproductive functions: (1) it receives the ejaculate during intercourse, (2) it provides an exit for menstrual fluid, and (3) it serves as the birth canal.

The entrance into the vagina has many nerve receptors; however, the inner two-thirds of the vagina is relatively insensitive to touch or pain. Recent attention has been given to an area located on the upper front wall of the vagina. This spot, the **Grafenberg Spot,** or **G-spot,** appears to be an area of erotic sensitivity for the female (illustrated in Figure 8–4.)

Hymen. The **hymen** is a thin connective-tissue membrane that partially covers the vaginal entrance of most women from birth until after first sexual intercourse. It has no known function. Hymens vary in shape and size. It was believed that the presence of an intact hymen was proof that a women had never had sexual intercourse. This is not a reliable indicator of virginity because other things, such as vigorous exercise, can rupture the hymen.

> ■ PROBLEM SITUATION   You have been in a monogamous relationship for several weeks, and the question of sexual intimacy has been raised. You are sexually inexperienced, and even though you care for the other person and feel a sexual attraction, you have been taught that sex before marriage is wrong. You feel confused, because part of you wants an intimate relationship, but the other part fears that intimacy will lead to loss of respect or rejection. What would you do at this point? Do you think that a male would prefer to marry a female who is a virgin or who is sexually experienced? What would a female prefer when selecting a marriage partner? What would be the advantages and disadvantages of marrying a virgin as compared to marrying a person who is sexually experienced?

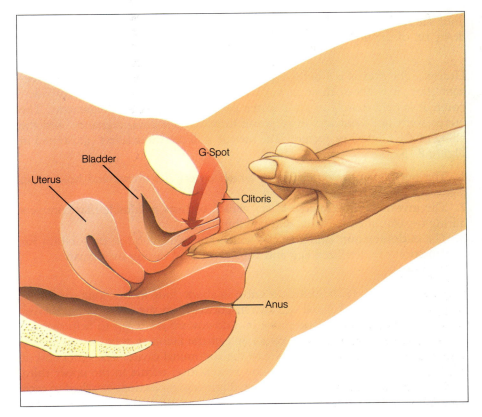

FIGURE 8–4 ■ **The Grafenberg Spot**

FIGURE Figure 8–5 ■ **Front View of the Female Reproductive Organs Showing the Relation of the Ovaries, Fallopian Tubes, Uterus, Cervix, and Vagina**

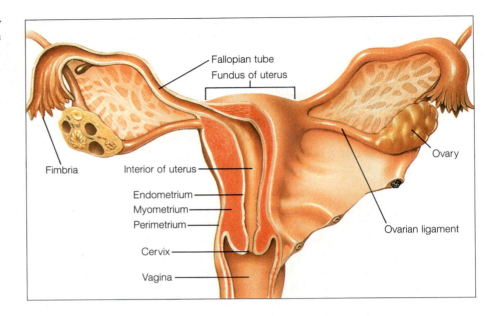

FAST FACTS

The cervix is one of the strongest muscles in the female body.

Cervix. The **cervix** is the lower end of the uterus that extends into the vagina. The opening of the cervix, which leads into the uterus, is called the cervical os. The cervix contains glands that secrete varying amounts of mucus. It is an extremely rigid muscle that cannot be penetrated by a penis during sexual intercourse. A woman can feel the cervix by inserting her finger into the vagina until she feels a firm, round projection. The feeling is similar to touching the fleshy tip of the nose.

Uterus. The **uterus** is a hollow, pear-shaped, muscular organ. In its nonpregnant state, it is about three inches long and two inches wide at its broadest point. It is held loosely in place in the pelvic cavity by several ligaments. The uterus shifts and contracts in response to sexual tension, pregnancy, and the filling of the bladder or rectum. The uterine wall has three layers (illustrated in Figure 8–5):

1. The **perimetrium** (outer layer), which covers the uterus and holds it in place.
2. The **myometrium** (middle layer), which consists of muscle that contracts during orgasm, menstruation, and childbirth.
3. The **endometrium** (inner layer), which fills with blood in preparation for implantation of a fertilized egg and is partially shed during menstruation.

Fallopian Tubes. Each **fallopian tube** is about four inches long, and it is through these tubes that the egg is transported from the ovary to the uterus. Cilia line the tube's walls and move in a downward direction to help the egg travel toward the uterus. The ovarian end of the fallopian tube is not directly connected to the ovary but opens into the abdominal cavity. The other end of the tube opens into the uterine cavity. Fertilization occurs in the upper third of the fallopian tube. **Fimbriae** are long, finger-like projections attached to each fallopian tube at the ovarian end. These projections hang over each ovary and act as a suction mechanism to direct the egg into the fallopian tube (see Figure 8–5).

Ovaries. The **ovaries** are the female gonads, or sex organs. These two small organs located on each side of the uterus are about the size and shape of an almond. They are held in place by connective tissue, which attaches to the broad ligament of the uterus. The ovaries have the dual function of producing eggs and the female sex hormones, estrogen and progesterone. (Figure 8–6 illustrates a side view of the female reproductive system.)

■ Hormones and Sexual Functioning

The production and secretion of hormones are essential for the normal development and functioning of the reproductive system in males and females. **Hormones** are chemicals produced by the endocrine glands. **Endocrine glands** are ductless glands that deliver their hormones directly into the bloodstream. There are six endocrine glands involved in sexual development and behavior: the **hypothalamus,** the **pituitary gland,** the **adrenal glands,** the testes, the ovaries, and the placenta. The hypothalamus is the primary controlling mechanism that triggers the production and secretion of sex hormones.

The hypothalamus releases a hormone called **gonadotropin-releasing factor** (GnRF). This hormone stimulates the pituitary gland to secrete two gonadotropins (hormones that affect only the testes and ovaries), which are called **follicle-stimulating hormone** (FSH) and **luteinizing hormone** (LH). Both FSH and LH are released cyclically in females and continuously in males. In males, FSH is responsible for causing the testes to produce sperm cells and LH

FAST FACTS

Each fallopian tube is approximately twice the thickness of a single strand of human hair.

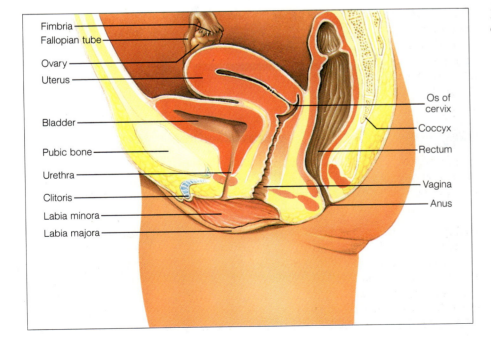

FIGURE Figure 8–6 ■ **Side View of the Female Reproductive Organs**

(also referred to as interstitial-cell-stimulating hormone (ICSH) in males) is responsible for inducing the production and secretion of testosterone. In females, FSH is responsible for stimulating follicle maturation and for causing the ovaries to produce estrogen; LH is responsible for triggering ovulation and for stimulating the empty follicle to produce progesterone. (Figure 8–7 summarizes this process.)

■ The Major Sex Hormones

The principal male sex hormone is testosterone, and the principal female sex hormones are estrogen and progesterone. Even though we frequently speak of these as being either male or female hormones, both sexes produce all three. It is the amount of each hormone produced that differentiates male from female.

Testosterone

Testosterone is a masculinizing sex hormone. It is present in both sexes; however, males produce substantially higher amounts. Testosterone is produced in

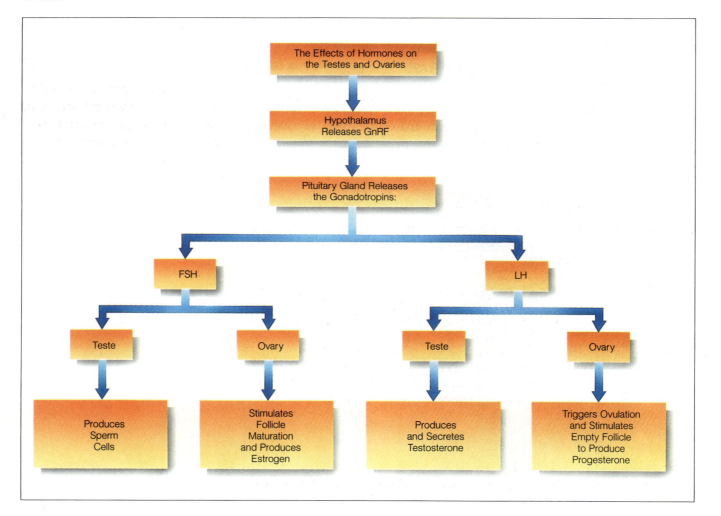

FIGURE Figure 8–7 ■ **The Effects of Hormones on the Testes and Ovaries**

the testes, and small amounts are produced in the ovaries and adrenal glands. In the male, testosterone stimulates the development of male primary and secondary sex characteristics. In the female, testosterone is responsible for the female patterns of body-hair development in the pubic and axillary (armpit) areas. Testosterone is responsible for sexual desire in both males and females. Without testosterone, there would be no sex drive.

Estrogen

Estrogen is a general name for feminizing sex hormones. Although it is present in both sexes, the amount produced in females is much higher. Estrogen is produced in the ovaries, and small amounts are produced in the testes and adrenal glands. In the female, estrogen maintains the elasticity of the vagina, produces vaginal lubrication, maintains the texture and function of the breasts, regulates the menstrual cycle, and stimulates the development of female primary and secondary sex characteristics. In the male, estrogen has no known function; however, it has been found that too much estrogen can decrease sexual desire, enlarge the breasts, and cause difficulties with erection.

Progesterone

Progesterone is a feminizing sex hormone. It is present in both sexes; but the amount produced in females is considerably higher. Progesterone is produced in the ovaries, and small amounts are produced in the testes and adrenal glands. In the female, progesterone stimulates the growth of the endometrium and prepares the endometrium for implantation of a fertilized egg. In the male, progesterone has no known function.

FAST FACTS

A female produces only about two tablespoons of estrogen and progesterone throughout her entire life span.

■ Sexual Preferences and Behaviors

The range of human sexual preferences and behaviors is quite diverse. This diversity has been the basis of many psychological, legal, and moral issues. Individuals seem to be concerned about knowing which sexual life-styles and behaviors are deemed normal, healthy, and morally and legally acceptable. As discussed in Chapter 7, what constitutes normal and healthy behavior depends on the standard from which you are judging that particular life-style. **Sexual preference** refers to erotic attraction toward people of the same gender, the opposite gender, or both genders. Americans often base "normalcy" on the statistical standard. According to this standard, whatever the majority of people engage in would be considered healthy and permissible; therefore, sexual intercourse between heterosexual individuals would be deemed acceptable. With heterosexuality and sexual intercourse established as the norm, other sexual preferences and behaviors are often considered to be abnormal, unhealthy, deviant, or perverse. Let's look at the types of sexual preferences that exist in our society.

- **Celibacy**—choosing not to share sexual activity with others.
- **Heterosexuality**—being sexually attracted to persons of the opposite sex.
- **Bisexuality**—being sexually attracted to members of both sexes.

- **Homosexuality**—being sexually attracted to persons of the same sex. The homosexual does not have a gender-identity conflict. For example, if the homosexual is anatomically a male, he perceives himself to be a male but is **psychosexually** attracted to persons of his own sex.
- **Transsexuality**—being sexually attracted to persons of the same sex. The transsexual's gender identity is different from his or her anatomical gender. For example, if the transsexual is biologically a male, even though he has male genitalia, he perceives himself to be a female who is *trapped* in a male's body. Therefore, although the transsexual cross-dresses and engages in sexual activities with persons of the same sex, the idea that a homosexual relationship is taking place does not exist in the transsexual's mind.

Whatever an individual's sexual preference may be, there are various ways of expressing oneself sexually. An individual may engage in *autoeroticism*, which involves solitary sexual activities. *Masturbation*, which is self-stimulation of the genitals, is the most common form of solitary sexual expression for the majority of Americans. *Mutual masturbation* involves sexual partners mutually stimulating each other's genitals. This behavior can serve as a prelude to other types of behaviors, such as *cunnilingus* (oral stimulation of the female genitals), *fellatio* (oral stimulation of the male genitals), *analingus*, (oral stimulation of the anus), anal intercourse, or sexual intercourse.

The Sexual Response Cycle

Whatever sexual preference a person has or whatever sexual behavior he or she decides to engage in, once aroused, all individuals tend to follow relatively predictable patterns of sexual response. Masters and Johnson were the first to provide an objective and detailed description of the human sexual response cycle. **Sexual response** refers to the series of changes in the body that take place as men and women become progressively more aroused. Masters and Johnson identified four phases in the sexual response cycle: *excitement, plateau, orgasm,* and *resolution*. Table 8–1 and Table 8–2 summarize the male and female responses, respectively, during each phase.

Masters and Johnson reported two major differences between male and female sexual responses. One was that men could ejaculate and women could not. The other was that females did not have the refractory period characteristic of males; women were capable of having a series of orgasms within a short period of time and men were not. Recent research now suggests that some women do ejaculate and some men are capable of multiple orgasms.

One of the most important conclusions of the Masters and Johnson data is that male and female sexual response patterns are fundamentally the same. In both sexes, the bodily changes that occur are due to **vasocongestion,** which is an increase of blood in the genital organs, and muscular tension.

When looking at the sexual response patterns of males and females, it is wise to remember the following considerations:

- Not everyone responds alike or neatly fits into this stereotypical model.
- An individual's day-to-day responses may vary according to internal and external factors.
- Although listed as four separate phases, the sexual response cycle should be viewed as a continuum with overlapping phases rather than as four distinct entities.

TABLE 8-1 ■ **Male Responses during the Sexual Response Cycle**

Excitement Phase

1. Vasocongestion (accumulation of blood) erects the penis.
2. Scrotal skin tightens.
3. Testes start to increase in size.
4. Testes and scrotum become elevated.
5. Nipples may become erect.
6. Some increase occurs in muscle tension, heart rate, and blood pressure.

Plateau Phase

1. There is a slight increase in the area of the glans penis.
2. Vasocongestion purples the glans.
3. Testes continue to elevate up into the scrotal sac until they are positioned close against the body.
4. Testes increase in size as much as 50 percent.
5. Cowper's glands secrete a few drops of fluid.
6. Possible **sex flush** and muscle tension are present, breathing is rapid, heart rate increases (100 to 160 beats per minute).

Orgasm

1. Contractions of the vas deferens, seminal vesicles, ejaculatory duct, and prostate gland cause semen to collect in the base of the urethra.
2. Collection of semen in the base of the urethra produces feelings of **ejaculatory inevitability.**
3. The internal sphincter in the prostate contracts, preventing passage of urine.
4. The external sphincter in the prostate relaxes, allowing passage of semen.
5. Contractions in the urethra propel the semen out of the penis. The contractions occur four or five times at intervals of eight-tenths of a second.
6. Muscles go into spasm throughout the body, respiration increases, blood pressure and heart rate reach a peak (about 180 beats per minute).

Resolution Phase

1. Body returns gradually to its prearoused state.
2. Male gradually loses his erection.
3. Testes and scrotum return to normal size.
4. Scrotum regains its wrinkled appearance.
5. Male enters a **refractory period** (unresponsive to further sexual stimulation).
6. Blood pressure, heart rate, and respiration become normal.
7. About one-third of males find their palms and soles or entire body covered with perspiration.

■ Sexual response patterns should not be evaluated from only a physiological and behavioral viewpoint. The emotional component must be included if we are to truly understand human sexual response.

■ A good sexual relationship should not be equated with the number of times an individual achieves orgasm. The *quality* of a mutually caring relationship is a far better indicator of a good sexual relationship than the *quantity* of orgasms achieved.

TABLE 8-2 ■ Female Responses during the Sexual Response Cycle

Excitement Phase

1. Vaginal lubrication begins.
2. Vasocongestion swells the external genitalia.
3. Labia majora flatten and retract from the vaginal opening.
4. Inner two-thirds of the vagina expands.
5. Vaginal walls thicken.
6. Breasts enlarge and blood vessels near the surface become more prominent.
7. Nipples become erect.
8. Muscle tension, heart rate, and blood pressure increase somewhat.

Plateau Phase

1. Vasocongestion produces a narrow vaginal pathway in the outer third of the vagina.
2. Inner part of the vagina expands fully.
3. Uterus becomes elevated.
4. Clitoris withdraws beneath the clitoral hood.
5. Rosy appearance may occur on the stomach, thighs, and back.
6. Nipples become more erect.
7. Muscles tense, breathing is rapid, and heart rate increases (100 to 160 beats per minute).

Orgasm

1. Swelling of the tissues of the outer part of the vagina constricts the vaginal opening.
2. Contractions begin in the outer third of the vagina. First contractions may last two to four seconds and later ones may last three to fifteen seconds. They occur at intervals of eight-tenths of a second.
3. Inner two-thirds of the vagina expands slightly.
4. Uterus contracts.
5. Muscles go into spasm throughout the body, respiration increases, blood pressure and heart rate reach a peak (about 180 beats per minute).

Resolution Phase

1. Blood is released from engorged areas.
2. Rosy appearance disappears.
3. Clitoris descends to normal position.
4. Vagina, uterus, and labia gradually shrink to normal size.
5. Blood pressure, heart rate, and respiration become normal.
6. About one-third of females find their palms and soles or entire body covered with perspiration.

■ The Menstrual Cycle

Menarche, or first menstruation, usually occurs between the ages of ten and eighteen, with the average age being twelve or thirteen. It is a normal part of the female reproductive cycle. Menstrual cycles usually end when a woman is between the ages of forty-eight and fifty-two. At this time, she is said to be experiencing menopause.

Most women think of menstruation as a three or four day occurrence that happens once a month. The word *menstruation* is derived from the Latin meaning "monthly." Menstruation, however, is just one phase of a woman's menstrual

CHAPTER 8 ■ SEXUAL BODYWORKS   211

cycle, which consists of a series of four overlapping processes: (a) *the follicular phase,* (b) *ovulation,* (c) *the luteal phase,* and (d) *menstruation.* (Figure 8–8 illustrates the four phases of the menstrual cycle.) Each of these phases is controlled by fluctuations in the amounts of estrogen and progesterone secreted into the bloodstream.

The length of each menstrual cycle varies among women. It can range from twenty-one to forty days, with the average being about twenty-eight days. Very few women are so regular that they can accurately and consistently predict the

FIGURE 8–8 ■ The Menstrual Cycle

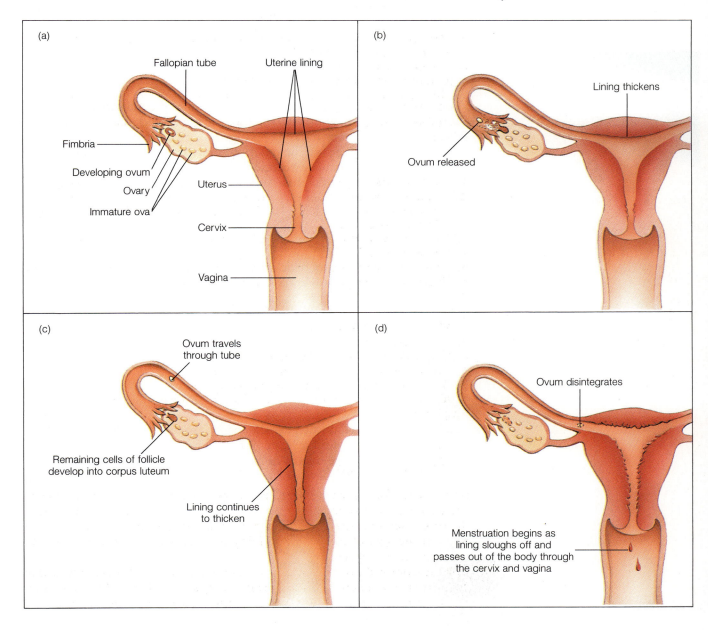

exact length of each cycle. Such factors as stress, poor diet, vigorous and excessive exercise, and illness can temporarily interfere with normal functioning of the menstrual cycle. When a female wants to calculate the number of days in her cycle, the first day of menstruation is usually counted as Day 1. The reason for this is that menstrual blood is a physical indicator that is simple and easy to detect. The other three phases do not have any tangible signs to indicate their occurrence.

Follicular Phase

The menstrual cycle begins when the pituitary gland secretes follicle-stimulating hormone (FSH), which in turn stimulates several follicles to ripen and mature within an ovary. This process of maturation occurs in the **follicular phase.** During this time, estrogen is being secreted from the follicles.

Ovulation

Toward the end of the follicular phase, the pituitary gland secretes luteinizing hormone (LH). This hormone triggers a mature follicle, called the Graafian follicle, to rupture, thus releasing an egg. This phase, called **ovulation,** occurs about fourteen days before the onset of menstruation. It is difficult to predict when a woman will ovulate because the number of days in each of her cycles can vary. It is during this phase that a woman can get pregnant if she is not using contraception.

Luteal Phase

After ovulation, the empty follicle, called the corpus luteum, secretes high levels of progesterone along with lower levels of estrogen. The progesterone stimulates the increased growth of the endometrium in preparation for the implantation of a fertilized egg. This is the **luteal phase.** If the egg does not implant in the endometrial wall within ten to twelve days, the corpus luteum disintegrates and stops producing hormones. As a result of the lower levels of progesterone, the endometrial lining degenerates.

Menstruation

The degeneration and discharge of the endometrial lining results in the shedding of blood, mucus, and dead cells; this is **menstruation.** Over the course of about four days, two or three ounces of menstrual fluid is shed. Toward the end of menstruation, the low levels of estrogen stimulate the production of FSH, thereby starting the cyclical process all over again.

> ■ *PROBLEM SITUATION* You are involved in a sexual relationship with your girlfriend. Would you be interested in learning about her menstrual cycle? If you feel awkward about asking questions, how might you approach the topic? Should the female initiate such a discussion?

Menstrual Synchrony

Pheromones are chemical substances externally secreted through the skin and other body openings. The presence of pheromones has been observed through the phenomenon of **menstrual synchrony.** It has been found that the menstrual cycles of females living or working in close proximity to one another begin to synchronize, so that after a few months, these females' menstrual cycles occur at the same time. In addition, those females who are close friends and who spend more time together develop menstrual synchronization within a shorter period of time. This suggests that odoriferous substances existing in one individual, not readily detectable on a conscious level, may trigger biological functions in another.

Other research suggests that females may vaginally secrete a pheromone called copulin during periods of sexual arousal and around the time of ovulation. This biological scent may be sexually arousing for males. Evidence is limited as to whether males secrete similar sexually arousing odors.

Menstrual Myths

The curse! How many times has a female heard this expression when she is menstruating? Much has been said about menstruation, and, unfortunately, most of it has been negative. Many primitive societies have attributed great powers to menstruation. For example:

> Menstrual blood has been known to cure leprosy, warts, birthmarks, gout, goiter, hemorrhoids, epilepsy, worms, and headache. It was effective as a love charm, could ward off river demons and other evil spirits, and was occasionally fit to be an honorific offering to a god. The first napkin worn by a virgin was to be saved for use as a cure for the plague. (Delaney, Lupton, and Toth, 1988)

In some primitive cultures, contact with a menstruating woman was thought to lead to bad luck in hunting. Therefore, during the fishing season, the men had to live in a canoe house and abstain from contact with women. Sound familiar? Today's hunting lodge, that "no-woman's-land of just being with the boys," may reflect this primitive taboo.

Now, you might be thinking to yourself how crazy this all sounds. No one could possibly believe these things! Well, equivalent beliefs persist to this day. Let's look at what modern men and women are saying about menstruation.

1. A woman cannot become pregnant if she has sexual intercourse while she is menstruating.
2. It is unhealthy for both partners to have sexual intercourse while the woman is menstruating.
3. A woman should not bathe while she is menstruating.
4. A woman must take an iron supplement to prevent anemia while she is menstruating.
5. A woman needs to rest and stay off her feet during menstruation.
6. A woman is less rational and more emotional during menstruation.

From the looks of things, modern men and women are not any more educated about the facts of menstruation than were primitive men and women. Let's briefly examine why each of the preceding statements is false.

1. Menstruation is not a reliable method of birth control. Some women ovulate while menstruating. Don't take foolish chances. It only takes one error in judgment to become pregnant.
2. There are no health reasons for avoiding intercourse while a woman is menstruating. The only issue is one of aesthetics. If one or both partners object to the blood, the couple may choose to abstain from sexual intercourse.
3. A woman's hygienic practices should not change just because she is menstruating. If anything, she should bathe more frequently to keep her genital area clean and free from odor.
4. The amount of iron lost in menstrual blood is minimal. If a woman is healthy and is eating a well-balanced diet, iron supplements are unnecessary. If, however, the woman is iron deficient to begin with, she should consult her physician about the need for supplements.
5. Unless there is an illness or health problem associated with menstruation, a healthy woman can continue doing all her usual activities. Remember, menstruation is not a sickness. It is a normal, healthy function.
6. Because of the fluctuations in hormonal levels, some women experience psychological distress just before or during menstruation. Treatment is available, however. To say that women are less rational and more emotional during menstruation is a generalization that does not apply to the majority of women.

It appears that the real "curse" has to do with the perpetuating ignorance associated with menstruation.

Toxic Shock Syndrome

Believed to be caused by a toxin produced by the bacterium *Staphylococcus aureus (S. aureus),* **toxic shock syndrome** (TSS) most frequently occurs in menstruating females who use highly absorbent tampons. Tampons are suspected of playing an important role in either helping the bacteria multiply or spreading its toxin. It is thought that the presence of the tampon in the vagina for a prolonged period of time may prevent air circulation, thus allowing the bacteria to proliferate. Also, menstrual blood provides a good medium for the growth and spread of the bacteria. Tampon use alone does not cause TSS. If a female who uses tampons doesn't have the bacteria present in the vagina, she is not at risk. It is the combination of menstruation, the presence of *S. aureus,* and the use of highly absorbent tampons that increases the risk of TSS. Characteristic warning signs of toxic shock syndrome may include a sudden fever of 102 degrees or higher, a sunburn-like rash, vomiting or diarrhea, a sudden drop in blood pressure, and possible shock. If any of these symptoms occur while a female is menstruating and using a tampon, she should remove the tampon immediately and contact her doctor.

Premenstrual Syndrome

Premenstrual syndrome (PMS), refers to the intense feelings of depression, irritability, tension, and fatigue that some women experience prior to menstruation. These symptoms occur several days before the onset of menstruation and usually subside by the time menstruation begins. Some physiological theories speculate that the causes of PMS include: low levels of progesterone in the bloodstream; increased fluid retention; a deficiency of B-complex vitamins; an

FAST FACTS

Alcohol is absorbed faster during the premenstrual phase of a female's cycle, so a female may find herself getting drunk faster right before menstruation.

GUIDELINES TO YOUR GOOD HEALTH

Wise precautionary measures that a female should follow when using tampons include the following:

1. Choose a tampon that is only as absorbent as you need. Some tampons are so absorbent that they dry the vagina, absorbing its normal secretions.
2. Change tampons every four to six hours, depending on need. Don't wear the same tampon all day and all night. This might encourage the growth of bacteria within the vagina. On the other hand, don't change tampons every half hour. This can be very irritating to the vagina.
3. Use a sanitary napkin instead of a tampon during bedtime hours.
4. Be wary of deodorant tampons. They may cause allergic reactions resulting in vaginal burning and itching. Also, it is unnecessary to "deodorize" the vagina. Menstrual blood has no odor until it reaches the air. Any internal vaginal odor may be a sign of infection; thus, instead of masking the odor, see your physician to determine the cause.
5. Don't use tampons when you are not menstruating. The tampon will absorb the normal vaginal secretions that are there to help protect your body from infection.

---

estrogen-progesterone imbalance; and an overproduction of prostaglandins. Some believe that the distress is linked to psychological factors. Negative attitudes toward menstruation and the expectation of menstrual discomfort may serve as a self-fulfilling prophecy. The specific cause of PMS is still unclear, and the number of women actually experiencing PMS is unknown.

Because the exact cause of PMS is not known, it is difficult to prescribe a treatment that will be effective for all women experiencing this syndrome. Some of the plausible treatment options include: low-dose combined oral contraceptives; minimizing salt, sugar, and fluid intake; taking diuretics; taking vitamin supplements; taking aspirin; reducing or eliminating caffeine intake; increasing exercise; and progesterone therapy. The FDA has approved only preliminary studies of progesterone therapy; more information is needed about its potential health hazards. To help determine the cause and possible treatment of PMS, a female experiencing major physical and psychological distress prior to menstruation should keep a record of the following information:

1. Her symptoms.
2. The number of days during which she has these symptoms.
3. What effect diet, exercise, and medications have on these symptoms.
4. The duration and severity of the menstrual period that follows.
5. The type of contraception used.

■ **PROBLEM SITUATION** You have a female friend who experiences PMS. What can you say and do to be supportive of her?

POSITIVE BEHAVIORS FOR MALES

I. *Place a check mark in front of each behavior that you now practice.*

_____ 1. I discourage negative jokes and comments about menstruation. (NEGATIVE COMMENTS)

_____ 2. I do not treat a female as if she is "ill" during the time she is menstruating. (ILL)

_____ 3. If I am having a sexual relationship with a female, I ask for information about her menstrual cycle. (MENSTRUAL CYCLE)

_____ 4. A method of birth control is used if I have sexual intercourse with a female during menstruation. (BIRTH CONTROL)

_____ 5. I encourage a female friend to contact her physician if she is experiencing major physical and psychological distress prior to menstruation. (DISTRESS)

_____ 6. I am sensitive to the problems of a female experiencing premenstrual syndrome. (PMS)

_____ 7. I do not judge my sexual ability on the basis of penis size. (SIZE)

_____ 8. I keep the glans area of the penis clean. (CLEAN)

_____ 9. If birth control is not being used, I avoid genital contact with a female when pre-ejaculatory fluid appears on the tip of the penis. (PRE-EJACULATORY FLUID)

_____ 10. I do routine self-examinations for testicular abnormalities. (SELF-EXAMS)

II. *For each behavior that you DO NOT ENGAGE IN, write the KEY WORD(S) located in the parentheses at the end of the statement in the column below. Then put a check mark in the appropriate column to indicate whether you are going to keep or change that behavior.*

Behaviors I Don't Engage In   KEEP/CHANGE

_____   _____/_____
_____   _____/_____
_____   _____/_____
_____   _____/_____
_____   _____/_____
_____   _____/_____
_____   _____/_____
_____   _____/_____
_____   _____/_____

III. *For each of the preceding behaviors that you choose to KEEP, write a statement indicating why you are choosing to keep that behavior.*

I choose to keep behavior _____ because:
                           KEY WORD

For each of the preceding behaviors that you choose to CHANGE, write a statement indicating how you plan to implement that change.

I will change behavior _____ by:
                         KEY WORD

POSITIVE BEHAVIORS FOR FEMALES

I. *Place a check mark in front of each behavior that you now practice.*

_____ 1. I do not use highly absorbent tampons. (HIGHLY ABSORBENT)

_____ 2. I use a sanitary napkin instead of a tampon during bedtime hours. (SANITARY NAPKIN)

_____ 3. I change tampons or sanitary napkins frequently during menstruation. (CHANGE FREQUENTLY)

_____ 4. I use birth control if I have sexual intercourse during menstruation. (BIRTH CONTROL)

_____ 5. I bathe more frequently during menstruation. (BATHE)

_____ 6. I continue doing all my usual activities during menstruation. (USUAL ACTIVITIES)

_____ 7. I keep a record of the length of each menstrual cycle. (RECORD)

_____ 8. I contact my physician if I experience major physical and psychological distress prior to menstruation. (DISTRESS)

_____ 9. I do not judge a male's sexual ability on the basis of penis size. (SIZE)

_____ 10. I have yearly gynecological examinations. (EXAMS)

II. *For each behavior that you DO NOT ENGAGE IN, write the KEY WORD(S) located in the parentheses at the end of the statement in the column below. Then put a check mark in the appropriate column to indicate whether you are going to keep or change that behavior.*

Behaviors I Don't Engage In   KEEP/CHANGE

_____/_____

_____/_____

_____/_____

_____/_____

_____/_____

_____/_____

_____/_____

_____/_____

_____/_____

_____/_____

III. *For each of the preceding behaviors that you choose to KEEP, write a statement indicating why you are choosing to keep that behavior.*

I choose to keep behavior _____ because:
KEY WORD

For each of the preceding behaviors that you choose to CHANGE, write a statement indicating how you plan to implement that change.

I will change behavior _____ by:
KEY WORD

Now You Know

1. **FALSE.** There is no correlation between penis size and sexual satisfaction.
2. **FALSE.** The testicles have the dual function of producing sperm and the male sex hormone, testosterone.
3. **FALSE.** The collective name for the female's external genitals is the vulva.
4. **TRUE.** The majority of vaginal nerve endings are located in the outer third of the vagina.
5. **TRUE.** Estrogen is present in both sexes; however, the amount produced in females is significantly higher.
6. **TRUE.** Without testosterone, there would be no sex drive.
7. **FALSE.** Ovulation occurs about fourteen days before the onset of menstruation, but the time of occurrence is variable.
8. **FALSE.** The hypothalamus is the primary controlling mechanism that triggers the production and secretion of sex hormones.
9. **FALSE.** Tampon use alone does not cause toxic shock syndrome. Tampons are suspected of playing an important role in either helping the bacteria multiply or spreading their toxin.
10. **TRUE.** PMS refers to premenstrual syndrome. Symptoms occur several days before the onset of menstruation and usually subside by the time menstruation begins.

Summary

1. The male reproductive system consists of both internal and external organs. The male's external genitals are the penis and scrotum. The male's internal reproductive organs are the testes and the epididymis. The testes are the male's gonads, or sex organs.
2. The male's genital ducts include the vas deferens, ejaculatory ducts, and urethra. The male's fluid-producing glands include the seminal vesicles, the prostate gland, and Cowper's glands.
3. The female reproductive system also consists of both internal and external organs. The collective name for the female's external genitals is the vulva. The vulva consists of the mons veneris, the labia majora, the labia minora, the vestibule, and the clitoris.
4. The female's internal organs are the vagina, uterus, fallopian tubes, and ovaries. The ovaries are the female's gonads, or sex organs.
5. Hormones are essential for the normal development and functioning of the reproductive system in males and females. Hormones are produced by the endocrine glands. The endocrine glands that are involved in sexual development and behavior include the hypothalamus, the pituitary gland, the adrenal glands, the testicles, the ovaries, and the placenta. The hypothalamus triggers the production and secretion of sex hormones.
6. The pituitary gland secretes FSH and LH. These two hormones affect only the testicles and ovaries. In males, FSH is responsible for causing the testes to produce sperm cells. In females, FSH is responsible for stimulating follicle maturation and for causing the ovaries to produce estrogen. In males, LH is responsible for causing the testes to produce and secrete testosterone. In females, LH is responsible for triggering ovulation and for stimulating the empty follicle to produce progesterone.
7. The major sex hormones are testosterone, estrogen, and progesterone. Testosterone is a masculinizing hormone. It is present in both sexes. The greatest amount is produced in the testicles, and smaller amounts are produced in the ovaries and adrenal glands. Testosterone is responsible for sexual desire in both males and females.
8. Estrogen is a general name for feminizing sex hormones and is present in both sexes. The greatest amount is produced in the ovaries, and smaller amounts are produced in the testicles and adrenal glands.
9. Sexual response refers to the series of changes that take place in the body as men and women become progressively more aroused. Masters and Johnson identified four phases in the sexual response cycle: excitement, plateau, orgasm, and resolution.
10. Menarche, or first menstruation, usually occurs between the ages of ten and eighteen. The menstrual cycle is a series of four overlapping processes consisting of the follicular phase, ovulation, the luteal phase, and menstruation. The length of each menstrual cycle varies among women, with the average being about twenty-eight days.
11. It has been found that the menstrual cycles of females living or working together begin to synchronize, so that after a few months, they occur at the same time. This phenomenon is known as menstrual synchrony. Pheromones, which are chemical substances externally secreted through pores and body openings, are responsible for this occurrence.

12. Toxic shock syndrome (TSS) is believed to be caused by a toxin that is produced by a bacteria. It most frequently occurs in menstruating females who use highly absorbent tampons.

13. Premenstrual syndrome (PMS) refers to the intense feelings of depression, irritability, tension, and fatigue that some women experience prior to menstruation.

References

1. Bell, Ruth, *Changing Bodies, Changing Lives*. New York: Vintage Books, 1988.
2. Bender, Stephanie DeGraff. *PMS: Questions and Answers*. Los Angeles: The Body Press, 1989.
3. Byer, Curtis O., Louis W. Shainberg, and Kenneth L. Jones. *Human Sexuality,* 2d ed. Dubuque, Ia.: William C. Brown, 1988.
4. Delaney, Janice, Mary Jane Lupton, and Emily Toth. *The Curse: A Cultural History of Menstruation*. Urbana, Il.: University of Illinois Press, 1988.
5. Greenberg, Jerrold S., Clint E. Bruess, Kathleen D. Mullen, and Doris W. Sands. *Sexuality: Insights and Issues,* 2d ed. Dubuque, Ia.: William C. Brown, 1989.
6. Haas, Kurt, and Adelaide Haas. *Understanding Sexuality*. St. Louis: Times Mirror/Mosby College Publishing, 1987.
7. Jones, Richard E. *Human Reproduction and Sexual Behavior*. Englewood Cliffs, N.J.: Prentice-Hall, 1984.
8. Katchadourian, Herant A. *Biological Aspects of Human Sexuality,* 3d ed. New York: Holt, Rinehart and Winston, 1987.
9. Kelly, Gary F. *Sexuality Today: The Human Perspective*. Guilford, Conn.: The Dushkin Publishing Group, 1988.
10. Masters, William H., Virginia E. Johnson, and Robert C. Kolodny. *Human Sexuality,* 3d ed. Glenview, Il.: Scott, Foresman and Co., 1988.
11. Masters, William H., and Virginia E. Johnson. *Human Sexual Response*. New York: Bantam Books, 1986.
12. Nass, Gilbert D., and Mary Pat Fisher. *Sexuality Today*. Boston: Jones and Bartlett, 1988.
13. Rice, Philip F. *Human Sexuality*. Dubuque, Ia.: William C. Brown, 1989.
14. Taguchi, Yosh. *Private Parts: A Doctor's Guide to the Male Anatomy*. New York: Doubleday, 1988.

Suggested Readings

Bell, Ruth. *Changing Bodies, Changing Lives*. New York: Vintage Books, 1988.

Bender, Stephanie DeGraff. *PMS: Questions and Answers*. Los Angeles: The Body Press, 1989.

Delaney, Janice, Mary Jane Lupton, and Emily Toth. *The Curse: A Cultural History of Menstruation*. Urbana, Il.: University of Illinois Press, 1988.

Hite, Shere. *The Hite Report: A Nationwide Study of Female Sexuality*. New York: Dell Publishing Co., 1987.

Hite, Shere. *The Hite Report on Male Sexuality*. New York: Ballantine Books, 1988.

Jovanovic, Lois, and Genell J. Subak-Sharpe. *Hormones: The Woman's Answerbook*. New York: Fawcett-Columbine, 1987.

CHAPTER 9

Family Planning

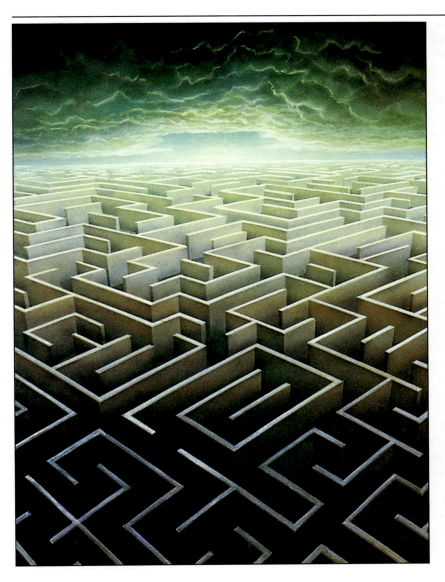

What Do You Know?

Are the following statements true or false?

1. Any technique, drug, or device used to prevent conception, implantation, or birth is considered to be contraception.
2. A vasectomy is a form of male sterilization that interferes with sperm production.
3. Estrogen, which is present in the combined birth-control pill, is responsible for inhibiting ovulation.
4. Petroleum jelly, such as vaseline, should never be used to lubricate a condom.
5. A diaphragm must be removed within six hours after the last act of sexual intercourse to minimize the risk of infection.
6. The contraceptive sponge should not be used during menstruation.
7. A spermicidal foam can be inserted into the vagina up to one hour before sexual intercourse occurs.
8. If you are looking for a 100-percent safe and effective method of birth control, it doesn't exist.
9. Severe chest pain, severe headaches, and leg pain in the calf or thigh may be early danger signals of problems caused by the birth-control pill.
10. Withdrawal is not considered to be a reliable birth-control alternative.

Are you reliable? Can you be trusted or depended on? Are you morally, legally, and mentally accountable for your actions? If you have answered "yes," then, by definition, you are a responsible individual. We are all quick to take the credit for being the one responsible when something good results from a situation, but when something negative occurs, we are quick to pass the buck and put the responsibility on someone else. A truly responsible individual has a sense of duty or obligation and stands accountable for his or her behaviors no matter what the consequences.

▰ Responsible Sexual Behavior

More than one million American teenage girls become pregnant each year. The United States has a higher rate of teenage pregnancies than anywhere in the developed world. If current trends continue, 40 percent of today's fourteen-year-old girls will be pregnant at least once before age twenty. Responsibility is extremely important in regard to sexuality. Along with greater sexual freedoms come greater sexual responsibilities. Are you prepared to take on such responsibilities?

> ▰ *PROBLEM SITUATION* You have decided that you want a sexual relationship. What would be your responsibilities to both yourself and your partner?

FAST FACTS

Only one in three sexually active young women in the United States always uses contraception.

Responsible sexual behavior could mean the difference between sickness and health, life and death. The best way to approach your sexual responsibility is with honesty and openness. Decide what your attitudes and feelings are, and be honest with yourself. Being honest means deciding what's best for you. That decision must come from within yourself. Decision making is often difficult. Every decision has some risks connected to it, but you have to weigh the advantages and disadvantages to decide what risks you are willing to take. What happens to you is ultimately a result of your own actions. Don't let others determine the destiny of your health and life. You must think for yourself, and even though you are faced with thousands of choices, you must act with the courage of your convictions to be a responsible individual.

Whether or not you are going to be sexually active is your decision. If you *are* going to be sexually active, however, it is important for you to acknowledge that decision. Acknowledgment is the first step toward sexual responsibility. The question of contraception is the next step. Talking about contraception with your partner is a way of sharing responsibility and intimacy. Don't be afraid to communicate your feelings to your partner. If you and your partner are mature enough to be involved in a sexual relationship, you should be mature enough to share all your questions, doubts, and anxieties with each other. If you are hesitant to talk these concerns over with your partner, maybe you need to reconsider your relationship.

If you feel awkward and uneasy about discussing contraception, it helps to sort out your own feelings before talking with your partner. Find out about what methods of contraception are available and the advantages and disadvantages of using each one. You'll find that each method has its good and bad points. The most important thing to ask yourself is, "Which method is best for me?" Don't be afraid to ask questions. Contact professionals at health-care clinics who can provide you with accurate information. You will be able to communicate more effectively with your partner when you know the facts.

Remember, if you decide to wait for the perfect, spontaneous moment to initiate such a discussion with your partner, that moment may never come. Plan to sit down with your partner in a private, nonthreatening atmosphere when there is sufficient time for both of you to discuss your feelings. Don't worry if bringing up the topic seems "unromantic" or "forward." Any honest, responsible relationship that includes sex also includes contraception. The contraceptive decisions you make now—or fail to make—may affect the rest of your life. All you need is one unprotected instance of sexual intercourse to change your life forever. Don't assume that your partner will be offended or angry if you want to discuss birth control. If you or your partner are too embarrassed, shy, or insecure to include contraception in your relationship, you had better postpone that relationship until both of you grow up.

Birth Control versus Contraception

Because "contra" means "against," **contraception** means "against conception." Conception occurs when a sperm fertilizes an egg. Therefore, a technique, drug, or device used to prevent conception is considered to be contraception. **Birth control,** however, means "to control the birth process." This encompasses a broader spectrum of options than just preventing conception. The birth process can be altered at any point from the time prior to conception up until the actual birth of the fetus. Therefore, any technique, drug, or device used to prevent conception, implantation, or birth is considered to be birth control. All contraceptive methods would be considered birth control; however, not all birth-control methods would qualify as contraception. The two terms have been used synonymously, but, as you can see, there is a difference by definition. This difference can be of major importance to an individual who believes that life begins at the time of conception. This particular individual may have no objections to using a contraceptive method but may strongly object to using a birth-control method that might interfere with the implantation or birth process. As we examine the various contraceptives available today, we will also identify which methods are actually birth control rather than contraception.

> *PROBLEM SITUATION* Suppose you had the ability and resources to invent the ideal method of birth control. What would it be? How would it differ from what is already available? Which sex would be responsible for using it? What would be its advantageous features?

Birth-Control Options

There are many methods of birth control available today. The one that a person chooses depends on personal and health considerations. An individual's decisions about birth control can depend on such factors as age, relationship status, religious beliefs, sexual attitudes, medical history, availability and convenience of various methods, and knowledge of and previous experiences with specific methods. The main reason for using birth control is to prevent an unintended pregnancy. With the high incidence of sexually transmitted diseases, certain methods are becoming increasingly popular because of their ability to afford protection against such diseases.

How do you go about choosing a method of birth control? If you are looking for a 100-percent safe and effective method, you'll never find it. Each method has its advantages and disadvantages. When determining which method is best for you, you should consider how effective it is, how safe it is, and if it can be easily incorporated into your life-style. Answering the following questions will help you in your decision-making process:

1. How does each method work?
2. How effective are the methods that I am considering?

SELF-INVENTORY 9.1

What Is Your Attitude about Birth Control?

Read the following statements and respond by placing a check mark in the column that expresses your current attitude about birth control.

Agree　Disagree　Unsure

1. I feel that using birth control takes the fun out of sex.
2. I feel that using birth control is the female's responsibility.
3. I feel that using birth control is the male's responsibility.
4. I feel that using birth control is the responsibility of both partners.
5. I feel that discussing birth control with my partner is uncomfortable and embarrassing.
6. I feel that a birth-control method should be used every time a couple is sexually intimate (unless pregnancy is the desired outcome).
7. I would not feel concerned if I or my female partner became pregnant.
8. I feel that it is important to have a backup method of birth control readily available.
9. I feel that one of the worst things that could happen to me or my female partner is to become pregnant.
10. I would not feel upset if I or my female partner became pregnant because I believe in abortion as a birth-control option.
11. I feel that there are enough adequate birth-control methods available to use.

3. What are the inherent dangers of each method?
4. Am I aware of the contraindications of the methods that I am considering?
5. Have I had difficulties with any methods in the past?
6. How might each method affect my sexuality?
7. How inconvenient are the methods that I am considering?
8. Is sexual spontaneity important to me?
9. Am I fearful of any methods?
10. How do I feel about touching my genital area?
11. How often do I have sexual intercourse?
12. How many sexual partners do I have?
13. How do my partner and I feel about an unplanned pregnancy?
14. How much cooperation can I expect from my partner?
15. Do I want children in the future?

12. I feel that using birth control is an act against nature. _____ _____ _____
13. I feel that there are no suitable methods of birth control available for my needs and lifestyle. _____ _____ _____
14. I feel that I keep myself well-informed about the different methods of birth control. _____ _____ _____
15. I feel that using birth control takes the spontaneity out of lovemaking. _____ _____ _____
16. I feel that adolescents should receive birth-control education. _____ _____ _____

Scoring:

If you answered "Agree" to questions 4, 6, 8, 9, 11, 14, and 16, this is the interpretation:

If you answered six to seven of these questions with "Agree" your attitude about birth control is "very responsible."

If you answered four to five of these questions with "Agree," your attitude about birth control is "responsible."

If you answered three or fewer of these questions with "Agree" or "Unsure," your attitude about birth control is "uncertain."

If you answered "Agree" to questions 1, 2, 3, 5, 7, 10, 12, 13, and 15, this the interpretation:

If you answered eight to nine of these questions with "Agree" your attitude about birth control is "very irresponsible."

If you answered five to seven of these questions with "Agree," your attitude about birth control is "irresponsible."

If you answered four or fewer of these questions with "Agree" or "Unsure," your attitude about birth control is "uncertain."

TABLE 9-1 ■ First-Year Failure Rates of Birth-Control Methods

Method	Theoretical Failure Rate(%)[a]	Actual Failure Rate(%)[b]
Tubal ligation	0.04	0.04
Vasectomy	0.1	0.15
Combined oral contraceptives	0.5	2.0
Progestin-only pill (mini-pill)	1.0	2.5
Intrauterine device (IUD)	1.5	6
Condom	2	12
Diaphragm (with spermicide)	3	18
Vaginal sponge	5–8	18–28
Cervical cap (with spermicide)	5	18
Spermicides (foams, creams, jellies, and vaginal suppositories	3	21
Coitus interruptus (withdrawal)	4	18
Fertility awareness techniques (basal body temperature, mucous method, and calendar method)	2–20	24
Douche	—[c]	40
Chance (no method of birth control)	89	89

[a]Designed to complete the sentence: "In one hundred women who use a given method and who use it correctly and consistently, the lowest percentage expected to experience an accidental pregnancy during the first year will be _____."

[b]Designed to complete the sentence: "In one hundred *typical* women who use a given method, the percentage who experience an accidental pregnancy during the first year will be _____."

[c]There is no theoretical failure rate data because douching is not considered to be a birth control method.

SOURCE: Data from Robert A. Hatcher, et al., *Contraceptive Technology* (New York: Irvington Publishers, 1988); Nancy W. Denney and David Quadagno, *Human Sexuality* (St. Louis: Times Mirror/Mosby College Publishing, 1988); and Albert Allgeier and Elizabeth Rice Allgeier, *Sexual Interactions* (Lexington, Mass.: D.C. Heath and Co., 1988).

Method effectiveness is a high priority when considering what method of birth control to use. Table 9–1 compares **theoretical failure rates** with **actual failure rates** for some of the most commonly used birth-control methods. If people were to use a method consistently and correctly at all times, the theoretical effectiveness rate would convey an accurate picture. Theoretical effectiveness, however, does not take into account human error. Lack of user knowledge of correct method use, negative attitudes about using the method, forgetting to use the method, or deciding that "just this once won't matter," greatly reduces effectiveness. A method of birth control is only as dependable as the person using it; therefore, the actual effectiveness rate portrays a more realistic picture.

▰ Method: Tubal Ligation

Theoretical Failure Rate: 0.04%
Actual Failure Rate: 0.04%

How Method Works: A small portion of each fallopian tube is cut out, and the ends are then either tied or cauterized. This prevents sperm from reaching the egg so that fertilization cannot occur (illustrated in Figure 9–1).

How to Use: This procedure usually involves an overnight hospital stay, anesthesia, and a recovery period. Postoperative recovery may take two to three days, but once coitus is resumed, there is no need to worry about birth-control protection.

Birth Control, Contraceptive, or Both? Because tubal ligation prevents the union of sperm and egg, it would be considered both a birth-control and a contraceptive method.

Advantages:
1. Is highly reliable.
2. The production of hormones and the menstrual cycle are unaffected.
3. Appears to have no physiological effect on sexual desire or response.
4. Allows spontaneity in lovemaking.

Disadvantages:
1. Is an irreversible procedure.
2. As with any surgical procedure and use of anesthesia, there is some risk involved.
3. Possible postoperative discomfort and/or infection may occur.
4. Is an expensive procedure.

Precautions: If there are postoperative complications, contact your physician immediately. Possible signs of infection would be fever, severe abdominal pain, hemorrhaging, yellowish vaginal discharge, or foul-smelling odor.

Contraindications: Tubal ligation is generally not recommended for women who are undecided about having children.

FAST FACTS

By 1982, sterilization had become the most prevalent method of contraception among married women in the United States.

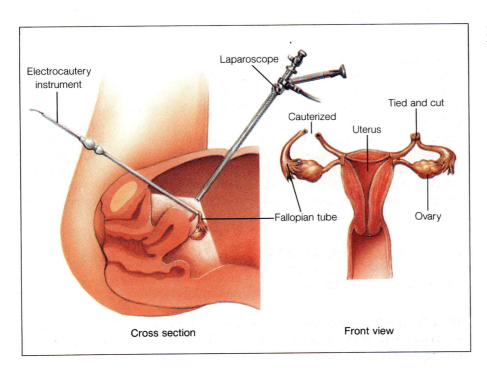

FIGURE 9–1 ■ **Tubal Ligation Using Laparoscope**

GUIDELINES TO YOUR GOOD HEALTH

Once you have chosen a contraceptive method, you can help to ensure maximum effectiveness by doing the following:

1. Making sure that you have selected a method that fits your life-style.
2. Using the method every time.
3. Always having a backup method readily available.
4. Consulting your physician if any problems occur.

Additional Comments about Tubal Ligation: The most commonly used method for tubal ligation is **laparoscopy**. A long, tubelike instrument called a **laparoscope** is inserted into the abdomen through an incision in the well of the navel. Through this instrument, the doctor is able to locate each fallopian tube and then cut and cauterize it. The incision is so small that only a Band-Aid is needed to cover it. That's why this procedure is often referred to as a "Band-Aid operation."

Method: Vasectomy

Theoretical Failure Rate: 0.1%
Actual Failure Rate: 0.15%

How Method Works: A small incision is made on each side of the scrotum. Through each incision, a section of the vas deferens is cut and then tied or cauterized (illustrated in Figure 9–2). Sperm are still produced, but they can no longer be transported by the vas deferens. Instead the sperm are absorbed and eliminated by the body. Since sperm account for only a small percentage of the total volume of semen, most men do not notice any difference when they ejaculate.

How to Use: This is a short procedure that is performed in the doctor's office. A local anesthetic is injected into the scrotum. Postoperative recovery is minimal. Another form of birth control should be used until two semen specimens have been confirmed to be sperm-free.

Birth Control, Contraceptive, or Both? Because a vasectomy prevents the union of sperm and egg, it would be considered both a birth-control and a contraceptive method.

Advantages:
1. Is highly reliable.
2. The production of hormones is not affected.
3. Does not affect erection or ejaculation.
4. Allows spontaneity in lovemaking.

Disadvantages:
1. Is an irreversible procedure.
2. As with any surgical procedure and use of anesthesia, there is some risk involved.

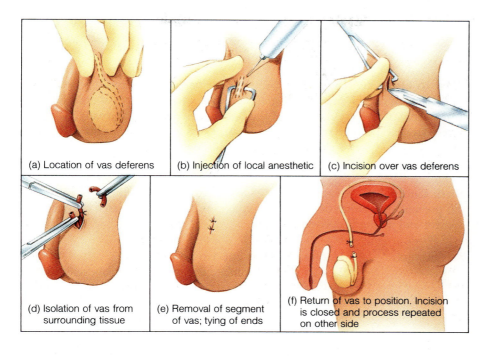

FIGURE 9-2 ■ Vasectomy

        3. Possible postoperative discomfort and/or infection may occur.
        4. Is an expensive procedure.

Precautions: 1. Immediately after the procedure, the male may experience pain and swelling in and around the testicles. Using ice packs may alleviate some of the discomfort.
        2. If there are signs of infection, contact your physician immediately.

Contraindications: A vasectomy is generally not recommended for men who are undecided about having children.

Additional Comments about Vasectomy: Even though there have been cases in which vasectomies were reversed so that males became fertile again, there is no guarantee of success. One of the major problems complicating reversibility is the tendency of many men to develop antibodies to their own sperm following a vasectomy. Until evidence proves to the contrary, a vasectomy should be considered a permanent, irreversible procedure.

▮ Method: Combined Oral Contraceptives

Theoretical Failure Rate: 0.5%
Actual Failure Rate: 2.0%

How Method Works: 1. Estrogen inhibits ovulation.
        2. Both estrogen and progestin alter the endometrium, thereby preventing implantation of any possible fertilized egg.
        3. Estrogen may accelerate ovum transport.

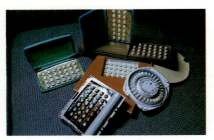

There are a variety of oral contraceptives available. A female's physician will prescribe the brand that is best suited to her.

4. Progestin causes thickening of cervical mucus, thereby hindering the transport of sperm from the vagina into the uterus.

How to Use: One pill is taken every day for twenty-one days. The first pill is usually taken on the fifth day of the menstrual cycle. The pill should be taken at the same time every day so that the hormone level remains steady. Then, for seven days, no pills are taken. (Some women prefer to take placebo pills during this time so that they won't get out of the pill-taking regimen.) Bleeding, similar to menstruation, occurs during this time.

Birth Control, Contraceptive, or Both? Because the combined birth-control pill prevents the union of sperm and egg, it would be considered both a birth-control and a contraceptive method.

Advantages:
1. Has very high effectiveness rate.
2. Can help to regulate irregular menstrual cycles.
3. Can help to reduce menstrual cramping.
4. Is convenient and easy to use.
5. Doesn't interrupt lovemaking.
6. Found to protect women from endometrial and epithelial ovarian cancers.

Disadvantages: User may experience some common side effects, such as nausea, weight gain, breast enlargement and tenderness, headaches, hypertension, spotty darkening of facial skin, fatigue, and depression.

Precautions:
1. Use an additional method of birth control during the first three weeks of taking the Pill.
2. There are many different brands of pills, and they are not all taken in exactly the same way. Be sure that you understand how to take your particular pills before leaving your doctor's office.
3. If you forget to take one pill, take it as soon as you remember and then continue taking the rest as scheduled.
4. If you forget to take two pills in a row, double up on your pills for the next two days and then continue taking the rest as scheduled. However, you must also use an additional method of birth control for the remainder of that cycle.
5. If you forget to take three or more pills in a row, don't try to catch up. Never take three birth-control pills at one time. Discard the package of pills and use another method of birth control for the remainder of that cycle. Missing three consecutive pills will probably trigger ovulation. At this point, you should reevaluate whether you are responsible enough to use the Pill as your method of birth control.
5. Because the Pill depletes the body of certain vitamins and minerals, increase your intake of B_2, B_6, B_{12}, folic acid, C, and zinc.
6. If you want to become pregnant, stop taking the Pill and use another method of birth control for three months

before trying to conceive. This gives the body a chance to return to normal hormonal levels.

7. If you experience any of the following early danger signals, contact your physician immediately:
    a. Severe abdominal pain.
    b. Severe chest pain, shortness of breath, or difficulty in breathing.
    c. Severe headaches.
    d. Eye problems (blurred vision, double vision, loss of vision, or flashing sensations)
    e. Leg pain in the calf or thigh.

Contraindications: The combined oral contraceptive is generally not recommended for a woman with the following characteristics:

1. Age 35 or over
2. Smokes cigarettes
3. Has a medical history of cancer, liver or heart disease, blood-clotting disorders, or high blood pressure.

(The more of the preceding characteristics a woman has, the greater her risk.)

Additional Comments about Combined Oral Contraceptives: In 1960, the FDA approved the use of estrogen and progestin for contraceptive purposes. These pills were called combined oral contraceptives. It became evident by the late 1960s that the amounts of estrogen and progestin found in the Pill were too high. Women taking these pills were experiencing side effects and complications. Most of the serious side effects were estrogen-related. Present brands of combined oral contraceptives contain lower and safer amounts of estrogen and progestin. Even though these lower-dose pills lessen the risk of complications, women need to be aware of the early danger signals associated with taking the Pill.

GUIDELINES TO YOUR GOOD HEALTH

It is inadvisable for females to use oral contraceptives if they have or previously had any of the following conditions:*

1. Blood clots in the legs, lungs, or elsewhere in the body
2. Chest pains on exertion
3. Known or suspected cancer of the breast or reproductive organs
4. Unusual vaginal bleeding that has not been diagnosed
5. Known or suspected pregnancy
6. Heart attack or stroke
7. Liver tumor

*If a female has a scanty or irregular menstrual period and decides to use oral contraceptives, she may have difficulty becoming pregnant after discontinuing the Pill.

> **FAST FACTS**
>
> Research on mini-pill users has shown that ovulation is prevented in only 15 to 40 percent of cycles.

Method: Progestin-Only Pill (Mini-Pill)

Theoretical Failure Rate: 1.0%
Actual Failure Rate: 2.5%

How Method Works: The mini-pill contains a smaller amount of the progestin used in combined birth-control pills but does not contain any estrogen.

1. Progestin alters the endometrium, thereby preventing implantation of any possible fertilized egg.
2. Progestin causes thickening of cervical mucus, thereby hindering the transport of sperm from the vagina into the uterus.
3. Ovulation may be inhibited by a disturbance in the hormonal cycle.

How To Use: One pill is taken each day of the month, even during menstruation. The first pill is taken on the day menstruation begins. A woman never stops taking mini-pills. When one packet of mini-pills is finished, the next packet is started the next day.

Birth Control, Contraceptive, or Both? Because ovulation may be inhibited and the thick, dry cervical mucus acts as a barrier to sperm, the union of sperm and egg is quite unlikely. The mini-pill would be considered both a birth-control and a contraceptive method.

Advantages:
1. Causes fewer side effects because it does not contain estrogen.
2. Other advantages are similar to those obtained from the combined pill.

Disadvantages:
1. Is not quite as effective as the combined pill.
2. User may experience such side effects as spotting between periods, irregular menses, edema, irritability, and depression.

Precautions:
1. Because ovulation may still occur, consider using a back-up method of birth control during mid-cycle.
2. If menstruation does not occur within forty-five days from last menstrual period, contact your physician.
3. The same early danger signals listed for the combined pill also pertain to the mini-pill. If you experience any of them, contact your physician immediately.

Contraindications: The mini-pill is generally not recommended for women with irregular vaginal bleeding, acute mononucleosis, and past histories of ectopic pregnancy.

Additional Comments about Mini-Pills: Mini-pills have been marketed in the United States since 1973. Many women are unable to use combined birth-control pills because of the negative effects estrogen has on their health. The mini-pill may be used by (1) women over the age of thirty-five; (2) women who smoke; (3) women with medical histories of headaches, hypertension, or **varicose veins;** and (4)**lactating** women.

Method: Intrauterine Device (IUD)

Theoretical Failure Rate: 1.5%
Actual Failure Rate: 6.0%

How Method Works:
1. May cause an inflammation within the uterus, thus preventing implantation of a fertilized egg.
2. May increase movement of the egg through the fallopian tube, reducing the chance of fertilization.
3. May immobilize sperm, reducing their chances of reaching the egg.

How to Use: IUDs are about one inch long and are made of plastic. They come in various shapes, such as loops and coils. All have a nylon string hanging from the end. A plastic tube, thinner than a drinking straw, is passed through the vagina and through the cervix into the uterus. The IUD, which is inside the tube, is gently pushed out of the tube and opens up inside the uterus. The tube is withdrawn and the IUD remains. A small nylon string hangs down from the IUD and extends into the top of the vagina. While a woman is using an IUD, she should check frequently to see if the string is extending out of the cervical os. If the string cannot be felt or if it seems to be hanging down farther into the vagina, it probably means that the IUD is not in place correctly, and the woman should contact her physician. Once the IUD is inserted, it can remain in place for several years (unless it contains copper or progesterone, which means that it must be replaced more frequently). When a woman wants to become pregnant, her physician removes the IUD.

Birth Control, Contraceptive, or Both? Because the most probable reason for the IUD's effectiveness is its ability to prevent implantation of a fertilized egg, the IUD would be considered a birth-control method.

Advantages:
1. Has high rate of effectiveness.
2. No preparation is required before intercourse.
3. Allows for complete spontaneity.

Disadvantages:
1. Initial insertion may be painful.
2. Heavier cramps and bleeding during menstruation may occur.
3. Risk of **pelvic inflammatory disease** and other uterine infections is increased.
4. Partial or complete expulsion of the IUD may occur.
5. Risk of ectopic pregnancy is increased.
6. Possible uterine perforation may occur.

Precautions:
1. Check the string once a week, especially after menstruation, to be sure that the IUD is still in place.
2. Use an additional method of birth control for the first three months after insertion (highest rate of expulsion during this time).

3. Contact your physician immediately if:
   a. you can't feel the string.
   b. the IUD comes out.
   c. you miss a menstrual period.
   d. you have fever, chills, vaginal discharge, abdominal pains or cramps, or excessive bleeding.

Contraindications: An IUD is generally not recommended for women who have had heavy or painful menstrual periods, pelvic inflammatory disease, a tubal pregnancy, an abnormal Pap smear, or an abnormally shaped uterus.

Additional Comments about IUDs: On January 31, 1986, G. D. Searle and Co. announced that it was taking its IUDs off the market. Searle was the major U.S manufacturer of IUDs. This decision came as a result of the many lawsuits filed against Searle, charging that the IUDs caused infections and infertility. Searle decided that it was no longer economically feasible to continue producing IUDs. A. H. Robins Co., manufacturer of the Dalkon Shield IUD, filed bankruptcy in August 1985 after being held legally responsible for at least twenty deaths and thousands of cases of infection and miscarriage caused from use of the Shield. As of 1986, only the Progestasert IUD was being manufactured in the United States. This is a T-shaped IUD that slowly releases small amounts of progesterone. The Progestasert must be replaced yearly, thus increasing the possible health risks. Just when it seemed as though the IUD was heading toward extinction, it was announced that a new, smaller, and updated version of the IUD would be available in the United States by the early 1990s. This new version—the Copper T-380A—has never been sold in the United States, but it has been available in Canada, where it appears to have high success rates and to cause few complications.

Method: Condom
Theoretical Failure Rate: 2.0%
Actual Failure Rate: 12.0%

How Method Works: Collects semen and prevents sperm from entering the vagina.

How to Use: A condom is a thin sheath of latex or animal membrane. It is put on an erect penis before any genital contact with a woman. If the condom does not have a nipple end, some space has to be left at the end of it to catch the semen. This can be done by holding the tip of the condom while rolling it onto the erect penis. Once the condom is on correctly, the penis can be inserted into the vagina until ejaculation. (Figure 9–3 illustrates the proper application of a condom).

Birth Control, Contraceptive, or Both? Because the condom prevents the union of sperm and egg, it would be considered both a birth-control and a contraceptive method.

Advantages:
1. May help to prevent the spread of sexually transmitted diseases (STDs).
2. May help to prevent cervical cancer.
3. Presents no known health risks.
4. Is a way for the male to share birth control responsibility.
5. Is available without a prescription.
6. Is easy to use.

Disadvantages:
1. May interrupt lovemaking.
2. May cause anxiety over possible breakage.
3. Some men believe that it reduces glans sensitivity.
4. Allergic reaction to latex rubber is possible.

Precautions:
1. When the condom is on, there should always be some slack at the end.
2. After ejaculation, the penis must be withdrawn from the vagina while it is still erect.
3. While withdrawing from the vagina, male must hold the rim of the condom against the penis to prevent condom slippage and sperm leakage.
4. A new condom must be used for each act of intercourse.
5. Petroleum jelly, such as Vaseline, should never be used to lubricate a condom. Its oily base deteriorates the rubber. Always use a water soluble lubricant.
6. Heat deteriorates rubber, so don't store in a warm, moist place. Store in a cool, dry place.
7. Condoms should be purchased at clinics or drugstores to assure that they are not an outdated supply.

FAST FACTS

Natural membrane or "skin" condoms appear to be somewhat less effective in preventing the spread of some infections than latex condoms.

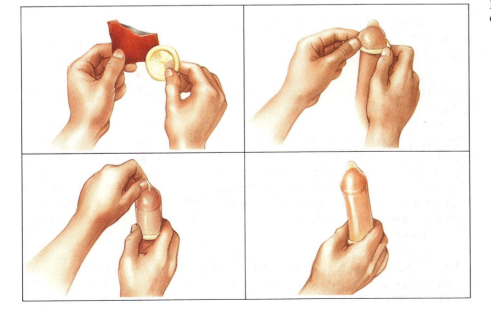

FIGURE 9–3 ■ Application of a Condom

With all the different types of condoms that can be purchased, it is important to read the information on each box and select the one that has the features you are looking for.

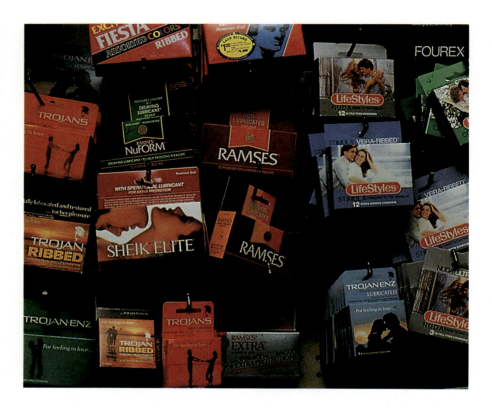

Contraindications: Condoms are generally not recommended for males who are not motivated to participate in contraceptive responsibilities.

Additional Comments about Condoms: There are many different types of condoms. Some are rounded on the end, whereas others have a nipple-like end to catch the semen. There are also unlubricated or lubricated (wet jelly or dry powder) condoms. Lubrication on a condom can make vaginal penetration easier. Spermicidal agents, a water soluble lubricant (such as K-Y jelly), or even saliva is a good lubricant for a condom that is not prelubricated. To increase the effectiveness of the condom, it can be used in combination with a spermicide or a diaphragm.

Today, condoms can be purchased that contain spermicidal agents inside and outside. This definitely increases condom effectiveness because two contraceptive measures are involved instead of just one. The Mentor condom, which contains a surgical adhesive within the condom, stays on the penis more securely, thus decreasing the chances of slippage and leakage. Recently, condom use has increased greatly. This new found popularity is not because people have suddenly realized that the condom is an effective birth-control device but because it is probably the only means of birth control known to afford some protection against certain sexually transmitted diseases.

■ *PROBLEM SITUATION* Suppose that you want to promote the use of condoms. What features would you emphasize? What strategies would you use to persuade both males and females to buy and use them?

Method: Diaphragm (with spermicide)

Theoretical Failure Rate: 3.0%
Actual Failure Rate: 18.0%

How Method Works: The diaphragm is a dome-shaped latex cup with a flexible rim. It is a barrier method of birth control that is only effective when used with a spermicide. The diaphragm provides a physical barrier between the penis and the cervix, and the spermicide kills the sperm.

How to Use: Use one to two teaspoons of spermicidal jelly or cream and spread it inside the dome and around the rim of the diaphragm. Squeeze the rim together and insert the diaphragm inside the vagina, up against the cervix. Be sure that the rim is tucked behind the pelvic bone (illustrated in Figure 9–4). The diaphragm can be inserted up to two hours prior to intercourse. For repeated intercourse, leave the diaphragm in place and insert another application of spermicide. The diaphragm must be left in place six to eight hours after the last act of intercourse. To remove the diaphragm, hook one finger up over its rim and pull it down and out of the vagina. Wash it with warm water and mild soap, dry thoroughly, and lightly dust with cornstarch. Place the diaphragm back in its container until its next use.

Birth Control, Contraceptive, or Both? Because the diaphragm prevents the union of sperm and egg, it would be considered both a birth-control and a contraceptive method.

Advantages:
1. Presents no major health risks.
2. Can be inserted up to two hours before intercourse.
3. Does not interrupt lovemaking.
4. Provides a mechanical barrier as well as a chemical barrier.
5. Spermicide may decrease the risk of contracting a STD.
6. May be used for intercourse during menstruation. Holds several hours worth of menstrual blood.
7. Can be reused.

Disadvantages:
1. Is not recommended for women who feel uncomfortable about touching their genital area.
2. Irritation from the spermicide is possible.
3. Is available by prescription only.
4. Is messy to insert and remove.

Precautions:
1. A woman must be properly fitted for a diaphragm. It must fit exactly over her cervix. Never use another woman's diaphragm.
2. Spermicidal jellies or creams, rather than foam, should be used on the diaphragm because they have a better "staying" capacity.
3. Never use vaseline on a diaphragm.
4. The diaphragm must be left in place for six to eight hours after the last act of intercourse. Douche or tampons should not be used during this time.

FIGURE 9–4 ■ **Insertion of the Diaphragm**

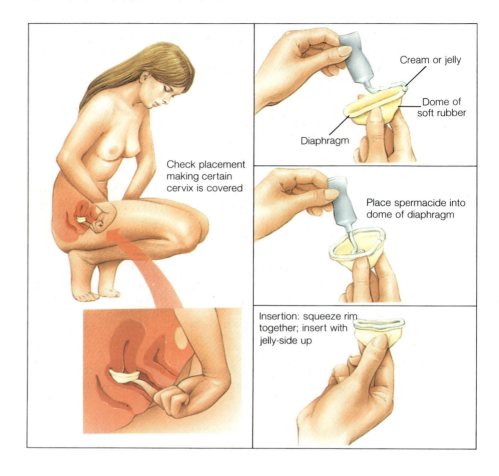

5. If intercourse occurs again before the six to eight hours pass, additional spermicide must be inserted into the vagina.
6. The diaphragm should not be left in place for more than a twenty-four-hour period. This may increase the risk of toxic shock syndrome or other infections. Leaving the diaphragm in place too long may also cause a foul-smelling vaginal discharge.

Contraindications: A diaphragm is generally not recommended for women who are allergic to the rubber the diaphragm is made of or to all spermicides. A woman may have poor support from the muscles surrounding the vagina and be unable to keep a diaphragm in place.

Additional Comments about Diaphragms: A well-cared-for diaphragm can last for several years. It should remain soft and flexible. A diaphragm should be checked after each use for holes or tears by holding it up to the light. Any tiny leaks can be detected by placing water in the dome and swishing it around. A woman needs to be refitted for a new diaphragm if she has a baby, has a miscarriage or abortion, or gains or loses substantial amounts of weight.

Method: Vaginal Sponge
Theoretical Failure Rate: 5.0–8.0%
Actual Failure Rate: 18.0–28.0%

How Method Works: The small, two-inch wide polyurethane sponge contains a spermicide that is released gradually once the sponge is moistened and inserted into the vagina. Similar to the diaphragm, this device works in three ways: it forms a barrier over the cervix, it releases a spermicide, and it absorbs semen.

How to Use: Hold the sponge with the dimple side up and wet it with a few drops of water. (Make sure to read and follow the directions carefully before insertion.) Squeeze gently to activate the spermicide contained within the sponge. Insert the sponge into the vagina with the string loop hanging down and the dimpled part up against the cervix (illustrated in Figure 9–5). It works by the same principles as the diaphragm; however, it can be inserted several hours before intercourse and can be effective for up to twenty-four hours. While it is

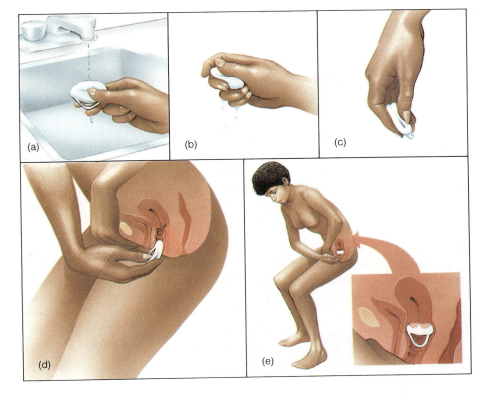

FIGURE 9–5 ■ **The Contraceptive Sponge and the Method of Its Placement**

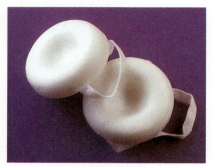

The vaginal contraceptive sponge is a "one-size-fits-all" barrier method of birth control.

in place, intercourse can occur as often as a couple desires without having to use additional spermicide. The sponge must be left in place for six to eight hours after the last act of intercourse. To remove the sponge, insert your finger through the string loop and pull it down and out of the vagina. Then throw it away.

Birth Control, Contraceptive, or Both? Because the sponge prevents the union of sperm and egg, it would be considered both a birth-control and a contraceptive method.

Advantages:
1. Is available without a prescription.
2. Spermicide does not need to be reapplied before each act of intercourse.
3. Is effective for about twenty-four hours.
4. Does not interrupt lovemaking.

Disadvantages:
1. May shift positions internally.
2. Can be inserted only one time. Once removed, it is thrown away and a new sponge must be used.
3. Is sometimes difficult to remove.
4. Is not recommended for women who object to touching their genital area.

Precautions:
1. Do not leave the sponge in place for more than twenty-four hours. It may increase the risk of toxic shock syndrome or other vaginal infections.
2. If the sponge creates an air suction, making it difficult to remove, squat and bear down and gently break the suction by inserting your finger between the sponge and the cervix. Pull down and out by holding the string loop.
3. Examine the sponge to be sure that it came out intact. If any of the sponge cannot be removed from the vagina, call your physician immediately for his or her advice.
4. Do not use the sponge during menstruation.

Contraindications: The sponge is generally not recommended for women who have had toxic shock syndrome. Also, women with lax pelvic muscle tone should not use the sponge.

Additional Comments about Sponges: The contraceptive sponge was given approval as a birth-control method by the FDA in 1983. It is marketed under the name "Today" contraceptive sponge. Although many women view the "one-size-fits-all" characteristic as an advantage for using the sponge, others view it as a disadvantage. These women ask, "Can one size really fit all? And am I willing to risk the consequences if the answer is no?" More studies are being conducted to determine the risk-to-benefit ratio.

Method: Cervical Cap (with spermicide)

Theoretical Failure Rate: 5.0%
Actual Failure Rate: 18.0%

How Method Works: The cervical cap is thimble-shaped and made from rubber or polyethylene. It fits tightly over the cervix to prevent sperm from entering into the uterus. Spermicidal cream or jelly is put inside the cap to kill sperm.

How to Use: The cap is currently available in only four sizes. Before inserting, the cap is filled one-third to one-half full with spermicidal jelly or cream. It is then pushed up into the vagina as far as it will go. It is held in place against the cervix by suction. The cap can be worn for up to twenty-four hours. The use of additional spermicide is optional. The cervical cap must not be removed for at least six to eight hours after the last act of intercourse. To remove the cap, the suction is broken by lifting the rim. It is then cleaned with soap and water and dried thoroughly.

Birth Control, Contraceptive, or Both? Because the cervical cap prevents the union of sperm and egg, it would be considered both a birth-control and a contraceptive method.

Advantages:
1. Does not require additional applications of spermicide with each act of intercourse.
2. Does not interrupt lovemaking.

Disadvantages:
1. Because there are only four sizes available, it is not possible to fit all women properly.
2. Cannot be used during menstruation.
3. Cannot be used for the first six to twelve weeks after childbirth.
4. Insertion and removal may be somewhat difficult.

Precautions:
1. The cap can be dislodged by intercourse when either the fit or the insertion is not quite right.
2. There is some question about the relationship between the cervical cap and toxic shock syndrome.
3. The cap may predispose females to cervical cell changes.

Contraindications: The cervical cap is generally not recommended for women with past or present histories of cervical disorders or infections or those who have a history of toxic shock syndrome.

Additional Comments about Cervical Caps: In May 1988, cervical caps were approved for marketing as contraceptives in the United States by the FDA.

Method: Spermicides (foams, creams, jellies, vaginal suppositories, and Vaginal Contraceptive Film)
Theoretical Failure Rate: 3.0%
Actual Failure Rate: 21.0%

How Method Works: A spermicide forms a chemical barrier over the cervix that kills sperm before they can enter the uterus.

How to Use: A spermicide is used before there is any genital contact between the male and female. Whatever type is used, all have applicators that allow the female to insert the chemical deep into the vagina, up against the cervix (illustrated in Figure 9–6). When using foam, cream, or jelly, it should be inserted a few minutes before sexual intercourse, but definitely no more than thirty minutes before. The newest form of spermicide is Vaginal Contraceptive Film (VCF), which became available in early 1988. VCF is a thin square of a translucent material composed of **nonoxynol-9.** When it dissolves in the vagina, it becomes a thickened gel. Once dissolved, it remains effective for two hours. When using **vaginal suppositories** or Film, one must remember to allow sufficient time for dissolution. For maximum effectiveness, therefore, it should be inserted at least five minutes (preferably fifteen minutes) before intercourse.

Birth Control, Contraceptive, or Both? Because a spermicide prevents the union of sperm and egg, it would be considered both a birth-control and a contraceptive method.

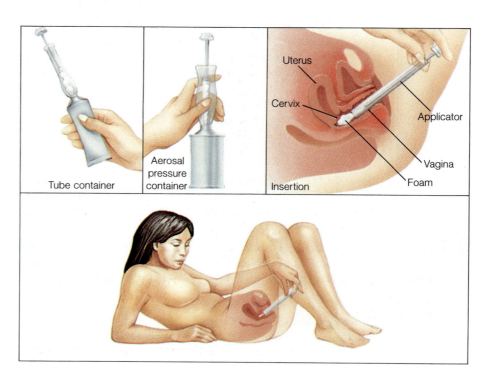

FIGURE 9–6 ■ Insertion of a Spermicidal Agent

Advantages:
1. May give some limited degree of protection against certain sexually transmitted diseases.
2. Presents no known health risks.
3. Is available without a prescription.
4. Is relatively inexpensive.

Disadvantages:
1. Has a lower effectiveness rate than other methods.
2. Application must be repeated before each act of intercourse.
3. Minor skin irritation can develop.
4. Is messy to use.
5. Takes advanced planning to use.
6. May interrupt lovemaking.

Precautions:
1. Do not douche or use tampons for at least six to eight hours after intercourse.
2. Reapply spermicide after thirty minutes if ejaculation has not yet occurred.
3. Buy name brands in reputable stores.
4. Read and follow the directions carefully before using. Many brands require two applications of spermicide before intercourse.
5. When using foam, shake the container vigorously before using.
6. Make sure applicator is put far enough into the vagina to provide adequate protection around the cervix.
7. When using a vaginal suppository, allow the required time for it to activate in the vagina before having intercourse.
8. Always be prepared with an extra supply.
9. If a particular brand is irritating, try another.
10. Do not mistake feminine hygiene products for spermicides. Be sure that the label specifically says it is for contraceptive use.

Contraindications: Spermicides are generally not recommended for women who are allergic to all brands or for those who are not motivated to use them each time they have intercourse.

Additional Comments about Spermicides: When using only a spermicide for contraception, foam is more effective than creams or jellies. Foam provides a better barrier. To increase effectiveness, use a spermicide in combination with a diaphragm or condom.

FAST FACTS

The staff of the Birth Defects Branch of the Centers for Disease Control do not believe that the use of spermicides is associated with an increased incidence of birth defects.

Method: Coitus Interruptus (withdrawal)

Theoretical Failure Rate: 4.0%
Actual Failure Rate: 18.0%

How Method Works: Withdrawal supposedly prevents sperm from entering the vagina.

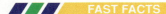

FAST FACTS

Sperm enter the cervical canal as soon as fifteen seconds after ejaculation.

How to Use: Remove the penis from the vagina before ejaculation occurs.

Birth Control, Contraceptive, or Both? Theoretically, withdrawal is supposed to prevent the union of sperm and egg. If it actually worked, withdrawal would be considered both a birth-control and a contraceptive method. In reality, however, withdrawal has such a low effectiveness rate that it would be wise not to consider it as either a reliable birth-control or contraceptive alternative.

Advantages:
1. Is always available to use.
2. Gives the male contraceptive responsibility.
3. Requires no devices or chemicals.
4. Has no side effects.
5. Costs nothing to use.

Disadvantages:
1. Has high failure rate.
2. Is frustrating for both sexes.

Precautions: Even if the male withdraws the penis before ejaculation, two or three drops of preejaculatory fluid contain enough sperm to impregnate a female.

Contraindications: Withdrawal is generally not recommended for any individual who can use a more effective method of birth control.

Additional Comments about Withdrawal: Withdrawal is not considered to be a reliable birth-control alternative. If you are engaging in sexual intercourse, however, and no other birth-control method is available at the time, withdrawal is still better than doing or using nothing at all. But always be prepared! Don't end up in a situation in which withdrawal is your only hope.

Method: Fertility-Awareness Techniques (basal body temperature [BBT], mucous method, and calendar method)
Theoretical Failure Rate: 2.0–20.0%
Actual Failure Rate: 24.0%

How BBT Method Works: This method consists of keeping a daily record of a woman's body temperature in an attempt to determine the time of ovulation.

How Mucous Method Works: This method consists of observing the daily changes in cervical mucus in an attempt to determine the time of ovulation.

How Calendar Method Works: This method consists of keeping track of the number of days in a woman's menstrual cycle in an attempt to determine the time of ovulation.

How to use the BBT Method: Every morning before arising, the woman must take her temperature with a special BBT thermometer. One to two days before ovulation, the body temperature will drop. At the time of ovulation, the temperature will rise and will remain raised through the remainder of that cycle. From the day the temperature drops to the third consecutive day of the higher body temperature, the woman should abstain from intercourse.

How to Use the Mucous Method: The woman must insert her finger into the vagina and withdraw cervical mucus. She then must examine the color and characteristics of the mucus. After menstruation, there is generally little or no mucus for a few days. As the mucus increases, it gets a thicker and stickier consistency and is white or yellow in color. Gradually the mucus changes to a watery and clearer state until there are one or two days when the mucus resembles raw egg whites (clear, slippery, and stretchable). This indicates ovulation. After ovulation occurs, the mucus becomes thick and sticky again. The woman should abstain from intercourse from the first day the mucus appears watery and clear until it becomes thick and sticky.

How to Use the Calendar Method: The woman must record the number of days in her menstrual cycle for eight to ten months before using this method. To determine her first "unsafe" day, she must subtract 18 from the number of days in her shortest menstrual cycle. To determine her last "unsafe" day, she must subtract 11 from the number of days in her longest cycle. For example, after eight months a woman records her shortest cycle as being twenty-eight days in length and her longest cycle as being thirty days. Her calculations would be as follows:

28 (shortest cycle)	30 (longest cycle)
−18	−11
10 (first "unsafe" day)	19 (last "unsafe" day)

Based on the preceding calculations, ovulation could occur between days 10 and 19. By using this method, the woman would have to abstain from intercourse from Day 10 to Day 19 of her menstrual cycle.

Birth Control, Contraceptive, or Both? Fertility-awareness techniques attempt to identify the time during which a woman is fertile so that she knows when to abstain from intercourse. If she doesn't have intercourse when she is ovulating, there can be no union of sperm and egg. For this reason, fertility-awareness techniques would be considered both birth-control and contraceptive methods.

Advantages of All Methods:
1. Are acceptable to religious groups that reject artificial methods of birth control.
2. Have no side effects.
3. No cost is involved (except minimal cost for a BBT thermometer).
4. Female becomes more aware of body changes.
5. Can also be used to increase chances of desired pregnancy.

Disadvantages of All Methods:
1. Require faithful monitoring of the menstrual cycle.
2. Are not highly reliable.
3. Period of abstinence may be frustrating for one or both partners.

4. Takes considerable time and effort to learn how to use these methods correctly.
5. May be an inconvenience or a bother to pursue.
6. Woman may object to touching the genital area and the cervical mucus.

Precautions for BBT Method: This method cannot tell you when ovulation WILL occur but that it HAS occurred. For this reason, successful use of this method depends on keeping a record of your body temperature for several months before attempting to interpret the results.

Precautions for Mucous Method: You must not confuse cervical mucus with other types of secretions, such as semen, lubricants, or discharges caused by infection. Cervical mucus should not have an offensive odor or cause genital itching or burning. These are signs of infection, and you should contact your doctor if they occur.

Precautions for Calendar Method: Successful use of this method requires that you keep an *updated* record of the lengths of your menstrual cycles. If the number of days in your shortest or longest cycle changes, so must your calculations.

Contraindications: Fertility-awareness methods are generally not recommended for women with irregular menstrual cycles or for women who are not motivated to consistently and accurately pursue the method chosen.

Additional Comments about Fertility-Awareness Methods: Since the failure rate for fertility-awareness methods is relatively high, it is strongly recommended that an individual or couple receive in-depth instruction from a trained clinician on how to use a particular method. To increase reliability, use at least two of the previously described methods in combination with each other.

FAST FACTS

Between 1.3 and 1.5 million legal abortions are performed each year in the U.S. Nearly one third are performed on teenagers, while another third are performed on women between the ages of 20 and 24.

Abortive Procedures

In 1973, the Supreme Court legalized **abortion** throughout the United States. The Court ruled that states were prohibited from interfering with a woman's decision to have an abortion during the first three months of pregnancy. The Court further ruled that states may regulate abortion during the second trimester only to protect the mother's health. During the last trimester, states may regulate or ban abortions altogether, unless the life or health of the woman is threatened.

On July 3, 1989, by a 5 to 4 vote, the United States Supreme Court gave states greater authority to regulate abortions. This decision came as a result of the Supreme Court's ruling on a Missouri abortion case, "Webster vs. Reproductive Health Services." Reproductive Health Services maintained that the right to privacy contained in the 14th Amendment of the United States Constitution protects a woman's right to terminate a pregnancy in the first trimester. Webster, the Attorney General of Missouri at that time, argued that children have "protectable interests in life, health and well-being" at any stage of a pregnancy. The United States Supreme Court upheld the Missouri law. It ruled that states could set new limits on abortions, but declined to reverse the landmark 1973 Roe vs. Wade decision. The immediate ramifications of this decision will allow states to stop public funding of abortions for the poor and to restrict abortions and counseling in publicly-funded hospitals and clinics. This ruling sets the stage for three more abortion rights cases that could possibly lead to the overturning of Roe vs. Wade.

On the last day of the Supreme Court's 1988–1989 term, Justice Harry A. Blackmun read from the bench portions of his opinion in "Webster vs. Reproductive Health Services:"

"For today at least, the law of abortion stands undisturbed. For today, the women of this nation will retain the liberty to control their destinies. But the signs are evident and very ominous, and a chill wind blows."

Since the Supreme Court has given the states more power to restrict or limit access to and performance of abortion, what will be the future fate of abortion in the United States? At this point, the only thing we know for certain is that the battle lines are drawn between pro-choice and anti-abortion groups, and the outcome rests in the hands of the state legislatures.

Since the 1973 Supreme Court ruling, termination of unwanted pregnancy has become the most common surgical procedure in the United States for women of reproductive age. Over one-and-a-half million American women choose to terminate their pregnancies via induced abortion every year. The method of abortion chosen is determined by the number of weeks the woman has been pregnant. This is measured from the first day of her last menstrual period or estimated from the date of probable conception.

The abortive procedures have been divided into four categories. The first category, postcoital methods, includes methods that are generally performed shortly after unprotected intercourse has occurred. The second category, first-trimester methods, includes methods that are performed during the first trimester of pregnancy. The third category, second-trimester methods, includes methods that are performed during the second trimester of pregnancy; and the fourth category, the abortion pill, includes a method not yet available for use in the United States.

Postcoital Methods

Methods are available to women who have had unprotected intercourse and who wish to terminate a possible pregnancy. These methods are generally used before a pregnancy test would indicate a positive test result. A woman choosing to use one of these methods may have been raped, may have had a contraceptive failure, or may believe that a possible pregnancy could pose a health risk. These methods are effective in preventing pregnancy because they either interfere with fertilization or prevent implantation. They should by no means be considered an acceptable alternative to contraceptive use. They should be thought of as emergency procedures.

Morning-After Pills. **Morning-after pills** contain synthetic female hormones and, when taken by a woman within seventy-two hours of unprotected intercourse, will prevent pregnancy. A pill that contains 50 mcg of ethinyl estradiol and .5 mg of dl-norgestrel (marketed in the United States as Ovral) is the most commonly used morning-after pill. In the past, **diethylstilbestrol (DES)**, a highly potent synthetic estrogen, was used. Because DES produced many negative side effects, it is no longer prescribed. Ovral has been found to be effective

FAST FACTS

In 1981, the International Planned Parenthood Federation endorsed the use of postcoital methods to avoid an unwanted pregnancy.

in preventing pregnancy, and it causes fewer negative side effects. Although the FDA has not approved postcoital methods of birth control, it does not prohibit using a drug for purposes other than those included in approved drug labeling. Since Ovral is an approved drug, its prescribed use is up to the discretion of individual physicians.

IUD Insertion. Postcoital insertion of a copper IUD, from one to seven days after unprotected intercourse, works by preventing implantation should an egg become fertilized. The advantage of IUD insertion is that it can be used up to seven days after unprotected intercourse, as compared with the three-day limitation for hormone administration. A disadvantage is that a woman may be more susceptible to pelvic inflammatory disease with an IUD in place.

Menstrual Extraction. If a woman's menstrual period is up to two weeks late, **menstrual extraction** can be performed. A long, hollow tube, which is inserted into the uterus, removes the menstrual blood and tissue from the endometrial walls. This procedure can be performed in an outpatient setting with minimal health risk.

First-Trimester Methods

Vacuum Aspiration or Suction Method. The most frequently performed type of abortion during the first trimester of pregnancy is **vacuum aspiration**. A thin tube, which is connected to a vacuum pump, is inserted through the cervix into the uterus. Gentle suction from the pump removes the uterine contents. The woman might feel some slight cramping during the procedure, which is generally done on an outpatient basis under local anesthesia. It takes about five to ten minutes to complete. Complications are rare but can include hemorrhage, uterine perforation, and infection. The following after-procedure care measures should be taken:

1. Rest for the remainder of the day.
2. Avoid strenuous activity for one to two days.
3. Avoid intercourse and douching for several weeks.
4. Since bleeding may continue for a number of days, use sanitary napkins instead of tampons.
5. Do not take medications containing aspirin, because its anticoagulating effect may increase the risk of hemorrhage.
6. Contact your physician immediately if there are any signs of complications.
7. Get a follow-up examination about two weeks after the abortion.

The advantages of vacuum aspiration are that the time involved in the procedure is shorter, recovery is quicker, and complications are fewer than in other first trimester methods.

> ■ *PROBLEM SITUATION* An unmarried female friend wants to have an abortion. She asks you to go with her, but you feel strongly against abortion. What would you do?

Dilation and Curettage (D&C). **Dilation and curettage** is similar to vacuum aspiration except that the cervix is dilated more and a curette is used to scrape out the contents of the uterus. The risks involved are somewhat greater for a D&C because there is cervical dilation and often the use of general anesthesia.

Second-Trimester Methods

Dilation and Evacuation (D&E). **Dilation and evacuation** is similar to a D&C, but because there is skeletal development in the second trimester, an instrument is used to break up and then extract the contents of the uterus through a vacuum curette.

Intraamniotic Injection (Saline or Prostaglandin). A procedure involving an **intraamniotic injection** requires several days in the hospital. A local anesthetic is first injected into the abdomen. Some amniotic fluid is then withdrawn from the amniotic sac, and it is replaced with an equal amount of saline solution. This kills the fetus and induces expulsion within two days. Instead of a saline solution, prostaglandins are sometimes used. Prostaglandins are hormones that induce uterine contractions and fetal expulsion. Possible complications from prostaglandins include nausea and vomiting, diarrhea, cervical tearing, and asthma-like symptoms. There has been much debate about the relative safety of prostaglandin use as compared to saline use. Prostaglandin use may pose ethical and medical issues, because the fetus may be alive when expelled from the uterus.

Hysterotomy. Considered to be a major surgical procedure, a **hysterotomy** is similar to a caesarean section. General anesthesia is used. A surgical incision is made in the abdomen through the uterine muscle, and the fetus is removed. Because there is greater risk and more complications involved with this procedure, a hysterotomy should be performed only under emergency conditions.

The Abortion Pill

Pro-choice groups have been investigating a method of abortion that is not used in the United States, but is popularly used in France. The French abortion pill, RU 486, was developed in 1982 by French scientist, Dr. Etienne Baulieu. RU 486, Mifepristone, is an antiprogestin which has been proven to be an effective and safe agent for fertility control. Its rate of effectiveness is 95 percent if taken in conjunction with a synthetic prostaglandin. The drug is administered under medical supervision yet, unlike a vacuum aspiration abortion, the procedure does not require even local anesthesia because it is a non-invasive procedure. Therefore, there is no risk of infection.

So far, the French pharmaceutical company, Roussel-Uclaf, that manufactures RU 486, has not licensed any pharmaceutical company to market RU 486 in the United States. Clinical tests on the drug, however, are under way at several institutions across the country. If RU 486 becomes available for use in the United States, pro-choice and anti-abortion groups will face a new issue of contention.

Future Trends

What kinds of birth control can we expect to be using within the next few years? Here are some ideas already in the developing or testing stages.

Long-Acting Progestin Injections. Contraceptive injections of long-acting progestins are now being used in many countries. The most commonly used is Depo-Provera. These injections only need to be given at three- or six-month intervals. Depo-Provera has not been approved for use in the United States because the FDA believes that the following issues still need to be investigated:

1. The relationship of Depo-Provera to breast and uterine cancer.
2. Whether Depo-Provera has teratogenic (birth defect-producing) effects.
3. The potential hazards that might require estrogen supplementation to curtail irregular bleeding.

Subdermal Implants. Small plastic tubes filled with progestin would be implanted under the skin of the upper arm. The progestin would slowly be released and absorbed by the body. Preliminary evaluations show that these implants may remain in place and be effective for five years. The side effects seem to be minimal. Subdermal implants have been successfully used in several countries, and they are currently undergoing clinical trials in the United States.

Vaginal Ring. A hormone-secreting rubber ring, shaped like a thin donut, would be worn in the vagina for twenty-one days and then removed for seven days to allow for menstrual bleeding.

A Female Condom. A vaginal shield, or Femshield, is currently undergoing acceptability trials in London, England. The shield is held in the vagina by two flexible rings inside the shield. When in place, the shield is not skin tight like a male condom. It covers the surface of the vagina but allows the penis to move freely. After intercourse, the shield is removed by pulling the outer ring, and the device is then thrown away.

Improved IUDs. Scientists are trying to develop a "tail-less" magnetic IUD. A magnet would be used to detect and remove the IUD. This tail-less version would be safer to use and would lower the risk of reproductive infection.

Safer Oral Contraceptives. Development of oral contraceptives with a high effectiveness rate and a low probability of side effects is an ongoing project.

Improved Barrier Contraceptives. More barrier contraceptives containing spermicides within them are being tested. A disposable diaphragm that slowly releases nonoxynol-9 is being considered.

Improved Ovulation-Detection Methods. A device has been developed that monitors basal body temperature. It contains an electronic remote-sensing thermometer, a computerized clock, and a light display. It reportedly monitors the cycles of women and accurately indicates fertile and infertile periods with a red or green light. Its level of reliability needs to be proved. There have been suggestions about developing a simple urine or saliva test that a woman could perform and interpret herself to determine when she is ovulating.

Oral Contraceptives for Males. Gossypol, a cottonseed derivative, has been found to interfere with sperm production. It is used in China and is reported to be highly effective when taken daily. Its only side effect seems to be fatigue. Gossypol has not been approved for use in the United States, but it is currently being tested to determine its safety and reversibility.

Vaccines for Females and Males. Scientists are trying to develop a vaccine for females that would interrupt the hormone action that supports a pregnancy and a vaccine for males that would interfere with sperm production.

Production of Temporary Sterility in Males. Research is being conducted to determine if valves can be implanted within the vas deferens to regulate sperm transportation. Also, methods are being investigated, such as ultrasound, that would elevate the temperature of the testicles, thus reducing sperm production.

How many of these experiments will actually become methods of birth control is not yet known. One thing is sure, however; there will always be the ongoing search for more innovative, effective, and safer methods of birth control.

SELF-INVENTORY 9.2

Which Method of Birth Control Should You Use?

Now that you have learned about the various methods of birth control, which methods are best for your particular needs and life-style? Place a check mark in the column that accurately describes your feelings or behaviors. Statements 1 through 12 should be answered by both males and females. Statements 13 through 20 should be answered only by females.

	Yes	No
1. I like sexual spontaneity.	___	___
2. I prefer not to touch my genital area.	___	___
3. I have sexual intercourse frequently.	___	___
4. I have more than one sexual partner.	___	___
5. I have or have had a sexually transmitted disease.	___	___
6. I have only one sexual partner.	___	___
7. I eventually want to have children.	___	___
8. I am forgetful.	___	___
9. I feel that the female should be the one to use birth control.	___	___
10. I feel that the male should be the one to use birth control.	___	___
11. I dislike swallowing pills.	___	___
12. I have sexual intercourse infrequently.	___	___

Continue responding ONLY if you are a female:

13. I am over 35 years of age.	___	___
14. I bleed heavily and usually have cramps during my menstrual period.	___	___
15. I want to have the option of conceiving immediately after discontinuing birth control.	___	___
16. I have had at least one previous pregnancy.	___	___
17. I get bladder infections.	___	___
18. I am presently breastfeeding.	___	___
19. I smoke cigarettes.	___	___
20. I have a medical history of cancer or liver or heart disease.	___	___

Interpretation:

If you answered "Yes" to the following statements:

1, 2, 3, 6, 7, 9, and 14 .... Consider using the Pill.

1, 3, 6, 8, 9, 11, 13, 16, 18, and 19 ..... Consider using the IUD.

6, 7, 9, 11, 12, 13, 14, 15, 18, 19, and 20 .... Consider using the diaphragm or cervical cap with spermicidal agent.

4, 5, 7, 8, 10, 11, 12, 13, 14, 15, and 17–20 .... Consider using the condom.

4, 7, 9, 11, 12, 13, 14, 15, and 17–20 .... Consider using spermicides.

As you can see, there is more than one recommended birth-control method to use, depending on your needs and life-style. Select the one that appeals to you. To maximize effectiveness, you may need to use a combination of methods.

POSITIVE BEHAVIORS

I. *Place a check mark in front of each behavior that you now practice.*

_____ 1. I use some method of birth control each time I have sexual intercourse. (BIRTH CONTROL)

_____ 2. A contraceptive method is used before I have any genital contact with my partner. (GENITAL CONTACT)

_____ 3. I approach my sexual responsibility with honesty and openness. (HONESTY)

_____ 4. I discuss birth-control options with my partner. (DISCUSS)

_____ 5. I use condoms to help prevent the transmission of STDs. (CONDOMS)

_____ 6. I feel comfortable going into a drugstore and purchasing contraceptives. (COMFORTABLE PURCHASING)

_____ 7. I always have a back-up method of birth control. (BACK-UP)

_____ 8. I use a highly effective method of birth control. (EFFECTIVE)

_____ 9. When I am in a sexual relationship, I am monogamous. (MONOGAMOUS).

_____ 10. I abstain from genital contact with my partner when I have signs of possible infection. (INFECTION)

II. *For each behavior that you DO NOT ENGAGE IN, write the key word(s) located in the parentheses at the end of the statements in the column below. Then put a check mark in the appropriate column to indicate whether you are going to keep or change that behavior.*

Behaviors I Don't Engage In   KEEP/CHANGE

_____   _____/_____
_____   _____/_____
_____   _____/_____
_____   _____/_____
_____   _____/_____
_____   _____/_____
_____   _____/_____
_____   _____/_____
_____   _____/_____

III. *For each of the preceding behaviors that you choose to KEEP, write a statement indicating why you are choosing to keep that behavior.*

I choose to keep behavior _____ because:
                            KEY WORD

For each of the preceding behaviors that you choose to CHANGE, write a statement indicating how you plan to implement that change.

I will change behavior _____ by:
                        KEY WORD

Now You Know

1. FALSE. Contraception means "against conception." It does not encompass the options of preventing implantation or birth.
2. FALSE. Sperm are still produced, but they can no longer be transported by the vas deferens.
3. TRUE. That is one of the reasons for the Pill's high effectiveness rate.
4. TRUE. Its oily base deteriorates the rubber.
5. FALSE. A diaphragm must be left in place for six to eight hours after the last act of sexual intercourse in order for the spermicide to kill the sperm.
6. TRUE. The sponge, in combination with the menstrual blood, may increase the risk of toxic shock syndrome or other infection.
7. FALSE. A spermicide should be inserted a few minutes before sexual intercourse occurs, but definitely no more than thirty minutes before.
8. TRUE. Each method of birth control has its advantages and disadvantages.
9. TRUE. Other early danger signals may include severe abdominal pain and eye problems such as blurred or double vision.
10. TRUE. Withdrawal has such a high failure rate that it is not considered to be a reliable birth-control alternative.

Summary

1. Responsibility is extremely important in regard to sexuality. A responsible person has a sense of duty or obligation and stands accountable for his or her behaviors no matter what the consequences.
2. *Contraception* means "against conception." Conception occurs when a sperm fertilizes an egg. A technique, drug, or device used to prevent conception is considered to be contraception.
3. *Birth control* means "to control the birth process." It encompasses a broader spectrum of options than just preventing conception. Any technique, drug, or device used to prevent conception, implantation, or birth is considered to be birth control.
4. Sterilization is a highly reliable but irreversible method of contraception. The most commonly used method of sterilization in the female is tubal ligation. The most commonly used method of male sterilization is vasectomy.
5. The combined birth-control pill is highly effective because it contains estrogen and progestin. Estrogen inhibits ovulation, and progestin alters the endometrium and causes thickening of the cervical mucus.
6. The mini-pill contains only progestin; it has no estrogen. It is not quite as effective as the combined pill, but it is still highly reliable. Because it does not contain estrogen, it causes fewer side effects.
7. The intrauterine device (IUD) may cause an inflammation in the uterus, thus preventing implantation of a fertilized egg. By definition, the IUD is a method of birth control, not contraception. Even though the IUD has a high effectiveness rate, it also has a high rate of expulsion and its use brings an increased risk of infection.
8. The condom collects semen and prevents sperm from entering the vagina. Condoms can be purchased that contain spermicidal agents on the inside and outside. This definitely increases effectiveness. The condom is the only means of birth control known to afford some protection against STDs.
9. The diaphragm and vaginal sponge are barrier methods of birth control. A female must be fitted for a diaphragm, and it is only effective when used with a spermicide. The sponge is a "one size fits all" device that can be purchased over-the-counter. The sponge contains a spermicidal agent.
10. A spermicide forms a chemical barrier over the cervix that kills sperm before they can enter the uterus. Spermicides come in the form of foams, creams, jellies, vaginal suppositories, and vaginal film. The active ingredient, nonoxynol-9, is thought to give some limited protection against STDs.
11. Coitus interruptus, or withdrawal, requires removing the penis from the vagina before ejaculation occurs. This method has a high failure rate. Withdrawal is not considered to be a reliable birth-control alternative.
12. Fertility-awareness techniques include the basal body temperature method, the mucous method, and the calendar method. They attempt to identify when a female is fertile so that she knows when to abstain from intercourse. The BBT method determines the time of ovulation by charting a female's body temperature. The mucous method determines the time of ovulation by the changes in the color and consistency of cervical mucus. The calendar method determines the time of ovulation by recording the number of days in a female's menstrual cycle over an eight- to ten-month period.
13. Abortion is the voluntary termination of a pregnancy. Over 1.5 million American women choose to terminate their pregnancies by means of induced abortion every year. The method of abortion chosen is determined

by the number of weeks the woman has been pregnant.

14. Postcoital methods of abortion are methods that are generally performed shortly after unprotected intercourse has occurred. They include morning-after pills, IUD insertion, and menstrual extraction.

15. First-trimester methods of abortion include vacuum aspiration and dilation and curettage (D&C). Vacuum aspiration is the most frequently performed type of abortion during the first trimester.

16. Second-trimester methods of abortion include dilation and evacuation (D&E), intraamniotic injection, and hysterotomy. There are greater risks and complications involved with second-trimester abortions. A hysterotomy should be performed only under emergency conditions.

17. The French abortion pill, RU 486, is a method of abortion not yet available for use in the United States. Clinical tests on the drug, however, are under way at several institutions across the country.

18. Future birth control methods currently in the development or testing stages include long-acting progestin injections, subdermal implants, a vaginal ring, a female condom, improved IUDs, safer oral contraceptives, improved ovulation-detection methods, oral contraceptives for males, vaccines for females and males, and production of temporary sterility in males.

References

1. Allgeier, Albert Richard, and Elizabeth Rice Allgeier. *Sexual Interactions*. Lexington, MA: D.C. Heath and Co., 1988.
2. Byer, Curtis O., Louis W. Shainberg, and Kenneth L. Jones. *Dimensions of Human Sexuality*. Dubuque, IA: William C. Brown Publishers, 1988.
3. "Can You Rely on Condoms?" *Consumer Reports,* March 1989, 135–141.
4. Denney, Nancy W., and David Quadagno. *Human Sexuality*. St. Louis: Times Mirror/Mosby College Publishing, 1988.
5. Greenberg, Jerrold S., Clint E. Bruess, Kathleen D. Mullen, and Doris W. Sands. *Sexuality: Insights and Issues*. Dubuque, IA: William C. Brown Publishers, 1989.
6. Hatcher, Robert A., et al. *Contraceptive Technology,* 14th ed. New York: Irvington Publishers, 1988.
7. "IUDS—A New Look." *Population Reports.* March 1988, B-5:1–25.
8. Lacayo, Richard. "Whose Life Is It?" *Time,* May 1, 1989, 133:20–24.
9. Rice, Philip F. *Human Sexuality*. Dubuque, IA: William C. Brown Publishers, 1989.
10. Terkel, Susan Neiburg. *Abortion: Facing the Issues*. New York: Franklin Watts, 1988.
11. "The Battle Over Abortion." *Newsweek,* May 1, 1989, 113:28–32.

Suggested Readings

"Can You Rely on Condoms?" *Consumer Reports,* March 1989, 135–141.

Hatcher, Robert A., et al. *Contraceptive Technology,* 14th ed. New York: Irvington Publishers, 1988.

Terkel, Susan Neiburg. *Abortion: Facing the Issues*. New York: Franklin Watts, 1988.

CHAPTER 10

Conception Through Birth

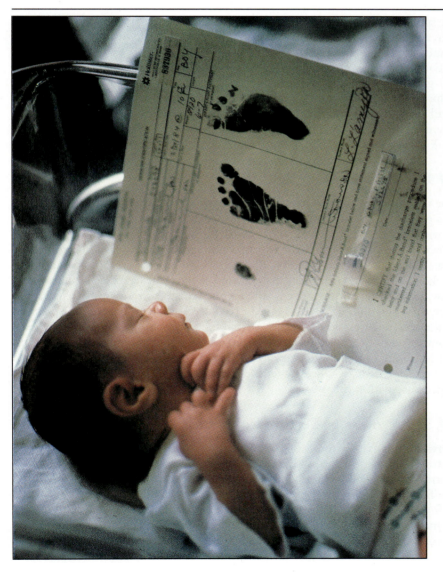

/////////

What Do You Know?

Are the following statements true or false?

1. The ovum, or egg, is one of the largest cells in the human body.
2. Fertilization has to occur during the first twenty-four hours that the egg is in the fallopian tube.
3. Sperm can live for up to 5 days in the female's reproductive tract.
4. It is the mother's chromosome that is ultimately responsible for sexual determination.
5. To increase the chances of conceiving a male, a couple should have sexual intercourse at the time of ovulation.
6. The first objective sign of pregnancy that is experienced by the majority of women is enlargement and tenderness of the abdomen.
7. A woman should gain about thirty pounds during her pregnancy.
8. A blood sample can detect pregnancy within a week after conception.
9. A pregnant woman should stop having sexual intercourse around the sixth month of pregnancy to avoid possible health risks to the fetus.
10. When a baby is born, a gentle slap on the behind is necessary to start the baby breathing on its own.

The Sexual Beginning

What does the word "sex" mean to you? Does it conjure up images of romance and lovemaking, or does it simply mean the actual act of sexual intercourse? Does it refer to the biological aspects of reproduction or the physical fact of being male or female? Depending on the context in which it is used, sex can mean all of these things. Whether it refers to "the act of doing" or "the fact of being," sex is just one part of an individual's sexuality. Sexuality involves the integration of biological, psychological, ethical, and cultural factors. Let's take a look at our sexual beginning.

Sperm Production

Spermatozoa, or sperm, are the male's reproductive cells. They are produced in the seminiferous tubules, which are located in the testes. The temperature of the testes must be several degrees below normal body temperature in order for sperm to be produced. Sperm production begins at puberty and continues into old age. Millions of sperm cells are produced daily, with the average male manufacturing billions of sperm annually.

Each mature sperm cell consists of a head, a midpiece, and a long tail. The tail gives the sperm its motility. The head contains a chemical antibody that helps dissolve the membrane of the egg and allows the sperm to enter. The head also contains the twenty-three **chromosomes** that will join with the egg's twenty-three chromosomes should fertilization occur. Each sperm cell has either an X **gynosperm** or Y **androsperm** sex-determining chromosome.

Egg Production

The **ova,** or eggs, are the female's reproductive cells. The egg is about the size of a grain of sand. It is the largest cell in the human body. At birth, the female's ovaries contain all of the potential eggs that she will ovulate throughout her reproductive years. The female is born with approximately 500,000 immature ova. When she reaches **puberty,** the eggs begin to mature in preparation for ovulation. Each maturing egg is surrounded by a cluster of cells. These cells provide nourishment for the egg and secrete female hormones. The egg, along with these surrounding cells, is called a **follicle.** As the egg matures, the pressure of the accumulating fluid increases within the follicle. Approximately once each month, one of the follicles ruptures from an ovary, releasing the egg along with the hormone-rich fluid. This process is called **ovulation.** Only about 400 to 500 eggs are ovulated during a female's reproductive years. The remaining eggs degenerate within the ovaries.

The Process of Fertilization and Implantation

Fertilization is the union of sperm and egg. For fertilization to occur, two factors must exist. One is that an egg must be released from the ovary and carried into the fallopian tube, and the second is that sperm must be present in the fallopian tube. During sexual intercourse, a male's **ejaculate** may contain 200 to 400 million sperm. Now, you may ask the logical question, "Why are so many sperm needed if it takes only one to fertilize an egg?" There are many factors responsible for reducing the number of sperm that actually reach the egg, such as the following:

FAST FACTS

Sperm are among the smallest cells in the human body.

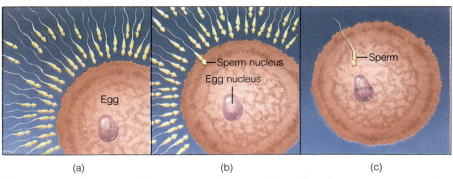

FIGURE 10–1 ■ **Fertilization**
Although many sperm reach an ovum, only one sperm will fertilize it.

- sperm spilling out of the vagina before reaching the cervix.
- the vagina's hostile acidic environment.
- the high percentage of defective sperm.
- the difficult journey encountered by the sperm traveling from the vagina to the fallopian tube.
- the sperm entering into the "eggless" fallopian tube.

Although several million sperm are ejaculated into the vagina, only a few thousand make their way to the fallopian tubes, and only a few hundred actually get near the egg.

Before fertilization can occur, several sperm are needed to secrete a chemical that dissolves the jellylike coating around the egg (see Figure 10–1). Once a sperm fertilizes an egg, the egg is impenetrable to the entrance of other sperm. Fertilization has to occur during the first twenty-four hours that the egg is in the fallopian tube. The egg is only viable for twenty-four hours; after that it degenerates. Sperm, however, can live in the female's reproductive tract for up to five days. If intercourse occurs within five days before ovulation, live sperm may be waiting in the fallopian tube to fertilize the egg.

The joining of sperm and egg produces a single-cell organism referred to as a **zygote.** As the zygote travels down the fallopian tube toward the uterus, rapid cell division begins. By the end of the first week, the zygote forms a hollow, spherical mass of cells referred to as a **blastocyst.** About seven or eight days after fertilization, the blastocyst attaches itself to the endometrial lining of the uterus. This process of attachment is called **implantation. Pregnancy** has now begun.

> ■ **PROBLEM SITUATION** If it was physiologically possible, do you think men could mentally and emotionally handle being pregnant? How might this affect stereotypical sex roles?

In some instances, the fertilized egg either remains in the fallopian tube or leaves the tube at the ovarian end, implanting itself in the abdominal cavity. This is called an **ectopic** (abnormal place) **pregnancy.** The most common type of ectopic pregnancy is a **tubal pregnancy,** which occurs when the fertilized egg implants in the fallopian tube. Ectopic pregnancies usually abort spontaneously. Those that do not can pose a life-threatening situation for the female. If the condition goes undiagnosed, the tube can rupture about six weeks after conception, causing internal hemorrhaging. The only symptoms of a tubal pregnancy may be the cessation of menstruation and abdominal pain.

FAST FACTS

If a woman with a ruptured fallopian tube does not receive medical treatment for the internal bleeding within thirty minutes, she may die.

Gender Differentiation: Prenatal Variables

There are four biological variables related to **gender** (the state of biologically being male or female) that are determined **prenatally.** They include:

- **genetic gender**—XX or XY chromosomes.
- **gonadal gender**—ovaries or testes.
- **hormonal gender**—high levels of estrogen or testosterone.
- **genital gender**—vulva (female's external genitalia) or penis and scrotum.

Genetic Gender

A person's sexuality begins with the determination of genetic gender, which occurs at the time of conception. At this time, the fertilized egg contains forty-six chromosomes, with the mother and father each contributing twenty-three chromosomes. The twenty-third pair are the sex chromosomes. This pair determines whether the internal sexual structures and the external genitalia will develop for a male or a female. The sex chromosomes are designated X and Y. The mother can only contribute an X chromosome, whereas the father can contribute either an X or a Y chromosome. If the twenty-third pair of chromosomes has an XX configuration, the zygote will develop into a female; if it has an XY configuration, it will develop into a male.

As you can see, it is the father's chromosome that is ultimately responsible for gender determination. It is interesting to note, however, that most of the genetic information is found on the X chromosome. The genes on the Y chromosome are mainly coded for "maleness" and little else. Humans cannot survive without at least one X chromosome.

Gonadal Gender

Even though the genetic gender of the embryo is already determined, the reproductive sex organs, or **gonads,** have not yet been established. The embryo contains tissue that is capable of forming either a male or a female reproductive system. If a Y chromosome is present, a signal is given for the gonads to develop into testes. If there is no Y chromosome, the gonads develop into ovaries. It is not until approximately six to eight weeks after conception that gonadal differentiation occurs.

Hormonal Gender

If the gonads develop into testes, the testes will produce and secrete androgens (male sex hormones). Androgens, with testosterone being the principal one, must be present in sufficient amounts for the normal development of the male internal reproductive system. If there is insufficient androgen production, development of the female internal reproductive system will occur instead. Thus, it is low levels of androgens rather than high levels of estrogens (female sex hormones) that are responsible for furthering female sexual development. The internal reproductive system is developed eight to twelve weeks after conception.

It is important to emphasize that even though there are male and female sex hormones, both sexes produce estrogen, progesterone, and testosterone. Gender differentiation depends on the relative proportions of androgens and estrogens secreted (see Chapter 8).

Genital Gender

Once the internal reproductive structures have developed, the external genitals begin to differentiate. If testes are present and are producing male sex hormones, a penis and scrotum will develop. The absence of male hormones will prompt the development of female external genitals. This includes the clitoris, the outer and inner folds of labial tissue, and the vaginal opening. By the end of the twelfth week, the fetus is clearly male or female in its sexual anatomy.

■ Determining Your Child's Sex

Have you given any thought to whether or not you want to have children? If you want children, how many would you like to have? Do you want sons, daughters, or both? If you could have a son and a daughter, which one would you want first? It is a couple's decision regarding the number of children they are going to have. As long as both partners are fertile and there are no health problems, a couple can choose to have one child or ten children. Can a couple also decide what gender their child is going to be? Is this a decision within the realm of possibility? It may surprise you to know that not only can a couple select the gender of their child but that the methods involved are relatively simple and easy to follow.

In this chapter, the section on genetic gender explained that the male sperm contains the sex-determining chromosome. The semen ejaculated during intercourse contains millions of sperm cells. Both X and Y chromosomes are present. Reliable gender-selection methods are based on knowing the differences between Y-bearing sperm and X-bearing sperm. If a couple wants a boy, they need to know what factors will increase the likelihood of getting the Y-bearing sperm to fertilize the egg; if a couple wants a girl, they need to know what factors will increase the likelihood of getting the X-bearing sperm to fertilize the egg. Let's consider some necessary information about androsperm (sperm carrying a Y chromosome) and gynosperm (sperm carrying an X chromosome).

Androsperm are not as hardy as gynosperm. They are less resistant to the vagina's acidic environment, which causes them to die more rapidly once deposited into the vagina. They are, however, more motile than gynosperm, so they are able to move faster. Gynosperm are hardier and are able to survive the vagina's acidity, but because they're less motile than androsperm, they do not travel as quickly. Using this information, how can a couple increase the chances of conceiving a male?

1. Because androsperm move quicker, the couple should have intercourse at the time of ovulation. By doing this, the androsperm will be the first to reach the egg in the fallopian tube.
2. To lessen the acidity of the vagina, the female should **douche** with a baking soda and water solution right before intercourse. Since baking soda is alkaline, it will make the vagina more hospitable for the androsperm.
3. Deep penetration in the vagina by the male at the time of ejaculation will help deposit the sperm close to the cervix. This will help the androsperm bypass the vagina's acidic environment.

The following would be done to increase the chances of conceiving a female:

FAST FACTS

There are laboratory procedures for treating a man's semen that may increase the chances of conceiving a child of the sex of choice. Artificial insemination, however, would then be required to achieve fertilization.

1. Because gynosperm are hardy but slower, the couple should have intercourse about two to three days before ovulation. By doing this, the gynosperm will be waiting in the fallopian tube when ovulation occurs.
2. To increase the acidity of the vagina, the female should douche with a vinegar and water solution right before intercourse. Since vinegar is acidic, it will increase the chances of immobilizing the androsperm.
3. Shallow penetration in the vagina by the male at the time of ejaculation will force the sperm to travel through the vagina's acidic environment.

The preceding suggestions can help increase the likelihood of conceiving a male or a female child. These methods are not foolproof, however. The couple must be certain that they want a child, regardless of what its gender will be. Once that is decided, trying any of the suggested methods will have no harmful effects on the male, female, or potential child. There is still controversy surrounding the use of gender-selection methods. Many people question their morality and wonder what the future ramifications might be.

> ■ *PROBLEM SITUATION* Suppose you could determine your child's sex? Would you want to? What advantages and disadvantages could you envision?

■ The Question of Parenthood

One of the most important, responsibility-laden decisions that you will make in your life is whether or not to have children. The outcome of this decision will have far-reaching effects that will last throughout your lifetime. Most people in our society become parents, yet an increasing number of people are choosing not to do so. It is important to decide for yourself if and when you should become a parent. Having children is not for everyone. Readiness for parenthood involves physical, psychological, emotional, intellectual, and financial factors. Some people may conclude that they are mature enough and ready for the responsibility of parenthood. Others may feel that they will not be ready to undertake such a commitment for several years. Then there are those people who, for whatever reason, choose never to become parents.

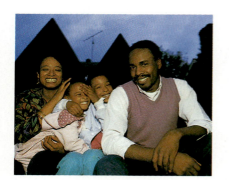

Happy parents make happy children!

If you want to become a responsible parent, the first step is to learn the realities of parenthood. Parenthood has been romanticized, glamorized, and idealized. On television, for example, children are pictured as being sweet, cute, cheerful, and clean. Parents are portrayed as being wise and understanding and as having infinite amounts of patience. If you put this combination together, you get perfect parents raising perfect children. Perfection, however, is a myth, not a reality. Children can be sweet and cute, but they can also be irritating and unpleasant. Even the most patient parent can be sorely tested after a stressful day. And you must realize that when raising children, there will be many stressful days.

To prepare for parenthood, you should obtain information about child care and development. Becoming aware of developmental patterns and child-care procedures will give you a better understanding of what to expect when raising a child. The care of a child necessitates high energy levels, especially during the early stages of parenthood. A child must be fed, bathed, clothed, nurtured, loved, played with, socialized, disciplined, and educated. Don't underestimate the amount of energy and patience you will need in order to meet a child's physical and emotional demands. A parent must be prepared to set aside his or her personal needs and make the child's needs top priority. This doesn't mean that parents must totally abandon their activities and interests, but many personal goals might have to be postponed. Financial considerations are also very important. The expense of having a child begins with pregnancy and continues through college and beyond. Government estimates of the cost of raising a child to age eighteen range from $81,000 to $117,000.

You may be wondering, after reading this information, why anyone would want to become a parent if it brings so many burdens. The reason is because parenthood also brings so much joy, love, excitement, enrichment, and fulfillment into a person's life. No one can decide for you whether or not you should have children. What makes another person happy may not make you happy. The two most important questions you must ask yourself are: Do I want to

GUIDELINES TO YOUR GOOD HEALTH

The following questions should be considered when deciding whether or not to have a child:

1. Does my partner want to have a child? Have we talked about our reasons?
2. Could we give a child a good home? Is our relationship a happy and strong one?
3. Are we both ready to give our time and energy to raising a child?
4. Do my partner and I understand each other's feelings about religion, work, family, child raising, and future goals? Do we feel pretty much the same way? Does having and raising a child fit the life-style I(we) want?
5. What would happen if we separated after having a child or if one of us should die?
6. Can I(we) afford to support a child? Do I(we) know how much it costs to raise a child?
7. Do I(we) like children? When I'm(we're) around children for a while, what do I(we) think or feel about having one around all of the time?
8. Do I(we) like doing things with children? Do I(we) enjoy activities that children can do?
9. Am I(we) patient enough to deal with the noise and the confusion and the twenty-four-hour-a-day responsibility? What kind of time and space do I(we) need?
10. How would I(we) take care of the child's health and safety?
11. What does discipline mean to me(us)? What does freedom, or setting limits, or giving space mean? Would I(we) want a perfect child?
12. Do I(we) want a boy or girl? What if I(we) don't get what I(we) want?
13. Do I(we) want a child in order to make my(our) life happier or better? Do I(we) see a child as someone to take care of me(us) in old age?
14. What if I(we) have a child and find out that I(we) made a wrong decision?

have a child? and Am I ready for the responsibility of parenthood? The more information you have about parenting, the easier it will be to make a responsible and appropriate decision.

> ■ *PROBLEM SITUATION* If you could be the "ideal" parent, what characteristics would you want to possess? What characteristics do you perceive as obstacles or weaknesses that might stand in your way of being a good parent?

■ Pregnancy

Once implantation of the blastocyst occurs, the endometrium remains intact in order to nourish the developing organism; therefore, one of the first signs of pregnancy is the cessation of menstruation. Other signs may include frequency of urination, enlargement and tenderness of the breasts, fatigue, and nausea. If any or all of these symptoms occur, a pregnancy test should be performed.

Pregnancy Testing

A pregnancy test is based on finding the hormone, **human chorionic gonadotropin** (HCG), in the blood or urine of a pregnant woman. HCG is secreted by the placenta. The presence of HCG may be detected in a blood sample within a week after conception. Many of today's do-it-yourself home pregnancy tests claim to be able to detect pregnancy within a day or two of the first missed menstrual period. At-home tests simply require a morning sample of urine. Because these tests can give misleading results, especially if the test is performed too early into the pregnancy, it is important to repeat the test after waiting a few days.

If the test results are positive (indicate pregnancy), the woman should seek confirmation by having a laboratory test and an internal pelvic examination performed. A **gynecologist** can usually detect pregnancy by an internal examination within two weeks of the first missed menstrual period. When a woman is pregnant, the cervix becomes softer and appears bluish in color. Also, the uterus expands and becomes rounder and softer.

If a woman is pregnant, she can figure out her expected date of delivery by adding seven days to the first day of her last menstrual period and then subtracting three months from that day. This predicted delivery date is called the **expected date of confinement** (EDC). Most women deliver their babies within two weeks of the EDC. The average length of human pregnancy is 266 days, or approximately nine months.

Pregnancy and Diet

The amount and kinds of food a woman eats during pregnancy are crucial for a healthy pregnancy and baby. A woman should gain about twenty to twenty-five pounds during her pregnancy (see Figure 10–2). Additional weight gain will consist of retained fluid and fat.

Many women overeat during pregnancy because they believe that they are "eating for two." Pregnancy should not be used as an excuse for overeating. A pregnant woman should expect a usual weight gain of about seventeen pounds.

FAST FACTS

Some men experience morning sickness and vomiting when their wives become pregnant.

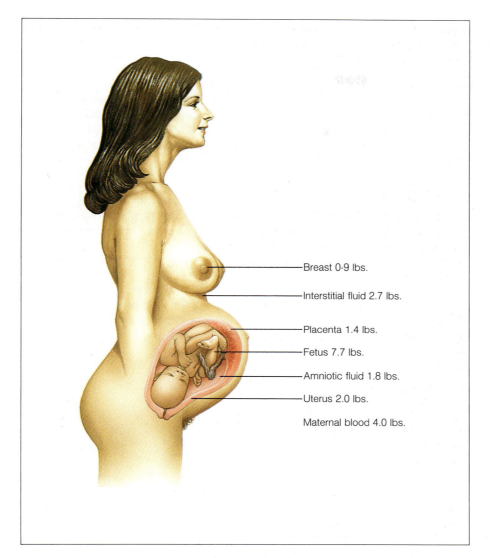

FIGURE 10–2 ■ Weight Gain in Pregnancy

This weight gain will account for the actual weight of the baby, the placenta, the amniotic fluid, the increase in the size of the breasts and uterus, and the additional blood in the system. Provided that the woman is not overweight when she conceives, an increase of five to ten pounds in her own weight is acceptable. Thus, a total weight gain in the area of twenty-five pounds is considered normal. If a woman is overweight at the beginning of her pregnancy, she is at a disadvantage, but her physician will probably not want her to try to lose any weight. A pregnant woman should never try any crash diets or fad diets while she is pregnant. She needs to eat well-balanced meals and nutritious foods. She should reduce or eliminate her intake of high-fat and high-sugar foods. During pregnancy, there is an increased need for many vitamins and minerals, such as calcium, iron, and B vitamins. A pregnant woman should consult with her physician about the amount and types of food she should be eating, the amount of fluid she should be drinking, and the types of dietary supplements she should be taking.

FAST FACTS

During pregnancy, a female's RDA for folic acid more than doubles; for iron, it doubles; but for calcium it remains the same.

SECTION III ■ UNDERSTANDING SEXUALITY

Pregnancy and Activity

A pregnant woman does not need to restrict her activities during most of her pregnancy. Unless there are complications, she can do everything she did before her pregnancy. She may set her own limits based on factors such as fatigue or physical discomfort. Exercise is important during pregnancy, but the woman must proceed with care and moderation. She should engage in activities that will improve her cardiovascular functioning and give her a feeling of well-being. She should avoid activities that are too strenuous and that might pose health risks to both her and the fetus.

> ■ **PROBLEM SITUATION** If you were pregnant and your physician told you that you must keep physically fit throughout your pregnancy, what kinds of activities would be healthy and beneficial for you? How might your needs change as you progress further into pregnancy?

During an uncomplicated pregnancy, sexual intercourse can continue right up until the last month of pregnancy. As the pregnancy progresses, however, the couple may need to modify their intercourse positions. Even when the couple decides to stop having intercourse, they can continue to give and receive sexual pleasure through other means.

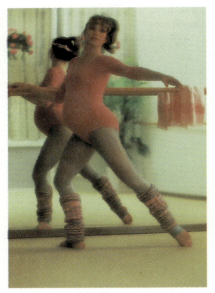

Dancing is an excellent way to exercise during pregnancy.

FIGURE 10–3 ■ **Fetus in Amniotic Sac with Placenta and Umbilical Cord**

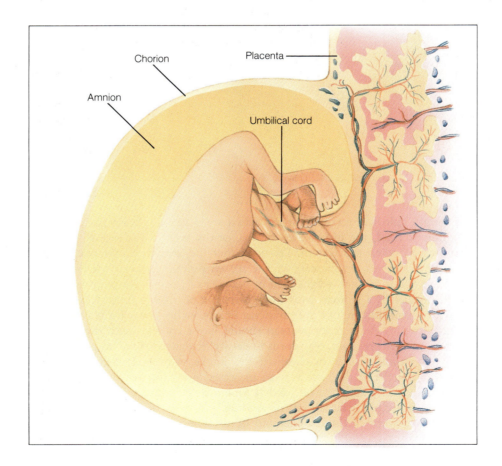

Fetal Development

After implantation occurs, the outer part of the cell mass develops into the placenta, umbilical cord, and amniotic sac (illustrated in Figure 10–3). The **placenta** is an organ that attaches to the uterine wall and exchanges nutrients and waste products between the mother and the fetus. The placenta also secretes enough progesterone and estrogen to maintain the pregnancy. The **umbilical cord** connects the fetus to the placenta. Through this cord the exchange of nourishment and body wastes between the mother and the fetus takes place. The **amniotic sac** is a fluid-filled membrane that surrounds and protects the fetus.

From the second week of pregnancy to the end of the eighth week, the developing organism is referred to as an **embryo**. From the beginning of the ninth week of pregnancy until birth, it is referred to as a **fetus**. Prenatal development is usually described in terms of trimesters. There are three trimesters, each one being three months in length.

First Trimester

The first trimester, weeks one through twelve, begins with implantation of the blastocyst. During the first month of pregnancy, many women are unaware that they are pregnant. The embryo, however, is developing its major systems and body parts. The heart and circulation have begun to function. The embryo's body is elongated, tapering off into a small, pointed tail.

During the second month, the head represents almost half the embryo's total bulk. The beginnings of facial features, such as eyes, ears, nose, and lips, can be seen. The small tail, which developed during the first month, will disappear by the eighth week. By the end of the second month, the embryo is starting to look like a tiny human being (illustrated in Figure 10–4).

When the third month begins, the embryo begins to be referred to as a fetus. Bone cells are now present. A backbone is clearly visible. All of the fetus's internal organs, such as the liver and kidneys, have begun limited functioning. The fetus can move, but its motions are not yet felt by the mother. The external

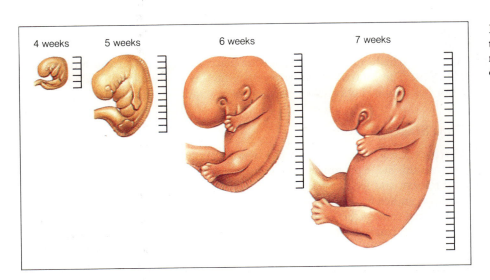

FIGURE 10–4 ■ **In the fifth through seventh weeks of development, the embryonic body and face develop a humanlike appearance.**

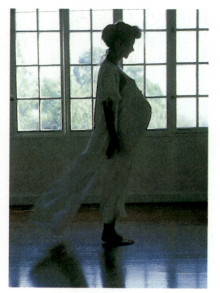

A woman's figure changes perhaps most obviously during the second trimester of pregnancy.

genitals can distinguish the fetus as being male or female. By the end of the first trimester, the fetus is three inches long and weighs about one ounce. During this three-month period, it is particularly vulnerable to damaging influences.

Second Trimester

The second trimester consists of weeks thirteen through twenty-four. All body systems and parts are developed. Everything is present in the fetus that will be found at birth. The body is growing increasingly larger, and the head is now about one-third the length of the body. By the end of the fourth month, the fetus's movements, called **quickening,** can be felt by the mother.

During the fifth month, the fetus first opens its eyes. It sleeps and wakes. The whole body is covered by a fine, downlike hair, called lanugo, that disappears before birth. The fetal heartbeat can be heard by pressing an ear to the mother's abdomen.

By the sixth month, fat deposits have formed, giving the fetus a more rounded shape. The skin is wrinkled and pink. The fetus is now about fourteen inches long and weighs over one pound. A fetus born at this stage probably would not survive.

Third Trimester

During the third trimester, weeks twenty-five through birth, the fetus primarily gains weight. The skin becomes less wrinkled as fat deposits continue to form. The fine body hair disappears, and hair often grows on the head. The testes of males descend into the scrotum during this time. The fetus can cry, breathe, and swallow. A fetus born in the seventh month is capable of survival.

Toward the end of this trimester, the fetus positions itself for birth by turning to a head-down position. At the end of the ninth month, the fetus is said to be full term. It is now about eighteen to twenty inches long and weighs an average of six to eight pounds. The fetus is now ready for delivery and birth.

■ Childbirth

Several hours before **labor** begins, a small amount of bloody vaginal discharge appears **(bloody show).** This results from the release of the mucous plug that had blocked the cervix. Labor seems to be triggered by hormones secreted by the fetus, which, in turn, stimulate the placenta and uterus to secrete **prostaglandins.** These prostaglandins produce uterine contractions. The process of labor has begun. Labor takes place in three stages (see Figure 10–5).

First Stage of Labor

Uterine contractions are felt by the woman about every fifteen to twenty minutes. As this stage progresses, the contractions come closer together, are longer in duration, and feel intensely uncomfortable. During the first stage, the cervix dilates completely. This stage of labor is the longest. Complete dilation, four inches (ten centimeters) across, usually takes an average of eight to twelve hours in a first pregnancy. During this time, the fetus's head is descending into the pelvic canal. If anesthesia is used, it is administered late in the first stage or during the second stage of labor.

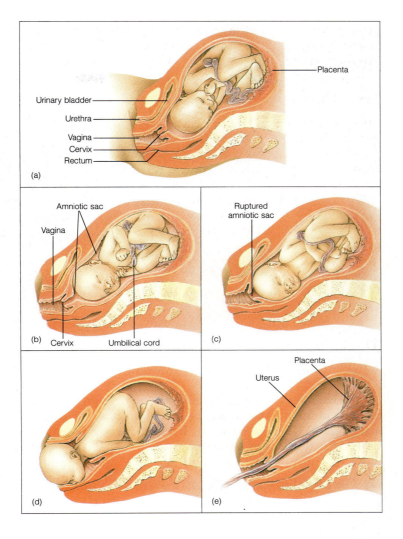

FIGURE 10-5 ■ **Birth**
(a) Fetal position prior to birth; (b and c) Stages of dilation; (d) Stage of expulsion; (e) Placental stage.

Second Stage of Labor

The second stage of labor involves the actual birth of the baby. It can last from a few minutes to about two hours. During this stage, the woman "bears down" with the abdominal muscles in order to assist the uterine contractions. When the baby's head is visible at the vaginal opening, crowning is said to have occurred. Sometimes an **episiotomy** is performed. An incision is made to enlarge the vaginal opening to provide a larger passageway for the baby and to prevent the tearing of vaginal tissue. An episiotomy should not be a routine procedure; it should be performed only when absolutely necessary. When the baby is born, it takes its first breath of air and cries spontaneously. The baby's mouth and nose are suctioned, the umbilical cord is cut and tied, and the baby is cleaned and examined.

Third Stage of Labor

The third stage of labor involves the expulsion of the **afterbirth.** The afterbirth consists of the placenta and the rest of the umbilical cord. This stage usually

FAST FACTS

In 1900, less than 5 percent of all American women delivered their babies in hospitals.

Giving birth to a child should be a shared experience.

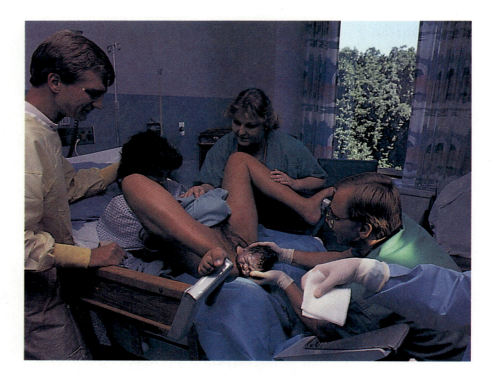

occurs about five to ten minutes after the baby is born. The placenta is examined carefully to make certain that it is intact. Any placental tissue left in the uterus may cause bleeding or infection. If an episiotomy was performed, it is sewn closed after the delivery of the placenta.

■ Gender Differentiation: Postnatal Variables

There are four variables relevant to gender that have their effect after birth. They include:

■ **Assigned gender**—the gender assigned to a newborn infant based on the appearance of the infant's external genitals.
■ **Gender identity**—the feeling that one is a male or a female.
■ **Gender role**—the traits and behaviors expected of males as compared to females in a give culture.
■ **Gender role identification**—the way in which a person incorporates into his or her personality the behavior expected of males and females in his or her culture.

At the time of birth, the newborn infant is assigned a gender. The assignment is based on the appearance of the infant's external genitals. The moment the doctor announces that the baby is a boy or a girl, other variables are set into action that will affect the baby's psychosexual development throughout his or her life.

When a baby is born, the selection of a name and the use of the male or female pronoun immediately begin the establishment of gender identity for the infant. Throughout the infant's development, boy-girl differences in clothing, toys, and activities reinforce specific gender. Sometime during childhood, the child realizes that he or she is of one gender and that some children are of another. Once gender identity is established, society has certain expectations of what male versus female traits and behaviors should be. This concept of gender role is culturally defined. In the American culture, males have been expected to be the strong, aggressive, brave, "take-charge-of" gender. Females, in contrast, have been expected to be the weak, passive, emotional, "take-care-of" gender.

Our society has deemed what makes a person masculine or feminine. Remember, however, that masculinity and femininity are just concepts. It is your right to choose those traits and behaviors that are appropriate and comfortable for you. You may choose to conform to those behaviors traditionally associated with your gender, or you may choose to reject them. You may feel that you want to experience and integrate a combination of traits and behaviors. The important thing is that you don't deprive yourself of being a fully functioning individual because of gender stereotypes.

POSITIVE BEHAVIORS

I. *Place a check mark in front of each behavior that you now practice.*

_____ 1. I don't perpetuate the stereotypical myths about male and female sex roles. (SEX ROLES)

_____ 2. I don't deprive myself of being a fully functioning individual because of gender stereotypes. (FULLY FUNCTIONING)

_____ 3. I am not a selfish person. (SELFISH)

_____ 4. I give of myself freely. (GIVE FREELY)

_____ 5. I don't feel that I would be less of a man or woman if I decided not to have children. (CHILDREN)

_____ 6. I am a patient person. (PATIENT)

_____ 7. I can cope with lots of noise and activity going on around me. (COPE)

_____ 8. I don't panic in crisis situations. (PANIC)

_____ 9. I can effectively handle conflict. (CONFLICT)

_____ 10. I value the rights of children. (RIGHTS)

II. *For each behavior that you DO NOT ENGAGE IN, write the KEY WORD(S) located in the parentheses at the end of the statement in the column below. Then put a check mark in the appropriate column to indicate whether you are going to keep or change that behavior.*

Behaviors I Don't Engage In   KEEP/CHANGE

_____   _____/_____
_____   _____/_____
_____   _____/_____
_____   _____/_____
_____   _____/_____
_____   _____/_____
_____   _____/_____
_____   _____/_____
_____   _____/_____
_____   _____/_____

III. *For each of the preceding behaviors that you choose to KEEP, write a statement indicating why you are choosing to keep that behavior.*

I choose to keep behavior _____ because:
                           KEY WORD

For each of the preceding behaviors that you choose to CHANGE, write a statement indicating how you plan to implement that change.

I will change behavior _____ by:
                        KEY WORD

Now You Know

1. TRUE. The ovum is about the size of a grain of sand.
2. TRUE. The egg is only viable for twenty-four hours; after that it degenerates.
3. TRUE. If intercourse occurs within five days before ovulation, live sperm may be waiting in the fallopian tube to fertilize the egg.
4. FALSE. The mother can only contribute an X chromosome, whereas the father can contribute either an X or a Y chromosome.
5. TRUE. A Y-bearing sperm has the ability to move faster than an X-bearing sperm. By having sexual intercourse at the time of ovulation, the Y-bearing sperm will be the first to reach the egg in the fallopian tube.
6. FALSE. The first objective sign of pregnancy is the stoppage of menstruation.
7. FALSE. A woman should gain about twenty to twenty-five pounds during her pregnancy.
8. TRUE. The hormone, human chorionic gonadotropin (HCG), which is secreted by the placenta, can be detected in the blood within a week after conception.
9. FALSE. During an uncomplicated pregnancy, sexual intercourse can continue right up until the last month of pregnancy.
10. FALSE. When a baby is born, it takes its first breath of air and cries spontaneously.

Summary

1. Sperm are the male's reproductive cells. They are produced in the seminiferous tubules, which are located in the testicles. The male starts producing sperm when he reaches puberty, manufacturing billions of sperm annually.

2. Each mature sperm cell consists of a head, a midpiece, and a long tail. The tail gives the sperm its motility. The head contains a chemical antibody that helps dissolve the membrane of the egg and allows the sperm to enter. The head also contains twenty-three chromosomes, with the twenty-third chromosome being the sex-determining chromosome.

3. Ova, or eggs, are the female's reproductive cells. At birth, the female's ovaries contain all of the potential eggs that she will ovulate throughout her reproductive years. The female is born with approximately 500,000 immature eggs. When she reaches puberty, the eggs begin to mature in preparation for ovulation. Only about 400 to 500 eggs are ovulated during a female's reproductive years. The remaining eggs degenerate within the ovaries.

4. Fertilization is the union of sperm and egg. Although several million sperm are ejaculated into the vagina, only a few hundred actually get near the egg. Factors responsible for reducing the number of sperm that reach the egg include sperm spilling out of the vagina, the hostile environment of the vagina, and the high percentage of defective sperm. Once a sperm fertilizes an egg, the egg is impenetrable to the entrance of other sperm. Fertilization has to occur during the first twenty-four hours that the egg is in the fallopian tube.

5. The joining of sperm and egg produces a zygote. By the end of the first week, the zygote forms a hollow, spherical mass of cells referred to as a blastocyst. About seven or eight days after fertilization, the blastocyst attaches itself to the endometrial lining of the uterus. This process of attachment is called implantation. Pregnancy has now begun.

6. The biological variables related to gender that evolve prenatally include genetic gender, gonadal gender, hormonal gender, and genital gender. Genetic gender determines whether the embryo will have an XY (male) or an XX (female) chromosomal configuration. Gonadal gender determines if the sex organs will develop into testicles or ovaries. Hormonal gender determines whether significant amounts of male or female sex hormones will be produced. Genital gender determines whether the external genitals will be a penis and scrotum or a vulva.

7. If a couple wants to conceive a boy, they should have intercourse at the time of ovulation, the female should douche with a baking soda and water solution right before sexual intercourse, and there should be deep penetration in the vagina by the male at the time of ejaculation.

8. To increase the chances of conceiving a girl, the couple should have intercourse about two to three days before ovulation, the female should douche with a vinegar and water solution right before sexual intercourse, and there should be shallow penetration in the vagina by the male at the time of ejaculation.

9. Whether or not to have children is an important, responsibility-laden decision. Readiness for parenthood involves physical, psychological, emotional, intellectual, and financial factors. You must ask yourself whether you want to have a child and whether you are ready for the responsibility of parenthood.

10. One of the first signs of pregnancy is the cessation of menstruation. Home pregnancy tests claim to be able to detect pregnancy within a day or two of the first missed menstrual period. If a woman is pregnant, she can figure

out her expected date of delivery by adding seven days to the first day of her last menstrual period and then subtracting three months from that day. This predicted date of delivery is called the expected date of confinement (EDC).

11. A woman should gain about twenty to twenty-five pounds during her pregnancy. Pregnancy should not be used as an excuse for overeating. If a woman is overweight at the beginning of her pregnancy, she is at a disadvantage, but her physician will probably not want her to lose any weight. A pregnant woman should never try any crash diets or fad diets while she is pregnant.

12. A healthy pregnant woman does not need to restrict her activities during most of her pregnancy. Exercise is important, but the woman must proceed with care and moderation. During an uncomplicated pregnancy, sexual intercourse can continue right up until the last month of pregnancy.

13. Prenatal development is usually described in terms of three trimesters, each one being three months in length. From the second week of pregnancy to the end of the eighth week, the developing organism is referred to as an embryo. From the beginning of the ninth week until birth, it is referred to as a fetus.

14. When a woman goes into labor, she knows the fetus is ready to be born. Labor takes place in three stages. During the first stage of labor, uterine contractions are felt by the woman and the cervix starts to dilate. Complete dilation usually takes an average of eight to twelve hours in a first pregnancy. This stage of labor is the longest. The second stage of labor involves the actual birth of the baby. This stage can last from a few minutes to about two hours. The third stage of labor involves the expulsion of the afterbirth, which consists of the placenta and the rest of the umbilical cord. This stage usually occurs about five to ten minutes after the baby is born.

15. The variables relevant to gender that have their effect postnatally include assigned gender, gender identity, gender role, and gender role identification. At the time of birth, the baby is assigned a gender (male or female). From that moment, other variables are set into action that will affect the baby's psychosexual development throughout his or her life.

References

1. Allgeier, Albert Richard, and Elizabeth Rice Allgeier. *Sexual Interactions.* Lexington, Massachusetts: D.C. Heath and Co., 1988.
2. Benderly, Beryl Lieff. *The Myth of Two Minds.* New York: Doubleday, 1987.
3. Doyle, James A. *The Male Experience,* 2d ed. Dubuque Iowa: William C. Brown, 1989.
4. Grabowski, Casimer T. *Human Reproduction and Development.* Philadelphia: Saunders College Publishing, 1983.
5. Haas, Kurt, and Adelaide Haas. *Understanding Sexuality.* St. Louis: Times Mirror/Mosby College Publishing, 1987.
6. Katchadourian, Herant A. *Biological Aspects of Human Sexuality,* 3d ed. New York: Holt, Rinehart and Winston, 1987.
7. Kelly, Gary F. *Sexuality Today: The Human Perspective.* Guilford, Connecticut: The Dushkin Publishing Group, 1988.
8. Nass, Gilbert D., and Mary Pat Fisher. *Sexuality Today.* Boston: Jones and Bartlett, 1988.
9. Schulz, David A. *Human Sexuality,* 3d ed. Englewood Cliffs, N.J.: Prentice-Hall, 1988.
10. Shettles, Landrum B., and David M. Rorvik. *How to Choose the Sex of Your Baby.* New York: Doubleday, 1984.
11. Stoppard, Miriam. *Pregnancy and Birth Book.* New York: Ballantine Books, 1985.
12. Strong, Bryan, and Christine DeVault. *The Marriage and Family Experience,* 4th ed. St. Paul: West Publishing Co., 1989.
13. Strong, Bryan, and Christine DeVault. *Understanding Our Sexuality,* 2d ed. St. Paul: West Publishing Co., 1988.
14. Whelan, Elizabeth. *Boy or Girl?* New York: Pocket Books, 1986.

Suggested Readings

Eisenberg, Arlene, Heidi Eisenberg Murkoff, and Sandee Eisenberg Hathaway. *What to Expect When You're Expecting.* New York: Workman Publishing Co., 1988.

Semchyshyn, Stefan, and Carol Colman. *How to Prevent Miscarriage and Other Crises of Pregnancy.* New York: MacMillan, 1989.

Shettles, Landrum B., and David M. Rorvik. *How to Choose the Sex of Your Baby.* New York: Doubleday, 1984.

Sussman, John R., and B. Blake Levitt. *Before You Conceive: The Complete Prepregnancy Guide.* New York: Bantam Books, 1989.

SECTION IV

Drugs and the Body

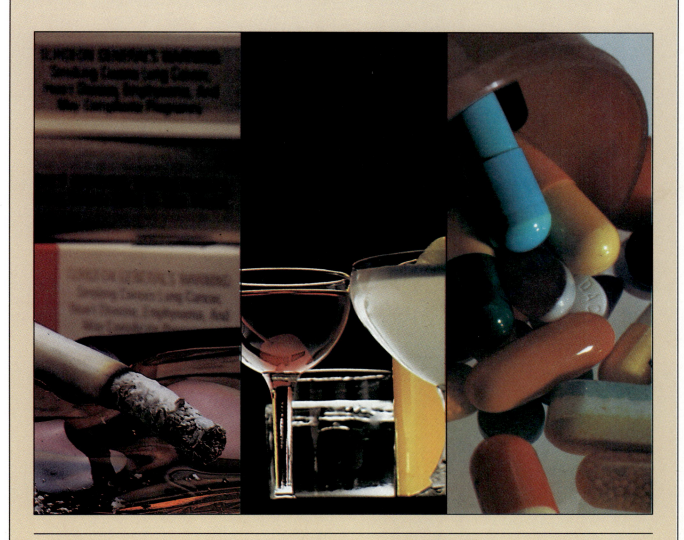

Chapter 11: The Tobacco Road
The Nervous System
Basic Facts About Smoking
Nicotine Addiction
The Major Constitutents of
Cigarette Smoke
Smoking and Health
Smoking Cessation Programs
The Benefits of Quitting Smoking
Involuntary Smoking

Smokeless Tobacco
Clove Cigarettes
Tobacco and the Law

Chapter 12: Alcohol Awareness
Basic Facts about Alcohol
Pharmacology
Alcohol and Disease
Alcohol and the Law
Fetal Alcohol Syndrome

Alcoholism

Chapter 13: Psychoactive Drugs
Deliriants
Depressants
Stimulants
Hallucinogens
Marijuana
Designer Drugs
The Xanthines

CHAPTER 11

The Tobacco Road

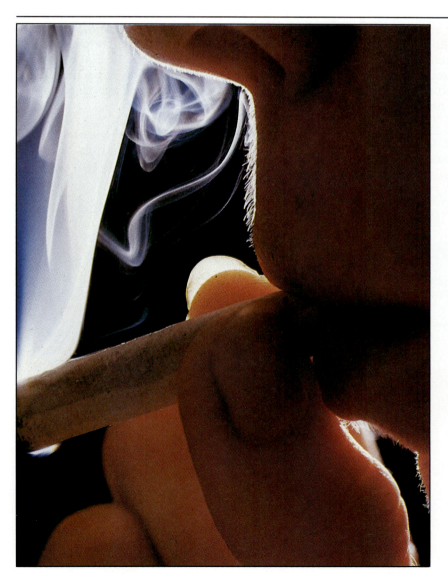

What Do You Know?

Are the following statements true or false?

1. Transmission of impulses through the nervous system is entirely electrical in nature.
2. Nicotine can increase heart rate and raise blood pressure.
3. Babies born to women who smoke during pregnancy are usually a little heavier than those born to nonsmoking women.
4. Smoking is a contributing factor in the development of wrinkles.
5. There are well-established relationships between exposure to second-hand smoke and disease.
6. The only type of cancer related to smoking is lung cancer.
7. Smokeless tobacco such as chewing tobacco is much safer than smoking itself.
8. Clove cigarettes are safer to smoke than tobacco cigarettes.
9. Tobacco use may be related to infertility in both men and women.
10. The most effective way to stop smoking is "cold turkey."

The Nervous System

To understand how drugs, including alcohol and tobacco, affect the body, it is important to have some understanding of the anatomy and physiology of the parts of the nervous system that they affect. Drugs, whether legal or illegal, are abused principally because of a desired effect on the central nervous system and, in particular, on the brain.

The nervous system is divided into the **central nervous system** (CNS), which consists of the brain and spinal cord, and the **peripheral nervous system** (PNS) (see Figure 11–1). The PNS is further divided into the **somatic nervous system** (SNS) and the **autonomic nervous system** (ANS). The ANS is still further divided into the **sympathetic** and **parasympathetic** systems. The sympathetic and parasympathetic systems generally have opposing effects on the parts of the body that they control—the visceral organs and the glandular and circulatory systems.

There are many billions of **neurons,** or nerve cells, in the body. Neurons may be as short as less than a millimeter or as long as a few feet. These specialized cells serve to transmit nerve impulses from one part of the body to another, electrically through the neurons and chemically from one neuron to another through a space known as a **synapse.** Impulse transmission across the synapse occurs through the action of a number of specific chemical substances known as **neurotransmitters.**

FIGURE 11–1 ■ **Organization of the Nervous System**

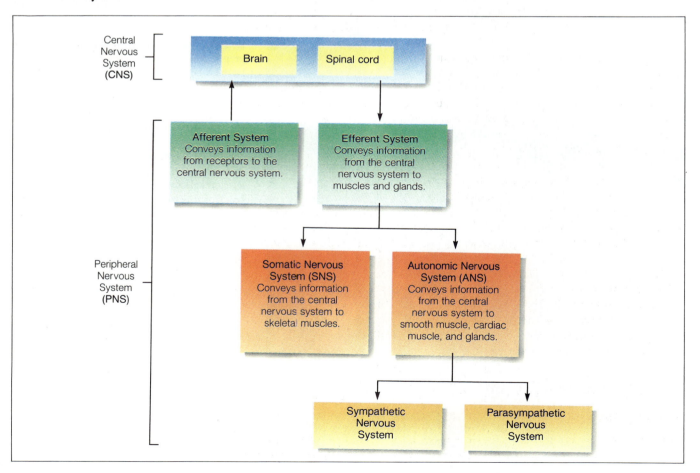

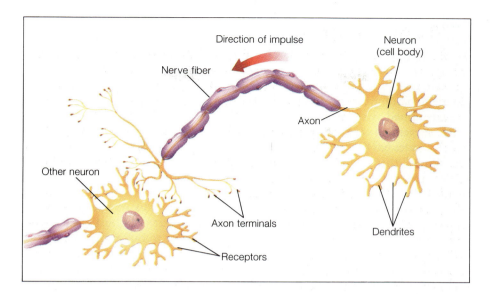

FIGURE 11-2 ■ **Diagram of a Neuron**

The neuron consists of the **cell body,** which directs the activities of the cell; the **dendrites,** which contain receptor sites that receive the information from the neurotransmitter; the **axon,** along which the impulse is transmitted electrically; and the **terminals,** from which the impulse is communicated chemically to the next synapse. Each neuron may synapse with thousands of other neurons. (See Figure 11-2.)

There are several chemical neurotransmitters. The four most often referred to are acetylcholine, serotonin, norepinephrine, and dopamine. Some experts believe that these are the only four neurotransmitters, whereas others think that there are more as yet undiscovered. The drugs we will discuss in the next three chapters act in some way on these neurotransmitters.

The receptor-site theory suggests that neurotransmitters act similarly to the way that a lock works with a key. The receptor site is the "lock" in which a specific neurotransmitter "key" must fit. When a nerve impulse reaches the terminals of a neuron, the appropriate neurotransmitter is released from vesicles in which it has been stored. In less than a thousandth of a second, the chemical crosses the synapse, binds to the receptor sites on the dendrites of the next neuron, and elicits an impulse in that cell. Then, as quickly as it was released, the neurotransmitter must either be destroyed or reabsorbed into the neuron from which it came.

Drugs, in some way, affect the release, action, breakdown, or reabsorption of the neurotransmitters. Some drugs may either increase or decrease the amount of neurotransmitter released. Others may mimic or block the action of a neurotransmitter. Some may inhibit the enzymes that break down the neurotransmitters, and still others may either increase or decrease the rate of the neurotransmitter's reabsorption back into the vesicles from which it was released.

■ Basic Facts About Smoking

Smoking and Life-style

At the turn of the century, most deaths were due to infectious diseases, and the average life expectancy was forty-seven years. Today life expectancy averages

FAST FACTS

Depression among teenagers is associated with increased frequency of cigarette smoking.

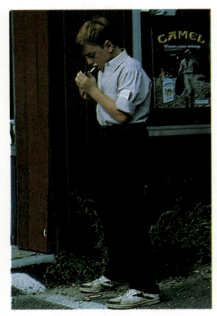

Although most smokers start at around 16 years of age, many start when they are much younger.

seventy-four years, and we no longer fear the diseases of the past such as smallpox, diphtheria, and typhoid. Now, chronic illnesses such as heart disease, cancer, emphysema, and diabetes present the major threats to health and longevity. Many of these diseases are related to our life-style habits and can be prevented to a great extent.

One habit of great concern throughout the world is cigarette smoking. It has been described by the director of the World Health Organization as the "largest single preventable cause of ill health in the world." The Surgeon General of the United States has reported that there are "more than 50,000 studies from dozens of cultures" that establish "cigarette smoking as the single largest preventable cause of premature death and disability in the United States." Table 11–1 notes the effects of nicotine on the body.

Approximately fifty million Americans smoke cigarettes regularly and consume more than 500 billion cigarettes per year. About one-third of all adults smoke, with a somewhat lower proportion of smokers among teenagers. Smokers represent about 30 percent of the population, down from over 42 percent in 1964. Until recently, the incidence of smoking was rising among young women and teenage girls. At present, the number of teenage girls who smoke exceeds the number of teenage boys who smoke. The overall rate of smoking has declined over the past twenty-five years, and many people have quit. Most of those giving up smoking have been well-educated older men, and most have quit *cold turkey*. The term "cold turkey" means that the individual has stopped smoking or some other behavior suddenly. At the present time, cigarette smoking is still decreasing in all groups (see Figure 11–3). About forty million Americans are ex-smokers.

Children whose parents smoke are more likely to become smokers, especially if they have brothers, sisters, or friends who smoke as well. Several studies have shown that children at lower educational and socioeconomic levels are more likely to smoke than those from higher educational and higher income levels. Those students who work while attending school are more likely to smoke than those who do not. Most smokers begin in the latter part of their high-school years at around sixteen years of age. Only about 10 to 15 percent of smokers

TABLE 11–1 ■ **Effects of Nicotine on the Body**

Short Term Effects	Long Term Effects
increases blood pressure	lung cancer
replaces oxygen in blood with carbon monoxide	heart disease
	stroke
paralyzes ciliary function	aortic aneurysm
decreases blood flow to the extremities	premature wrinkling
causes bad breath	chronic obstructive pulmonary disease
causes yellowing of fingernails and teeth	contributes to impotence and infertility
increases heart rate	
increases mucous	
dulls taste buds	

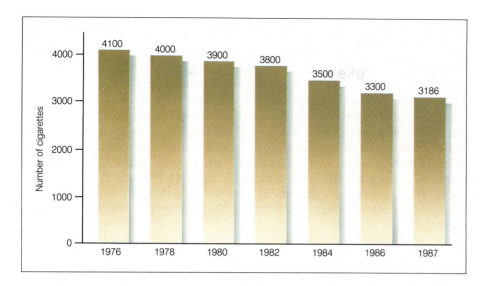

FIGURE 11-3 ■ Annual U.S. per Capita Consumption of Cigarettes by People 18 and Older

SOURCE: U.S. Department of Agriculture

begin after the age of nineteen. It is considered rare for anyone to begin smoking after the age of twenty-five.

Data about ethnic differences in patterns of cigarette smoking are limited, but recent evidence reported by the Centers for Disease Control suggests that certain minority groups, particularly Mexican-Americans, have shown a rise in the number of beginning smokers and "that minority groups may be at relatively high risk for lung cancer and other smoking-related diseases." Donald Garner of Southern Illinois University reported in his study that approximately 25 percent of white-collar workers and 50 percent of blue-collar workers smoke.

A government study published in May 1988 reported that smokers tend to snack more than nonsmokers. Smokers also tend to be less physically active, sleep less than six hours each night, skip breakfast more often than nonsmokers, and drink alcoholic beverages more heavily. Men who smoke heavily are more likely to be overweight, although that is not the case for smokers in general. Heavy smoking was defined in the study as smoking thirty-five or more cigarettes per day.

Nearly 22.5 percent of those who smoke heavily reported drinking two or more drinks per day as compared to only 3.6 percent of those who never smoked. Nearly half of the heavy smokers reported never eating breakfast. Approximately 65 percent of heavy smokers led a sedentary life-style. The study reported that "additional evidence has indicated that combining smoking with other unhealthy behaviors can multiply the probability of serious illness, . . . increase their probability of succumbing to serious illness, disability, and even death."

Economics of Tobacco

Tobacco is grown for profit in sixteen states and is the principal crop of several of them. Over $7 billion are collected each year in federal and state cigarette taxes. Tobacco companies spend nearly $900 million per year promoting smoking. Overall, tobacco growing is a $35 billion a year industry, with 90 percent of the money being spent on cigarettes. A one-pack-a-day smoker will spend over $400 per year on cigarettes.

FAST FACTS

The negative effects of smoking on blood vessels begin soon after a person begins smoking and are not easily reversed.

FAST FACTS

Nicotine gum helps suppress the withdrawal symptoms of smoking but does not reduce the craving.

As restrictions on tobacco advertising in the United States increase and as the number of smokers decrease, tobacco companies spend a great deal of time and money seeking new markets for their products. Dr. Gregory Connolly of the World Health Organization has criticized American tobacco companies for unleashing an advertising campaign directed specifically at the one billion females in the Orient who do not smoke. He condemned the companies for trying to create a "new demand among Oriental females and youth to offset the people that have quit in the United States" and for targeting "2 billion female lungs that haven't been contaminated by tobacco." Many foreign countries do not require warning labels on cigarette packs and allow tobacco products to be labeled with misleading information. A *Los Angeles Times* article in May 1988 reported that Marlboro cigarettes sold in the Phillipines as Marlboro Lights "actually have 50% higher tar content than the same product sold in the United States."

A September 1987 report from the Centers for Disease Control, U.S. Public Health Service, estimated the annual cost of smoking-related illness at between $39 billion and $55 billion. Other facts reported by the American Lung Association, but not always considered when discussing smoking, include the following: there are more than 130,000 fires each year related to smoking; smoking causes 20 percent of all work loss caused by illness; and smoking women spend 17 percent more sick days in bed than nonsmoking women. The American Council on Science and Health reports that over $930 billion was spent for cigarette-induced major illnesses between 1964 and 1983. According to Congress's Office of Technology Assessment, the total cost of combined health care and lost productivity caused by smoking is about $65 billion per year. That averages to approximately $2.17 per pack of cigarettes sold in the United States.

Nicotine Addiction

Horace Greeley, famous newspaper editor, once said that a cigarette had a fire on one end and a fool on the other. In the 1988 report, *The Health Consequences of Smoking: Nicotine Addiction,* C. Everett Koop, the Surgeon General of the United States, stated, "This report shows conclusively that cigarettes and other forms of tobacco are addicting in the same sense as are drugs such as heroin and cocaine." He also reported that tobacco-related deaths (300,000 per year) far outnumber those from alcohol (125,000), heroin (4,000), and cocaine (2,000).

At the Addiction Research Center in Baltimore, studies showed that monkeys taught to inject themselves with nicotine and cocaine would be equally anxious to get either drug. Another study at the University of Vermont College of Medicine showed that **withdrawal** from nicotine takes up to six weeks, whereas heroin withdrawal takes only a few days.

The Major Constituents of Cigarette Smoke

The major constituents of cigarette smoke are nicotine, carbon monoxide, and tars, although more than 1,200 toxic chemicals have been identified in it. Some of these include acrolein, nitrogen dioxide, formaldehyde, hydrogen sulfide, ammonia, and hydrocyanic acid. Some researchers estimate that there may be as many as 4,000 toxic materials in cigarette smoke.

SELF-INVENTORY 11.1

Why Do You Smoke?

Here are some statements made by people to describe what they get out of smoking cigarettes. How *often* do you feel this way when smoking them? Circle one number for each statement.

Important: Answer every question.

A. I smoke cigarettes in order to keep myself from slowing down. *Always* (5), *Frequently* (4), *Occasionally* (3), *Seldom* (2), *Never* (1).

B. Handling a cigarette is part of the enjoyment of smoking it. *Always* (5), *Frequently* (4), *Occasionally* (3), *Seldom* (2), *Never* (1).

C. Smoking cigarettes is pleasant and relaxing. *Always* (5), *Frequently* (4), *Occasionally* (3), *Seldom* (2), *Never* (1).

D. I light up a cigarette when I feel angry about something. *Always* (5), *Frequently* (4), *Occasionally* (3), *Seldom* (2), *Never* (1).

E. When I have run out of cigarettes I find it almost unbearable until I can get them. *Always* (5), *Frequently* (4), *Occasionally* (3), *Seldom* (2), *Never* (1).

F. I smoke cigarettes automatically without even being aware of it. *Always* (5), *Frequently* (4), *Occasionally* (3), *Seldom* (2), *Never* (1).

G. I smoke cigarettes to stimulate me, to perk myself up. *Always* (5), *Frequently* (4), *Occasionally* (3), *Seldom* (2), *Never* (1).

H. Part of the enjoyment of smoking a cigarette comes from the steps I take to light up. *Always* (5), *Frequently* (4), *Occasionally* (3), *Seldom* (2), *Never* (1).

I. I find cigarettes pleasurable. *Always* (5), *Frequently* (4), *Occasionally* (3), *Seldom* (2), *Never* (1).

J. When I feel uncomfortable or upset about something, I light up a cigarette. *Always* (5), *Frequently* (4), *Occasionally* (3), *Seldom* (2), *Never* (1).

K. I am very much aware of the fact when I am not smoking a cigarette. *Always* (5), *Frequently* (4), *Occasionally* (3), *Seldom* (2), *Never* (1).

L. I light up a cigarette without realizing I still have one burning in the ashtray. *Always* (5), *Frequently* (4), *Occasionally* (3), *Seldom* (2), *Never* (1).

M. I smoke cigarettes to give me a "lift." *Always* (5), *Frequently* (4), *Occasionally* (3), *Seldom* (2), *Never* (1).

N. When I smoke a cigarette, part of the enjoyment is watching the smoke as I exhale it. *Always* (5), *Frequently* (4), *Occasionally* (3), *Seldom* (2), *Never* (1).

O. I want a cigarette most when I am comfortable and relaxed. *Always* (5), *Frequently* (4), *Occasionally* (3), *Seldom* (2), *Never* (1).

P. When I feel "blue" or want to take my mind off cares and worries, I smoke cigarettes. *Always* (5), *Frequently* (4), *Occasionally* (3), *Seldom* (2), *Never* (1).

Q. I get a real gnawing hunger for a cigarette when I haven't smoked for a while. *Always* (5), *Frequently* (4), *Occasionally* (3), *Seldom* (2), *Never* (1).

R. I've found a cigarette in my mouth and didn't remember putting it there. *Always* (5), *Frequently* (4), *Occasionally* (3), *Seldom* (2), *Never* (1).

How To Score

1. Enter the numbers you have circled to the questions in the spaces below, putting the number you have circled to question A over line A, to question B over line B, and so on.

2. Total the 3 scores on each line to get your totals. For example, the sum of your scores over lines A, G, and M gives you your score on *Stimulation*—lines B, H, and N give the score on *Handling,* etc.

			Totals
___ + ___ + ___ =			_____
A G M			Stimulation
___ + ___ + ___ =			_____
B H N			Handling
___ + ___ + ___ =			_____
C I O			Pleasurable relaxation
___ + ___ + ___ =			_____
D J P			Crutch: tension reduction
___ + ___ + ___ =			_____
E K Q			Craving: psychological addiction
___ + ___ + ___ =			_____
F L R			Habit

Scores can vary from 3 to 15. Any score 11 and above is *high;* any score 7 and below is *low.*

SOURCE: National Clearinghouse for Smoking and Health (USPHS)

Nicotine

Nicotine is a very powerful chemical. It is found in no other plant except tobacco. Nicotine interferes with the neurotransmitter acetylcholine. It first excites the neurons for which acetylcholine is the neurotransmitter by attaching to the receptor sites; then it remains attached, thereby blocking further transmission. Ultimately, nicotine soothes and relaxes the smoker without diminishing alertness. People who smoke more than twenty cigarettes per day are considered to be addicted to the chemical. There are some indications that nicotine may cause stimulation of the pleasure centers in the brain.

Physiological effects of nicotine include constriction of the peripheral blood vessels (those near the surface of the body), which causes a five- to six-degree drop in skin temperature. A recent study suggested that the presence of nicotine in cigarettes increases the rate of development of lung cancers. Heart rate may increase as much as fifteen to twenty-five beats per minute with just one or two cigarettes, and blood pressure may rise as much as twenty points.

Evidence indicates that nicotine and other chemicals found in cigarette smoke increase the rate at which fatty materials—particularly cholesterol—are deposited along the inner linings of arteries. The development of these deposits may cause obstruction that leads to heart attack, stroke, and tissue damage in the extremities (see Chapter 16).

Carbon Monoxide

Carbon monoxide is a poisonous substance. It interferes with the transport of oxygen by attaching to the **hemoglobin** of the red blood cells in an almost irreversible reaction. Hemoglobin has a 200-times greater affinity for carbon monoxide than for oxygen. Smokers find themselves short of breath when extra

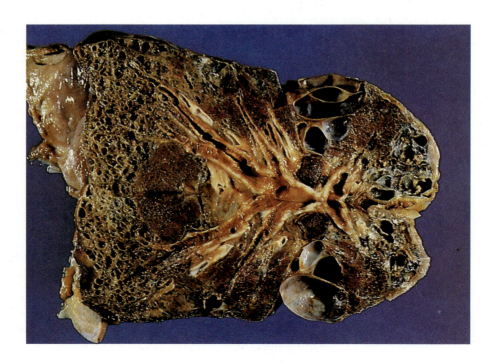

Both lung cancer and emphysema are evident in this lung from a smoker.

demands for oxygen are placed on the body, such as during athletic activities, because so much of their hemoglobin is made unavailable to oxygen as a result of their carbon monoxide levels.

Tars

Tars, as well as a variety of other chemicals found in cigarette smoke, are known **carcinogens.** Others include 4-aminobiphenyl, 2-naphthylamine, and polonium-210. These chemicals set up an irritative process in the bronchial tree that causes the epithelial cells (the cells lining the bronchial tubes) to become atypical and, in many cases, malignant. See Chapter 17 for a discussion of lung cancer.

Tars and damaged tissue may obstruct the air passages that lead to the tiny air sacs in the lungs. This can subsequently cause emphysema, a disease brought about by the gradual stretching of the walls of the alveoli, resulting ultimately in their rupture. Nicotine may also contribute to the changes that lead to this disease.

Cigarette smoking is the major cause of chronic bronchitis and emphysema, both of which are discussed in Chapter 17. It is estimated that ten to twelve million people in the United States are susceptible to the destructive effects of cigarette smoke that can lead to emphysema. Stopping smoking can not reverse the progress of emphysema, but it can prevent further damage.

> ■ *PROBLEM SITUATION* You have caught your eleven-year-old brother smoking a cigarette with his friends. How should you handle this situation? How can you discourage him from developing the smoking habit?

FAST FACTS

Recent evidence indicates that people who die due to smoking die an average of 23 years prematurely.

■ Smoking and Health

Smoking and Cancer

The American Cancer Society reports that there are about 150,000 new cases of lung cancer annually in the United States, 83 percent of which are caused by smoking. Smokers have a ten-fold greater chance of developing lung cancer than nonsmokers. Once a smoker gives up smoking, it takes the lungs ten to fifteen years to completely heal. At that point, the ex-smoker will have reduced his or her risk of lung cancer to that of a nonsmoker. The age at which a person begins to smoke, how long he or she has smoked, the depth of inhalation, and the amount smoked are all related to the chances of developing lung cancer.

Cigarette smoking is also related to cancer of the mouth, larynx, esophagus, bladder, and kidneys. In addition, the incidence of peptic ulcers is increased in smokers. Two studies reported in 1983, one in the *Journal of the American Medical Association* and the other in *American Journal of Public Health,* linked cigarette smoking to **dysplasia**—the growth of abnormal cells—and cancer of the cervix. (See Figure 11–4).

Smoking and Respiratory Disease

A smoker has a six times greater chance of dying from chronic bronchitis and emphysema than a nonsmoker. Smoking leads to excessive mucous production and paralysis of the hairlike cilia lining the bronchi. Studies show that cigarette

FIGURE 11-4 ■ Risks of Smoking and Cancer

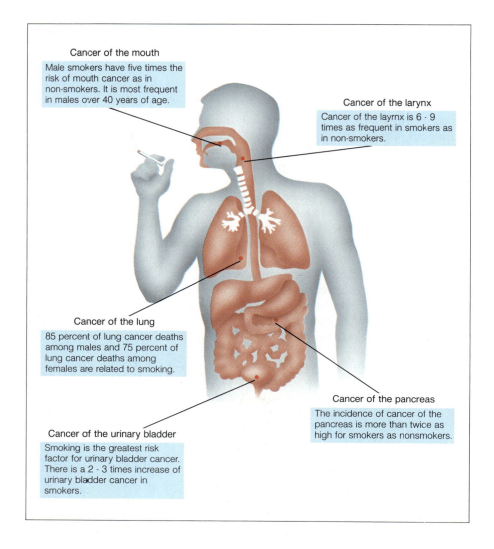

smoking is a more important factor in the development of lung disease than environmental pollution and that pollution has a much greater effect on the lungs of a smoker than those of a nonsmoker.

Smokers are more vulnerable to a variety of respiratory infections because of smoking's effect on the cilia. Tars and other substances in tobacco smoke interfere with the lungs' natural cleaning system.

Smoking and Cardiovascular Disease

Most studies on cardiovascular disease and its relation to smoke have shown that cigarette smokers have approximately twice the mortality rate from this disease as nonsmokers. Circulating free fatty acids in the blood are increased, which may increase the risk of atherosclerotic disease (see Chapter 16) and heart attack. The tendency for blood to clot also increases, possibly because of an increase in the stickiness of blood **platelets.** Clot formation can lead to heart attack.

There is a ten-fold increase in risk of heart attack in women who both smoke heavily and take oral contraceptives (heavy cigarette smoking is considered to be fifteen or more cigarettes per day). *Health Tips,* a publication of the California Medical Association, has reported that "a 25-year-old smoker faces the same risks from the pill as a 35-year-old nonsmoker."

Smoking and Other Diseases

Many studies have linked smoking to a variety of other diseases and conditions. In 1986, Dr. Michael Condra of Queens University in Ontario reported that cigarette smoking may be a significant risk factor in impotence. Dr. Condra's study showed that penile blood pressure in smokers was considerably less than in nonsmokers. In another experiment, the results of which were published in *Urology* in August 1987, dogs were exposed to cigarette smoke by natural inhalation. After inhaling the smoke of from two to three cigarettes, five of the six experimental animals were unable to achieve full erections.

Fertility and Sterility, August 1987, reported that studies of ejaculate volume, sperm density, and total sperm count showed that tobacco users had lower values for all three parameters than nonusers. Users included both smokers and those who chewed tobacco. Other studies have shown a relation between smoking and certain types of female infertility.

A 1987 study reported in *The Journal of Clinical Gastroenterology* that the recurrence of ulcers is more common in patients who smoke than in those who do not. This occurs because nicotine negatively affects the body's ability to counteract the effects of stomach acid. Other studies of patients with ulcers have shown that drugs used to treat the condition are more effective in nonsmokers than in smokers and that ulcers in nonsmokers tend to heal more quickly than in smokers.

An article in *The Journal of Clinical Periodontology,* April 1986, reported that smoking may negatively affect the healing of gum disease. Other studies have shown relations between smoking and increased incidence of Alzheimer's disease, increased numbers of kidney lesions in diabetic patients, increased hip fractures in elderly women, and more complications during general anesthesia.

Smoking and Pregnancy

Although it has been known for centuries that smoking during pregnancy can have a harmful effect on the unborn baby, serious studies of the subject did not take place until the 1950s. Recent evidence shows that cigarette smoking by a pregnant woman can have devastating effects on the unborn baby. Babies born to women who smoke tend to be of lower birth weight, show a higher incidence of prematurity, and show a higher incidence of stillbirths than babies born to nonsmoking mothers. Low birth weight is the leading cause of death during the first year of life. Babies born to smoking mothers have twice the death rate from sudden infant death syndrome (SIDS) as those born to nonsmoking mothers. They also have a higher incidence of respiratory problems as children.

Babies born to smoking women show a two- to three-times greater rate of prematurity than would normally occur. There is also a higher rate of spontaneous abortions among smoking mothers. The specific reasons for these oc-

FAST FACTS

Babies with low birth weight are approximately forty times more likely to die in the first month of life than babies of normal weight.

currences are not known. Theories relate to the carbon monoxide in cigarette smoke, which could possibly poison the blood of the fetus, or to nicotine, which reduces blood flow across the placenta.

Nearly fifty studies done since 1957 have confirmed that babies born to smoking mothers have an average birth weight 200 grams lower than that of babies born to nonsmoking mothers. As early as 1971, the report of the Surgeon General of the United States, *The Health Consequences of Smoking,* confirmed that the more a woman smokes during pregnancy, the greater are her chances of having a low-weight baby. In a study of newborn babies done in Sweden, researchers found that as maternal smoking increased, the baby's length, head circumference, and shoulder circumference decreased. The National Research Council has stated that babies born to nonsmoking women whose husbands smoke have a higher incidence of low birth weight than those born to nonsmoking parents. The March of Dimes has produced a button that states, "babies don't thrive in smoke filled wombs."

Studies of six- to seven-year-old children showed that those born to smoking mothers were, on the average, smaller for all measurements than children born to nonsmoking mothers. Other studies have shown that children of nonsmoking mothers have higher IQ scores than those whose mothers smoked during pregnancy.

The developing fetus, although immersed in fluid, needs to exercise its lungs so that it will be able to breathe on its own after birth. When a pregnant woman lights up a cigarette, the nicotine that enters her blood stream also enters the bloodstream of the fetus. That nicotine will temporarily stop the muscular activity of the baby's lungs. The more cigarettes the mother smokes, the less time the fetus's muscles get to exercise. This is thought to be a contributing factor in the higher incidence of respiratory problems, stillbirths, and sudden infant death syndrome among the infants born to smoking women.

> **PROBLEM SITUATION** Your sister is pregnant. Both she and her husband smoke. What can you tell them to discourage them from smoking during her pregnancy? Where can they go for help?

Smoking and Aging

A California study conducted more than ten years ago was the first to indicate that smoking accelerates the development of wrinkles. Because nicotine causes constriction of blood vessels near the skin surface, there is reduced circulation to that area. This makes the skin more susceptible to the damaging rays of the sun. The California study also showed that heavy cigarette smokers are as wrinkled as nonsmokers ten to twenty years older. Next time you are people-watching, see if you can tell the smokers from the nonsmokers just by looking at their skin.

Dr. Kay-Tee Khaw of the University of California at San Diego reported in June 1988 that higher levels of certain male hormones are found in older women who smoke cigarettes, which may explain why they have twice the risk for heart disease. Women who smoked had a 50 percent higher level of these hormones than those who did not smoke. The more a woman smoked, the higher the levels. One hypothesis is that smoking stimulates the adrenal glands to produce

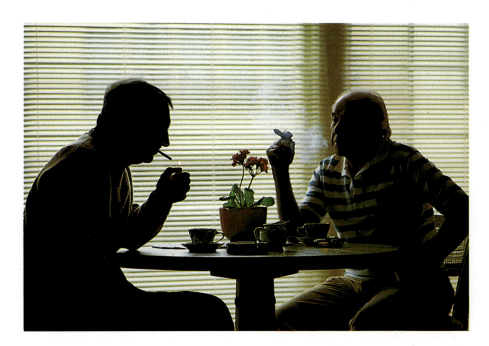

Cigarette smoking is responsible for a reduction in life expectancy of over 8 years in a 2-pack a day smoker.

larger amounts of these hormones. A second is that the proper metabolism of the hormones is prevented by some as-yet unidentified chemical found in cigarette smoke.

Older women may suffer from the effects of osteoporosis, a bone disease associated with frequent fractures. It is often treated with the female sex hormone estrogen. Studies have shown that smoking aggravates this disease. A report in *Health Tips* states that smoking "seems to increase the effects of osteoporosis in women who don't take estrogen and reduces the benefits of the hormone in those women who take it."

GUIDELINES TO YOUR GOOD HEALTH

To reduce the risk of cancer, cardiovascular disease, and other smoking-related illnesses for yourself and others:

1. Do not smoke any tobacco products.
2. Do not use smokeless tobacco or clove cigarettes.
3. Always ask for seating in the "No Smoking" section of a restaurant, airplane, or other public place.
4. Do not allow smoking in your home, car, or office.
5. Help educate others who smoke on the dangers of smoking.
6. Become involved in community campaigns against smoking in public places.
7. Adopt a smoker during the next Great American Smokeout and help him or her break the habit.

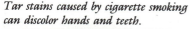

FAST FACTS

Only about 20 percent of those entering a smoking-cessation program continue to refrain from tobacco use one year after the program has ended.

Tar stains caused by cigarette smoking can discolor hands and teeth.

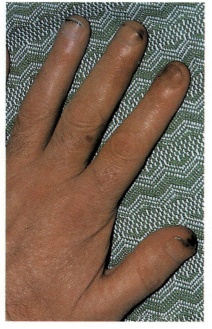

Smoking and Life Expectancy

The effect of smoking on life expectancy is significant. A fifteen-year-old nonsmoker has double the chance of living to age seventy-five than a fifteen-year-old smoker. The American Lung Association states that a twenty-five-year-old smoker of two packs per day will reduce his or her life expectancy by approximately eight years. Over 300,000 deaths per year—approximately 15 percent of all deaths—are directly related to smoking. A German study reported in 1986 that the health consequences of smoking can be seen soon after a person begins to smoke. In teenagers who had smoked only moderately for less than two years, abnormal white blood cell counts, lower-than-normal levels of high density lipoproteins in the blood, and reduced pulmonary function were detected. Approximately 40 percent of male smokers and 28 percent of female smokers will die prematurely.

■ Smoking-Cessation Programs

Many smokers say they would like to quit but can't. Ninety percent of teenagers who smoke say they want to quit. Each November, the American Cancer Society conducts the Great American Smokeout, during which time many thousands of smokers quit smoking for twenty-four hours. Nonsmokers are asked to "adopt a smoker" for the day to help him or her quit smoking (see Figure 11–5). Only about 6 to 7 percent of those who quit for the day are able to permanently break the habit. See Table 11–3 for a list of agencies that can supply materials to help a smoker quit.

Hypnotism, acupuncture, biofeedback, negative reinforcement, and many other stop-smoking products and programs are available. Over-the-counter medications sold in pharmacies and other retail stores are ineffective. Cigarette substitutes are also sold, many by mail order. They, too, do not work. (See Table 11–2 for information on quitting.) Nicorette, a prescription chewing gum containing nicotine, is now available. Chewing a piece of the gum instead of lighting a cigarette provides the nicotine without the dangers of inhaling smoke. It is easier to wean someone off nicotine chewing gum than cigarettes themselves. A recent study reported that Nicorette was the most successful method of stopping smoking other than quitting "cold turkey." Dr. Murray Jarvik of UCLA has suggested that only substitution therapy—the substitution of nicotine gum for smoking—has been successful.

Patrick Reynolds, grandson of R. J. Reynolds, the founder of the R. J. Reynolds Tobacco Company, has developed the "Reynolds Stop Smoking Program." It consists of two 60-minute audiocassette tapes narrated by Reynolds, a booklet, and a 60-day supply of beta carotene tablets. Beta carotene is the precursor of vitamin A, which Reynolds says rebuilds body tissue damaged by smoking. Reynolds' father died at age 58 of emphysema. Several other relatives also died of smoking-related illnesses. After smoking cigarettes and trying to give them up for sixteen years, Patrick Reynolds finally quit smoking, divested himself of all of his holdings in the tobacco fortune, and began traveling the country on an anti-smoking campaign. His message to all smokers is "Butts Out."

The best way to reduce the numbers of people who smoke is through prevention. Many schools have educational programs conducted by student ex-smokers, who can relate well to those the programs are trying to reach. Similar

FIGURE 11–5 ■ Adopt a Smoker

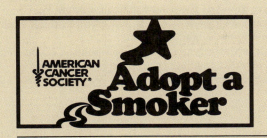

Courtesy the American Cancer Society

TABLE 11–2 ■ Tips for Smokers Who Want to Quit

When thinking about quitting . . .
- ☐ List all the reasons why you want to quit. Every night before going to bed, repeat one of the reasons 10 times.
- ☐ Decide positively that you want to quit. Try to avoid negative thoughts about how difficult it might be.
- ☐ Develop strong personal reasons in addition to your health and obligations to others. For example, think of all the time you waste taking cigarette breaks, rushing out to buy a pack, hunting for a light, etc.
- ☐ Set a target date for quitting—perhaps a special day like your birthday, your anniversary, a holiday. If you smoke heavily at work, quit during your vacation. Make the date sacred, and don't let anything change it.
- ☐ Begin to condition yourself physically: start a modest exercise regimen; drink more fluids; get plenty of rest and avoid fatigue.

Involve someone else . . .
- ☐ Bet a friend you can quit on your target date. Put your cigarette money aside every day, and forfeit it if you smoke.
- ☐ Ask your spouse or a friend to quit with you.

Switch brands . . .
- ☐ Switch to a brand you find distasteful.
- ☐ Change to a brand that's low in tar and nicotine a couple of weeks before your target date. This will help lessen your physical dependence on cigarettes if you *do not* smoke more cigarettes, inhale them more deeply or place your fingertips over the holes in the filters.

Cut down the number of cigarettes you smoke . . .
- ☐ Smoke only half of each cigarette.
- ☐ Each day, postpone lighting your first cigarette one hour.
- ☐ Decide you will smoke only during odd or even hours of the day.
- ☐ Decide beforehand how many cigarettes you'll smoke during the day. For each additional smoke, give a dollar to your favorite charity.
- ☐ Don't smoke when you first experience a craving. Wait several minutes; and during this time, change your activity or talk to someone.
- ☐ Stop buying cigarettes by the carton. Wait until one pack is empty before buying another.
- ☐ Stop carrying cigarettes with you at home and at work. Make them difficult to get to.
- ☐ Smoke only under circumstances which are not especially pleasurable for you. If you like to smoke with others, smoke alone.
- ☐ Make yourself aware of each cigarette by using the opposite hand, or putting cigarettes in an unfamiliar location or different pocket to break the automatic reach.
- ☐ If you light up many times during the day without even thinking about it, try to look in a mirror each time you put a match to your cigarette—you may decide you don't need it.
- ☐ Don't smoke "automatically." Smoke only those you *really* want.
- ☐ Reward yourself in some way other than smoking.
- ☐ Reach for a glass of juice instead of a cigarette for a "pick-me-up."
- ☐ Change your eating habits to aid in cutting down. For example, drink milk, which is frequently considered incompatible with smoking. End meals or snacks with something which won't lead to a cigarette.
- ☐ Don't empty your ashtrays. This will not only remind you of how many cigarettes you have smoked each day, the sight and smell of stale butts will be very unpleasant.

Just before quitting . . .
- ☐ Smoke more heavily than usual so the experience becomes distasteful.
- ☐ Collect all your cigarette butts in one large glass container as a visual reminder of the filth smoking represents.
- ☐ Practice going without cigarettes. Don't think of *never* smoking again. Think of quitting in terms of one day at a time. Tell yourself you won't smoke today and then don't.

On the day you quit . . .
- ☐ Throw away all cigarettes and matches. Hide lighters and ashtrays.
- ☐ Visit the dentist, and have your teeth cleaned to get rid of tobacco stains. Notice how nice they look, and resolve to keep them that way.

(continued on page 293)

TABLE 11-2 ■ Tips for Smokers Who Want to Quit, continued

- ☐ Make a list of things you'd like to buy yourself or someone else. Estimate the cost in terms of packs of cigarettes, and put the money aside to buy these presents.
- ☐ Keep very busy on the big day. Go to the movies, exercise, take long walks, go bike riding.
- ☐ Buy yourself a treat, or do something special to celebrate.

Immediately after quitting . . .
- ☐ The first few days after you quit, spend as much free time as possible in places where smoking is prohibited, e.g. libraries, museums, theaters, department stores, churches. etc.
- ☐ Drink large quantities of water and fruit juice.
- ☐ Try to avoid alcohol, coffee, and other beverages with which you associate cigarette smoking.
- ☐ Strike up a conversation with someone instead of a match for a cigarette.
- ☐ If you miss the sensation of having a cigarette in your hand, play with something else—a pencil, a paper clip, a marble.
- ☐ If you miss having something in your mouth, try toothpicks or a fake cigarette.

Avoid temptation . . .
- ☐ Instead of smoking after meals, get up from the table and brush your teeth or go for a walk.
- ☐ If you always smoke while driving, take public transportation for a while.
- ☐ Temporarily avoid situations you strongly associate with the pleasurable aspects of smoking, e.g., watching your favorite TV program, sitting in your favorite chair, having a cocktail before dinner, etc.
- ☐ Develop a clean, fresh non-smoking environment around yourself—at work and at home.
- ☐ Until you are confident of your ability to stay off cigarettes, limit your socializing to healthful, outdoor activities or situations where smoking is prohibited.
- ☐ If you must be in a situation where you'll be tempted to smoke (such as a cocktail or dinner party), try to associate with the non-smokers there.
- ☐ Look at cigarette ads more critically to better understand the attempts to make individual brands appealing.

Find new habits . . .
- ☐ Change your habits to make smoking difficult, impossible, or unnecessary. Try activities such as swimming, jogging, tennis or handball. Wash your hands or the dishes when the desire for a cigarette is intense.
- ☐ Do things to maintain a clean mouth taste, such as brushing your teeth frequently, and using a mouthwash.
- ☐ Do things that require you to use your hands. Try crossword puzzles, needlework, gardening, or household chores. Go bike riding; take the dog for a walk; give yourself a manicure; write letters; try new recipes.
- ☐ Stretch a lot.
- ☐ Get plenty of rest.
- ☐ Pay attention to your appearance. Look and feel sharp.
- ☐ Absorb yourself with activities which are the most meaningful, satisfying and important to you.
- ☐ Add more spontaneity and excitement to your daily routine.

When you get the "crazies" . . .
- ☐ Keep oral substitutes handy—things like carrots, pickles, sun-flower seeds, apples, celery, raisins, sugarless gum, and so on.
- ☐ Take 10 deep breaths, and hold the last one while lighting a match. Exhale slowly, and blow out the match. Pretend it is a cigarette, and crush it out in an ashtray.
- ☐ Take a shower or bath if possible.
- ☐ Learn to relax quickly and deeply. Make yourself limp, visualize a soothing, pleasing situation, and get away from it all for a moment. Concentrate on that peaceful image and nothing else.
- ☐ Light incense or a candle, instead of cigarette.
- ☐ Never allow yourself to think that "one won't hurt"—it will.

Marking progress . . .
- ☐ Each month, on the anniversary of your quit date, plan a special celebration.
- ☐ Periodically, write down new reasons why you are glad you quit, and post these reasons where you'll be sure to see them.
- ☐ Make up a calendar for the first 90 days. Cross off each day and indicate the money saved by not smoking.
- ☐ Set other intermediate target dates, and do something special with the money you've saved.

SOURCE: Adapted from "Clearing the Air," U.S. Department of Health and Human Services.

TABLE 11-3 ■ Sources of Information on Quitting Smoking

American Cancer Society*
777 3rd Avenue
New York, New York 10017
(212) 371-2900

American Heart Association*
7320 Greenville Avenue
Dallas, Texas 75231
(214) 750-5300

American Lung Association*
1740 Broadway
New York, New York 10019
(212) 245-8000

General Headquarters
5 Day Plan To Stop Smoking
Seventh Day Adventist Church*
Narcotics Education Division
6840 Eastern Avenue, N.W.
Washington, D.C. 20012
(202) 722-6000

Office on Smoking and Health
U.S. Department of Health and Human Services
5600 Fishers Lane
Parklawn Bldg.,
Room 1-58
Rockville, MD 20857
(301) 443-5287

National Interagency Council on Smoking and Health
7320 Greenville Ave.
Dallas, Texas 75231
(214) 750-5359

Schick Laboratories
1901 Avenue of the Stars, Suite 1530
Los Angeles, CA 90067
(213) 553-9771

smokEnders
37 N. Third St.
Easton, PA 18042
(215) 250-0700

Office of Cancer Communications
National Cancer Institute
National Institutes of Health
Bethesda, Maryland 20205
(800) 638-6694

*Consult your local telephone directory for listings of local chapters.
SOURCE: Adapted from "Clearing the Air," U.S. Department of Health and Human Services.

programs by and for adult smokers are conducted by various health agencies, such as the American Heart Association, American Cancer Society, and American Lung Association.

The Benefits of Quitting Smoking

The American Lung Association lists the following benefits of quitting smoking:

1. There is a consistent decline in the death rate of male smokers related to the time elapsed since quitting.
2. Death rates for ex-smokers who have not smoked for ten years or more are close to those of nonsmokers.
3. Your food will taste better.
4. If you have "smokers cough," it will probably clear up soon after you quit.
5. You'll have more money to spend on things that you really want.
6. You'll have an improved self image.
7. You'll probably have more energy and you'll just feel better.
8. You'll decrease the possibility of burn damage to clothing and furniture in your home caused by cigarettes.
9. You'll probably spend fewer "sick" days at home out of work.
10. You'll join 40 million other ex-smokers who have "kicked the habit."

Involuntary Smoking

There has been much discussion about the health consequences of involuntary smoking, also known as passive smoking. This involves the inhalation of smoke by others sharing air space with a smoker.

In the 1986 report, *The Health Consequences of Involuntary Smoking*, the Surgeon General of the United States stated:

1. Involuntary smoking is a cause of disease, including lung cancer in healthy nonsmokers.
2. The children of parents who smoke, compared with the children of nonsmoking parents, have an increased frequency of respiratory infections, increased respiratory symptoms, and slightly smaller rates of increase in lung function as the lung matures.
3. Simple separation of smokers and nonsmokers within the same air space may reduce, but does not eliminate, exposure of nonsmokers to environmental tobacco smoke.

Data in the report clearly establish a link between exposure to environmental tobacco smoke and lung cancer. The respiratory health of infants and children under two years of age is negatively affected by parents' smoking, especially if both parents smoke. The report does not show any relation between environmental tobacco smoke and other cancers or cardiovascular disease. It is also not known what effects exposure to smoke will have on children later in life.

The National Research Council has stated that "children and spouses of smokers have an increased risk for developing respiratory ailments and lung cancer." Pneumonia, bronchitis, and hospitalization for other respiratory infections are "significantly increased" in children whose parents smoke. The incidence of lung cancer among nonsmoking spouses of smokers is 30 percent greater than among nonsmoking spouses of nonsmokers.

FAST FACTS

An opinion poll indicates that two-thirds of smokers believe that involuntary smoking is hazardous to the health of nonsmokers.

> ■ **PROBLEM SITUATION** You are now aware of the potential problems of involuntary smoking. What can you do to reduce your exposure to these hazards?

■ Smokeless Tobacco

Smokeless tobacco, also known as chewing tobacco or snuff, has been used in the United States far longer than smoking tobacco. In fact, in the 1860s there were many more tobacco companies producing chewing tobacco than smoking tobacco. Approximately twelve million Americans use smokeless tobacco. Snuff use in the United States is up 60 percent since 1978. One form of snuff consists of powdered tobacco, which is inhaled into the nose. Dipping snuff involves placing a wad of moist snuff between the cheek and gum and sucking on it. It is estimated that 20 to 40 percent of all smokeless tobacco users are adolescent males. One survey showed that in the northeast, 10 percent of boys age twelve to seventeen used smokeless tobacco. In southern states, this figure jumped to 27 percent. The average age for a beginning user is twelve years.

In 1985, the National Household Survey conducted by the National Institute on Drug Abuse showed that 19 percent of men and 3 percent of women twenty-one years of age or older used smokeless tobacco. Again, highest use was in the south and lowest use was in the northeast. In the past, much of the advertising for smokeless tobacco has used well-known sports figures, especially baseball players, to sell the products. Carlton Fisk (a famous baseball player) and Walt Garrison (a football player) have been featured in television ads for smokeless tobacco. Athletes have been known to fall prey to the myth that the use of smokeless tobacco increases reaction time, when evidence indicates that it has the opposite effect.

Long-term use of smokeless tobacco has been associated with cancer of the mouth, nicotine addiction, early tooth loss, decreased sense of taste and smell, bad breath, tooth discoloration, and periodontal disease. Carcinogens known as nitrosamines are found in both chewing tobacco and snuff. Users of smokeless tobacco have four times the risk of developing mouth and throat cancers as

GUIDELINES TO YOUR GOOD HEALTH

The following suggestions can help you avoid exposure to second-hand smoke if you are invited to a party or you are at some other public place where people are smoking around you.

1. Leave and go home or go to some other place where smoking is not permitted.
2. If you are at a sporting event or concert where you are seated near a smoker, change your seat.
3. Carry a battery-operated fan and use it to blow the smoke away from yourself.
4. Ask the smoker to refrain from smoking near you.

nonusers. The effects of nicotine on the cardiovascular system that result from smoking tobacco, such as increased blood pressure and heart rate, can also be expected from using smokeless tobacco. *Leukoplakia,* or white leathery patches appearing on the soft tissues of the mouth, is a condition that often results from using chewing tobacco and may precede the development of oral cancers. In research done at East Carolina University, Elbert Glover reported that "the nicotine level in the blood is higher in smokeless-tobacco users than smokers." He has also found that some users could not "stop for even half a day."

A young man from Oklahoma, Sean Marsee, began using smokeless tobacco when he was twelve years old by picking up free samples at a local rodeo. He was a track star at school and, like many of the other athletes, took up the habit of chewing a wad of smokeless tobacco to get a buzz. He was using between seven and ten cans a week by the time he reached high school. In his senior year, Sean was diagnosed as having oral cancer. Between that time and his death less than a year later, he endured four operations and a series of radiation treatments. He had been voted the most valuable athlete in his school but never had the opportunity to develop his potential because of his untimely death.

FAST FACTS

Clove cigarettes possess all of the hazards associated with smoking regular cigarettes.

Clove Cigarettes

During the past several years, clove cigarettes have gained in popularity, especially among young people. Most of these cigarettes are imported from Indonesia and are composed of approximately 60 percent tobacco and 40 percent ground cloves and other additives. Tar, nicotine, and carbon monoxide are all produced by smoking clove cigarettes and in quantities similar to smoking regular tobacco. The American Lung Association reports that smokers of clove cigarettes have reported such symptoms as coughing up blood, nosebleeds, severe sore throats, and frequent upper respiratory infections. Deaths have been reported from smoking clove cigarettes, but a specific cause-and-effect relationship has not yet been established.

The number of clove cigarettes imported into the United States is approaching 150 million per year. Many smokers believe, erroneously, that these cigarettes are safer or that they produce a high not found in tobacco cigarettes. The truth is that clove cigarettes are at least as dangerous and can cause the same addiction as regular cigarettes.

> *PROBLEM SITUATION* Because of all the negative publicity about smoking, your younger brother has bought a pack of clove cigarettes. He has heard that they are much safer than regular cigarettes. What can you tell him about their contents and their effects?

Tobacco and the Law

As of this date, forty-two states have passed laws restricting smoking in public places. Laws vary greatly from place to place. One town, city, or county might have a ban on smoking in public places while a neighboring municipality might not. In many places, restaurants must have separate sections for smokers and nonsmokers, and laws limiting smoking in the workplace are becoming more and more common. Utah bans any billboard advertising of cigarettes, and California prohibits smoking in planes, trains, and buses (see Table 11–4).

TABLE 11-4 ■ Federal Government Actions on Smoking

1966—As of January 1, 1966, cigarette packs must be labeled "Caution: Cigarette Smoking May Be Hazardous To Your Health."

1967—The Federal Communications Commission requires that radio and TV stations carrying cigarette advertising must also carry antismoking messages.

1970—Federal law requires that the warning on cigarette packages be changed to "The Surgeon General Has Determined That Cigarette Smoking Is Dangerous To Your Health".

1971—As of January 2, 1971, radio and television advertising are no longer permitted.

1972—The warning required on cigarette packs is also required on all cigarette advertising. Advertising must also indicate tar and nicotine content.

1978—Cigar and pipe smoking is banned on American commercial airlines.

1985—As of October 12, 1985, cigarette packs and advertising must contain four rotating warnings.
1. Smoking Causes Lung Cancer, Heart Disease and Emphysema and May Complicate Pregnancy.
2. Smoking By Pregnant Women May Result in Fetal Injury, Premature Birth and Low Birth Weight.
3. Cigarette Smoke Contains Carbon Monoxide.
4. Quitting Smoking Now Greatly Reduces Serious Risks To Your Health.

1988—Smoking is banned on domestic airline flights of two hours or less.
1989—Smoking is banned on almost all domestic airline flights (certain flights over six hours in duration are excepted).

In 1988, Canada passed some of the strictest legislation in the world controlling smoking and tobacco advertising. By 1993, all newspaper, magazine, and billboard advertising will be prohibited. The use of tobacco brand names in association with sports and cultural events will not be allowed. Also prohibited will be such items as tee shirts, cigarette lighters, and other products that show brand names or picture packs of cigarettes. Heavy penalties will be enforced against violators. In addition, smoking in federal workplaces and on federally regulated ships, planes, and trains will be limited to specially designated areas.

Approximately 300 lawsuits related to smoker deaths have been filed against tobacco companies since the 1950s. Not one had been settled or lost by the companies until June 1988, when the family of a New Jersey woman who died of lung, liver, and brain cancer sued three tobacco companies. The family sued on the grounds that the companies knew of the dangers of cigarette smoking as early as 1946 but continued to advertise their products as being safe. The jury found in favor of the family and awarded $400,000 to the woman's husband. It stated that the tobacco companies had a duty to warn smokers of the dangers of smoking before 1966, the year that warnings were first required on cigarette packs. In the 1950s, cigarette ads contained phrases such as "Play Safe—Smoke Chesterfield," "Just What the Doctor Ordered," and "Nose, Throat and Accessory Organs Not Adversely Affected by Smoking Chesterfields." It is expected that the result of this case will encourage others who have been harmed by tobacco to file similar lawsuits.

POSITIVE BEHAVIORS

I. *Place a check mark in front of each behavior that you now practice.*

_____ 1. I do not smoke. (SMOKE)
_____ 2. I encourage smokers I know to stop smoking. (STOP SMOKING)
_____ 3. I avoid exposure to second-hand smoke. (SECOND-HAND SMOKE)
_____ 4. I do not use clove cigarettes. (CLOVE CIGARETTES)
_____ 5. I do not use smokeless tobacco. (SMOKELESS TOBACCO)
_____ 6. I do not buy tobacco products for others, such as younger brothers and sisters, to use. (BUY FOR OTHERS)
_____ 7. I volunteer to assist agencies such as the American Cancer Society and American Lung Association in promoting smoking prevention or intervention programs. (VOLUNTEER)
_____ 8. I eat only at restaurants that provide non-smoking sections. (RESTAURANTS)
_____ 9. I purchase only those magazines that do not advertise tobacco products. (MAGAZINES)

II. *For each behavior that you DO NOT ENGAGE IN, write in the appropriate space below the KEY WORD(S) located in the parentheses at the end of the statement. Then indicate whether you intend to keep or change that behavior.*

Behaviors I Don't Engage In   KEEP/CHANGE

_____ / _____
_____ / _____
_____ / _____
_____ / _____
_____ / _____
_____ / _____
_____ / _____
_____ / _____

III. *For each of the preceding behaviors that you choose to KEEP, write a statement indicating why you are choosing to keep that behavior.*

I choose to keep behavior _____ because:
                           KEY WORD

For each of the preceding behaviors that you choose to CHANGE, write a statement indicating how you plan to implement that change.

I will change behavior _____ by:
                        KEY WORD

Now You Know

1. FALSE. Transmission through the nerves themselves is electrical; however, transmission across the synapses is chemical and is accomplished by neurotransmitters.

2. TRUE. Heart rate may increase as much as twenty-five beats per minute and blood pressure may rise as much as twenty points after just one or two cigarettes.

3. FALSE. Babies born to women who smoke during pregnancy are likely to be of lower birth weight. They also show a higher incidence of premature births and stillbirths.

4. TRUE. Evidence indicates that smoking causes wrinkles, probably because of constriction of peripheral blood vessels, which, in turn, makes the skin more susceptible to the damaging effects of the sun.

5. TRUE. A 1986 report from the Surgeon General of the United States establishes a link between exposure to second-hand smoke and both lung cancer and the respiratory health of children under two years of age.

6. FALSE. Smoking is also related to cancer of the mouth, larynx, esophagus, cervix, bladder, and kidneys.

7. FALSE. The nicotine in smokeless tobacco still causes harmful effects. In addition, smokeless tobacco is associated with periodontal disease and cancer of the mouth.

8. FALSE. Smoking clove cigarettes produces tar, nicotine, and carbon monoxide. Smokers have reported coughing up blood, nosebleeds, severe sore throats, and respiratory infections.

9. TRUE. Studies have shown that experimental animals are unable to achieve full erections after being exposed to tobacco smoke and that ejaculate volume, sperm density, and total sperm count are lower in male smokers than in male nonsmokers. Other studies have shown that smoking may contribute to infertility in women.

10. TRUE. Studies of ex-smokers have shown that the majority have successfully quit "cold turkey."

Summary

1. Nerve impulses are conducted electrically through the many billions of neurons in the body and chemically by the neurotransmitters across the synapses between the nerve cells.

2. The neurotransmitters fit specific receptor sites and trigger impulses in the neurons to which they attach. These chemicals are then either metabolized or reabsorbed to prevent further transmission.

3. Most psychoactive drugs work by affecting the release, breakdown, or reabsorption of neurotransmitters.

4. At the turn of the century, most deaths were due to infectious diseases. Today, most deaths are due to chronic diseases and may, to some degree, be controlled by changes in life-style.

5. About fifty million Americans consume over 500 billion cigarettes per year. The most successful method of quitting is going "cold turkey."

6. Over $7 billion are collected each year from cigarette taxes. Tobacco production is a $35 billion a year industry in the United States. The annual cost of smoking-related illness is estimated to be around $65 billion.

7. Nicotine is a powerful chemical constituent of cigarette smoke. It is highly addicting and is a leading cause of heart attack and stroke. Recent studies have implicated it as a contributing factor in a variety of cancers.

8. The carbon monoxide in smoke has a strong affinity for the hemoglobin of the red blood cells, reducing their oxygen-carrying capacity. This tends to cause smokers to become short of breath more easily than nonsmokers.

9. The tars in smoke are known carcinogens and are responsible for over 90 percent of the lung cancers in the United States. They also contribute to the development of emphysema and chronic bronchitis.

10. In addition to lung cancer, cancers of the mouth, larynx, esophagus, cervix, bladder, and kidneys have all been related to cigarette smoking.

11. Smoking has been shown to be related to many other health problems, including impotence, infertility in both men and women, ulcers, cardiovascular disease, the development of premature wrinkles, hip fractures in elderly women, and Alzheimer's disease.

12. Babies born to women who smoke during pregnancy are twice as likely to be stillborn, to have lower birth weight, or to be premature than those born to nonsmoking women. Respiratory problems are more common among infants and young children born to smoking women.

13. A variety of programs designed to help the smoker quit are available through both involuntary and private health agencies. Hypnotism, biofeedback, acupuncture, and negative reinforcement have also been used. Nicotine chewing gum is available by prescription.

14. Nonsmokers exposed to involuntary smoking are at greater risk for lung cancer than those not exposed. Further investigation is underway to determine other long-term effects of exposure to second-hand smoke.

15. Smokeless tobacco and clove cigarettes have been substituted by many for regular cigarettes. Their use can lead to serious health problems.

16. Many municipalities have passed laws controlling smoking in public places and in the workplace. Federal law requires that four specific health warnings be printed on cigarette packages.

References

1. American Lung Association. *Chronic Obstructive Pulmonary Disease,* New York, N.Y., 5th ed. American Lung Association and American Thoracic Society, 1977.
2. California Medical Association. "Smoking and Women." Health Tips. San Francisco: California Medical Association, October 1984.
3. Condra, M.; Morales, A.; Owen, J. A., et al. "Prevalence and Significance of Tobacco Smoking in Impotence" Urology. 27(6):495–498, June 1986.
4. Dikshit, R. K.; Buch, J. G.; Mansuri, S. M. "Effect of Tobacco Consumption on Semen Quality" Fertility and Sterility. 48(2):334–336, August 1987.
5. Jarvik, M E.; Henningfield, J. E. "Pharmacological Treatment of Tobacco Dependence" Pharmacology Biochemistry and Behavior. 30(1):279–294, May 1988.
6. Juenemann, K. P.; Lue, T. F.; Luo, J. A., et al. "The Effect of Cigarette Smoking on Penile Erection" Journal of Urology. 138(2):438–441, August 1987.
7. Khaw, K. T.; Tazuke, S.; Barrett-Connor, E. "Cigarette Smoking and Levels of Adrenal Androgens in Postmenopausal Women" New England Journal of Medicine. 318(26):1705–1709, June 30, 1988.
8. Orlando, R. C. "Peptic Ulcer: Factors Influencing Recurrence" Journal of Clinical Gastroenterology. 9(Supplement 1):2–7, 1987.
9. Preber, H.; Bergstrom, J. "Effect of Non-Surgical Treatment on Periodontal Pockets in Smokers and Non-Smokers" Journal of Clinical Periodontology. 13(4):319–323, April 1986.
10. Report of the Advisory Committee to the Surgeon General. *The Health Consequences of Using Smokeless Tobacco.* U.S. Department of Health and Human Services, NIH Publication No. 86-2874, April 1986.
11. Report of the Surgeon General: *The Health Consequences of Cigarette Smoking: Nicotine Addiction.* Washington, D.C.: U.S. Department of Health and Human Services, 1988.
12. Report of the Surgeon General. *The Health Consequences of Involuntary Smoking.* Washington, D.C.: U.S. Department of Health and Human Services, 1986.
13. Report of the Surgeon General. *The Health Consequences of Smoking: Chronic Obstructive Lung Disease.* Washington, D.C.: U.S. Department of Health and Human Services, 1984.
14. U.S. Department of Health and Human Services. "Psychosocial Predictors of Smoking among Adolescents." *Morbidity and Mortality Weekly Report* 36 (1987).
15. U.S. Department of Health and Human Services, Centers for Disease Control. *Smoking and Health Bulletin.* Public Health Service, Center for Health Promotion and Education, Office on Smoking and Health, September–October 1987; November–December 1987; January–February 1988; March–April 1988; and May–June 1988.

Suggested Readings

Blum, Alan, ed. *The Cigarette Underworld—A Front Line Report on the War Against Your Lungs,* New York: Lyle Stuart, 1985.

Carroll, Charles R. *Drugs in Modern Society.* Dubuque, Iowa: William C. Brown Publishers, 1985.

Julien, Robert. *A Primer of Drug Action.* San Francisco: W. H. Freeman and Co., 1981.

Rucker, William B., ed. *Drugs, Society and Behavior.* Guilford, Conn.: The Dushkin Publishing Group, 1987.

The Health Consequences of Involuntary Smoking: A Report of the Surgeon General. Washington, D.C.: Department of Health and Human Services, U.S. Government Printing Office, 1986.

Witters, Weldon, and Peter Venturelli. *Drugs and Society.* Boston: Jones and Bartlett Publishers, 1988.

CHAPTER 12

Alcohol Awareness

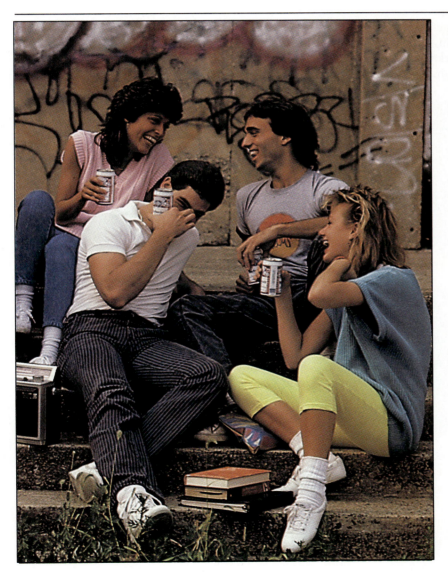

////////

What Do You Know?

Are the following statements true or false?

1. There is approximately the same amount of pure ethyl alcohol in a twelve ounce can of beer as in a mixed drink made with scotch, rye, or vodka.
2. Ethyl alcohol is a central nervous system stimulant.
3. Consuming alcoholic beverages in cold weather will cause you to lose body heat.
4. Alcohol does not produce calories; therefore it will not have any affect on body weight.
5. Alcohol consumed by a pregnant woman can damage her unborn baby.
6. In addition to ethyl alcohol, it is safe to consume other types of alcohol.
7. Alcohol must be digested before it can be absorbed into the bloodstream.
8. Alcohol consumption can lead to physical dependence and cause severe withdrawal when the drinker stops "cold turkey."
9. Some types of cancer have been associated with excessive alcohol consumption.
10. Most experts agree that an alcoholic can give up heavy drinking and still be able to drink moderately without problems.

Basic Facts about Alcohol

Throughout history, it has been known that fruit juices, as well as several other substances, undergo a change when they are left in a warm place and are exposed to air. This change is known as **fermentation.** Fermentation is due to the action of an enzyme from a tiny yeast organism and results in the production of carbon dioxide, water, and ethyl alcohol. Almost all societies have consumed alcoholic beverages, primarily for their intoxicating effects. These beverages have also played a role in the religious ceremonies of many societies. Wine has been used since as early as 4,000 B.C.

Ethyl alcohol, also known as ethanol or grain alcohol, is the type of alcohol that we consume as a beverage. There are actually many chemicals in the group known as alcohols. It is important to realize that the term *alcohol* does not relate only to the type we drink. The group includes methyl alcohol, isopropyl alcohol, propyl alcohol, butyl alcohol, and hundreds of others.

Most alcoholic beverages are manufactured by the fermentation of fruits or vegetables containing carbohydrates. For example, vodka is made from potatoes, rum from molasses, wines from different varieties of grapes, and beer from barley, malt, and hops. Wines and beers are undistilled beverages, whereas brandies and hard liquors are distilled.

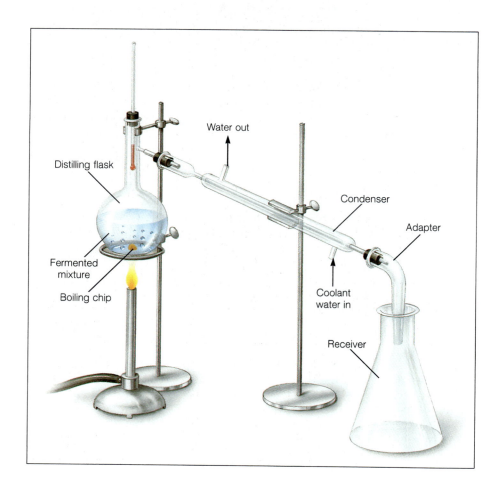

FIGURE 12–1 ■ **Distillation Process**

It is relatively easy to make an alcoholic beverage (although some home brews might not be as palatable as the commercial products). To do so, place about two ounces of crushed fruit such as grapes, strawberries, or peaches in an eight-ounce container. Add about four ounces of water and one-half packet of yeast (available in any grocery store). Close the container with a cotton plug or similar cover but be sure not to make it airtight. Fermentation produces carbon dioxide gas, which can build up pressure inside the container and cause it to burst. Set the container aside. After about two days, you will easily be able to tell by smelling the product that alcohol has been produced. If you would like to seriously make alcoholic beverages for your own consumption, you should purchase a reference book that describes the proper techniques for making products that taste good and are safe to drink. Federal and state laws generally allow individuals to manufacture alcoholic beverages for their own consumption. It is important to check the laws of your state for specific information.

Yeast cannot survive in concentrations of alcohol greater than about 14 percent, so the yeast will die as the fermentation process continues. Distillation is necessary to produce a beverage with a stronger concentration of alcohol. The distillation process involves the use of heat to separate the ethyl alcohol from water and other impurities in the mixture. (See Figure 12–1 for an example of the distillation process.)

The percentage of alcohol in a specific alcoholic beverage is expressed in terms of **proof**. Proof is double the percentage. A beverage that is 80 proof is 40 percent alcohol. "Absolute" alcohol is 100 percent alcohol, or 200 proof. In reality, the strongest alcohol is 190 proof, or 95 percent alcohol, because absolute alcohol tends to absorb small amounts of water from the air once the container is opened.

There is approximately the same amount of alcohol in a twelve-ounce container of beer, about four to six ounces of wine, and one mixed drink (see Table 12–1). Therefore, six beers will make you just as intoxicated as six bourbon and waters or six Bloody Marys.

Pharmacology

Absorption and Elimination

Ethyl alcohol is a very potent drug. Pharmacologically, it is a central nervous system depressant. Absorption of alcohol takes place primarily in the small

FAST FACTS

Alcohol abuse costs our society more than $117 billion per year.

TABLE 12–1 ■ **Amount of Alcohol in Selected Beverages**

Beverage	Quantity	Alcohol Content	Amount of Pure Alcohol
1 can of beer	12 oz.	4%	.48 oz.
1 can of beer	12 oz.	6%	.72 oz.
1 glass of wine	4 oz.	12%	.48 oz.
1 glass of wine	6 oz.	12%	.72 oz.
1 shot of scotch	1 oz.	40%	.40 oz.
1 shot of scotch	1 oz.	50%	.50 oz.
1 glass of sherry	2 oz.	20%	.40 oz.

FAST FACTS

Being a host means that you are responsible for the safe recovery of anyone who drinks too much at your party.

intestine, although some is absorbed from the stomach. As much as 30 to 40 percent of the alcohol in a drink may be absorbed directly through the stomach wall if the drinker has not eaten and the stomach is empty. It is one of the few substances that is absorbed into the bloodstream without the need for any digestion to take place. Once absorbed, alcohol is quickly distributed to every part of the body.

The rate at which alcohol is absorbed depends on a variety of factors, including the type of beverage consumed, the percentage of alcohol it contains, the rate at which it is drunk, and the amount of food in the stomach. Body weight as a factor in determining how fast a person can become intoxicated will be discussed later. Research has shown that women become more intoxicated on the same amount of alcohol at the time of the month just prior to their menstrual period than at other times. This effect may be related to altered levels of sex hormones.

Alcohol is eliminated from the body directly and through metabolism by the liver. The metabolism of alcohol involves the chemical conversion of alcohol to carbon dioxide and water. About 10 to 20 percent is removed directly through sweat, saliva, urine, and breath (see Figure 12–2). The rest is metabolized in the liver at a fairly constant rate of about ten milliliters or one-third of an ounce of absolute alcohol per hour. The rate of metabolism of alcohol is constant, irrespective of the concentration of alcohol in the blood. This differs from the metabolism of most other drugs, for which the rate of metabolism is directly related to the drug's concentration in the bloodstream. Intoxication occurs when alcohol builds up in the bloodstream as a result of its being drunk at a faster rate than it can be eliminated from the body. We presently have no way to increase alcohol's rate of metabolism by the liver and reduce the level of intoxication of someone who has consumed too much alcohol.

The symptoms we know as hangover are caused by a variety of conditions. First, alcohol is a gastric irritant. This causes an unpleasant reaction in the gastrointestinal tract, which can lead to nausea and diarrhea. In addition, alcoholic beverages contain impurities known as **congeners**—chemicals that are by-products of the manufacture of the alcoholic beverage. These substances can be quite toxic and can cause the drinker to experience extremely unpleasant reactions, such as nausea and headache. In the metabolism of alcohol in the body, a substance known as acetaldehyde is produced (see Figure 12–2). This too is extremely toxic and contributes to the ill effects a person feels after drinking too much.

Many attempts have been made to reduce the feelings of a hangover but with little success. Vitamin B_6 has been recommended because of its antinauseant properties. Such things as a cold shower and a cup of coffee have been used, but, as it has been said, this produces nothing more than a "clean and wide-awake drunk." There really isn't much a person can do except try to sleep it off and, of course, avoid letting it happen again.

FIGURE 12–2 ■ **Equation for the Metabolism of Alcohol**

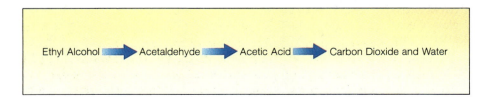

TABLE 12–2 ■ Breath Alcohol Content and Its Effects

	Approximate Breath Alcohol Concentration (in grams)[a]								Effects on Feeling and Behavior	Effects on Driving Ability
Drinks[b] in Body	**Body Weight in Pounds**									
	100	120	140	160	180	200	220	240		
1	.04	.03	.03	.03	.02	.02	.02	.02	Absence of observable effects. Mild alteration of feelings, slight intensification of existing moods.	Mild changes. Most drivers seem a bit moody. Bad driving habits slightly pronounced.
2	.08	.06	.05	.05	.04	.04	.03	.03		
3	.11	.09	.08	.07	.06	.06	.05	.05		
4	.15	.12	.11	.09	.08	.08	.07	.06		
5	.19	.16	.13	.12	.11	.09	.09	.08	Feeling of relaxation. Mild sedation. Exaggeration of emotions and behavior. Slight impairment of motor skills. Increase in reaction time.	Drivers take too long to decide and act. Motor skills (such as braking) are impaired. Reaction time is increased.
6	.23	.19	.16	.14	.13	.11	.10	.09		
7	.26	.22	.19	.16	.15	.13	.12	.11		
8	.30	.25	.21	.19	.17	.15	.14	.13		
9	.34	.28	.24	.21	.19	.17	.15	.14		
10	.38	.31	.27	.23	.21	.19	.17	.16		
11		.40	.34	.30	.27	.24	.22	.20	Difficulty performing gross motor skills. Uncoordinated behavior. Definite impairment of mental abilities, judgment, and memory.	Judgment seriously affected. Physical and mental coordination impaired. Physical difficulty in driving a vehicle.
12			.38	.33	.29	.26	.24	.22		
13			.40	.36	.32	.29	.26	.24		
14				.38	.34	.31	.28	.26		
15					.37	.33	.30	.28		
									Major impairment of all physical and mental functions. Irresponsible behavior. Euphoria. Some difficulty standing, walking, and talking.	Distortion of all perception and judgment. Driving erratic. Driver in a daze.
									At .40, most people have passed out. Hospitalization is probable at BALs of .40 and above, and death is imminent.	It is hoped that the driver passed out before trying to get into vehicle.

[a]Alcohol concentration is expressed here as grams of alcohol per 210 liters of breath. A reading of ".10" on a breath-testing instrument indicates 10 one-hundredths (10/100) grams of alcohol per 210 liters of breath.
[b]A drink is defined as: 1½ oz. of 80 proof liquor or 12 oz of beer or 5 oz. of table wine. Subtract one drink, from the number consumed, for each hour of drinking after the first hour.
SOURCE: National Safety Council.

Physiological Effects

Alcohol has a variety of physiological effects (see Table 12–2). It has an irritant action on the nervous system, similar to that of smelling salts, that results in an increase in the heart and breathing rates. As the blood alcohol level (BAL) rises, there are disturbances in higher intellectual functions such as judgment, discrimination, and inhibitions. These changes result from mild depression of the cortex of the brain. Impairment of muscular coordination, especially in movement and speech, follows. Loss of consciousness would occur in higher doses, and death, if it should happen, would result from alcohol's effect on the medulla, which controls respiration and heartbeat.

Another physiological effect of alcohol is irritation of the gastrointestinal tract. Individuals with conditions such as ulcers or colitis could seriously worsen their problems through consumption of even small amounts of alcohol.

Alcohol is a *dehydrating agent;* that is, it tends to remove water from the body's cells. Have you ever noticed that your mouth becomes dry after consuming moderate amounts of alcohol? Don't you almost always have to urinate after drinking even small amounts of alcohol?

Dilation (expansion) of peripheral blood vessels takes place after consumption of alcohol, giving the drinker a feeling of warmth. In reality, however, the body is losing heat because of the increased circulation near the skin surface. Drinking alcoholic beverages when a person is in a cold environment, such as when skiing, can actually lead to frostbite.

Alcohol produces 7 calories of energy per gram, or approximately 150 calories per drink (remember, one drink is twelve ounces of beer, four to six ounces of wine, or one mixed drink). This is in contrast to protein and carbohydrate, which produce 4 calories per gram, and fat, which produces 9. Light beer contains about 105 calories per twelve-ounce can or bottle. Since alcoholic beverages have little or no other nutritional value, the calories in what a person drinks will simply be burned and used by the body as energy. For moderate drinkers, these extra calories can lead to weight gain if added to their normal daily caloric intake.

Drinking moderate amounts of alcohol can also indirectly lead to weight gain. Alcohol increases the flow of saliva and causes an increase in secretions from the gastric mucosa, which in turn leads to a greater appetite. The impact of emotional problems, which can inhibit normal appetite and digestion, also tends to be reduced.

Tolerance

Alcohol is metabolized by **enzymes** in the liver. As the drinker consumes more and more alcohol, these enzymes get better and better at metabolizing away the alcohol. Thus, the drinker needs to increase his or her consumption to get the desired effect. The more alcohol that is consumed and the more frequent the drinking, the faster tolerance is likely to build. Tolerance does not necessarily build at the same rate for all of a given drug's effects. For example, the lethal dose of alcohol does not appreciably change, even though tolerance to other effects may increase considerably in a heavy drinker. In other words, as a drinker consumes more and more to get the desired effect, he or she gets closer and closer to the lethal dose, which remains the same.

Physiological or pharmacological tolerance, which is defined as the reduced sensitivity to the effects of a given drug, builds toward alcohol in the regular drinker. It may occur as the result of reduced concentrations of the drug at the **receptor sites,** known as *dispositional tolerance,* or from the drug's effects on the availability of certain neurotransmitters, known as *pharmacodynamic tolerance.*

The same enzymes that are responsible for the metabolism of alcohol are also responsible for the metabolism of the male hormone testosterone. In the regular drinker, as physiological tolerance toward alcohol builds, so does tolerance toward testosterone. This phenomenon is known as **cross tolerance.** Therefore, male heavy drinkers may become impotent as a result of the liver eliminating testosterone from the body too rapidly. Some research suggests that alcohol may also have a direct effect on the cells that produce testosterone, reducing their activity.

Behavioral or learned-behavior tolerance is also associated with alcohol consumption. The drinker learns what sensations to expect from drinking and is able to control them to some degree.

Dependence

Excessive alcohol consumption may lead to **physiological dependence,** or addiction. Dependence of this type does not generally occur in the individual who drinks moderately or drinks even larger amounts intermittently. It is usually seen in those who drink heavily over long periods of time.

If an alcoholic stops drinking suddenly, withdrawal will occur. Withdrawal from alcohol is characterized by a period during which the individual shows hyperexcitability, including symptoms such as tremors, profuse sweating, hallucinations, disorientation, and confusion. Subsequently, withdrawal can lead to delerium tremens (the dt's), convulsions, coma, and death.

Synergism

When two or more drugs are combined, a multiplication of effect can occur, which is called **synergism.** *Taber's Medical Dictionary* defines synergism as "the harmonious action of two agents, . . . producing an effect which neither could produce alone or an effect which is greater than the total effects of each agent operating by itself." Central nervous system depressants such as alcohol tend to exhibit this effect when combined with other central nervous system depressants. An example of this would be the combination of alcohol and barbiturate drugs. Instead of the effects of the drug combination being simply added together, they are multiplied; that is, each agent increases the potency of the other. Many deaths have been attributed to the inadvertent mixing of such drugs, each in a dose considered safe by itself but leading to a fatal combination.

Synergism would occur if alcohol was combined with barbiturates, minor tranquilizers such as diazepam (Valium), marijuana, or opiates such as morphine or codeine. To reach a lethal dose, one might need to have a blood alcohol level of between 0.4 and 0.6 or to take as many as twenty capsules of a given barbiturate. Yet a combination of as few as three or four capsules of the barbiturate with a blood alcohol level of 0.15 or so might be fatal because of synergism. It is difficult to predict the degree of synergism with various combinations of alcohol and other drugs because of the extreme variation in effects from one individual to another. Some effects of combining alcohol with common drugs are highlighted in Table 12–3 on the following page.

> ■ *PROBLEM SITUATION* Your mom takes sleeping pills on a regular basis to help her sleep at night. Tonight, she and your dad went to a party and had a little too much to drink. Now, before she goes to bed, she is about to take her usual sleeping medication. Will this cause her any problems? What should you tell her about taking sleeping pills along with alcohol?

FAST FACTS

Several studies have shown a rise in estrogen levels in chronic users of alcohol leading to feminization in male drinkers.

TABLE 12–3 ■ Effects of Combining Alcohol With Common Drugs

Drug	Interaction
Analgesics	
Narcotics	
codeine	Heightened central nervous system (CNS) and respiratory depression
heroin	Exaggeration of CNS depressant effect
Nonnarcotics	
acetylsalicytic acid (aspirin; Excedrin)	Enhanced gastointestinal blood loss and damage to stomach lining
Antidiabetic Drugs	
insulin	Alcohol use by itself may cause hypoglycemia; alcohol taken with insulin may result in heightening this effect
Antihistamines	
diphenhydramine (Benadryl)	Increased drowsiness, which makes driving more dangerous
chlorpheniramine (Chlor-Trimeton)	Enhanced sedative effects
Anti-infective Agents	
penicillin	No reported drug interaction
Central Nervous System Stimulants	
cocaine	No interaction
amphetamines (Benzedrine)	Heightens CNS depression
nicotine	Drug interaction not established
Hallucinogens	
cannabis (Marijuana)	Increases effect of alcohol
lysergic acid diethylamide (LSD)	Reported stimulus of LSD flashbacks
Oral Contraceptives	
"The Pill"	Extends blood-alcohol levels; decreases rate of alcohol elimination
Sedative-Hypnotics	
barbiturates	
"Downers"	
secobarbital (Seconal)	Nausea
nonbarbiturates	
methaqualone (Quaalude)	vomiting
Tranquilizers	
Minor	
chlordiazepoxide (Librium)	Slurred speech, impaired motor skills, possible coma, respiratory depression, death
Major	
chlorpromazine (Thorazine)	Decreased muscle coordination and judgment; careful when operating machinery

(continued on page 311)

TABLE 12–3 ■ **Effects of Combining Alcohol With Common Drugs, continued**

Drug	Interaction
Vitamins	Drug interaction not reported; malnutrition is often a result of alcohol abuse

SOURCE: Adapted from the National Center for Alcohol Education, National Institute on Alcohol Abuse and Alcoholism.

Alcohol and Other Drugs

The use of tetrahydrocannabinol, the active ingredient in marijuana, as an antinauseant has been known for many years. Recently, concern has been mounting over the combined use of marijuana and alcohol by young people. One of the reasons for the widespread use of this combination is that marijuana tends to reduce the nausea caused by the alcohol. When marijuana is used with alcohol in this manner, the user tends to drink more alcohol, because the negative feelings of this excess consumption are alleviated by the marijuana. Cases of alcohol overdose have been reported in a number of instances in which this combination has been used. Keep in mind that synergism as just described also occurs with the combination of alcohol and marijuana.

Alcohol interacts with a variety of other drugs. Metronidazole, a drug commonly used in treating vaginitis and pelvic inflammatory disease (see Chapter 15), prevents the proper metabolism of alcohol, which leads to a buildup of acetaldehyde. This causes severe nausea and vomiting in the individual who combines these drugs. Alcohol, being an irritant to the gastrointestinal tract, may increase the irritating properties of drugs such as aspirin and may cause gastric bleeding. Individuals who drink alcohol and are taking antidiabetic medications may feel flushing, headache, and dizziness and have unpredictable changes in blood-sugar levels. When combined with antihistamines, alcohol can lead to excessive drowsiness.

Psychological Effects

Alcohol reduces the brain's ability to process information. It also negatively affects decision making and judgment. One's ability to concentrate on driving is impaired and the ability to judge distance and speed is reduced. Behavior changes that occur with increased consumption of alcohol include increased risk taking and aggressiveness.

■ Alcohol and Disease

Alcohol and the Liver

Excessive consumption of alcohol can lead to cirrhosis of the liver, fatty liver, heart disease, malnutrition, and other disorders. Cirrhosis is a chronic liver disease in which there is progressive loss of function of the liver cells and reduced blood flow through the liver. It results from heavy alcohol consumption and poor nutrition in alcoholics. It is not the result of alcohol alone. Fatty liver occurs when fat infiltrates normal liver cells. In reality, it is also a type of cirrhosis. Alcohol may also lead to inflammation of the liver, sometimes referred to as **alcoholic hepatitis.**

Alcohol and Circulation

Alcohol in low doses causes blood vessels near the skin surface to dilate. A common characteristic of alcoholics, a red nose, is caused by chronic dilation of the blood vessels near the nose, which causes them to rupture. Congestive heart failure may result from damage to heart-muscle tissue after long-term heavy drinking. There have been many studies on alcohol's effects on levels of high-density lipoproteins (HDLs). Early studies suggested that alcohol consumption induces favorable levels of these protective lipoproteins, but more recent information refutes this theory.

Alcohol and Cancer

Cancer of the mouth occurs two and one-half times more frequently in persons who consume two drinks per day than in nondrinkers. Among persons who drink two drinks a day and smoke two packs of cigarettes a day, the risk of cancer of the mouth is increased fifteen times. Cancers of the esophagus, pharynx, and larynx have also been associated with heavy alcohol consumption. A recent study has also suggested a link between moderate alcohol consumption and breast cancer incidence.

Alcohol and Nutrition

As mentioned earlier, alcohol produces 7 calories per gram. When alcohol is oxidized in the body, these calories become available as energy. Unfortunately, no other appreciable amounts of nutrients are associated with alcoholic beverages; therefore, the calories derived from alcohol are "empty" calories. A fifth of 80-proof liquor will produce approximately 2,200 calories, with higher-proof beverages yielding even more. The body of the drinker then burns these calories for energy, making it less likely that he or she will eat the required nutrients in food. In the United States, alcoholism is considered to be the principal cause of vitamin deficiency.

■ Alcohol and the Law

Learn The Law

As of 1988, all fifty states have limited the purchase of alcoholic beverages to people 21 years of age or older. Some state legislatures are considering lowering the drinking age to 19, but pressure is being exerted by the federal government to maintain the 21-year-old limit. In some states, drivers are permitted to drink while driving, whereas in others they are not. Some states have open container laws, which prohibit the possession of an open container of an alcoholic beverage in the passenger compartment of a vehicle even if the driver or passengers have had nothing to drink. There are many places where the possession of an open container on a public street, even by a pedestrian, is illegal. Most states require drivers to have proof of adequate insurance in case of accidents. It is important that you learn the law in your locality.

Drinking and Driving

The leading cause of death for persons in the fifteen- to twenty-four-year-old age group is motor vehicle accidents (see Figure 12–3). Many of us have been

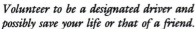

Volunteer to be a designated driver and possibly save your life or that of a friend.

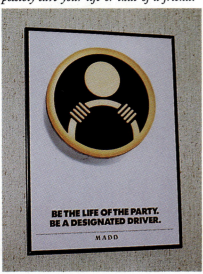

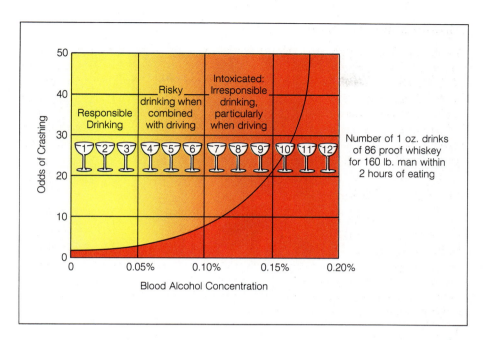

FIGURE 12–3 ■ **Drinking and Highway Safety: Odds of a Crash after Drinking.**

SOURCE: National Highway Traffic Safety Administration.

to a party where someone has had enough to drink to impair his or her ability to drive. What do we do in such situations? One solution is to choose a designated driver, someone who is willing to not drink at the party, to drive everyone home. Certainly, we would not get into a car as a passenger with someone who has been drinking. Students Against Driving Drunk (SADD) has developed a contract for young people to sign with their parents or friends in which the young person agrees to call the parent or friend if he or she is incapable of driving and the parent or friend agrees to pick the young person up and bring him or her home with no questions asked at the time. The college "Contract for Life" is illustrated in Figure 12–4.

The amount of alcohol in a person's bloodstream is expressed as the blood alcohol level (BAL) or blood alcohol concentration (BAC). There is one drop of alcohol per thousand drops of blood for each 0.1 percent increase in BAL. It takes approximately three drinks in a one-hour period to cause a 110-pound person to reach a BAL of 0.1 percent. For a 150-pound person, it would take approximately four drinks, and for a 200-pound person, approximately six drinks (see Table 12–2). The BAL is affected by how much alcohol is consumed, the time that has elapsed since the first drink, the time that has elapsed since the last drink, and the drinker's body weight. The amount of alcohol that is considered to be lethal is a BAL of 0.4 to 0.6.

As the blood alcohol level increases, visual acuity decreases, making it more difficult for the driver to see. Glare recovery time after passing the headlights of an oncoming car increases. Coordination is impaired and reaction time increases, making the driver less able to respond quickly to an emergency. Peripheral or side vision decreases so that the driver may not see things such as a car entering an intersection from the right or left or a child running into the street. Refer to Table 12–2 to see how drinking can affect your driving.

FAST FACTS

The Maryland Institute for Emergency Medical Services in Baltimore reported that 67 percent of all young people treated in its center have been involved in alcohol- or drug-related traffic accidents.

FIGURE 12-4 ■ SADD "Contract for Life"

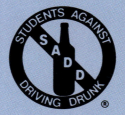

SOURCE: Reprinted with permission of Students Against Driving Drunk.

CHAPTER 12 ■ ALCOHOL AWARENESS

FIGURE 12–5 ■ Tips to Help Avoid "Driving Under the Influence of Alcohol" (DUI)

There is no safe way to drive after drinking. These charts show that a few drinks can make you an unsafe driver. They show that drinking affects your **Blood Alcohol Concentration (BAC)**. The **BAC** zones for various numbers of drinks and time periods are printed in yellow, orange, and red. **How to use these charts:** First, find the chart that includes your weight. For example, if you weigh 160 lbs., use the "150 to 169" chart. Then look under "Total Drinks" at the "2" on this "150 to 169" chart. Now look below the "2" drinks, in the row for 1 hour. You'll see your **BAC** is in the orange shaded zone. This means that if you drive after 2 drinks in 1 hour, you could be arrested. In the orange zone, your chances of having an accident are 5 times higher than if you had no drinks. But, if you had 4 drinks in 1 hour, your **BAC** would be in the red shaded area, and your chances of having an accident, 25 times higher. What's more, it is illegal to drive at this **BAC** (.10% or greater). After 3 drinks in 1 hour, the chart shows you would need 3 more hours, with no more drinks, to reach the yellow **BAC** zone again.

- Set a safe limit in advance and don't go above it.
- Space your drinks, try not to have more than one drink per hour.
- Taper off and STOP DRINKING at least one hour before you drive.
- Eat before and during drinking.
- Don't drink alcohol if you're taking medicine or drugs.

By strictly following these tips, you can greatly lower your chances of being arrested or having an accident.

Remember, coffee can't help, ONLY TIME CAN LOWER YOUR BLOOD ALCOHOL CONCENTRATION (**BAC**). Some drivers can even be under the influence at .03% **BAC**.

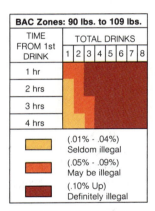

REMEMBER: "One drink" is a 12-ounce glass of beer, or a 4-ounce glass of wine, or a 1¼-ounce shot of 80-proof liquor (even if it's mixed with non-alcoholic drinks). If you have larger or stronger drinks, or drink on an empty stomach, or if you are tired, sick, upset, or have taken medicines or drugs, you can be unsafe with fewer drinks.

TECHNICAL NOTE: These charts are intended to be guides and are not legal evidence. Although it is possible for anyone to exceed the designated limits, the charts have been constructed so that fewer than 5 persons in 100 will exceed these limits when drinking the stated amounts on an empty stomach. Actual values can vary by body-type, sex, health status, and other factors.

Distributed by the Department of Motor Vehicles and prepared in cooperation with the California Highway Patrol, The Office of Traffic Safety, the Department of Alcohol and Drug Programs and the Department of Justice.

SECTION IV ■ DRUGS AND YOUR BODY

TABLE 12–4 ■ Years of Potential Life Lost (YPLL) before Age 65 and YPLL Rates from Total and Alcohol-Related Motor Vehicle Traffic (MVT) Fatalities, by Sex—United States, 1987

| | YPLL[a] | | |
MVT Fatalities	Number	Percent	Rate[b]
Total[a]	1,416,806	100.0	663
Male	1,027,956	72.6	966
Female	388,780	27.4	363
Alcohol-related[c]	783,304	100.0	367
Male	603,944	77.1	568
Female	179,333	22.9	167
Alcohol intoxication–related[c]	609,346	100.0	285
Male	476,662	78.2	448
Female	132,661	21.8	124

[a]Estimates provided by the Fatal Accident Reporting System. Infants dying before age 1 year were assigned age 0. Total YPLL includes a few persons of unknown sex.

[b]Rate per 100,000 persons under age 65. 1987 population estimates obtained from the Bureau of the Census Current Population Reports.

[c]Blood alcohol concentration of ≥0.01% for alcohol-related and ≥0.10% for alcohol intoxication–related fatalities.

SOURCE: *Morbidity and Mortality Weekly Report* 37 (December 16, 1988).

More than half of all highway deaths—approximately 25,000 each year—are related to drinking and driving (See Table 12–4). Although, in most states, it takes a BAL of 0.10 percent for a person to be considered legally drunk, many people are not capable of driving a car with far less alcohol in their bloodstreams. At a BAL of 0.10 percent, a driver is ten times more likely to have an accident than a nondrinker. At a BAL of 0.15 percent, the likelihood of an accident increases by twenty-five times and at 0.20 percent by one hundred times. Most drunk-driving accidents occur at about midnight on weekdays and at about 2 A.M. on Friday and Saturday nights (See Figure 12–6). Beer is the beverage most frequently associated with drinking and driving. Accidents not involving motor vehicles are also significantly higher when alcohol is involved.

■ *PROBLEM SITUATION* You are at a party with several of your friends. The person you drove with has had too much to drink. He refuses to give you or anyone else the keys to his car and intends to drive home. Since no one else at the party is going in your direction, he is your only way back. What do you do?

FAST FACTS

Among women who abuse alcohol, there are approximately twenty-three to twenty-nine cases of fetal alcohol syndrome per one thousand live births in the United States.

■ Fetal Alcohol Syndrome

It has been known for some time that an unborn baby can be seriously damaged by drugs taken by a pregnant woman, especially during the first trimester of the pregnancy, when the woman might not yet be aware that she is pregnant. Alcohol is one of these damaging drugs. Even the Bible has warnings against a pregnant woman consuming alcohol. Some experts believe that as many as

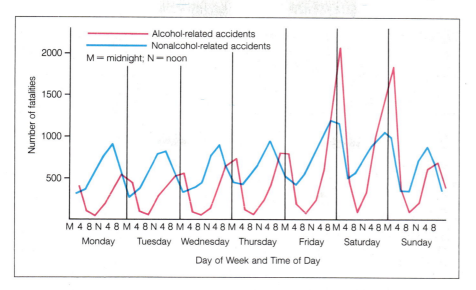

FIGURE 12–6 ■ **Number of Highway Fatalities by Day of Week, Time of Day, and Alcohol Involvement, 1981.**

SOURCE: Fifth Special Report to the U.S. Congress on Alcohol and Health, U.S. Department of Health and Human Services, December 1983.)

two drinks per day is safe, whereas others think that a pregnant woman should consume no alcohol whatsoever. A study reported in September 1987 by the National Institute of Child Health and Development analyzed the drinking habits and pregnancy outcomes of 32,870 women. The study determined that a woman drinking two drinks a day or less had the same risk of having a baby with birth defects as a woman who didn't drink at all. However, the same study reported that defects in the genital and urinary systems were directly proportional to the amount of alcohol consumed, "even in light amounts." Because of the potentially serious consequences to the baby, it seems that no drinking is the safest choice. It is also important that pregnant women be aware of the alcohol contained in some food and drugs and avoid those products.

Alcohol readily passes through the placenta into the infant's bloodstream. However, because the infant has an undeveloped liver, the alcohol cannot be easily metabolized. One theory suggests that it is a build-up of acetaldehyde (see the equation for the metabolism of alcohol) that damages the infant rather than the ethanol itself. The group of symptoms that may occur in an infant born to a drinking mother was first identified in 1973 and is called *fetal alcohol syndrome (FAS)*. The symptoms of FAS include mental retardation, defects in the face and limbs, and fine-motor impairment. Drinking is a more common cause of retardation than Down's Syndrome. Physical defects include small head; an indistinct groove between the nose and mouth; low-set, unparallel ears; heart and kidney disorders; hip dislocation; and many other problems. More than fifty separate signs and symptoms have been associated with fetal alcohol syndrome.

FAS is the third most common birth defect and the second most common cause of mental retardation in the United States. It is completely preventable by not drinking. The incidence of FAS today is about 1 in 750 live births. Approximately 40 percent of babies born to alcoholic mothers are diagnosed as having FAS.

■ *PROBLEM SITUATION*   Your friend has become pregnant. You have always known her to be a regular drinker of alcoholic beverages. Sometimes, at parties, she even drinks a little too much. What will you tell her about how alcohol can affect her pregnancy?

FAST FACTS

A study conducted by the University of California at Irvine School of Medicine showed that two-thirds of children in grades four through twelve drink. Of those, 11 percent can be considered alcoholics.

■ Alcoholism

Why People Drink

People drink alcohol for many reasons. Drinking is encouraged in our society. Some people are unable to engage in social relationships without the disinhibiting effects of alcohol. It has been called by some a "social lubricant." It helps to release tension. Many young people begin to drink as a result of peer pressure or as a behavior learned from their parents. Television commercials glamorize drinking as something done by anyone who is macho, sexy, stylish, or heroic. One advertisement for beer tells us to "go for the gusto."

Alcohol and Teenagers

Alcohol use is considered to be the number-one drug problem for young people in our country today. Studies show that over 90 percent of twelfth-grade girls and over 80 percent of twelfth-grade boys have tried alcohol. One study showed that over half of all seventh graders had consumed alcohol at least once during the previous year.

Most young people take their first drink in the home, served by their parents or relatives at some special occasion. Do you remember when you had your first taste of alcohol? Many young people begin drinking in order to appear grown-up or because they associate drinking with being an adult, although most say that curiosity is the primary motivator. Parental influence is a very strong factor in determining the drinking patterns of young people. Adolescents tend to view alcohol as a beverage, not as a drug.

Adolescent drinkers tend to do most of their drinking at unsupervised parties, at school activities such as dances and athletic events, and with their friends in secret in cars, empty lots, and fields. Beer is the most popular drink for boys, whereas wine is the most popular for girls. Hard liquors are the least popular. Adolescent problem drinkers tend to fit a certain profile. They are usually male, from an urban setting, and either of high or low socioeconomic status.

Each year nearly 8,000 young people die in alcohol-related automobile accidents and another 40,000 are crippled or disfigured for life.

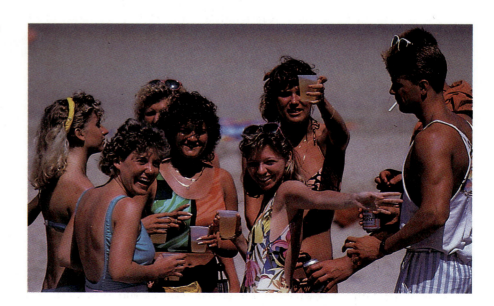

GUIDELINES TO YOUR GOOD HEALTH

The following are things that you can do to encourage responsible use of alcohol by you and those around you:

1. Do not drink alcoholic beverages in excess.
2. Do not serve alcoholic beverages to anyone under the legal drinking age.
3. Be aware of the interactions between alcohol and other drugs.
4. Do not drink and drive.
5. Volunteer to be the designated driver when going out with friends who wish to drink.
6. Do not drink alcohol if you are pregnant, and make others aware of the dangers of alcohol use during pregnancy.
7. Encourage friends and relatives with drinking problems to seek help.

What Is Alcoholism?

Alcoholism has been defined simply as the tendency to drink too much alcohol. What is too much? It is generally accepted that too much is any amount that interferes with normal activities. Alcoholics are classified as mild, moderate, or severe, depending on the degree to which normal functioning is impaired.

Is alcoholism an illness or just a bad habit that is hard to break? There are many theories about why an individual becomes an alcoholic. Some alcoholics are among a group people defined by psychologists as "antisocial personalities." If alcoholics are antisocial personalities, which came first—the alcoholism or the antisocial personality? Alcoholism may be related to family life, peer pressure, emotional factors, and anxiety. Many believe that it is an inherited disease. Studies have shown higher rates of alcoholism among children and siblings of alcoholics. At this time, however, no gene or other specific mode of inheritance has been discovered.

It is generally accepted today that alcoholism is an illness and should be treated as such. Studies show that alcoholism tends to run in families. Children of alcoholics have a 30 to 50 percent higher incidence of alcoholism than those of nonalcoholics. Even those children of alcoholics who grow up separated from their parents show a higher tendency toward alcoholism.

Several theories have been introduced to explain alcoholism. One of the more widely accepted theories is that alcoholism is genetically determined. Individuals inherit a tendency towards alcoholism that then manifests itself if certain social factors occur. Another theory suggests that alcoholism results from dysfunctions in the endocrine system.

It is estimated that there are at least ten to twelve million people in the United States with a dependency on alcohol. To some degree, these individuals exhibit a wide variety of behaviors associated with excessive drinking. These include impaired judgment, high suicide rate, child neglect and abuse, incest, and spousal abuse. Fifty percent of all violent crimes and more than 50 percent of all highway deaths are associated with alcohol.

There are as many female alcoholics as male alcoholics. Most alcoholics are not the skid row bums that we picture in our minds when we think of alcoholism. They are average men and women with families, homes, and jobs. Generally,

FAST FACTS

Only 7.2 percent of adolescent alcoholics will enter treatment programs.

SELF-INVENTORY 12.1

Do You Have A Drinking Problem?

Check the appropriate space after each question.

	Yes	No
1. Do you think about drinking often?	___	___
2. Do you drink more now than you used to?	___	___
3. Do you sometimes gulp your drinks?	___	___
4. Do you often take a drink to help you relax?	___	___
5. Do you drink often when you are alone?	___	___
6. Do you sometimes forget what happened while you were drinking?	___	___
7. Do you keep a bottle hidden somewhere—at home or at work—for a quick pick-me-up?	___	___
8. Do you need a drink to have fun?	___	___
9. Do you ever just start drinking without really thinking about it?	___	___
10. Do you drink in the morning to relieve a hangover?	___	___
11. Have you ever embarrassed your friends or family because of your drinking?	___	___
12. Have you ever been in trouble with the law because of your drinking?	___	___
13. Do you regularly drink more than six drinks per week?	___	___
14. Do you drink and then drive a car or operate machinery of any kind?	___	___

According to the National Institute on Alcohol Abuse and Alcoholism, if you had four or more "yes" answers on questions 1 through 10, you may be one of the 10 million Americans with a drinking problem. If you answered "yes" to any of questions 11 through 14, you should consider a change in your drinking habits.

they are not willing to recognize that they have a drinking problem and are not, therefore, willing to seek help.

Once an alcoholic recognizes his or her problem, there are many organizations that can help. One of the best known is Alcoholics Anonymous (A.A.), founded in 1935 by two alcoholics, but there are many others. Several large corporations have developed alcoholism recovery programs for employees. Alanon and Alateen are agencies dedicated to helping the family members of alcoholics.

Alcoholism is a disease that is with the alcoholic for his or her lifetime, but it can be controlled. Most experts believe that an alcoholic can never go back to being a social drinker but must refrain from *all* alcohol consumption.

■ **PROBLEM SITUATION** Your best friend drinks about fifteen to twenty beers each weekend. He doesn't drink during the week, doesn't miss classes, and gets average grades. But from Friday night until Sunday night, he always has a cold beer nearby. Is he an alcoholic? Does he need help? If so, what can you do to help him?

If you are concerned about someone close to you that you feel may have a problem with alcohol and need direction about dealing with the situation, refer to Table 12–5 below.

TABLE 12–5 ■ What to Do When Someone Close Drinks Too Much

Help is usually given in three stages:

1. Learning about the illness of alcoholism and various sources of treatment.
2. Guiding the "someone close" to treatment.
3. Supporting the person during and after treatment.

Do

Try to remain calm, unemotional, and factually honest in speaking with the problem drinker about his or her behavior and its day-to-day consequences.

Let the problem drinker know that you are reading and learning about alcoholism, attending Al-Anon or Alateen, and the like.

Discuss the situation with someone you trust—a clergyperson, a social worker, a friend, or some individual who has experienced alcoholism either personally or as a family member.

Establish and maintain a healthy atmosphere in the home and try to include the alcoholic member in family life.

Explain the nature of alcoholism as an illness to the children of the family.

Encourage new interests and participate in leisure-time activities that the problem drinker enjoys. Encourage him or her to see old friends in nondrinking situations.

Be patient and live one day at a time. Alcoholism generally takes a long time to develop, and recovery does not occur overnight. Try to accept setbacks and relapses with calm and understanding.

Refuse to ride with the alcoholic person if he or she insists on drinking and driving.

Do Not

Attempt to punish, threaten, bribe, preach, or try to be a martyr. Avoid emotional appeals that may only increase feelings of guilt and the compulsion to drink.

Allow yourself to cover up or make excuses for the alcoholic person or shield the person from the realistic consequences of his or her behavior.

Take over his or her responsibilities, leaving the person with no sense of importance or dignity.

Hide or dump bottles, or shelter the problem drinker from situations where alcohol is present.

Argue with the alcoholic person when he or she is drunk.

Try to drink along with the problem drinker.

Accept, above all, guilt for another's behavior.

SOURCE: National Institute on Alcohol Abuse and Alcoholism.

Alcoholics Anonymous

Alcoholics Anonymous (A.A.) began in June 1935 in Akron, Ohio. The first group developed from the recovery efforts of a New York stockbroker and an alcoholic physician in Akron. The first book published by the members of Alcoholics Anonymous for the benefit of other alcoholics was published in 1939. At the time, the organization's membership was somewhere around one hundred people. By the time the second edition was published in 1955, membership had grown to over 150,000, and chapters could be found in every state and in fifty foreign countries. A.A. boasts that 50 percent of the alcoholics who come to an A.A. group sober up immediately and another 25 percent do so after repeated efforts.

Alcoholics Anonymous has no religious affiliation, and men and women of all religions are welcome. Today, the membership is composed of about one-third women. There are more than 58,000 groups in 114 countries, and membership totals well over one million. About one-fifth of the members are under thirty years of age.

Alcoholics Anonymous treats alcoholism as an illness. It bases its approach on the notion that an "ex–problem drinker who has found (the) solution, who is properly armed with facts about himself, can generally win the entire confidence of another alcoholic in a few hours." No fees are charged by A.A., and the alcoholic who wishes to recover doesn't have to endure endless lectures and preaching. The concept is based on recovered alcoholics helping others to recover. Those who work in A.A. groups do not do it as a vocation, nor are they paid for their efforts. They devote virtually all of their spare time to A.A.

Most alcoholics are unwilling to admit that they have a drinking problem. They attempt over and over again to demonstrate to themselves and to others that they can drink like anyone else. They even quit periodically just to demonstrate to themselves that they can. Most believe that they could control their drinking if they wanted to do so. A.A. states emphatically that they can not. Alcoholics "are in the grip of a progressive illness." A.A. believes that "no real alcoholic ever recovers control." An alcoholic can never be like everyone else.

Alcoholics try a variety of maneuvers to prove that they can drink like other people. According to Alcoholics Anonymous, they try "drinking beer only, limiting the number of drinks, never drinking in the morning, drinking only at parties, drinking only natural wines," and so on. They try to exercise, become more religious, swear off alcohol, and more. None of these methods work. Do you know anyone who has tried any of these?

Alcoholics Anonymous believes that most drinkers could have stopped had they been willing to admit to their problem earlier in their drinking careers. Most drinkers, of course, deny that there is a problem until it is too late to stop on their own. Many alcoholics never recognize that they have a drinking problem. A.A. suggests that if a drinker wants to prove that he or she is not an alcoholic, that person should "try leaving liquor alone for one year."

Alcoholics find it virtually impossible to give up drinking without help, no matter how much they might want or need to. There is "an utter inability to leave it alone." A.A. describes the all-consuming desire for alcohol as being "strangely insane."

Alcoholics Anonymous teaches that there is a greater power than ourselves—in other words, God. It also asserts that God is whatever each individual's

---

FAST FACTS

Separated, single, and divorced individuals are more likely to have problems with alcoholism than married or widowed individuals.

FAST FACTS

A severely alcoholic person must go through a 5 to 8 day detoxification before alcoholism treatment can begin.

conception of that higher power might be. According to A.A., an alcoholic must believe in that higher power before he or she can be on the road to recovery.

Alcoholics Anonymous has twelve steps to recovery. They are the following:

1. We admitted that we were powerless over alcohol—that our lives had become unmanageable.
2. Came to believe that a Power greater than ourselves could restore us to sanity.
3. Made a decision to turn our will and our lives over to the care of God as we understood Him.
4. Made a searching and fearless moral inventory of ourselves.
5. Admitted to God, to ourselves, and to another human being the exact nature of our wrongs.
6. Were entirely ready to have God remove all these defects of character.
7. Humbly ask Him to remove our shortcomings.
8. Made a list of all persons we had harmed and became willing to make amends to them all.
9. Made direct amends to such people wherever possible, except when to do so would injure them or others.
10. Continued to take personal inventory and when we were wrong, promptly admitted it.
11. Sought through prayer and meditation to improve our conscious contact with God, as we understood him, praying only for knowledge of His will for us and the power to carry that out.
12. Having had a spiritual awakening as a result of these steps, we tried to carry this message to others, and to practice these principles in all our affairs.

There are also several organizations dedicated to helping those who live with or whose lives are affected by another's drinking. They include Alanon, Alateen, and Adult Children of Alcoholics (A.C.A.). Alanon is designed to serve those whose lives are affected by an alcoholic and is primarily for adults, whereas

GUIDELINES TO YOUR GOOD HEALTH

If someone you care about drinks too much, the following suggestions can help you cope with the problem:

1. Do not make excuses for the drinker when he or she is unable to meet social or work obligations because of drinking.
2. Do not hide the drinker's alcoholic beverages.
3. Do not throw away or otherwise discard the drinker's alcoholic beverages.
4. Do not scold or nag the drinker.
5. Do not try to punish the drinker by withholding money from him or her.
6. Attend meetings of Alanon, Alateen, Adult Children of Alcoholics, or some other comparable organization.

Alateen serves the same purpose for teenagers. A.C.A. utilizes the same twelve steps that A.A. uses in its recovery program, but these steps are applied to the person who is the nondrinker. A.C.A. describes itself as "spiritual though not religious; . . . emotional but not group therapy; . . . individual though practiced with and through the help of others; . . . entirely voluntary, and the only requirement is to be willing to try; . . . costs little or nothing monetarily or as much as we can afford; . . . based on love, caring, and understanding."

Alcoholics learn to manipulate those around them. They get others to cover up for them, make excuses for them, lie for them, and more to protect their drinking. In many cases, they victimize those who love them the most. Those us of who had our lives touched by an alcoholic know that it does no good to yell at them, preach to them, hide or throw away their liquor, and so on. An alcoholic can stop only if he or she wants to and with help from A.A. or a similar organization.

POSITIVE BEHAVIORS

I. *Place a check mark in front of each behavior that you now practice.*

_____ 1. I do not drink alcoholic beverages. (DRINK)
_____ 2. I do not drink more than six alcoholic drinks per week. (SIX DRINKS)
_____ 3. I do not serve alcohol to anyone under the legal age limit. (LEGAL AGE)
_____ 4. I do not drink and drive. (DRINK AND DRIVE)
_____ 5. I do not ride as a passenger in a car with a driver who has been drinking. (PASSENGER)
_____ 6. I encourage women who are pregnant not to drink during their pregnancy. (PREGNANCY)
_____ 7. I encourage anyone I know who is an alcoholic to seek professional help. (ALCOHOLIC)
_____ 8. I do not combine alcohol with other drugs. (COMBINE)

II. *For each behavior that you DO NOT ENGAGE IN, write in the appropriate space below the KEY WORD(S) located in the parentheses at the end of the statement. Then indicate whether you intend to keep or change that behavior.*

Behaviors I Don't Engage In	KEEP/CHANGE
	_____ / _____
	_____ / _____
	_____ / _____
	_____ / _____
	_____ / _____
	_____ / _____
	_____ / _____
	_____ / _____

III. *For each of the preceding behaviors that you choose to KEEP, write a statement indicating why you are choosing to keep that behavior.*

I choose to keep behavior _____ because:
                              KEY WORD

For each of the preceding behaviors that you choose to CHANGE, write a statement indicating how you plan to implement that change.

I will change behavior _____ by:
                          KEY WORD

Now You Know

1. TRUE. A twelve-ounce can of beer, four to six ounces of wine, and one mixed drink all contain approximately the same amount of alcohol.
2. FALSE. Ethyl alcohol depresses the central nervous system. Drinkers feel stimulated because of depression of the centers in the brain that control inhibitions.
3. TRUE. Alcohol causes the blood vessels near the skin surface to dilate, leading to a loss of body heat. Drinking alcohol in cold weather will cause more rapid heat loss and could possibly lead to frostbite.
4. FALSE. Alcohol produces seven calories per gram (almost twice the amount produced by protein or carbohydrate). Approximately 150 calories is supplied by the alcohol in one drink.
5. TRUE. A variety of physical and mental symptoms can occur in children born to women who drink during pregnancy. Collectively, these symptoms are known as the fetal alcohol syndrome.
6. FALSE. Other alcohols, such as methyl alcohol, are highly toxic, and their consumption can lead to death or other serious health problems.
7. FALSE. Alcohol is one of the few substances that is absorbed directly into the blood stream in its undigested form.
8. TRUE. Physical dependence is possible with long-term use of alcohol. Withdrawal symptoms may include hallucinations, delerium tremens, convulsions, coma, and death.
9. TRUE. Cancers of the mouth, esophagus, pharynx, and larynx have all been associated with excessive alcohol consumption.
10. FALSE. Most experts believe very strongly that an alcoholic must stop drinking completely if he or she is to successfully recover.

Summary

1. Alcoholic beverages are made through the fermentation of fruits, vegetables, and other sources of carbohydrates. Wines and beers are undistilled, whereas brandies and hard liquors are either distilled or have additional alcohol added.
2. The concentration of alcohol in a beverage is measured by its proof. The proof is double the percentage of alcohol. For example, a beverage that is 40 percent alcohol would be 80 proof.
3. Ethyl alcohol is absorbed directly into the bloodstream without first being digested. The rate of absorption may be affected by food in the stomach as well as a number of other factors.
4. Alcohol is metabolized by the liver at a fairly constant rate of about ten milliliters of absolute alcohol per hour. This rate is constant irrespective of the concentration of alcohol in the bloodstream.
5. A hangover is due to the gastric irritation caused by alcohol, congeners present in the beverage, and the accumulation of acetaldehyde during the metabolism of alcohol.
6. Other physiological effects of drinking alcohol include dehydration, dilation of peripheral blood vessels, increased flow of saliva, and irritation of ulcers.
7. Ethyl alcohol is a central nervous system depressant. It causes a release of inhibitions, impairment of muscular coordination, and visual disturbances.
8. Physiological dependence and tolerance may result from excessive alcohol consumption. Withdrawal may be severe and include delerium tremens, hallucinations, coma, and death.
9. Alcohol interacts with a variety of other drugs. Combined with other central nervous system depressants, alcohol's effect can be synergistic and can possibly lead to death.
10. Alcohol consumption has been associated with disorders of the liver, circulatory diseases, several types of cancer, and nutritional problems.
11. In most states, a person with a blood alcohol level of 0.1 percent or greater is considered legally drunk. At this level, a drinker's chances of having an automobile accident are ten times that of a nondrinker.
12. Fetal alcohol syndrome (FAS) is a group of physical and mental symptoms that can occur in a baby born to a woman who drinks alcohol during pregnancy. It is the third most common birth defect.
13. Alcohol is the number-one drug problem among young people in the United States. Most first-time use of alcohol takes place in the home. Most adolescent drinking takes place at unsupervised parties, at school events, and with friends.
14. Alcoholism is sometimes defined as simply the tendency to drink too much alcohol. It is generally accepted by the medical community that alcoholism is a disease.
15. There are several theories about why certain individuals become alcoholics. Alcoholism may be genetically determined because it tends to run in families. Another theory is that it is due to a malfunction of the endocrine system.
16. Alcoholics Anonymous is one of several organizations available to help the alcoholic stop drinking. Founded in 1935, it today has a membership of over a million men and women in 114 countries. About 20 percent of its members are under thirty years of age.

References

1. Alcoholics Anonymous. *Alcoholics Anonymous: The Story of How Many Thousands of Men and Women Have Recovered from Alcoholism* 3d ed., New York: Alcoholics Anonymous World Services, 1976.
2. Alcoholics Anonymous. *The Twelve steps for Everyone ... Who Really Wants Them*. Minneapolis: CompCare Publications, 1977.
3. Alcoholics Anonymous. *Twelve Steps and Twelve Traditions*. New York: Alcoholics Anonymous World Services, 1986.
4. President's Commission on Law Enforcement and Administration of Justice. *Task Force Report: Drunkenness*. Washington, D.C.: U.S. Government Printing Office, 1967.
5. Rittenhouse, Joan Dunne, ed. *Consequences of Alcohol and Marijuana Use*. Washington, D.C.: U. S. Department of Health, Education, and Welfare, 1979.
6. Secretary of Health and Human Services. *Fourth Special Report to the U. S. Congress on Alcohol and Health*. Washington, D.C.: U. S. Department of Health and Human Services, 1981.

Suggested Readings

Alcoholics Anonymous. New York: Alcoholics Anonymous World Services, 1986.

Blane, H. T., and K. E. Leonard, *Psychological Theories of Drinking and Alcoholism*. New York: The Guilford Press, 1987.

Carroll, Charles R. *Drugs in Modern Society*. Dubuque, Iowa: William C. Brown Publishers, 1985

Julien, Robert, *A Primer of Drug Action*. San Francisco: W. H. Freeman and Co., 1981.

Pinkham, M. E. *How to Stop the One You Love from Drinking*. New York: The Putnam Publishing Group, 1986.

Rucker, William B., ed. *Drugs, Society and Behavior*. Guilford, Conn.: The Dushkin Publishing Group, 1987.

Alcoholics Anonymous. Twelve Steps and Twelve Traditions. New York: Alcoholics Anonymous World Services, 1986.

Witters, Weldon, and Peter Venturelli. *Drugs and Society*. Boston: Jones and Barlett Publishers, 1988.

Woititz, J. G. *Adult Children of Alcoholics*. Pompano Beach, Florida: Health Communications, 1983.

CHAPTER 13

Psychoactive Drugs

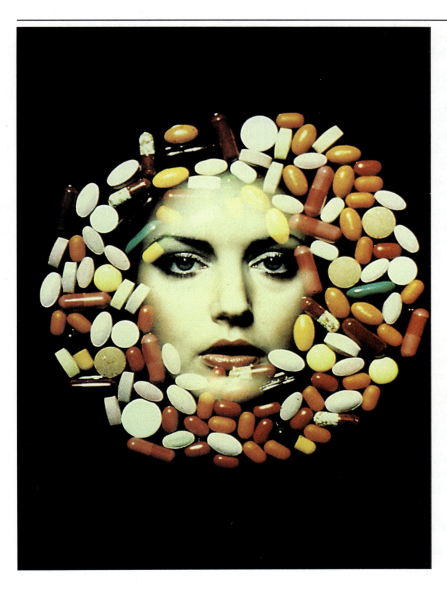

What Do You Know?

Are the following statements true or false?

1. Inhalation of volatile solvents such as glue and paint thinner can cause kidney and liver damage.
2. Withdrawal from physiological dependence on barbiturates is not as dangerous as withdrawal from heroin.
3. Life-threatening synergism can occur between barbiturates and alcohol.
4. Barbiturates are the principal drugs used for suicide in the United States.
5. The minor tranquilizers such as Valium do not cause physiological dependence.
6. The only two naturally occurring opiates are morphine and codeine.
7. Methadone is useful in treating heroin addiction because it does not cause the physiological dependence that occurs with heroin.
8. Only about 10 percent of addicts who enter methadone maintenance programs will remain drug free.
9. Cocaine is slowly metabolized in the body, so its effects can be felt for several hours.
10. Both regular and decaffeinated coffee can cause irritation to a person with ulcers.

Deliriants

Volatile Solvents

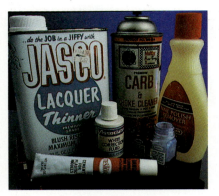

Many common household products contain volatile solvents and, therefore, have a potential for abuse.

Volatile solvents have been inhaled for their euphoric or deliriant effects for many years. Deliriants are substances that cause disorientation, confusion, and hallucinations. These include chemicals such as ether, benzene, gasoline, and so on. Laws governing the sale of commercial products containing volatile solvents such as glues, typewriter correction fluids, and paint removers have been passed in many states. These products have been readily available in the past, especially to young people, who could purchase them in hobby shops and hardware stores.

When inhaled, these substances rapidly enter the bloodstream and are quickly delivered to the brain. Effects include intoxication, **euphoria,** hyperactivity, and hallucinations. Many other effects may also occur. Overdose can depress breathing and lead to convulsions, and death. Long-term effects include kidney and liver damage, depression of bone-marrow function, and appetite suppression.

Poppers

Poppers contain drugs in a class known as volatile nitrites, principally amyl nitrite and butyl nitrite. In medicine, amyl nitrite is used to relieve the severe chest pain of angina pectoris. The name "poppers" comes from the nature of the unique dosage form. The drug is in liquid form and is contained in a small glass tube encased in an absorbent material such as gauze. When the medication is needed, the glass tube is broken (popped), and the liquid soaks onto the gauze. It is then inhaled by the user. You may have seen this method of drug administration before as it is used in ammonia inhalants given to people who faint.

Poppers used at the moment of orgasm are said by some users to significantly enhance the experience. Some of the drugs used in poppers require a prescription, but others are sold freely in head shops and other such establishments. They are dangerous drugs and cause dilation of blood vessels in the heart and brain. Side effects, therefore, may include headache and chest pain. Many studies have suggested that the drugs in poppers reduce the body's immune capabilities. A 1987 study showed a statistically significant relationship between the use of poppers and the rate of sexually transmitted diseases in gay men.

> ■ **PROBLEM SITUATION** Your best friend tells you that he has tried poppers for the first time. He believes that they are safe because the ones he used were bought in a store without a prescription. He plans to use them again. What advice should you give him?

Depressants

In this section, we will look at those drugs that depress activity in the central nervous system—the brain and spinal cord. They include barbiturates, nonbarbiturate sedative-hypnotics, minor tranquilizers, opiates, and marijuana.

Barbiturates

Barbiturates are derivatives of a chemical known as barbituric acid, discovered in 1864 by a German chemist, Adolph von Baeyer. Thousands of barbiturates have been synthesized over the years, but only a few have been marketed, most of which are still available today. Because of their potential for abuse, barbiturates are tightly controlled and are not widely used.

These drugs are classified as sedative-hypnotics. In low doses, they serve to tranquilize, or sedate, an individual. In larger doses, they are hypnotics; that is, they induce sleep. The first barbiturate to be marketed commercially, in 1903, was barbital (generic name) or Veronal (brand name). Phenobarbital was the next compound to be made commercially available (1912), and it is probably the most widely used of the barbiturates today.

The barbiturates act primarily on the central nervous system. In doses that have either sedative or hypnotic effect on the CNS, there is little or no effect on other body systems. The exact mechanism by which barbiturates act is unknown, but it is thought that they inhibit the release of neurotransmitters that are responsible for excitatory activity. Barbiturates cause relaxation, lowered inhibitions, and a reduction in muscular coordination in lower doses.

Barbiturates are used in medicine to treat convulsive disorders, insomnia, and anxiety. For convulsive disorders such as epilepsy, the principal drug used is phenobarbital, primarily because of its long duration of action. For insomnia, the barbiturate chosen would depend on the specific sleep problems of the patient. For example, a physician might choose a short-acting barbiturate if the patient had a difficult time getting to sleep but not staying asleep. A longer-acting drug might be needed for someone unable to stay asleep. Barbiturates are also effective in treating anxiety, but they have been replaced for the most part by the minor tranquilizers.

Although barbiturates are effective for the treatment of insomnia, it must be noted that they do not induce REM (rapid eye movement) sleep. REM sleep is a deep level of sleep in which the individual dreams, and it is considered unhealthy for a person to sleep without some degree of dreaming. Patients using barbiturates to treat insomnia for long periods of time often complain of excessive dreaming and nightmares when the drugs are no longer used. In addition, many barbiturate users suffer from drug hangover the next day.

A variety of potential problems can occur with use of barbiturates. These drugs are known to cause **physiological dependence,** leading to **withdrawal** when the drug is stopped. In fact, withdrawal from these drugs is far more dangerous than from any other physically addicting drug, and it should be attempted only under appropriate medical supervision. Suddenly stopping the use of a barbiturate, known as "cold turkey" withdrawal, is not considered safe and could result in convulsions, coma, and death. During withdrawal, it is often necessary to give the patient other medications to reduce the danger of convulsions. If you know anyone who is hooked on barbiturates and wants to stop using them, be sure to encourage him or her to seek medical care.

Barbiturates build moderate physiological **tolerance.** The liver enzymes responsible for metabolizing barbiturates increase in ability with continued exposure to the drug, so the individual must take more and more of the barbiturate to get the desired effect. **Cross tolerance** to all barbiturates develops in a person taking any one of these drugs. In other words, as the user becomes tolerant to one barbiturate, he or she becomes tolerant to all other barbiturates at the same time. It is important to note that even though physiological tolerance to barbiturates develops, the dose that could potentially be fatal does not change. Therefore, the dose needed for the desired therapeutic results tends to get closer and closer to the dose that could cause death.

> **FAST FACTS**
>
> Psychotic behavior has resulted from some cases of deliriant use.

FAST FACTS

Reasons for drug abuse include alienation, low self esteem, peer pressure, and the need for a coping mechanism.

Synergism—the multiplication of effect when two or more drugs are combined—occurs with barbiturates and all other central nervous system depressants. As indicated in Chapter 12, synergism between alcohol and drugs such as barbiturates can be fatal. Consider an individual who for a long period of time has been taking barbiturates to induce sleep. He or she goes to a party and has a few drinks, not even enough to become legally drunk. After the party, the individual goes home and takes the usual dose of sleeping pills. The next morning, someone finds the person dead. Neither the dose of alcohol nor the dose of barbiturate was enough to be fatal but in combination, because of synergism, death resulted.

Three-fourths of all drug-related suicides in the United States involve the use of barbiturates. Death results from depression of the centers of the brain that control respiration and heartbeat. In this country, most barbiturates are classified as controlled substances under special drug laws (see Chapter 18).

> **PROBLEM SITUATION** A friend has been using barbiturates regularly for several years. She wants to quit and plans on stopping "cold turkey." What dangers does she face if she tries to stop? How can she stop without risking her life?

Minor Tranquilizers

The group of drugs known as the minor tranquilizers consists primarily of drugs in a class called the benzodiazepines. The most popular of these drugs is Valium, although many new drugs in this group developed during the last few years are gaining in popularity. Benzodiazepines are used to reduce anxiety in patients exhibiting neurosis, as anticonvulsants, and as muscle relaxants in conditions such as multiple sclerosis and degenerative diseases of the spine. Flurazepam is a benzodiazepine that has become the most commonly prescribed drug for insomnia in this country. It does not depress REM sleep, as would occur with barbiturates.

Benzodiazepines are no more effective as anti-anxiety drugs than barbiturates, but they are safer in terms of the possibilities of drug overdose and suicide. They do not depress respiration to any appreciable degree. They do, however, lead to physiological dependence and tolerance. Withdrawal symptoms have been reported, but in very few cases have they been severe. Synergism does occur between alcohol and benzodiazepines.

Other Sedative-Hypnotics

Ever since the barbiturates were first used, drug manufacturers have sought to develop new drugs that have the positive qualities of the barbiturates without the negative effects. Many sedative-hypnotics have been developed as a result of this research. Examples of these are glutethimide, methaqualone, and methyprylon (Noludar).

Methaqualone (generic name) has been manufactured under several brand names, including Quaalude, Sopor, and Parest. It was developed as a sedative-hypnotic and was introduced into the United States in the mid-1960s. It quickly became a very popular drug with physicians, who thought that it had all the advantages of the barbiturates but was not dangerous or physically addicting.

It also quickly became a popular drug of abuse. By 1973, it had been placed in schedule II of controlled substances, and in 1984, it was removed from the legal marketplace.

Methaqualone is highly physically addicting, causes severe and potentially fatal withdrawal symptoms when abruptly discontinued, and can readily be used to commit suicide. When compared to other drugs with similar therapeutic uses, its negative effects far outweigh its positive effects.

Opiates

The source of opium and its natural **alkaloids** is the opium poppy plant, which is usually grown in Asia. Raw opium is obtained from the unripened seed capsule after the flower's petals have dropped off. Codeine and morphine naturally occur in the plant, whereas heroin is a semi-synthetic drug made from morphine.

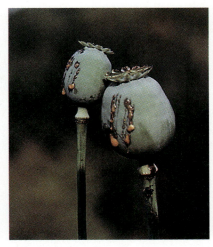

Opium is derived from the unripened seed capsule of the poppy plant.

Opium has been used as an intoxicant and pain reliever for thousands of years. Morphine was isolated from crude opium in 1803 and codeine in 1832. First thought to be a cure for morphine addiction, heroin has been used in medicine since 1898. There are many synthetic opiate drugs available on the market today, principally prescribed either as analgesics (pain relievers) or as cough suppressants. They include dolophine, meperidine, oxycodone, hydrocodone, and a number of others.

The natural and synthetic opiate drugs are classified as narcotics; that is, they induce narcosis, or central nervous system depression. Morphine, meperidine, dolophine, and codeine are used as pain relievers. They reduce pain without causing loss of consciousness. Codeine, however, is principally used for its cough-suppressing properties. Most of us have probably taken a cough syrup containing codeine at some time in our lives (unless you are allergic to it, of course). Because narcotics reduce **peristalsis** in the gastrointestinal tract, they can be used to treat diarrhea. Side effects of opiate use include drowsiness, decrease in body temperature, constipation, nausea, and vomiting.

An opiate overdose is characterized by pinpoint pupils, coma, and depression of respiration, which can lead to death. Tolerance results from continued use of opiates, and physiological as well as **psychological dependence** occurs. Withdrawal from opiates causes a variety of symptoms, including fever, chills, stomach cramps, muscle aches, nausea, vomiting, tremors, and runny nose. Rarely does withdrawal from these drugs result in death. Synergism occurs between the opiates and other central nervous system depressants.

Addicts inject heroin most often using unsterile needles and syringes and in unclean surroundings.

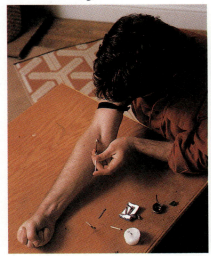

In the United States, heroin use is illegal. This is not the case in all countries, some of which use heroin in medical practice in the same way that we use morphine. Heroin addiction is related to violent crime in this country because of the addict's need for the drug and the expense of maintaining his or her habit. Some addicts will spend hundreds of dollars per day in order to obtain sufficient quantities of the drug to prevent withdrawal. Programs aimed at reducing addict populations, estimated at approximately 500,000, have largely been unsuccessful. It is estimated that less than 2 percent of addicts have the potential for rehabilitation.

Methadone is a synthetic narcotic drug with properties similar to morphine. It has been used as a substitute for heroin in treatment programs designed to maintain the user and reduce his or her need for heroin itself. Methadone's advantages in such programs are its longer duration of action and the fact that

> **FAST FACTS**
>
> Instead of getting high on drugs, get high on activities such as sailing, running, meditation, volunteer work, and listening to music.

it can be administered by mouth. Some programs are designed to switch the user from heroin to methadone and then gradually wean him or her off the methadone. Others assume that the user will have to be maintained on methadone indefinitely.

Methadone treatment programs have been very controversial. Proponents say that such programs maintain the addicts and reduce the risk of their committing crimes to obtain their drug supply. Opponents believe that methadone programs simply substitute one addiction for another. Maintenance programs with heroin itself, as well as with other opiates, have been tried in the United States and other countries. In any case, best estimates are that only about 10 percent of addicts who enter and complete methadone maintenance programs will remain drug free.

Therapeutic communities such as Synanon, Harmony House, and Phoenix House have been established to treat addicts in a residential setting with other addicts. These programs have been successful only as long as the ex-addicts stay in close association with the therapeutic community. Very few of them have remained drug free after leaving and going out on their own.

Naturally occurring chemicals in the brain called endorphins and enkephalins fit the same receptor sites as opiates. These substances are responsible for pain-relieving, pleasure-producing, and euphoriant effects. Studies have shown that they are produced in the brain in response to sexual activity, physical exercise, music, and a variety of other pleasurable activities. A great deal of research is being conducted with these materials in order to better understand how the brain works, how pleasure is induced, and how drug addiction takes place, as well as to explain various other brain functions. In addition to human beings, endorphins have been discovered in many animals.

■ Stimulants

Cocaine

Cocaine is a naturally occurring stimulant derived from the leaves of the plant *Erythroxylon coca*. The plant is found in many of the mountainous areas of Central and South America. It has long been used for its stimulant properties by natives of the regions in which it grows. Until the late 1800s, when cocaine was first isolated from the plant, it was obtained principally by chewing coca leaves. Sigmund Freud used cocaine extensively with psychiatric patients and thought it to be a panacea until he later realized the serious consequences of its use and discontinued working with it completely. It is still widely used today as a stimulant and in native rituals in South America.

Prior to 1906, cocaine was identified as an ingredient in Coca Cola, originally marketed as a tonic, not a soft drink. A popular recreational drug in the early 1900s, cocaine was referred to in a Cole Porter song, "I Get A Kick Out Of You." The fictional detective Sherlock Holmes was depicted as a user of cocaine.

In the United States today, cocaine is used by people in virtually every sector of society. It is estimated that five to six million Americans use it regularly. Nearly one out of five high-school seniors report having tried it. In the last ten years, cocaine use among teenagers has doubled.

Cocaine is an extremely effective local **anesthetic** for mucous membranes as well as a strong central nervous system stimulant. It has been widely used medically for its local anesthetic properties, especially to relieve pain following nasal surgery. It is also combined with morphine in an oral liquid medication called Brompton's solution, which is given to terminally ill cancer patients. The morphine is for pain relief, and the cocaine reduces the side effects of the morphine.

Cocaine acts at the synapses for which norepinephrine and dopamine are the neurotransmitters, blocking their **reuptake** into the vesicles and thereby producing stimulation of the brain. The strong psychological dependence that results from use of cocaine is thought to be brought about by stimulation of the pleasure centers of the brain through dopamine synapses (see Chapter 11). The drug also stimulates the sympathetic nervous system.

Cocaine is very rapidly metabolized in the body, its effects lasting less than thirty minutes to an hour. Methods of administration include inhalation (snorting), smoking, and intravenous injection. When cocaine is injected, the effects of the drug can be felt within a few seconds, whereas with snorting or smoking, it may take a few minutes. The degree of the drug's absorption through smoking or injection may be as much as ten times greater than from snorting. When the drug is snorted, factors such as what it has been adulterated with and how much mucous the individual has in his or her nose will affect the rate of absorption.

Physiological effects of moderate doses of cocaine include increases in the rate of breathing, heart rate, motor activity, and body temperature. A notable increase in blood pressure may occur initially. A feeling of well being and euphoria results from stimulation of the brain's pleasure centers. Users often report reduced appetites, increased sex drive, increased sociability, reduced fatigue, and increased mental alertness. A rebound depression frequently follows use of the drug.

Long-term use can lead to a drug-induced **psychosis,** including **paranoia** and hallucinations. Some users believe that they have bugs crawling under their skin, and cases have occurred in which individuals have literally torn away their own flesh trying to destroy the "bugs." The irritating effect of constant exposure to cocaine can damage nasal and lung tissue. High doses have been associated with seizures potentially leading to death, irregular heart rhythms, and heart attack.

An overdose may lead to hallucinations, dilated pupils, a heart rate of well over 100 beats per minute, muscular spasms, abdominal pain, vomiting, and other symptoms. Death can result within a few minutes from intravenous doses as low as 20 milligrams (mg.) and is due to convulsions, coma, and circulatory failure. Fatal doses when cocaine is taken by mouth have ranged from 500 mg. to 1.2 grams. (One gram is equal to 1,000 mg.)

Cocaine has not been classified as a physiologically addicting drug because physiological withdrawal, as we define it for other drugs, does not occur when the drug is stopped. However, experts agree that the psychological dependence that occurs is stronger than with any other drug. Tolerance does occur with prolonged use of cocaine.

The drug is manufactured as a white crystalline powder and is rather inexpensive on the legal market. A retail pharmacy can probably buy an ounce of pure pharmaceutical-grade cocaine today for less than $200. On the illegal market, an ounce of cocaine, probably **adulterated** more than 50 percent with other white crystalline substances, will cost well over $2,000. Street cocaine may, in fact, contain no cocaine at all. Sellers frequently sell amphetamines mixed with local anesthetics such as procaine or benzocaine as cocaine. These local anesthetics are used to produce the numbness that a cocaine user expects from the drug.

FAST FACTS

A recent survey by the National Institute on Drug Abuse showed that for the first time since the surveys began, cocaine use by high-school students in the United States has declined.

Snorting of cocaine hydrochloride powder is still the most popular method of administration. The hydrochloride salt cannot be smoked because it is decomposed by heat. Smoking of the freebase (or alkaloidal) cocaine and of "crack" or rock cocaine is also widespread. Fewer users inject the drug. "Freebasing," the chemical conversion of cocaine hydrochloride to plain alkaloidal cocaine, involves the use of volatile solvents such as ether. It is a highly dangerous process. Deaths and injuries from explosions and fires associated with freebasing have been reported many times.

The procedure for making crack is much simpler and safer and uses ordinary ingredients such as ammonia and baking soda. The name "rock" cocaine comes from the physical appearance of the chunks and the name "crack" from the popping sound made by the burning crystals when they are smoked. Crack is an extremely pure form of cocaine and cannot be cut with impurities as cocaine hydrochloride powder can. Smoking the drug is also a very effective method of drug delivery and leads to blood levels almost as high as if the drug were injected intravenously. Because of its high level of purity and its comparatively lower cost, crack is a popular and extremely dangerous form of cocaine.

At present, there is a toll-free hotline that you can call if you or someone you know is dependent on cocaine and needs help. The number is 1-800-Cocaine. The hotline's founder is Dr. Mark Gold of Fair Oaks Hospital in Summit, New Jersey. Dr. Gold, one of the country's foremost experts in the field of substance abuse, established the hotline in 1983. As many as 1,200 calls per day are received by the hotline.

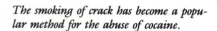

The smoking of crack has become a popular method for the abuse of cocaine.

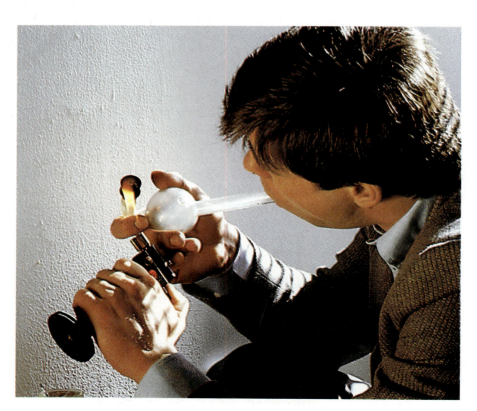

Amphetamines

Amphetamine was first discovered in the early 1930s and was marketed as a bronchodilator in an inhaler in 1932. Bronchodilators are drugs that cause dilation of the bronchial tubes and are often used to treat asthma. That inhaler, known today as a Benzedrex inhaler, no longer contains any amphetamine. The drug was also used in its early history to treat narcolepsy, a condition characterized by attacks of spontaneous deep sleep. Since the 1930s, amphetamines have also been used as stimulants, as appetite suppressants, and to treat hyperactive children.

Amphetamines have been used by armies to keep soldiers awake for extended periods of time, by astronauts to increase alertness, by truck drivers to maintain wakefulness during long trips, and by college students studying for exams.

In the 1960s, when the use of amphetamines obtained through legal prescriptions was probably at its height, these drugs were used principally as antidepressants and for long-term weight control. Today, there are far better drugs on the market to treat depression, and we are well aware of the inadequacy of drugs in treating obesity and overweight. It is well documented that amphetamines are not at all useful in long-term weight control. They might be helpful to a prizefighter who has to lose a few pounds to weigh in for a big bout in a couple of weeks but not for those of us who need to lose pounds and keep them off.

All amphetamine-containing products require a prescription. The commercially available amphetamines include amphetamine (Benzedrine), methamphetamine (Methedrine, Desoxyn), and dextroamphetamine (Dexedrine). Methamphetamine (speed, crystal, meth) is the drug of choice in the illegal market. It is taken principally by intravenous injection (mainlining).

Amphetamines are central nervous system stimulants and are believed to function principally by affecting the synapses for which norepinephrine and dopamine are the neurotransmitters. These drugs cause an increase in blood pressure and pulse rate, lower appetite, cause dilation of the bronchi, raise blood-sugar levels, and lead to restlessness and increased alertness.

High tolerance to amphetamines develops, although they do not cause physiological dependence. Of course, psychological dependence can become very strong. Severe depression and fatigue (crashing) can follow amphetamine use.

Overdose and long-term use of amphetamines can lead to serious consequences. Psychological effects such as paranoia, delusions, and hallucinations may occur. Drug-induced psychosis or schizophrenia has been reported.

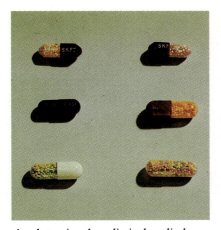

Amphetamines have limited medical use and are not widely prescribed by physicians.

> ■ **PROBLEM SITUATION** You are twenty pounds overweight and want to lose those extra pounds. A neighbor suggests amphetamines as a diet aid. Will they work? What would be a better suggestion?

■ Hallucinogens

Webster's New International Dictionary, second edition, defines *hallucination* as "perception of objects with no reality or experience of sensations with no external cause." Drugs that induce these effects are termed *hallucinogens.*

> **FAST FACTS**
>
> One kilogram (2.2 pounds) of LSD will contain about 10 million doses of the drug.

LSD

IN 1938, LSD, (or d-lysergic acid diethylamide) was developed as a derivative of lysergic acid, which is obtained from the ergot fungus that grows on rye grain. In 1943, purely by accident, Dr. Albert Hoffman, the developer of LSD, either inhaled the drug or absorbed some of it through his skin and experienced the first LSD trip. Further experimentation with LSD showed that a user could experience the hallucinogenic effects of the drug with a dose as small as 100 to 200 micrograms. Very few drugs produce their desired effects in such small doses. Evidence indicates that LSD works at the synapses in the brain for which serotonin is the neurotransmitter.

Physical effects of LSD can be felt within twenty minutes of ingesting the drug and include increased heart rate, blood pressure, and body temperature; dryness of the mouth; dilation of the pupils; nausea; and headaches. Much of this effect is due to stimulation of the sympathetic nervous system. Psychological effects take about an hour to reach their peak and include intoxication, visual disturbances, visual and auditory hallucinations, and synesthesia. Synesthesia is the transformation of one type of sensory experience into another, such as "seeing sounds" or "hearing smells." Physical and psychological effects of LSD last approximately six hours, though sometimes more.

Tolerance develops rapidly to most hallucinogenic drugs, and there is cross tolerance between LSD, mescaline, and psilocybin. Such cross tolerance is not unexpected because of these compounds' similar chemical structures. As with most drugs, LSD is metabolized in the liver. Physiological dependence does not occur, but psychological dependence may become quite strong.

"Bad trips" have been reported by many users. The setting in which the drug is used, the user's frame of mind at the time of use, and other environmental influences appear to have an effect on the positive or negative nature of the experience. Individuals having bad trips must be talked down as the drug wears off. Sometimes drugs such as Valium can be helpful under appropriate medical supervision. Flashbacks have also occurred with some LSD users; weeks, months, or possibly even years later, the past user will experience a recurrence of the effects of the drug. Some suicides have resulted from a panic reaction associated with the flashback experience.

Psychotic reactions have occurred following the use of LSD, and fetal abnormalities have been found in women who have used LSD during pregnancy. Studies have indicated that LSD causes chromosomal damage in some body cells, but thus far there has been no relationship established between this damage and birth defects.

Some experimentation is being conducted with LSD. Research has included work with cancer patients, treatment of alcoholism, and treatment of mental illness. To date, there has been little evidence that LSD is of any medical value. The use of LSD had declined since the 1960s, as it has been replaced by a variety of other mind-altering drugs. One of those is PCP (phencyclidine).

Peyote

Some hallucinogenic drugs occur naturally in plants, whereas many others are man-made. The peyote cactus produces a drug known as mescaline, long known by natives of North, Central, and South America for its hallucinogenic effects. The cactus itself has been used in the form of mescal buttons, made by slicing off the top of the cactus and drying the slices. The buttons are chewed and swallowed, although they have an extremely bitter taste, often as part of religious rituals. The effects of the drug are similar to those of LSD and generally last for about twelve hours after ingestion.

Mescaline

Mescaline, the active ingredient in peyote, is not widely used in the illicit market. The buyer is often sold other hallucinogenic agents, such as LSD or PCP, as a substitute for mescaline. Mescal buttons, however, are readily available. Although some native American groups are legally able to use peyote in religious rituals, both peyote and mescaline are listed as schedule I (illegal) controlled substances.

Psilocybin

For many hundreds (and possibly thousands) of years, some Central American natives have used hallucinogenic mushrooms containing the drugs psilocin and psilocybin. "Shrooms," as they have been called in the illegal market, are widely used today, although most samples purchased on the street are regular edible mushrooms laced with some other psychedelic agent. The effects of psilocybin are similar to those of LSD and may last up to eight hours.

Ololiuqui

The seeds of the morning glory plant, known as ololiuqui, had been long used by the Aztecs for their psychedelic effect. The hallucinogenic drug in this plant is related to the man-made drug LSD. Several other plants contain similar agents and have been used throughout history by a variety of groups.

PCP

Phencyclidine, or PCP, was first patented by Parke-Davis and evaluated under the brand name Sernyl until it was withdrawn for human use in 1965. It was later reintroduced under the name Sernylan as an animal anesthetic. All legal use of the drug was discontinued in 1979. PCP's first reported use as a recreational drug was in San Francisco in 1967. In its early days, it was generally unpopular because of its negative effects, which many users found to be unpleasant. Today it is widely used, often unknowingly by people who are given it as a substitute for some other drug.

Also known as angel dust, PCP is sold as a powder and may be made into tablets or capsules to be ingested, sprinkled on marijuana and smoked, snorted, or injected. It is readily and inexpensively manufactured in illegal laboratories.

The effects of smoking PCP can be felt in just a few minutes, with its peak effect occurring in less than half an hour. The duration of action may be up to six hours. Users report visual and perceptual distortions and a variety of psychological effects, such as feelings of depression, despair, apathy, and isolation. Violent and aggressive behavior, incredible physical strength, periods of psychosis, and seizures may occur. Often, the user does not remember these events. In addition to its hallucinogenic effects, PCP can cause stimulation, depression, analgesia (pain relief), and anesthesia. Adverse reactions occur in about one-third of PCP users.

FAST FACTS

PCP has been known as "The Peace Pill," "HOG," and more recently as "Angel Dust."

SECTION IV ■ DRUGS AND YOUR BODY

> **FAST FACTS**
> The marijuana of today is as much as fifteen times stronger than the marijuana of the sixties.

Symptoms associated with an overdose of PCP include a blank stare, nystagmus (jerky eye movements), inability to walk, excessive salivation, disorientation, and agitation. Higher doses result in other symptoms including muscular rigidity, vomiting, hypertension, numbness, blurred vision, increased heart rate, and profuse sweating. Deaths have been reported, some from the drug itself but many others from violent behavior or accidents associated with its use.

Long-term users report periods of anxiety and depression, violent behavior, flashbacks, and a variety of mental disturbances affecting memory, judgment, and concentration. These appear to be due to long-term fat tissue storage of the drug in the body. Drug-induced psychosis from PCP can last as long as two years.

■ Marijuana

Marijuana is one of the oldest and most widely used mind-altering drugs. References to it appear in Chinese literature dating to more than 5,000 years ago. Worldwide, it is second in popularity only to alcohol. It has been widely used throughout history for its medicinal properties, as an intoxicant, and in religious rituals. It was first introduced in Europe in the late 1700s. Today, it is estimated by some experts that more than $25 billion worth of marijuana is sold in the United States annually and over thirty million people use the drug regularly. Approximately 25 percent of all Americans have used it at least once.

Marijuana is derived from the plant *Cannabis sativa*. Other varieties include *Cannabis americana* and *Cannabis indica*. Cannabis grows wild in many areas, but the varieties that produce the highest quantity of drug come from the hotter climates. The plant, also known as hemp, has been used to provide fibers for the manufacture of rope and cloth. Prior to the mid-1930s, marijuana preparations were manufactured and sold by several major American drug manufacturers.

The active ingredient in marijuana, tetrahydrocannabinol (THC), is found in most of the parts of the plant, including the seeds, leaves, stems, and flowers. Hashish is a resin extracted from the flowering tops of the plant and has ap-

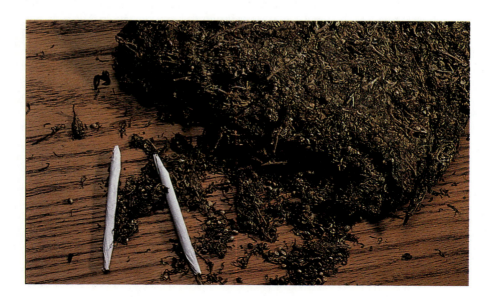

Marijuana cigarettes contain more carcinogens than the highest tar-containing regular cigarettes.

GUIDELINES TO YOUR GOOD HEALTH

On occasion, you may find yourselves in situations in which drugs are being used illegally. The following suggestions can help you to avoid such situations.

1. Choose your friends and companions carefully.
2. Ask those who invite you out socially if they use drugs or condone their use.
3. Do not attend parties at the homes of people who you know use drugs illegally.
4. Watch for changes in behavior that might suggest the use of illegal drugs among your friends and companions.
5. Don't yield to peer pressure to use drugs illegally.
6. If you find yourself in a situation in which drugs are being used illegally, leave!

proximately 10 to 20 percent THC. An even stronger preparation, hash oil, is a resin derived from the leaves.

Although the physical effects of marijuana are minimal, in many smokers THC causes a slight rise in blood pressure and pulse rate and a reddening of the eyes caused by dilation of blood vessels. It may increase frequency of urination and tends to increase appetite. Orthostatic or postural hypotension may occur (this is what happens when you get dizzy on standing up from a sitting or lying position). Dilation of the bronchial tubes and dryness of the mouth also occurs.

Within a few minutes after smoking marijuana, a feeling of euphoria, relaxation, and well-being follows. Users describe other experiences, such as reduced anxiety, reduced inhibitions, increased sense of taste and touch, and emotional closeness to others. Short-term memory loss is frequently reported. Time and space perception is impaired, and attention span is shortened (making such activities as driving a car extremely hazardous). Hallucinations may occur in higher doses, and anxiety or panic reactions have been reported in some users. When the drug is smoked, these effects may last up to four hours. None of these effects are permanent or long lasting.

A specific cause-and-effect relationship between marijuana smoking and lung cancer has not been established; however, it is known that the tar level in marijuana smoke is many times higher than that in regular cigarettes. In addition, marijuana smoke is inhaled much more deeply and is held in the lungs longer than regular cigarette smoke. This information, coupled with studies of lung abnormalities among heavy marijuana (pot) smokers, would tend to indicate that the risk of lung cancer is probably much greater for pot smokers than for regular cigarette smokers. Of course, as with regular cigarettes, the risk is related to the frequency and degree of exposure. Studies have shown that chronic marijuana smoking does impair lung function.

Studies to determine if there are any associations between marijuana use and what is termed *amotivational syndrome* have been inconclusive. Amotivational syndrome refers to the lack of motivation noted in some studies of regular

> **FAST FACTS**
>
> Studies show that the drug MDMA damages certain nerve cells in the brains of rodents and primates.

marijuana users. Other studies indicate that regular male users of marijuana tend to have reduced testosterone levels, increased numbers of abnormal sperm, and lower sperm counts. These effects are reversed when the drug is discontinued. Synergism occurs with marijuana and central nervous system depressant drugs such as alcohol and barbiturates.

Tolerance to THC does develop, but the drug does not create a physiological dependence. Psychological dependence does occur, however. There is no evidence that marijuana leads to sterility, has a negative effect on the immune system, or causes any chromosomal damage. As with all other drugs, pregnant women should not use marijuana. Marijuana has been listed as a schedule I controlled substance. Recent changes in federal and some state laws now allow THC to be used legally to treat **glaucoma.** Other studies are underway to determine its efficacy in other areas of medicine, such as an antinauseant in cancer chemotherapy.

Urine testing for the breakdown products of THC has become quite common, as has other drug testing, and is required in the military and by many civilian and government employers. Because THC is highly fat soluble, it may remain stored in the body for extended periods of time, leading to positive test results as long as thirty days or more after the last time marijuana was smoked.

Designer Drugs

A designer drug is a drug developed and manufactured in an illegal laboratory and that has a chemical structure and **pharmacology** closely related to some other legal or illegal substance. For example, in late 1979 in California, a drug dealer began selling a drug that he described as a new heroin. A second heroin substitute became available a couple of years later. Since the introduction of these drugs, several dozen people have died and many others have been severely disabled as a result of their use.

Although the manufacture and use of a new drug is not legal until it has been tested and approved by the federal Food and Drug Administration (FDA), these designer drugs are less risky to manufacture and sell than a drug already identified and classified as a controlled substance. Penalties for the manufacture and sale of designer drugs are far less severe than those for controlled substances. As the FDA identifies and classifies new designer drugs as controlled substances, the clandestine inventors simply invent a new drug not yet identified or controlled.

Designer drugs are generally inexpensive to make, costing far less than the drugs for which they are substitutes. Many of these drugs can be made by chemists with limited experience from raw materials that are easy to obtain.

MDMA

MDMA, also known as *ecstasy,* is a designer drug with both stimulant and hallucinogenic properties. It is one of a group of drugs known as hallucinogenic amphetamines. Other names for it are Adam and XTC. Derived from an amphetamine, MDMA has been classified as a schedule I (illegal) controlled substance since July 1985. Many psychiatrists have been using MDMA in approved research studies with their patients, and they find that the drug improves communication, promotes emotional closeness (it has been called the "hug drug"), appears to improve ability to remember past events, and reverses depression.

MDMA has been touted as an **aphrodisiac,** providing the user with a better sexual experience. This has not been documented and has been disputed by some experts.

MDEA

MDEA, or Eve, is closely related to MDMA. Also an amphetamine derivative, its effects closely parallel those of ecstasy. Other drugs in this group are MDA, TMA, and STP (DOM).

China White

China White is the name given to a designer drug made as a substitute for heroin. It, and several other heroin substitutes, are chemically related to the legal drug, fentanyl, a powerful anesthetic and pain reliever used in surgical procedures.

MPPP

MPPP is chemically related to the legal synthetic opiate meperidine. Meperidine is made under the brand name Demerol and is a widely used pain reliever. There have been several cases of a **Parkinson's disease**—like occurrence in MPPP users over the past few years. This effect has been associated with another chemical, MPTP, found as a contaminent in a number of street samples of MPPP.

A Final Note

There is a great risk involved in purchasing and using illegal drugs and designer drugs because of the lack of quality control. No one is watching the manufacturer of an illegal drug to determine the safety of the product. No one is making

GUIDELINES TO YOUR GOOD HEALTH

The following are some suggestions to help you develop a healthy attitude toward the responsible use of drugs:

1. Do not use drugs purchased from other than legitimate sources.
2. Do not use prescription drugs prescribed for someone else.
3. Keep volatile solvents out of the reach of children.
4. Do not mix central nervous system depressant drugs.
5. Do not take drugs for other than their intended purpose.
6. If you have become physiologically dependent on a drug, withdraw from it under a doctor's supervision.
7. Reduce your daily caffeine intake to the amount found in two cups of coffee.

sure that there are no harmful substances mixed in with the drug. Keep in mind that many deaths related to drug abuse are not caused by the drug itself but by other substances substituted for it or by adulterants.

The Xanthines

The methylated xanthines are among the most commonly used social drugs. They include caffeine, found in a variety of plants; theophylline, found principally in tea; and theobromine, found in cocoa and tea.

Caffeine has been used as a stimulant for thousands of years. One legend tells us that the coffee plant was discovered by an Arabian clergyman who had some difficulty staying alert during his prayers and who noticed that goats who ate the berries from the local plant would be restless and sleepless for many hours. In addition to the coffee plant, caffeine is found in tea, kola, and guarana plants, with only a trace amount found in cocoa (see Table 13–1). Of the three methylated xanthines, caffeine is the strongest stimulant of the central nervous system and the skeletal muscles. Theobromine comes in a poor third in these categories.

Numerous studies have been conducted to either prove or disprove that caffeine is harmful. Research has been done into its effect on the cardiovascular system relative to heart attack and stroke, its potential for causing birth defects, and its potential for leading to some types of cancer, but, to this date, no conclusive evidence of its harmful effects has been found. Caffeine has been shown to intensify certain psychiatric and emotional problems in some people.

As with all drugs, it is advisable for pregnant women to refrain from consuming caffeine. This recommendation is supported by the Food and Drug

TABLE 13–1 ■ Caffeine Content of Beverages or Preparations (approximate)

Beverage or Preparation	Caffeine Content (mg.)
Coffee, one cup, drip or percolated	100–150
Coffee, one cup, instant	50–70
Tea, one cup	30–60
Coffee, decaffeinated, one cup	1–6[a]
Cola beverage, 12 fluid ounces	72 maximum[b]
Sunkist orange soda, 12 fluid ounces	42
Chocolate, one ounce	20
Hot cocoa, one cup	5[c]
No-Doz, one tablet	100
Excedrin, one dosage unit	65
OTC combinations of aspirin, phenacetin, and caffeine	15–32

[a]Some years ago, a process was developed to remove up to 97% of the caffeine from unprocessed coffee beans. FDA tests on decaffeinated coffee, both ground and instant, have confirmed the claims of the low caffeine content of such products

[b]Federal regulations permit a 0.02% maximum caffeine content in any soda-water drink with the words "cola" or "pepper" in the name when such beverage is obtained from kola nut extracts or other natural extracts. Manufacturers routinely add enough additional caffeine to bring the concentration up to a range of 33–52 mg/12 fluid ounces; they use some of the 200 tons of caffeine obtained in the process of decaffeinating coffee.

[c]One cup of cocoa may contain up to 200 mg. of theobromine, a chemical relative to caffeine.

SOURCE: Reprinted with permission of MacMillan Publishing Company from *Drugs and the Human Body*, 2nd ed. by Ken Liska. Copyright © 1986 by Ken Liska.

Administration in light of some animal studies suggesting that caffeine may be **teratogenic** (cause birth defects). There has been an association suggested between caffeine consumption and the symptoms of **premenstrual syndrome** (PMS), so many practitioners recommend that women not use caffeine around the time of their menstrual periods. Caffeine may also increase the symptoms of benign **fibrocystic breast disease,** although one recent study at Ohio State University indicated that other chemicals in coffee might be the culprits.

Because coffee increases the production of stomach acid, it may aggravate conditions such as ulcers, although this effect has never been documented. Decaffeinated coffee has almost the same effect as caffeinated coffee in increasing gastric secretions. Most physicians will recommend that no caffeine-containing beverages be consumed during an acute ulcer attack. The xanthines also increase the production of urine.

Caffeinism, commonly known as coffee nerves, may result from long-term chronic use of coffee in high doses (ten cups or more per day). Symptoms may

---

SELF-INVENTORY 13.1

Responsible Drug Use

How do you feel about each of the following statements as it relates to you? Respond to each statement by placing a check mark under the appropriate column to the right of the statement.

	Yes	No	Not Sure
1. Is it acceptable to use medications prescribed for someone else?			
2. Would you buy prescription drugs in a country such as Mexico, where no prescription is required?			
3. Would you allow your younger brothers or sisters to use volatile solvents to get high?			
4. Would you buy alcoholic beverages for your underage brother or sister?			
5. Do you drink alcoholic beverages or take other mind-altering drugs and then drive a car?			
6. Would you use drugs such as aspirin on a regular basis even if you had no symptoms?			
7. Would you drink alcohol to reduce stress after a hard day at work or school?			
8. Would you try cocaine or marijuana just once if it was offered to you at a party?			
9. Would you use poppers or cocaine to increase sexual pleasure?			
10. Would you supply drug addicts with clean needles to reduce the spread of AIDS?			
11. Do you believe that it is appropriate to treat heroin addicts with methadone?			
12. Would you use drugs legally to reduce anxiety?			

If you answered "Yes" or "Not Sure" for any of the questions 1 through 9, you may have a problem with drugs.

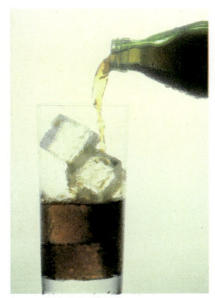

Cola beverages and coffee are the principal sources of dietary caffeine in the U.S.

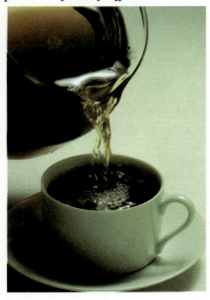

resemble those of an anxiety neurosis. Irregular heart beat, diarrhea, visual hallucinations, restlessness, and sleeplessness are also potential effects. Although several symptoms are associated with suddenly stopping caffeine intake, such as headaches, constipation, or nausea, caffeine is not generally considered to be an addictive drug. However, if you were to suddenly stop consuming caffeine after long-term use, you would probably suffer from what is termed "rebound headache." Caffeinism can also occur in children who consume a large amount of the drug (comparable to the amounts consumed by adults), often in soft drinks and iced tea.

High doses of caffeine can lead to convulsions, but deaths from the drug have been very rare. It has been estimated that it would take over one hundred cups of coffee to supply enough caffeine (10 grams) for a fatal dose. Other estimates suggest that it might take as much as 50 grams orally to cause death. A lethal intravenous dose of 3.2 grams has been reported. Caffeine creates tolerance and is cross tolerant with the other xanthines.

Caffeine can inhibit fatigue and increase wakefulness in a dose of about 200 mg., approximately the amount found in two cups of coffee. The drug increases **basal metabolic rate,** and heart rate and respiration may also be increased. Dilation of blood vessels occurs, except in the brain, where the vessels constrict. Because of this effect, caffeine is frequently used in both prescription and over-the-counter preparations for the treatment of headache. Headaches are often caused by dilation of blood vessels, placing pressure on surrounding brain tissue. Caffeine reverses this. A 1984 study indicated that pain relievers combining caffeine with either aspirin or acetaminophen (Tylenol, for example) worked better than either aspirin or acetaminophen alone. When caffeine is take orally, peak blood levels are reached in about two hours.

Caffeine is a central nervous system and skeletal-muscle stimulant. It specifically acts on the cortex of the brain and enhances conscious mental processes. The user feels more alert and demonstrates increased physical activity. Caffeine can reduce the loss of performance that occurs when you become fatigued. It can also increase the length of time that you can do physically demanding work before becoming exhausted, in part by increasing the tone of skeletal muscles. Levels of attention are increased, and boredom is minimized. Caffeine will not reverse the effects of alcohol intoxication or a hangover.

The xanthines act directly on heart muscle, causing an increase in heart rate, heart force, and blood flow. Although large doses may cause irregular heartbeats and slow the heart rate by acting on the control centers in the medulla of the brain, they do not appear to have any notable effect on blood pressure.

Theophylline is the principal xanthine found in tea (although a fair amount of caffeine is also present). Theophylline is the strongest of the three xanthines in the areas of smooth-muscle relaxation, diuresis, and cardiac stimulation, with caffeine placing third in all three categories. Diuresis is an increase in the rate at which water is removed from the body through urination. Because of theophylline's effects as a bronchodilator (a drug that causes opening of the bronchial tubes), it is widely used in prescription preparations for the treatment of asthma.

> ■ **PROBLEM SITUATION** Your roommate has been somewhat jittery and hasn't been able to sleep lately. She tells you that she is drinking about seven to eight cups of coffee per day. Would you suggest that she should drink less coffee? What can she do to cut back without getting a rebound headache?

POSITIVE BEHAVIORS

I. *Place a check mark in front of each behavior that you now practice.*

_____ 1. I do not use volatile solvents except for their intended purposes. (VOLATILE SOLVENTS)

_____ 2. I do not use poppers. (POPPERS)

_____ 3. I use barbiturates, minor tranquilizers, or opiates only if they have been prescribed for me by my physician or dentist. (PRESCRIBED FOR ME)

_____ 4. I do not mix central nervous system depressants because of synergism. (SYNERGISM)

_____ 5. I do not use cocaine illegally, and I encourage my friends not to use it. (COCAINE)

_____ 6. I do not use amphetamines illegally, and I encourage my friends not to use them. (AMPHETAMINES)

_____ 7. I would not use amphetamines for weight control, even if they had been prescribed legally for that purpose. (WEIGHT CONTROL)

_____ 8. I do not use hallucinogens, and I encourage my friends not to use them. (HALLUCINOGENS)

_____ 9. I do not smoke marijuana, and I encourage my friends not to smoke it. (MARIJUANA)

_____ 10. I would not drive a car after smoking marijuana, nor would I be a passenger in a car with any driver who has smoked marijuana. (DRIVING)

_____ 11. I do not use designer drugs, and I encourage my friends not to use them. (DESIGNER DRUGS)

_____ 12. I do not drink excessive amounts of coffee. (COFFEE)

II. *For each behavior that you DO NOT ENGAGE IN, write in the appropriate space below the KEY WORD(S) located in the parentheses at the end of the statement. Then indicate whether you intend to keep or change that behavior.*

Behaviors I Don't Engage In   KEEP/CHANGE

_____/_____
_____/_____
_____/_____
_____/_____
_____/_____
_____/_____
_____/_____
_____/_____
_____/_____
_____/_____
_____/_____
_____/_____

III. *For each of the preceding behaviors that you choose to KEEP, write a statement indicating why you are choosing to keep that behavior.*

I choose to keep behavior _____ because:
                           KEY WORD

For each of the above behaviors that you choose to CHANGE, write a statement indicating how you plan to implement that change.

I will change behavior _____ by:
                        KEY WORD

346 SECTION IV ■ DRUGS AND YOUR BODY

▰▰▰▰▰ Now You Know

1. TRUE. Kidney and liver damage may result from long-term abuse of volatile solvents. Respiratory depression, convulsions, and death may occur as a result of an overdose.

2. FALSE. Withdrawal from barbiturates may be life-threatening and should be accomplished only under appropriate medical supervision. Convulsions followed by coma and death may occur during barbiturate withdrawal.

3. TRUE. Synergism occurs between barbiturates and alcohol, as well as with other combinations of central nervous system depressant drugs. It can lead to overdose and death and has been responsible for many fatalities among drug users.

4. TRUE. More people commit suicide with barbiturates than with any other drugs.

5. FALSE. The minor tranquilizers are known to cause physiological dependence and tolerance. Withdrawal from minor tranquilizers, however, is less dangerous than from barbiturates.

6. TRUE. Morphine and codeine are found in the opium poppy. Heroin is made from opium and is termed "semi-synthetic." All other opiates in use today are synthetic.

7. FALSE. Methadone is a synthetic opiate and leads to physiological dependence, as do other opiates. The advantages of methadone are that it can be given by mouth and it is long acting.

8. TRUE. Approximately 90 percent of addicts entering methadone maintenance programs will return to their drug habit.

9. FALSE. Cocaine is a very rapidly metabolized drug. Its effects can be felt for only about thirty minutes to an hour.

10. TRUE. Coffee, whether decaffeinated or not, causes increased gastric secretions and can irritate existing ulcers.

■ Summary

1. Volatile solvents such as paint thinner and glue are inhaled for their euphoric effects. Long-term use can lead to kidney and liver damage. Overdose can lead to respiratory depression, convulsions, and death.

2. Poppers contain volatile nitrites, some of which are used medically to treat angina pectoris. They can cause headache and chest pains and dilation of the blood vessels in the heart and brain. Studies indicate that they reduce the body's immune capabilities.

3. Central nervous system depressants include the barbiturates, the minor tranquilizers, the opiates, and a variety of other sedative-hypnotic drugs.

4. The barbiturates are used in medicine primarily for inducing sleep, although they have some other medical uses. Long-term use leads to physiological dependence and tolerance. Withdrawal from barbiturates can be life-threatening and should be attempted only under competent medical supervision.

5. Minor tranquilizers are used to treat anxiety, to relax muscles, and to induce sleep. With respect to the problems of drug overdose and suicide, they are safer than barbiturates, but they may also lead to physiological dependence and tolerance.

6. Methaqualone was originally developed as a sedative-hypnotic drug. Its negative effects far outweighed its positive effects, and it was ultimately withdrawn from the market in 1984.

7. Opiates are used primarily for pain relief and cough suppression. Naturally occurring opiates are morphine and codeine. Heroin is semi-synthetic, and there are several synthetic drugs in the class.

8. Physiological dependence and tolerance occur with opiate drugs. It is estimated that there are approximately 500,000 opiate addicts in the United States.

9. Methadone is used as a means of maintaining the heroin addict. It is a synthetic opiate and therefore also leads to physiological dependence, but it is longer acting than heroin and can be taken by mouth. Most methadone maintenance programs report that only about 10 percent of their clients remain drug free.

10. Cocaine is a short-acting, naturally occurring stimulant drug. It is used medically as a local anesthetic on mucous membranes. When used recreationally, it can lead to a very strong psychological dependence. Serious side effects and death from heart attack have occurred with its use.

11. Most cocaine is snorted; however, it can be injected or smoked as the freebase form or in the form known as "crack" or rock cocaine. These forms of cocaine are extremely dangerous because they lead to very high blood levels.

12. Amphetamines are synthetic drugs used for their stimulant properties. They have been used for weight control but are not effective for this purpose. They do not lead to physiological dependence, but a user will develop tolerance to them.

13. Natural hallucinogens include mescaline, psilocybin, and ololiuqui. LSD and PCP are examples of synthetic hallucinogens. There are no current medical uses for these drugs.

14. Hallucinogens do not lead to physiological dependence, but users will develop tolerance to them. A variety of effects can occur with their use, including psychotic reactions, flashbacks, and panic reactions.

15. PCP is an extremely dangerous drug that causes adverse reactions in about one-third of users. Muscular rigidity, vomiting, numbness, blurred vision, depression, despair, and aggressive behavior, as well as a variety of other symptoms, may occur.

16. Tolerance may result from the use of marijuana, but physiological dependence does not occur. Smoking marijuana produces high levels of tar, leading to lung irritation. Driving an automobile under the influence of marijuana can be dangerous. Effects of pot smoking include reddening of the eyes, reduced inhibitions, increased sense of taste and touch, and increased frequency of urination.

17. Designer drugs are manufactured in clandestine laboratories to replace other drugs that have been listed as controlled substances. These drugs may be very dangerous to the user, because their effects are unknown and their quality is highly questionable. Examples include MDMA (ecstasy), MDEA (Eve), and China White.

18. The methylated xanthines include caffeine, theophylline, and theobromine and are found in a variety of plants. They are central nervous system and skeletal-muscle stimulants, diuretics, and bronchodilators.

19. The xanthines can cause irregular heartbeat, diarrhea, restlessness, and sleeplessness. Their use may be related to fibrocystic breast disease, premenstrual syndrome, and several other disorders. Withdrawal headaches may occur if they are suddenly stopped after long-term use.

■ References

1. Dusek, Dorothy, and Daniel A. Girdano. *Drugs: A Factual Account*. 4th ed. New York: Random House, 1987.
2. Huff, Barbara B., ed. *Physician's Desk Reference,* 14th ed. Des Moines, Iowa: Medical Economics Co., 1988.
3. Huff, Barbara B., ed. *Physician's Desk Reference for Nonprescription Drugs,* 7th ed. Des Moines, Iowa: Medical Economics Co., 1986.
4. Julien, Robert M. *A Primer of Drug Action*. San Francisco: W. H. Freeman and Co., 1981.
5. Kakis, Frederic J. *Drugs: Facts and Fictions*. New York: Franklin Watts, 1982.
6. Kastrup, Erwin K., ed. *Drug Facts and Comparisons*. St. Louis: J. B. Lippincott Co., 1985.
7. Knoben, James E., Philip O. Anderson, and Arthur S. Watanabe. *Handbook of Clinical Drug Data,* 4th ed. Hamilton, Ill.: Drug Intelligence Publications, 1978.
8. Leavitt, Fred. *Drugs and Behavior*. Philadelphia: W. B. Saunders, 1974.
9. Lingeman, Richard R. *Drugs from A to Z: A Dictionary*. New York: McGraw-Hill, 1969.
10. Liska, Ken. *Drugs and the Human Body,* 2d ed. New York: MacMillan, 1981.
11. Marin, Peter, and Allan Cohen. *Understanding Drug Use*. New York: Harper and Row, 1971.
12. Schlaadt, Richard G., and Peter T. Shannon, *Drugs of Choice: Current Perspectives on Drug Use,* 2d ed. Englewood Cliffs, NJ: McGraw-Hill, 1986.

■ Suggested Readings

Carroll, Charles R. *Drugs in Modern Society*. Dubuque, Iowa: William C. Brown Publishers, 1985.

Dusek, D. E., D. A. Girdano. *Drugs: A Factual Account,* 4th ed. New York: Random House, 1987.

Julien, Robert. *A Primer of Drug Action*. San Francisco: W. H. Freeman and Co., 1981.

Liska, Kenneth, *Drugs and the Human Body*. 2d ed. New York: MacMillan, 1986.

Ray, O., and C. Ksir. *Drugs, Society, and Human Behavior,* 4th ed. St. Louis: Times Mirror/Mosby Publishing Co., 1987.

Rucker, William B., ed. *Drugs, Society and Behavior*. Guilford, Conn.: The Dushkin Publishing Group, 1987.

Witters, Weldon, and Peter Venturelli. *Drugs and Society*. Boston: Jones and Bartlett Publishers, 1988.

SECTION V

Coping With Disease

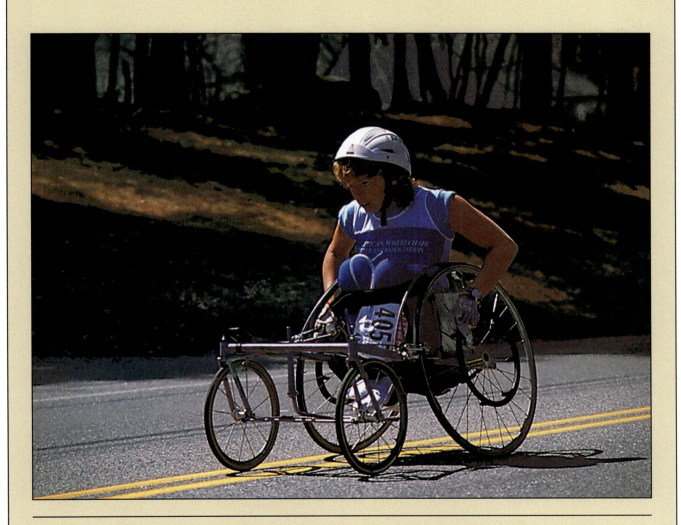

Chapter 14: Understanding the Disease Process and Infectious Diseases
Disease Organisms
Disease Transmission
Stages of Communicable Disease
Prevention of Communicable Disease
Miscellaneous Communicable Diseases

Chapter 15: Sexually Transmitted Disease
The Scope of the Problem
Bacterial Diseases
Viral Diseases
Other Sexually Transmitted Diseases
Prevention of Sexually Transmitted Disease

Chapter 16: Becoming Heart Smart
Risk Factors and Their Relationship to Chronic Disease
Cardiovascular Disease

Chapter 17: Dealing With Chronic Disease
Cancer
Arthritis
Diabetes Mellitus
Other Chronic Diseases
Genetic Disorders

CHAPTER 14

Understanding the Disease Process and Infectious Diseases

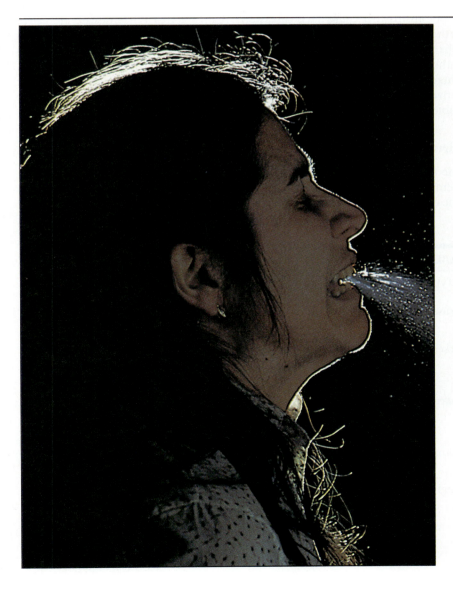

What Do You Know?

Are the following statements true or false?

1. Antibiotics are effective in the treatment of viral infections.
2. Ringworm is caused by a parasitic worm.
3. Some bacteria produce toxins (biological poisons) that actually poison the person who acquires the disease.
4. Salmonella is a food-borne disease that can be transmitted through raw milk.
5. Diseases cannot be transmitted to others during the incubation period.
6. Tears contain an antibacterial substance that helps immobilize and destroy bacteria.
7. Immunizations are available for more than one hundred diseases that affect humans.
8. As many as 20 percent of babies born to women who were infected with German measles during the early part of their pregnancy may be born with birth defects or retardation.
9. Mumps can cause sterility in both males and females if the disease occurs after puberty.
10. The immunization for tetanus provides lifelong immunity.

Disease Organisms

At the turn of the century, contagious disease was the principal cause of premature death. Since then, the advent of **immunizations** and **antibiotics** has reduced the risk from such diseases considerably. Today, we do not have to fear a widespread epidemic of smallpox, influenza, tuberculosis, or many other communicable diseases. Even so, communicable diseases still take their toll in human life and suffering. Gonorrhea and chlamydia, common sexually transmitted diseases, remain principal causes of sterility in the United States. Thousands of people are in institutions for the mentally retarded as a result of measles encephalitis, an inflammation of the brain caused by the measles virus. Millions of people suffer from the effects of herpes infections, the common cold, and a variety of other common diseases. Thousands have died from acquired immunodeficiency syndrome (AIDS).

Let us begin our discussion of communicable disease with a look at the types of organisms that cause such diseases. Organisms that cause disease are called **pathogens.** Some organisms are always pathogenic (disease producing), whereas others are never pathogenic. In addition, many organisms are ordinarily nonpathogenic but become pathogens under certain circumstances and conditions. There are many ways in which to classify disease-producing organisms. For convenience, we will classify them by size, beginning with the smallest (see Table 14–1).

Viruses

The smallest organisms are the viruses. They are so small that we cannot see them with an ordinary light microscope. An **electron microscope** is necessary. The question is often asked, "Are viruses living or nonliving?" This is a somewhat

TABLE 14–1 ■ **Pathogenic Organisms**

Type	Description	Diseases
Viruses	Semiliving particles consisting primarily of DNA or RNA	AIDS, mumps, measles, polio, chicken pox, colds, influenza
Rickettsia	Somewhat in between viruses and bacteria in their characteristics	Typhus, trench fever, Q fever, Rocky Mountain spotted fever
Bacteria	Single-celled, plantlike organisms	Syphilis, gonorrhea, tuberculosis, tetanus, strep throat, toxic shock syndrome
Protozoa	Single-celled animals	Trichomonas, amoebic dysentary, giardiasis
Fungi	Described either as plantlike or as plants lacking chlorophyll	Athletes foot, ringworm, yeast vaginitis, tinea versicolor
Worms	Animals classified as either flatworms or roundworms	Trichinosis, hookworm, tapeworm, roundworm, pinworm

tricky question, because at times they meet the biological definition of life and at other times they do not. For this reason, they are sometimes referred to as "semiliving." Viruses are intracellular parasites; that is, they must enter the cells of the **host** organism in order to reproduce. They take over the reproductive mechanism of the host's cells and direct the cells to produce more virus instead of more cells. Each virus has a specific target cell that it attacks in the host. In AIDS, for example, the virus responsible for the disease takes over the T-4 lymphocyte, an important cell in the immune system, thereby damaging or destroying the person's ability to resist disease. This results in the host ultimately dying of some opportunistic infection that his or her body is unable to defend against. An opportunistic infection is one that results from an infecting organism taking advantage of the host's reduced immune capacity.

Antibiotics are ineffective against viral infections. In certain circumstances, however, we may take them when we have a viral infection in order to protect ourselves from secondary infection from bacteria. For example, if a child had chicken pox (a viral infection), he or she might be given an antibiotic to prevent a secondary skin infection that may result from scratching the rash. Treatment generally consists of measures to reduce the discomfort or pain the patient might be experiencing and to prevent secondary infection. The best defense against viral infections is a strong immune system, another reason for all of us to maintain a high level of wellness.

Many common diseases are caused by viruses, including AIDS, measles, chicken pox, German measles, mumps, herpes simplex types I and II, hepatitis, influenza, and the common cold. Although many of these are self-limiting, others pose substantial risks.

FAST FACTS

Researchers have successfully transplanted parts of the human immune system into mice, enabling scientists to use the mice instead of humans in research on AIDS.

> ■ **PROBLEM SITUATION** Your brother comes home from school with a sore throat and upper respiratory congestion. There is a bottle of antibiotics in the medicine chest left over from the last time you had a skin infection. Is it appropriate to give your brother this antibiotic until you are able to take him to the doctor? Why or why not?

Bacteria

The next largest in size of the organisms that can produce disease are the bacteria. Bacteria are large enough to be seen using the ordinary light microscope but not large enough to be seen by the naked eye. They are considered to be plantlike in nature. Bacteria are divided into classifications based on their shapes. The cocci are round, bacilli are rod shaped, and spirilla (also known as spirochetes) are corkscrew shaped. Cocci are further identified by the way they group together. They may be seen in pairs (diplococci), chains (streptococci), or clusters (staphylococci). Figure 14–1 shows the different shapes of bacteria.

One of the most widespread of the diseases caused by a diplococcus is gonorrhea. Nearly one million cases are reported in the United States each year. (Further discussion of gonorrhea will be found in Chapter 15.) Streptococcal infections include strep throat and rheumatic fever. Staphylococci are responsible for boils, staph food poisoning, and toxic shock syndrome. Diseases caused by bacilli include tuberculosis, tetanus, and botulism, a type of food poisoning. In the United States, the principal disease resulting from spirilla is syphilis. Another is Lyme disease, caused by a spirochete transmitted by ticks.

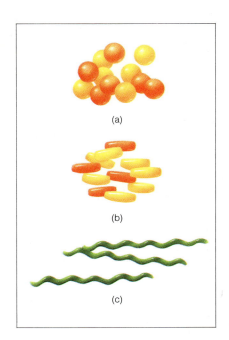

FIGURE 14–1 ■ **The Three Basic Shapes of Bacteria**
(a) Cocci
(b) Bacilli
(c) Spirilla

> **FAST FACTS**
>
> The major cause of waterborne gastrointestinal illness in the United States is *Giardia*.

Most bacterial infections respond favorably to treatment with antibiotics. It is important to recognize, however, that many bacterial infections respond only to specific antibiotics. It can not be assumed that an antibiotic used to treat a urinary tract infection can also be used to treat a sore throat or a skin infection. When dealing with a bacterial infection, it is important for us to seek professional medical care to ensure that the specific disease-producing organism will be identified and, subsequently, the correct antibiotic chosen.

Not all bacterial diseases are infections; some are intoxications. An intoxication is caused when a bacteria introduces a poison (toxin) into the bloodstream of the host. In this situation, not only must the organism itself be treated but the effects of the poison must also be counteracted. For many intoxications, medical science has been able to develop **antitoxins,** or chemicals that can serve as antidotes to the bacterial toxins. For other intoxications, we have not been so fortunate. For example, there is no antitoxin to the toxin produced by the staphylococcus of toxic shock syndrome. That is why it is so important to seek immediate medical care for this life-threatening problem. If treatment doesn't begin soon enough, the patient may die as a result of the toxin, even with the best that modern medicine has to offer.

Bacterial toxins are classified as either *exotoxins* or *endotoxins*. Exotoxins are produced by living bacteria, whereas endotoxins are produced by the death of certain bacteria. It is fortunate that medical science has been able to successfully combat a number of diseases in which exotoxins are produced, because some of them are among the most poisonous substances on earth. Diseases in which exotoxins are produced include botulism and tetanus.

Rickettsia

There has been much debate about the correct classification for the rickettsias. Some people have thought that they should be classified as bacteria and others have thought as viruses. Today, most experts agree that the rickettsias more closely resemble bacteria. Most rickettsial diseases are transmitted through **arthropod vectors** and include typhus, trench fever, Rocky Mountain spotted fever, and rickettsialpox. Q fever is a rickettsial disease that can be transmitted through infected animal products and is often contracted through inhalation.

Rocky Mountain spotted fever is probably the most common of the rickettsial diseases in the United States. Although it was first discovered around the turn of the century in the Rocky Mountain region, most cases today occur in the eastern part of the nation. The disease is transmitted by ticks and occurs most frequently in children. Although tetracyclines and other antibiotics are effective in treating Rocky Mountain spotted fever, about one out of twenty cases is fatal. The high death rate is generally blamed on practitioners' failure to diagnose and treat the disease early.

Protozoa

Protozoa are single-celled animals. You may remember seeing them under the microscope in high-school biology. Protozoa are widely found in bodies of water such as lakes, streams, and rivers. Most protozoa are microscopic, but a few are large enough to be seen with the naked eye. Some species of protozoa live in human intestines and are part of the normal fauna and flora—natural

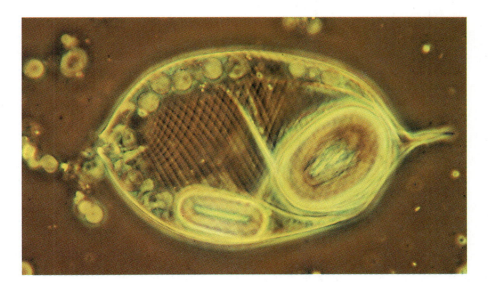

Protozoa are responsible for a number of diseases in humans including malaria and trichomonas.

plant and animal life—found there. Most of these do not cause disease and, in fact, help prevent disease by consuming certain disease-producing bacteria.

Protozoa cause a number of fairly common diseases, including malaria, trichomonas (a vaginal infection), and gastrointestinal infections such as amoebic dysentary (caused by *Entamoeba histolytica*) and giardiasis. There are several anti-infective drugs and antibiotics that are effective against these organisms.

Fungi

There are many microscopic fungi, but some reach extremely large sizes and include the common mushrooms and toadstools. Fungi are usually defined as plants without chlorophyll, but some authors choose to call them plantlike.

External fungal infections include athlete's foot, ringworm, and monilial vaginitis. External infections are generally treated with topically applied ointments or creams. Coccidioidomycosis (valley fever) and histoplasmosis are examples of systemic fungal infections. A systemic infection is one that can spread throughout the body. In very serious fungal infections, special antifungal agents may be given by mouth or **intravenously** under hospital conditions.

Parasitic Worms

Parasitic worms may vary in size from as short as a fraction of an inch to as long as fifty or sixty feet. The two major classifications of worms are roundworms, which include pinworms and *Trichinella*, and flatworms such as tapeworms.

One of the most common types of worm infestation found in this country is caused by the pinworm. Some of you may have had pinworms at some time during your childhood. These white worms infect only humans and are more commonly found in children than adults. They are about half an inch long and can often be seen around the rectum, especially at night. Treatment is simple but requires a physician's prescription. Treatment of all household members and careful attention to the decontamination of clothing and bed linens is essential to effectively eliminate the worms.

FAST FACTS

Children under four years of age are most often the victims of the common roundworms of dogs and cats as well as certain other intestinal worms that can cause serious harm to humans if the eggs, found in dirt, are accidentally swallowed.

Trichinosis is caused by a worm *(Trichinella)* found in animal meat. Many people think, incorrectly, that pork is the only meat that presents a hazard, but this is not the case. Almost any kind of meat may be infected. However, most of the approximately forty cases that occur each year in the United States are associated with the meat of wild animals, such as bear.

■ Disease Transmission

Most organisms do not produce disease. The actual number of pathogens is quite small. However, we are exposed to disease-producing organisms virtually all the time. As mentioned before, some organisms are generally nonpathogenic but may cause disease under certain conditions. If we come in contact with a pathogenic organism at a time when our body is unable to defend against it, we may become ill.

How are these pathogenic organisms transmitted? That generally depends on the specific organism. Some pathogens, such as the spirochete of syphilis or the virus of herpes, are transmitted almost solely by *direct contact*. This means that you must make direct contact with the infected individual to contract the disease. Because these pathogens are unable to live outside of the host for more than a few seconds, they must be directly transmitted from host to host in order to survive. Making direct contact with an infected individual doesn't always result in transmission, however. Many other factors, such as your body's defensive capabilities, environmental conditions, and the specific part of the body making contact, will influence the potential for transmission.

With *indirect contact,* the infectious organism is transmitted from one individual to another through some type of intermediary. The intermediary may be another person, an animal, or an inanimate object (known as a **fomite**). Many diseases, such as measles, hepatitis A, and chickenpox, are transmitted this way. To become infected, you must come in contact with something that the infected individual had come in contact with previously. (See Figure 14–2.) This method of transmission generally involves organisms that can live outside of the host for extended periods of time.

Airborne transmission is the method by which many upper respiratory diseases are passed from person to person. A cough or a sneeze may put millions of infectious organisms into the air. These organisms often are found in tiny airborne droplets of water or on dust particles, which are later inhaled by other individuals.

Many diseases are transmitted by *water, milk,* or *food*. These include botulism, staphylococcal food poisoning, typhoid fever, and a variety of others. Giardiasis is an intestinal illness, caused by a protozoa, that is associated with the drinking of water from streams and lakes. It has become quite common among people who enjoy outdoor recreation such as camping and among international travelers. Giardiasis is largely preventable through the use of iodine tablets and water filters or by boiling to treat contaminated drinking water. Another example is salmonella. Several outbreaks of salmonella in recent years have been associated with the consumption of raw milk or poor sanitary conditions in dairies.

Arthropod vectors are often associated with disease transmission. A vector is an organism, such as an insect, that carries a disease from one animal host to another, usually through a bite. Rocky Mountain spotted fever is transmitted

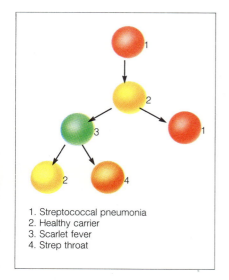

1. Streptococcal pneumonia
2. Healthy carrier
3. Scarlet fever
4. Strep throat

FIGURE 14–2 ■ Transmission of Typical Streptococcal Infections (Type SH I)

SOURCE: *Childrens' Infectious Diseases,* A. Kuzmicheva and I. Sharlal, *Medicine,* Moscow, 1978.

from host to host by a tick. Several years ago, an outbreak of eastern equine encephalitis occurred in New Jersey and was responsible for several deaths. The disease was transmitted by a mosquito from horses to humans.

Stages of a Communicable Disease

Once you come in contact with an infectious organism, the disease begins its *incubation* period. If your body is able to successfully defend against the invading organism, you will not develop the illness. If, however, the organism is able to gain a foothold, you will become ill.

The incubation period is the time from contact with the disease-producing organism until the onset of symptoms. How long does the incubation period last? You will notice that the incubation periods for the diseases discussed in the subsequent sections vary greatly and that each has a range of time. For example, the incubation period for gonorrhea is three to five days, whereas the incubation period for syphilis is ten to ninety days. Leprosy has an incubation period that may be as long as nine years.

It seems obvious that the specific disease organism is one of the factors in determining the length of the incubation period. The second factor is you; that is, your body's ability to defend against the disease. If all of the students in your class were exposed at the same time to a student with a cold, only some of the students would become ill. Among those, some would become ill within a day or two whereas others might not show signs for as long as a week. Again, your body's ability to defend against disease is an important factor in determining into which group of students you would fall. (See Table 14–2 for some common incubation periods.)

Following the incubation period, the disease enters the *prodromal stage*. During this stage, you experience nonspecific symptoms—symptoms not easily identifiable with the specific illness. It's during this period of time that you feel you are getting sick but you aren't really certain what the specific problem is. Symptoms often include muscle aches, headache, upper respiratory congestion, and general weakness.

FAST FACTS

Psittacosis (ornithosis) is a serious disease transmitted to humans through the droppings of birds such as parakeets, pigeons, seagulls, chickens, and turkeys.

TABLE 14–2 ■ Incubation Periods of Some Common Diseases

Disease	Average	Minimum	Maximum
Hepatitis A	20–30 days	15 days	45 days
Hepatitis B	90 days	30 days	180 days
Influenza	1 day	12 hours	2 days
Pertussis	5–7 days	2 days	14 days
Measles	10 days	9 days	21 days
German Measles	16–20 days	11 days	24 days
Mononucleosis	6–8 days	4 days	15 days
Chicken Pox	13–17 days	10 days	21 days
Mumps	15–19 days	11 days	23 days
Salmonellosis	1 day	6–8 hours	3 days
Scarlet Fever	3–6 days	1 day	12 days
Tetanus	7–10 days	3 days	30 days

SOURCE: *Childrens' Infectious Diseases*, A. Kuzmicheva and I. Sharlal, *Medicine*, Moscow, 1978.

The *fastigium,* or typical illness stage, follows. During this stage, the specific symptoms of the illness are at their peak, and temperature is at its highest. As with the other stages, the length of time you will be ill depends in part on the nature of the specific disease and on your body's ability to defend against the illness.

The *defervescence* is the next period. During this stage, temperature returns to normal and symptoms begin to subside. Generally, you begin to feel much better. It is usually during this period that you lose the capability of transmitting your illness to others.

Hopefully, the *convalescence* stage is next. The length of the convalescence may vary greatly from disease to disease and from person to person. During this period, care must be taken not to allow the infecting organism to gain a new foothold. Such an event could lead to relapsing back into the illness stage, often with more severe symptoms than before. The reason for the greater severity of symptoms during a relapse is the already weakened state of the body.

Generally, diseases are communicable from near the end of the incubation period through the end of the defervescence. Obviously, the period before the end of incubation, when symptoms are not yet apparent, is the time during which it is easiest to transmit a disease to someone without being aware of the potential risk.

Prevention of Communicable Disease

The Body's Defense Mechanisms

The body has a number of defense mechanisms that come into play when it is faced with an infectious disease. The first of these are the physical barriers created by the skin and mucous membranes. Intact skin serves as an excellent defense against a variety of organisms. Mucous membranes also provide a similar barrier, although not as effectively as the skin. For example, the spirochete of syphilis will not penetrate unbroken skin, but it can easily pass through mucous membranes.

Tears not only lubricate the eyes but also wash out dust particles and organisms that can potentially cause infection. Human tears contain an antibacterial substance that helps immobilize and destroy certain organisms.

Interferon is an antiviral chemical produced by the body's cells. Scientists are working to develop ways of synthesizing human interferon and have developed other similar chemicals. These newly discovered substances are being tested as antiviral drugs and in the treatment of cancers. A major drawback to the use of interferon will be its cost.

Cilia—the hairlike projections in the respiratory tract—aid the body's defenses by sweeping out foreign substances and invading organisms.

White blood cells actively seek out and destroy organisms that have entered the body. The principal types of white blood cells are the B lymphocytes, T lymphocytes, and macrophages. The B lymphocytes, derived from bone marrow, are responsible for the production of **antibodies,** whereas the T lymphocytes, derived from the thymus gland, provide what is known as cell-mediated immunity. When they come in contact with an **antigen** (foreign substance), T cells produce chemicals that assist in the destruction of the invading organism. Macrophages participate in phagocytosis, the process of destroying foreign materials.

FAST FACTS

An October 1989 article reported that a UCLA researcher has developed two vaccines that may be effective in preventing Legionnaires Disease.

Does the body produce antibodies for every type of invading organism? Yes, but many of the antibodies are short-lived and do not afford any long-lasting protection against disease. The antibodies against the spirochete of syphilis last for only a few months or more, and those against gonorrhea may last only a few weeks at most. Antibodies to other diseases, such as measles and mumps, may last a lifetime. Variance exists from person to person as well as from disease to disease. Some individuals will get a disease like measles only once in their lifetime, whereas others will get the disease a second or even a third time.

Immunizations

How can we protect ourselves from the organisms that cause measles, mumps, diphtheria, tetanus, and other diseases? Can we develop long-term **immunity** without having to experience the disease itself? The answer, of course, is yes. Medical science has developed immunizations to protect us against a variety of diseases. Keep in mind, however, that there are far more diseases for which there are no immunizations. We can protect against only about two dozen diseases in this manner. These include measles, German measles, mumps, tetanus, whooping cough, and diphtheria.

What does an immunization contain? How does it work to protect us? How long does it last? These are all important questions for which you should know and understand the answers.

Immunizations provide *active immunity*—that is, immunity developed by your own body to protect itself. This is the same type of immunity that your body develops when you have the disease itself. When you are given an active immunization, you are being injected with either the killed organism or a live organism that has been weakened (attenuated) so that it is unable to produce disease. Your body responds to this organism in the same way that it would respond to the virulent, disease-causing organism—it produces antibodies against the disease (see Table 14–3).

GUIDELINES TO YOUR GOOD HEALTH

To reduce your risk and the risk to those around you of exposure to a communicable disease:

1. Cook all meat properly and completely to kill potentially harmful organisms.
2. Avoid contact with anyone showing signs of illness.
3. Cover your mouth and nose when coughing or sneezing.
4. Drink only pasteurized milk.
5. Obtain a tetanus booster if you haven't had one in the last ten years.
6. Obtain a measles vaccination if you haven't had measles or if you were originally immunized with the killed vaccine.
7. Obtain a rubella immunization if you are a female of childbearing age.
8. Obtain an influenza immunization annually if you are in any of the groups for which it is recommended.
9. Don't swim in contaminated water.
10. Wash your hands after using the toilet.

TABLE 14–3 ■ **Childhood Immunization Checklist**

At This Age:	A Child Should Have Received
2 months old	1 DTP immunization 1 polio immunization
4 months old	2 DTP immunizations 2 polio immunizations
6 months old	3 DTP immunizations 2 polio immunizations
12 months old	3 DTP immunizations 3 polio immunizations
15 months old	3 DTP immunizations 3 polio immunizations 1 measles immunization[a] 1 rubella immunization[a] 1 mumps immunization[a]
18 months and older	4 DTP immunizations 3 polio immunizations (If your child has not already received measles, rubella, and mumps immunizations, they are needed.)
4 to 6 years, before starting school	A DTP booster (the 5th immunization) A polio booster (the 4th immunization) (If your child has not already received measles, rubella, and mumps immunizations, they are needed.)
Thereafter	Tetanus-diptheria (Td) booster should be given every 10 years or following a dirty wound if a booster has not been given in the preceding 5 years.

[a]Only one shot needed. Some doctors combine these vaccines in a single injection (MMR).
SOURCE: Department of Health, Education and Welfare, Public Health Service, Centers for Disease Control.

Some immunizations, such as those for measles and German measles, last a lifetime in the majority of individuals. Others are somewhat less effective, such as the mumps vaccine, which has an effectiveness rate of about 90 percent. Others, such as the immunizations for chicken pox and Rocky Mountain spotted fever, are not very useful and are not widely used.

What do you do if you are exposed to a disease that you have never had and have never been immunized against? Can you go for an immunization after your exposure? In most cases, you can not. Active immunity takes time to develop after you have been immunized. If you have already been exposed to a disease, you do not have that time, because the infectious organism is already working to gain a foothold in your body. Fortunately, there are techniques to protect you in such situations.

Passive immunity, or immunity not developed by your own body, is a means by which you can acquire temporary protection against a disease after exposure. Antibodies against certain diseases can be obtained from the blood of previously infected individuals or from certain animal sources and injected into you after you are exposed to a disease. These antibodies will provide you with short-term immunity to the disease—short-term because the injected material is foreign to your body and will be rejected. Such immunity may last from three to six months.

Materials containing antibodies for use as passive immunity are called globulins. Some are specific for specific diseases (such as hepatitis B immune globulin), whereas others afford protection to a variety of diseases. Immune serum globulin, for example, can be used against measles, German measles, hepatitis A, and other diseases.

Congenital immunity is a form of passive immunity passed from mother to unborn baby through the placenta. Some congenital immunity is also received through breast feeding. Like other passive immunity, congenital immunity is not long lasting. The infant is protected for only a short period of time after birth and needs to be vaccinated to develop active immunity. For some diseases, however, the initiation of active immunity in the child must wait until the congenital immunity wears off. If sufficient time is not allowed, the baby's active immunity will be ineffective.

Miscellaneous Communicable Diseases

Viral Diseases

General Information. The majority of viral diseases are spread through airborne or droplet transmission. They are usually epidemic at different times of the year but may occur anytime. For most viral diseases, one attack of the disease will provide lifetime immunity.

Chicken Pox (Varicella). Chicken pox is one of the milder diseases occurring during childhood. Most cases usually occur between the ages of two and eight years. The disease may be contracted through either direct or indirect contact and has an incubation period of about two weeks. The prodromal period is characterized by a fever, loss of appetite, headache, and upper respiratory symptoms.

FAST FACTS

In October 1979, the World Health Organization declared smallpox eradicated throughout the world. Therefore, routine vaccination for civilians is no longer recommended.

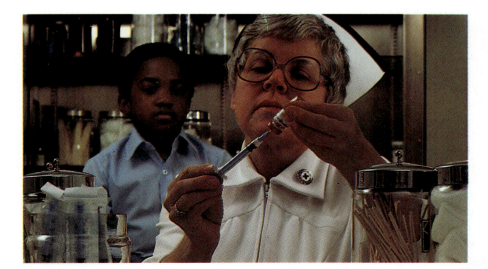

Vaccines are available for about two dozen human diseases affording a wide range of health protection.

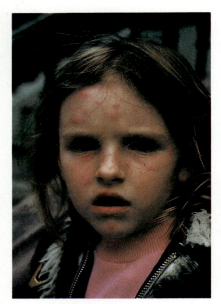

The rash of chicken pox causes intense itching. Scratching, however, may lead to secondary infection and scarring.

The rash of chicken pox begins with rose-colored spots, which become crops of small blisters, or **vesicles,** that break open, form scabs, and heal in a few days. The rash is generally accompanied by intense itching. Vesicles appear in successive crops, some appearing while others are disappearing. Scarring may occur if secondary infection develops from scratching. The disease can be transmitted from about twenty-four hours before the rash appears until about seven days after symptoms began, or until the last lesion becomes crusted over. After crusting of the lesions has occurred, the patient is no longer contagious, even though the rash is not completely gone.

There are no antibiotics that are effective against viral infections such as chicken pox. However, antibiotics are sometimes given by mouth and used topically in ointment form to prevent secondary bacterial infection from developing. The use of antibiotics by mouth, however, is not generally considered good medical practice unless some signs of secondary infection are apparent. Thorough washing with soap and water and the use of antibiotic ointments is best. Calamine lotion and antihistamines may be used to relieve the itching. Muscle aches, fever, and other discomforts can be relieved with acetaminophen. Aspirin should never be used in children or teenagers recovering from viral illness because of the danger of Reye's syndrome.

Herpes zoster (shingles) is a disease characterized by painful inflammation of the **ganglia** of certain spinal and cranial nerves. Inflammation of the skin also commonly occurs. It has a higher incidence in adults than in children. Herpes zoster (not to be confused with the sexually transmitted disease herpes simplex) is indistinguishable in viral cultures from varicella, and most medical experts believe it to be the same virus. Adults exposed to chicken pox will often develop shingles, sometimes years after exposure.

Although a vaccine for chicken pox has been developed recently, it is not widely used and is not considered to be particularly effective.

> ■ **PROBLEM SITUATION** Your child is recovering from chicken pox. The sores left by the rash are healed over and have formed scabs. When is it all right to allow your child to return to school?

Measles (Rubeola). Measles is an extremely contagious disease. The average incubation period is about seven to fourteen days and is followed by a prodromal period characterized by **lethargy,** headache, fever, irritability, and upper respiratory symptoms. Inflammation of the eyes is a typical characteristic of measles. The eyes may become bloodshot and swollen, and the patient may show an extreme sensitivity to light. If you have ever had measles, you probably remember the discomfort.

The rash follows in about two to five days, first on the lining of the mouth and throat, then behind the ears and on the forehead, and then spreading over the trunk and extremities. The initial rash on the lining of the mouth and throat resembles grains of white sand against a red background and is known as Koplik's spots.

Measles is an extremely dangerous disease because of the complications that may follow the primary illness. Secondary infection may occur in the respiratory tract, brain, or kidneys. Measles encephalitis may result from brain inflammation and the victim may be left permanently retarded. Deafness may also occur. How the rash of measles progresses is illustrated in Figure 14–3.

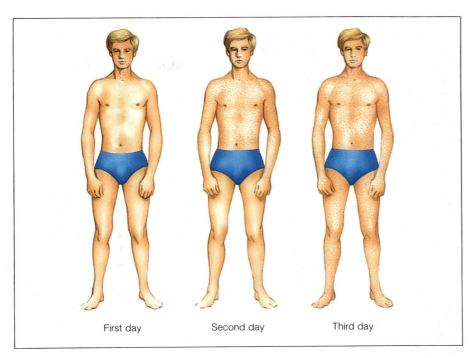

FIGURE 14-3 ■ The Rash of Measles

ADAPTED FROM—*Childrens' Infectious Diseases,* A. Kuzmicheva and I. Sharlal, *Medicine,* Moscow, 1978.

Treatment of symptoms includes using calamine lotion and antihistamines for the reduction of itching. As in chicken pox, good hygiene techniques are the best medicine for the prevention of secondary bacterial infection. The room should be kept dark because of the inflammation of the patient's eyes, and a humidifier can be used to reduce the severity of respiratory symptoms.

Live attenuated measles vaccine is available and should be given at around the age of fifteen months to anyone who has not been immunized. Many young people who were immunized prior to 1972 (which may include some of you using this text) with the older killed virus vaccines are not adequately protected and should be reimmunized with the newer vaccines. Children must be older than one year of age before they are immunized to allow adequate time for congenital immunity to disappear.

■ *PROBLEM SITUATION* You are thirty years old and received your immunization for measles in 1971. Are you adequately protected, or do you need to be immunized again?

Many public school systems and universities require measles immunization before admission. Several measles outbreaks have occurred on university campuses during the past few years. Immune serum globulin is available for passive immunity should exposure occur in an unprotected individual.

■ *PROBLEM SITUATION* A neighbor's child has just been diagnosed as having measles. Your five-year-old nephew has not yet had the disease and has not been immunized. Your sister thinks that she should allow her son to be exposed to the neighbor's child so that he can acquire the disease and have permanent immunity for the future. Should your nephew be exposed?

German Measles (Rubella). German measles is a highly contagious disease with an associated rash that can be confused with other rash diseases. Transmission can occur through direct or indirect contact as well as through airborne particles. An incubation period of two to three weeks is followed by a prodromal period that may include swollen glands and other mild symptoms such as fever and lethargy. The infected individual may be **asymptomatic,** however.

The rash first appears on the face but ultimately spreads over the entire body. (See Figure 14–4.) The **lymph nodes** of the neck are usually swollen and tender. The disease is generally self-limiting, lasting about three days.

The treatment for German measles is similar to that of other viral rash diseases and is directed at prevention of secondary infection and the reduction of itching. A vaccine is available and can be administered concurrently with the measles immunization, but it cannot be used once a person is infected with the disease.

German measles immunization is especially important for women of childbearing age because of the danger to an infected mother's unborn baby. The greatest danger is during the first trimester of pregnancy, with the incidence of deformity, hearing impairment, and mental retardation being as high as 10 to 20 percent. The vaccine should be given at least ninety days prior to conception and is not used once pregnancy occurs. If a pregnant woman is exposed to German measles, immune serum globulin can be used. Many states require that a woman applying for a marriage license be tested for her level of rubella antibodies at the same time that the blood test for syphilis is done.

Mumps (Parotitis). The main characteristics of infection by the mumps virus is swelling and inflammation of the parotid salivary glands, the salivary glands near the ears. In older children and adults, the testes, ovaries, and pancreas may become involved. The majority of cases occur between the ages of five and fifteen years. Long-term immunity usually results from having the disease.

Although the majority of infected patients show symptoms, as many as 40 percent do not. These asymptomatic victims can, however, pass on the highly infectious virus. After an incubation period of two to four weeks, a prodromal period begins with a low-grade fever, upper respiratory distress such as a sore

FIGURE 14–4 ■ **Localization of Rash of German Measles**

SOURCE: *Childrens' Infectious Diseases*, A. Kuzmicheva and I. Sharlal, *Medicine,* Moscow, 1978.

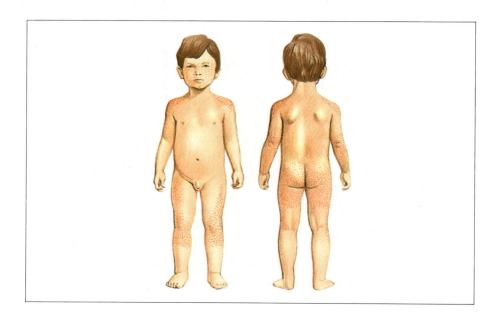

throat, and pain when chewing. Swelling on both sides of the jaw follows, although in a small percentage of cases, only one parotid salivary gland swells. Fevers as high as 103 to 104 degrees Fahrenheit usually follow.

The most serious consequence of mumps is sterility, which may occur in patients past the age of puberty if the testes or ovaries become involved. Other complications, including encephalitis, may also occur. Figure 14–5 illustrates how mumps affects certain body systems.

Treatment includes bed rest and relief of pain. A soft bland diet is best, as highly seasoned foods will increase pain.

A live attenuated mumps vaccine is available and can be combined with measles and German measles vaccines into one injection. The vaccine is specifically recommended for adolescent and adult males who have not had the disease. A skin test is available for evaluating past exposure and antibody response.

The Common Cold. More than one hundred different viruses have been associated with the set of symptoms we call the common cold. The symptoms include upper respiratory congestion, sore throat, fever, headache, and a variety of other discomforts.

Colds are not dangerous for most individuals and are usually self-limiting. The real danger is the possibility of secondary bacterial infections, which can be very serious. A high fever greater than 102.5 degrees Fahrenheit can be a sign of such a complication.

We have no way of preventing the common cold other than by maintaining our immune systems and avoiding exposure to people who are ill. Many practitioners suggest the use of vitamin C to prevent or reduce the incidence of colds, but to this date, there is no definitive scientific evidence to either prove or refute this claim. There is no vaccine and no long-term immunity.

There are literally thousands of remedies available to treat the common cold. Always keep in mind that these products do nothing but treat the symptoms.

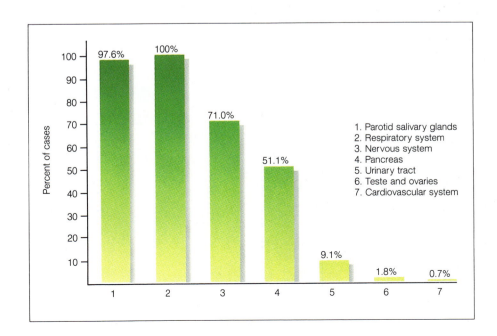

FIGURE 14–5 ■ How Mumps Affect Various Body Systems

SOURCE: *Childrens' Infectious Diseases*, A. Kuzmicheva and I. Sharlal, *Medicine*, Moscow, 1978.

There is no cure. Please see Chapter 18 for a thorough discussion of over-the-counter drugs. The best things that you can do are to rest, drink plenty of fluids, use warm salt-water gargles for sore throat if necessary, take medication for symptomatic relief, and give your body a chance to fight off the virus.

Influenza. The "flu," or influenza, is not one disease but a group of viral diseases that primarily affect the upper respiratory tract. Symptoms are typical of such infections and may be confused with those of a cold or other similar problem. Fever, chills, muscular aches, coughing, sore throat, and headache all may occur.

Influenza viruses can be transmitted through airborne transmission and fomites. Many individuals are exposed to influenza viruses and do not come down with the disease. Again, a strong immune system is the best defense against becoming ill.

Treatment of influenza's symptoms is the same as for the common cold. Possible complications are sinusitis, bronchitis, and middle ear infections.

Influenza viruses are divided into classes A, B, and C and are further identified by where they were first discovered. For example, there is a Type A New Jersey virus, a Type B Hong Kong virus, and a Type A Victoria virus, as well as many others that have been identified.

Immunizations are available for active immunity against the flu. Each year, the World Health Organization and other health agencies try to determine which strains of virus are most likely to cause a problem in the coming flu season. Vaccines are made up of those strains and are then made available to the public. Vaccines can be made up of just one or of several strains of virus. Of course, even with immunization, there is always the possibility that a strain other than the ones in the vaccine will strike you.

Vaccinations must be taken annually because of the variety of influenza viruses and the fact that immunity is not particularly long lasting. Generally, immunizations are recommended for those people who would be most susceptible to the disease, such as the elderly, medical personnel, and pregnant women. Usually, military personnel, police officers, and firefighters are also immunized.

Infectious Mononucleosis. Caused by the Epstein-Barr virus, infectious mononucleosis is, in some areas, the most common cause of fever, sore throat,

GUIDELINES TO YOUR GOOD HEALTH

If you do become ill with a communicable disease, the following suggestions can help you to have a speedier recovery:

1. Do not take antibiotics except those prescribed for your specific illness.
2. Get plenty of rest.
3. Follow your physician's instructions.
4. Avoid the use of unnecessary drugs, especially those that have a negative effect on the immune system.
5. Avoid contact with others so that you do not expose yourself to other illnesses while your immune system is in an already weakened state.

and swollen lymph nodes in the college-age group. The disease is rarely fatal but does cause a sometimes severe generalized weakness that can last from one week to several weeks. Mononucleosis has been called "the kissing disease," because it can be transmitted by the oral route through either direct contact or airborne particles and can often be detected in the throat of a previously infected individual many months after the symptoms of the disease have gone. Symptoms generally last from one to three weeks but may occur for up to two to three months.

There is no known method of prevention and no specific cure. Treatment includes bed rest, although recent information indicates that many physicians overtreat their patients with excessively prolonged convalescence, resulting in slower recovery from the disease. It is important to avoid contact sports during recovery and convalescence because of the possibility of damage to the spleen, which may become congested during the course of the illness.

Hepatitis A. The form of viral hepatitis generally known as infectious hepatitis is also known as hepatitis A. Hepatitis B, or serum hepatitis, will be discussed in Chapter 15.

Transmission of hepatitis A can be by direct contact, by indirect contact, through the fecal-oral route, or through contaminated water or food products. Outbreaks are often traced to food handlers. Onset is sudden following an incubation period of about two to six weeks. The patient usually has a fever, nausea, loss of appetite, generalized weakness, and **jaundice** (a yellowing of the skin, eyes, and other tissues). Hepatitis causes an inflammation of the liver.

There is presently no vaccine for hepatitis A, although passive immunity can be obtained through the use of immune serum globulin within two weeks after exposure. Treatment involves bedrest and frequently a long convalescence, although usually not as long as with other forms of hepatitis. Hepatitis A is less severe than hepatitis B and rarely causes death.

FAST FACTS

Many cases of Hepatitis A are traced to swimming in contaminated water and to eating contaminated seafood.

Bacterial Diseases

Whooping Cough (Pertussis). Whooping cough is a disease that is not heard about very often, even though it is a very serious illness and has been on the increase in recent years. In 1984, 2,218 cases were reported nationwide, and in 1985, 3,239 cases occurred. A substantial increase to 4,195 was reported in 1986. Reported cases declined 33% to 2,823 in 1987 but increased to 3,450 in 1988. Although it may occur in any age group, most deaths are among children under one year of age.

Whooping cough can be transmitted through direct contact, indirect contact, and airborne transmission. The incubation period is generally about one week but may last up to three weeks. The course of the disease is about six weeks.

The disease is caused by a bacillus and is characterized by a severe upper respiratory infection with excessive production of mucous. Severe coughing spells occur in which the victim cannot breathe because of the rapid succession of the coughs. After each series of coughs, the victim gasps for air, causing a whooping sound that gives the disease its name. Whooping cough is a dangerous disease and deaths can occur even with the best care that modern medicine has to offer. It is one of the principal causes of infant mortality in the United States.

An immunization for whooping cough is available and is part of the DPT series given at approximately two, four, and six months of age. The DPT immunizations protect the child against diphtheria, pertussis, and tetanus. There has been much debate during the last few years about the safety of the pertussis vaccine, and some parents have elected not to have their children immunized. This has contributed to the marked increase in cases from 1984 to 1986.

Tetanus. The toxin of tetanus is one of the most poisonous substances known to humankind. Tetanus is an *intoxication* caused by a bacillus. It acts on the central nervous system, causing a constant flow of electrical impulses through the nerves to various muscles causing them to be continuously stimulated. The first muscles to be affected are those of the jaw—hence the other name for the disease, lockjaw. The muscles of respiration may ultimately become paralyzed, which causes death. The incubation period for tetanus is from two to fifty days but usually averages from five to ten days.

Tetanus **toxoid** is available for active immunity. Like pertussis, tetanus is part of the DPT series of immunizations given during infancy. It is believed that protection against tetanus gained through immunization is good for about ten years. Therefore, periodic booster shots are essential.

Many people think, erroneously, that only a cut with a rusty nail is dangerous with regards to tetanus. That is not true. Any wound presents a risk for tetanus. The **spores** of the bacteria may be found in the soil and on many objects. The organism is **anaerobic;** that is, it grows and develops in the absence of oxygen. For this reason, deep puncture wounds are more dangerous than other types of wounds.

Because of the extreme danger of tetanus in many types of wounds and the fact that the disease may be fatal as often as 50 percent of the time, even with the best medical care, it is important that everyone maintains active immunity by getting booster shots regularly. Again, tetanus immunization should be repeated at least once every ten years.

Tuberculosis. In 1988, the Centers for Disease Control reported 22,436 new cases of tuberculosis (TB) nationwide. TB is caused by a bacillus that is very resistant to environmental factors such as heat and disinfectants. Transmission is usually through airborne particles but can also occur through the milk of infected cows. The incubation period is from four to twelve weeks. The principal site of infection is the lungs, but other parts of the body may also become infected. Many tuberculosis patients carry the bacillus for years after the initial infection and can have relapses of the disease if they become weak and unable to resist the organism.

Periodic skin tests are used to detect tuberculosis. A small amount of antigen is injected under the skin. The skin test is "read" forty-eight hours later, and a raised red area is indicative of a positive test. Skin tests can detect tuberculosis anywhere in the body but cannot distinguish between active cases and inactive cases. Once you have had a positive skin test, there is no need to have the test done again, because it will probably remain positive for your entire lifetime. Many employers require regular TB skin testing as a condition of employment. Chest x-rays are usually indicated in patients with a positive skin test.

There are several drugs used to treat tuberculosis. Treatment generally takes a year or more, although patients are unable to transmit the disease within several weeks after beginning therapy.

POSITIVE BEHAVIORS

I. *Place a check mark in front of each behavior that you now practice.*

_____ 1. I do not take any antibiotics unless they have been prescribed specifically for me and for my current illness. (ANTIBIOTICS)

_____ 2. I do my best to maintain a healthy immune system, thereby protecting myself against disease. (IMMUNE SYSTEM)

_____ 3. I am careful to avoid close contact with any persons showing the signs or symptoms of a communicable disease. (CONTACT)

_____ 4. When I become ill, I avoid contact with others to keep from transmitting my disease to them. (TRANSMITTING)

_____ 5. When recovering from an illness, I follow my physician's advice in order to achieve a successful convalescence. (PHYSICIAN'S ADVICE)

_____ 6. I obtain immunizations for all diseases in accordance with my physician's recommendations. (IMMUNIZATIONS)

_____ 7. When exposed to a communicable disease, I immediately seek medical advice and passive immunity if available. (PASSIVE IMMUNITY)

_____ 8. I encourage others to obtain immunizations against all diseases for which they are available. (ENCOURAGE OTHERS)

_____ 9. I obtain a tetanus booster immunization at least every ten years. (TETANUS)

II. *For each behavior that you DO NOT ENGAGE IN, write in the appropriate space below the KEY WORD(S) located in the parentheses at the end of the statement. Then indicate whether you intend to keep or change that behavior.*

Behaviors I Don't Engage In   KEEP/CHANGE

_____ / _____
_____ / _____
_____ / _____
_____ / _____
_____ / _____
_____ / _____
_____ / _____
_____ / _____

III. *For each of the preceding behaviors that you choose to KEEP, write a statement indicating why you are choosing to keep that behavior.*

I choose to keep behavior _____ because:
                                    KEY WORD

For each of the preceding behaviors that you choose to CHANGE, write a statement indicating how you plan to implement that change.

I will change behavior _____ by:
                           KEY WORD

Now You Know

1. FALSE. Antibiotics are ineffective against viral infections. Taking antibiotics when they are not necessary contributes to the development of resistant strains of bacteria.
2. FALSE. Ringworm is a fungal infection and is not caused by a worm. It is actually the name for a variety of fungal diseases that can affect the scalp, body, feet, nails, and so on.
3. TRUE. Toxins are produced by the bacteria of tetanus, botulism, toxic shock syndrome, and a number of other diseases. Some bacterial toxins are among the most poisonous substances known.
4. TRUE. Several outbreaks of salmonella have been associated with the consumption of raw milk. There are no important nutritional differences between raw milk and pasteurized milk; therefore, the consumption of raw milk should be avoided.
5. FALSE. Many diseases can be transmitted to others before the end of the incubation period, when the individual with the disease has not yet shown any symptoms. This is an especially dangerous time for others coming in contact with the person about to become ill.
6. TRUE. Tears do contain an antibacterial substance to help defend against organisms that may come in contact with the eyes.
7. FALSE. There are only about twenty diseases for which immunizations are available. It is important that you be immunized against all diseases for which you are at risk.
8. TRUE. As many as 10 to 20 percent of babies born to women who contract German measles during their pregnancy may be born with birth defects or mental retardation. Because of the extreme danger, it is essential that all women of childbearing age be immunized against this disease.
9. TRUE. The mumps virus can infect both the testes in males and the ovaries in females and can lead to sterility. All adults, male and female alike, should be certain that they are immunized against this disease.
10. FALSE. Active immunity from the vaccine for tetanus lasts approximately ten years; however, this may vary greatly from individual to individual. Booster shots are recommended at least every ten years or when there is an injury that has a high risk of exposure.

■ Summary

1. Although certain diseases, such as influenza and tuberculosis, no longer pose the threat that they did at the turn of the century, many other communicable diseases, such as AIDS, are still serious public-health hazards.
2. The viruses are the smallest of the pathogenic organisms and are responsible for diseases such as measles, mumps, chicken pox, and AIDS. They generally do not respond to treatment with antibiotics.
3. Bacteria are responsible for a variety of human diseases, including both infections and intoxications. Most bacterial diseases respond favorably to specific antibiotics.
4. Organisms such as rickettsia, protozoa, fungi, and parasitic worms are responsible for a number of human diseases.
5. Exposure to a disease-producing organism does not necessarily mean that you will acquire that disease. The strength of your immune system is extremely important in this respect.
6. Disease organisms can be transmitted through direct contact, indirect contact, airborne particles, food or water, and arthropod vectors.
7. The stages of a communicable disease include an incubation period, the prodromal period, the fastigium, a defervescence stage, and convalescence. Generally, diseases are communicable from the latter part of the incubation period through the defervescence stage.
8. The body's defense mechanisms against disease include the skin, mucous membranes, tears, white blood cells, cilia, interferon, and the production of antibodies.
9. We can protect ourselves against about twenty diseases through immunization, which produces active immunity.
10. Passive immunity can be used against some diseases following exposure. This involves the injection of antibodies from another source into the person exposed to the disease organism. These preparations are known as globulins.
11. Congenital immunity is passed through the placenta and breast milk to the newborn baby, but this is passive immunity to the infant and will last for only a short time. Active immunity through immunization at the appropriate time is essential to the child's health and well-being.
12. Chicken pox is one of the mildest of the childhood diseases and generally does not lead to serious consequences. It is, however, associated with a painful disease in adults known as shingles.
13. Measles is an extremely dangerous disease with the potential for causing mental retardation in those who contract it. Immunization against measles is essential for everyone.
14. German measles can lead to birth defects and mental retardation in children born to mothers exposed to the

virus during pregnancy. Women of childbearing age should be immunized against this disease.

15. Mumps can cause sterility in both males and females past the age of puberty. For this reason, immunization against this disease is important for all adults.

16. There are more than one hundred different viruses that cause the symptoms of the common cold. A strong immune system is the best defense against colds.

17. Influenza is caused by a number of related viruses. Immunizations are available and should be obtained by high-risk individuals such as the elderly, pregnant women, and medical personnel.

18. Whooping cough is an extremely hazardous childhood disease. Immunization is part of the DPT series and is very important for all children.

19. Immunization for tetanus, an often deadly bacterial intoxication, must be renewed at least every ten years. Any break in the skin, especially a deep puncture wound, may lead to tetanus.

References

1. Benenson, Abram S., ed. *Control of Communicable Diseases in Man,* 14th ed. Washington, D.C.: American Public Health Association, 1985.
2. California State Department of Health. *A Manual for the Control of Communicable Diseases in California,* 7th ed. Sacramento: California State Department of Health, 1977.
3. Friedman, Gary D. *Primer of Epidemiology,* 2d ed. New York: McGraw-Hill, 1980.
4. Jones, Kenneth L., Louis W. Shainberg, and Curtis O. Byer. *Disease.* Sacramento: Canfield Press, 1975.
5. Mausner, Judith S., and Anita K. Bahn. *Epidemiology: An Introductory Text.* Philadelphia: W. B. Saunders Co., 1974.
6. Purtillo, David T. *A Survey of Human Diseases.* Menlo Park, Calif.: Addison-Wesley, 1978.
7. Youmans, Guy P., Philip Y. Paterson, and Herbert M. Sommers. *The Biologic and Clinical Basis of Infectious Diseases,* 2d ed. Philadelphia: W. B. Saunders Co., 1974.

Suggested Readings

Benenson, Abram S., ed. *Control of Communicable Diseases in Man.* Washington, D.C.: American Public Health Association, 1985.

Cousins, Norman. *Anatomy of an Illness.* New York: Bantam Books, 1979.

Friedman, Gary D. *Primer of Epidemiology.* New York: McGraw-Hill, 1980.

Hansen, G. R. *Common Medicines,* 2d ed. Salt Lake City: 1987.

Purtilo, David T. *A Survey of Human Diseases.* Menlo Park, Calif.: Addison-Wesley, 1978.

Weiner, A. *Maximum Immunity.* New York: Pocket Books, 1987.

CHAPTER 15

Sexually Transmitted Disease

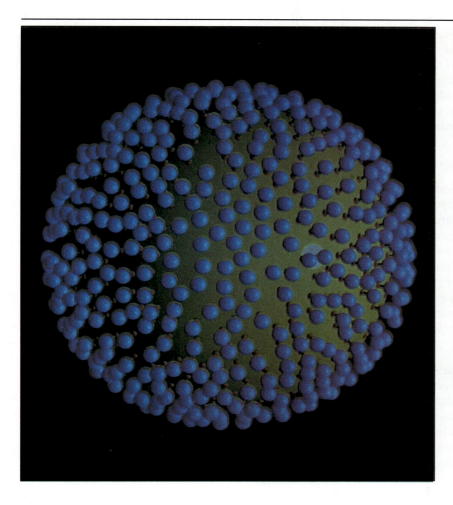

What Do You Know?

Are the following statements true or false?

1. There are more than twenty sexually transmitted diseases.
2. Sexually transmitted disease rates are on the rise.
3. The greatest risk factor in sexually related disease transmission is having multiple sex partners.
4. There are several sexually transmitted diseases for which immunizations are available.
5. If you acquire a sexually transmitted disease, you will know it because of the symptoms.
6. Syphilis and gonorrhea are both caused by bacteria and are easily treated with appropriate antibiotics.
7. The use of condoms will effectively prevent the transmission of gonorrhea.
8. Most organisms that cause vaginal infections in women do not affect the male partner.
9. There is no risk of getting AIDS through sexual contact unless you are a gay male.
10. Once treated, herpes simplex virus is eliminated from the body and subsequent infection is prevented through active immunity.

The Scope of the Problem

Sexually Transmitted Diseases Defined

Did you realize that there are more than twenty diseases grouped under the heading of sexually transmitted diseases (STDs)? Many of these diseases can be transmitted by other than intimate contact, but some are contracted solely through intimacy. A few of the sexually transmitted diseases are reportable; that is, federal law requires that medical practitioners report cases to their local health department. These include AIDS, syphilis, gonorrhea, and hepatitis B. Many others, such as chlamydia, bacterial vaginosis, and herpes, do not require reporting. One can take only educated guesses at the number of cases of the nonreportable diseases.

The lowest ebb in case rates of sexually transmitted diseases was reported in 1957. Whether this was due to truly low case rates or simply to poor reporting is anybody's guess. Since 1957, however, the incidence of sexually transmitted diseases has been rising at an alarming rate. At the end of 1988, the *Morbidity and Mortality Weekly Report* listed 719,536 cases of gonorrhea, 32,663 cases of AIDS, and 103,437 cases of syphilis nationwide (see Table 15–1). For a disease like gonorrhea, the reported cases represent just the tip of the iceberg. Some **epidemiologists** suggest that the actual number of cases could be as much as ten times the number reported because of the failure of many physicians and medical facilities to meet the reporting requirements.

Factors Affecting Disease Transmission

Because most of the sexually transmitted diseases (other than diseases such as herpes simplex, AIDS, and hepatitis B) are readily treated, why does the problem continue to be of such great magnitude? There are a number of contributing factors, not the least of which is frequency of sexual contact. It is a well-known fact that the greater the number of sexual partners, the greater the potential for acquiring an STD. The so-called "sexual revolution" brought sexual freedoms not previously accepted by society. As sexual activity became less of a taboo, people became more sexually active. Multiple-partner relationships became more commonplace, and with them came a more rapid rise in sexually transmitted diseases.

The Pill. The birth control pill is one factor that has spawned the sexual revolution. One of the effects of the advent of birth control pills was a substantial reduction in the use of condoms for birth control. Because condoms afford some degree of protection against the transmission of several STDs, this led to an increase in the spread of these diseases. Birth control pills also increase a woman's susceptibility to candidiasis, a vaginal yeast infection. The pill provides a degree of sexual freedom never known before and, along with that freedom, a higher risk of contracting sexually transmitted diseases.

Impulsive Behavior. Have you ever looked back on something you had done and wondered why you did it? We all behave irrationally once in a while. However, irrational decisions in sexual practice can be the direct cause of STD transmission. It has been said that, at the time of sexual arousal, some of us

---

FAST FACTS

It is estimated by experts at the Centers for Disease Control that as many as 20 million Americans have genital herpes.

TABLE 15-1 ■ Selected STD Rates, United States, 1983–1988

Year	AIDS	Chancroid[b]	Gonorrhea	Hepatitis B	Syphilis
1983	Not reported	847	900,435	24,318	74,637
1984	4,445	665	878,556	26,115	69,888
1985	8,249	2,067	911,419	26,611	67,563
1986	13,055	3,756	900,868	26,107	68,215
1987	20,740	4,998	780,905	25,916	86,545
1988[a]	32,663	5,001	719,536	22,233	103,437

[a]Updated through 8–31–89
[b]Cases of Chancroid are only those that are reported—reporting not required for this disease.
SOURCE: U.S. Dept. of Health and Human Services, Centers for Disease Control, Atlanta, GA, 1989.

> **FAST FACTS**
>
> Each year, more than $1 billion is expended in direct and indirect costs due to chlamydial infection.

think with our genitals instead of our brains. In part, sexual arousal acts as a narcotic on the reasoning centers in the brain. Intelligent, rational behavior can go a long way to protect us from actions that lead toward acquiring these diseases.

Ignorance. How good was the sex education you received as a child and adolescent? Ignorance is another important factor in the spread of sexually transmitted diseases. There is not enough education about STDs at age levels at which such information is of great importance. Society is not willing to recognize that adolescents are becoming sexually active at younger ages than in the past, and we aren't providing them with the information they need to make intelligent decisions about their sexual behaviors. One California sex educator has stated that a student entering the ninth grade in a California high school has a statistically better chance of getting gonorrhea during high school than graduating. True or not, sexually transmitted diseases are spreading among adolescents at an alarming rate.

Denial. Many of us develop a myth of invulnerability when it comes to sexually transmitted diseases. We function under the delusion that we will not come in contact with one of these diseases and therefore will not become infected. Some of us think that we can tell if someone is infected simply by looking at him or her. This may lead us to take chances that we would otherwise not take.

Irresponsibility. Some people who have STDs fail to tell their sexual partners about their disease and the associated risks. Others may fail to follow instructions for the treatment of their disease. This kind of irresponsible behavior is another contributing factor in disease transmission. One state, Georgia, has passed legislation making this failure to inform sexual partners a crime. It is not always easy to talk about such things with your partner, but you must do the best you can if you know that you have a sexually transmitted disease.

> **FAST FACTS**
>
> As many as 60 percent of cases of herpes simplex in neonates will result in death.

Lack of Reporting. As mentioned earlier, the law requires the reporting of a number of diseases, among them several of the STDs (see Figure 15–1). Many physicians and clinics fail to make these reports on a regular basis, often trying to protect a long-time patient or family friend from the embarrassment. This prevents adequate follow up of sexual partners and makes it impossible to break the chain of infection.

Lack of Vaccines. There is a vaccine for only one sexually transmitted disease—hepatitis B. Immunization is recommended for practicing male homosexuals and persons working in the health field for whom exposure to potentially infected body fluids is likely. There are no vaccines at present for any other STD.

Asymptomatic Victims. Many victims of sexually transmitted diseases are asymptomatic; that is, they have the disease but have no visible symptoms. Asymptomatic carriers can transmit their disease to others without being aware that they have it themselves. Gonorrhea in females and nonspecific urethritis in males are examples of diseases that more often than not exhibit no symptoms whatsoever. You may also recall from our discussion of the stages of a communicable disease in Chapter 14 that many diseases can be transmitted to others during the latter part of the incubation period. This holds true for STDs such as herpes and gonorrhea as well.

Bacterial Diseases

Syphilis

The first reports of syphilis as a new disease can be traced back to the time of Christopher Columbus. Although scientists of the time soon came to realize that syphilis was a sexually transmitted disease, an effective cure was not to be developed until Alexander Fleming discovered penicillin in 1928, over 400 years later. During the Renaissance, many physicians thought that they had cured their patients with some ointment, salve, or internal medication, not knowing that the spirochete of syphilis continues to live in its victim, destroying virtually every organ of his or her body.

For hundreds of years, syphilis claimed thousands of lives, sent thousands of others to institutions for the insane, and maimed and crippled countless others. It was known as "the great imitator" because of the many different ways in which it would ultimately kill its victim, often imitating other diseases. Not until 1905 was the corkscrew-shaped **spirochete** of syphilis seen under a microscope for the first time. About the same time, Wasserman developed the first blood test for syphilis. Although Fleming discovered penicillin in 1928, the drug was not tested on syphilis until 1941. Finally, a safe, effective cure was available (yet we still see more than 25,000 cases of primary and secondary syphilis per year in the United States today).

To contract syphilis, direct contact with the syphilitic **lesion** of an infected individual is required. The spirochete readily penetrates mucous membranes and broken or abraded skin. When contact is made, the spirochete enters the body, and the disease process begins with an incubation period of ten to ninety days. As with any disease, some individuals will remain uninfected even after direct contact with syphilis.

Primary Stage. At the end of the incubation period, the *primary stage* of syphilis begins. A sore called a chancre (pronounced "shanker") will appear at the site

---

FAST FACTS

The blood test for syphilis does not become positive until about four weeks into the infection.

CHAPTER 15 ■ SEXUALLY TRANSMITTED DISEASE   377

FIGURE 15–1 ■ Example of Confidential Reporting Card Including Some STDs.

SOURCE: State of California, Department of Health Services.

FAST FACTS

The blood test used for syphilis screening can be positive for reasons other than syphilis.

where the spirochete entered. The chancre, although quite unpleasant looking, is generally painless and does not contain pus. Multiple chancres may develop, but that is usually not the case. Chancres can develop on any part of the body. Common sites include the penis, cervix, anus, and lips.

What would you be likely to do if you developed a painless sore of this type? What would most people do? Most people would do nothing and wait to see what happens. If nothing is done at this point in the disease, the chancre will heal like any other sore and disappear.

Secondary Stage. For a period of time after the chancre clears, the infected individual appears to be free of disease. But such is not the case. The spirochete now spreads throughout the person's body. After a period that might be as short as a few weeks or as long as a few months, the disease enters the *secondary stage* of syphilis. Usually, the secondary stage involves a generalized rash. This stage is the most contagious because the many sores of the rash contain spirochetes, and anyone coming into direct contact with them could become in-

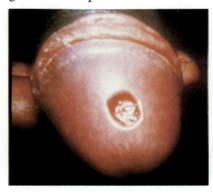

The principal sign of primary syphilis is the chancre which may appear as a single sore or multiple sores.

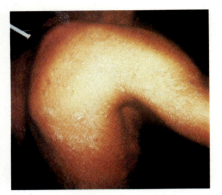
Secondary syphilis usually involves the presence of a generalized rash.

fected. Other manifestations of the secondary stage include loss of hair (alopecia), white patches on the underside of the tongue, and a bloodshot appearance in the eyes.

Many people seek medical care during the secondary stage. Most of these people do not realize that they have syphilis. They go to their physician or other health-care provider thinking that they have an allergic rash or a contact **dermatitis** (skin inflammation) of some type. They are usually quite surprised to learn the truth about their illness. Many people will pass through the secondary stage without seeking treatment, especially if their symptoms are mild.

Latent Stage. Even without treatment, the symptoms of the secondary stage eventually disappear and do not return. The disease now enters the *latent stage,* during which there are no outward symptoms or signs of infection. The individual is not able to transmit the disease to sexual partners, as there are no sores or rashes. The latent stage may last ten, twenty, thirty years or longer. During this time, the spirochete attacks virtually any and all organs of the patient's body. The brain can be affected, leaving the person insane. Bone, cartilage, and connective tissue can be damaged, causing severe disfigurement. Other internal organs can be destroyed, leading to the victim's death from an apparent heart attack, kidney failure, or other disorder.

The Late Stage. As mentioned earlier, syphilis has been called "the great imitator" because the eventual death of the infected person from the damage done by the spirochete can often resemble other problems such as heart disease, kidney disease, liver disease, and so on. If the individual survives the latent stage, he or she may then enter the final stage known as the *late stage*. During this period, all the manifestations of the damage done during the latent stage begin to show. Disfiguring sores known as gummas are often seen. Bone destruction may be extensive.

Pregnancy. From the fourth month of pregnancy on, the spirochete will readily pass through the placenta into the bloodstream of the fetus. Should this occur, the fetus will be placed in extreme danger. Fifty percent of syphilitic babies will die before birth or shortly thereafter. The remainder may be born severely deformed or as latent syphilitics, unaware of their disease and destined to face the same fate as other latent syphilitics.

Gummas are lesions associated with late syphilis.

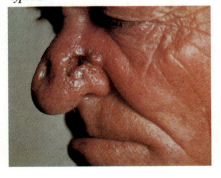

Treatment. Treatment for syphilis is relatively simple, especially in the earlier stages. Syphilis of less than one year's duration can generally be treated with a single injection of a long-acting form of penicillin. For those persons allergic to penicillin, an appropriate regimen of tetracycline can be used. At any time during the progress of the disease, the process can be arrested with appropriate antibiotic therapy. Of course, the physical damage done by the spirochete in a patient with the later stages of the disease will not be reversed by the antibiotics.

> ■ *PROBLEM SITUATION* You have a single sore on your penis. It is not painful and doesn't seem to be filled with pus. In fact, it has already started to heal. What should you do? Why?

Gonorrhea

Gonorrhea is the most widespread of the reportable sexually transmitted diseases. Cases of gonorrhea in the United States outnumber all other reportable diseases combined. Just under one million cases are reported nationwide each year. Gonorrhea is found in large cities at about eight times the rate of cases in rural areas.

Gonorrhea is caused by a diplococcus, *Neisseria gonorrhea*. Because it is a bacterial infection, it is readily treated with antibiotics. The incubation period is relatively short, only three to five days. In males, the infection is most often found in the urethra, although it can also be found in the rectum, throat, and conjunctiva, depending on the type of sexual activity. In females, the cervix is usually the site of infection, although the urethra, rectum, throat, and conjunctiva are also possible sites. Gay males often are found to have rectal gonorrhea resulting from anal intercourse. Gonorrhea in the throat is the result of transmission through oral sex.

Approximately 80 to 90 percent of males with gonorrhea will be symptomatic. Symptoms include a **purulent** discharge from the penis and painful and frequent urination. In contrast, only 10 to 20 percent of females will show symptoms. The most common symptom in the female is a vaginal discharge, which can often go unnoticed. The large number of asymptomatic patients is a major contributing factor in the spread of gonorrhea. These patients are often completely unaware of their disease and yet are capable of transmitting it to unsuspecting sexual partners.

Gonorrhea is one of the major causes of sterility in females in the United States. In the female reproductive system, the fallopian tubes are at risk of being damaged if the infection spreads upward from the cervix. In rare instances, infections in the male reproductive system can lead to the formation of scar tissue in such areas as the seminal vesicles, vas deferens, and prostate gland. In either case, sterility can result. Although it rarely occurs, the gonorrhea bacteria can enter the patient's bloodstream and cause a systemic infection that results in arthritis, heart damage, and kidney damage.

FAST FACTS

About five percent of women in their sexually active years show positive cultures for gonorrhea.

Treatment. Gonorrhea can be treated with antibiotics such as penicillin, tetracycline, spectinomycin, and Rocephin. The drug of choice is Rocephin. These drugs must either be given by injection or be obtained through a physician's prescription. Some strains of *Neiserria gonorrhea* have developed resistance to certain antibiotics, particularly to penicillin. These strains are known as *penicillinase-producing Neiserria gonorrhea* (PPNG), because they have developed the capability to produce an enzyme known as penicillinase that can destroy penicillin.

Infection in Newborns. Babies born to mothers with gonorrhea are at risk of developing the disease in their eyes, which can lead to permanent blindness. In all states, the law requires that the eyes of every newborn baby be treated within a few hours after birth with an antibiotic eye preparation to prevent gonorrhea.

> ■ *PROBLEM SITUATION* Your roommate comes home and tells you that her sexual partner has gonorrhea. She mentions that she is going to wait to see if she comes down with symptoms. What advice should you give to her?

> **FAST FACTS**
>
> Chlamydia infection strikes about three to four million Americans and causes sterility in about 11,000 women each year.

Nongonococcal Urethritis

Nongonococcal **urethritis** (NGU) or nonspecific urethritis (NSU) is a disease of the male urethra. The causative organism is usually ureaplasma or *Chlamydia*.

Symptoms of nonspecific urethritis include a colorless discharge from the penis and painful and frequent urination. The discharge is somewhat different in appearance to that of gonorrhea; it is generally not yellowish in color and is thinner.

Treatment of most nongonococcal urethritis cases is accomplished with the use of the antibiotics tetracycline, doxycycline, or erythromycin. Nongonococcal urethritis should never be ignored because it, like gonorrhea, can lead to permanent sterility if left untreated. Be sure to seek medical care at once should any symptoms of NGU occur.

Chlamydia Infection

Genital chlamydia infection is not a new disease, but the identifiable cases of it have increased substantially during the past few years. Although chlamydia infection is not a reportable disease, it is estimated that the number of cases outnumbers any other STD, including gonorrhea and herpes. Whether the disease is spreading more rapidly or we are simply getting better at identifying it is not known. The *Chlamydia* bacteria, which does not fall into any of the usual categories of bacteria, has been known for many years as the leading cause of eye disease in third-world countries and is responsible for blindness in about two million people today.

In the male, chlamydia infection causes a urethritis (inflammation of the urethra) with symptoms including painful urination and a thin watery discharge from the penis. About 10 percent of males with chlamydia infection show no symptoms. Complications include *epididymitis* (inflammation of the epididymis) and **prostatitis** (inflammation of the prostate gland).

In females, chlamydia infection causes a cervicitis, or inflammation of the uterine cervix (neck of the uterus), with the symptoms including vaginal discharge, an itching and burning sensation in the genital area, and pain in the pelvic area. Symptoms respond well to treatment with tetracycline or doxycycline. As many as 80 percent of women with chlamydia infection show no symptoms.

Untreated chlamydia infections can lead to a variety of potential problems for a baby exposed to the organism during prenatal development or birth. Possibilities include spontaneous abortion, stillbirth, or eye infection and pneumonia in the newborn.

There are appropriate laboratory tests to identify chlamydia infection. Many practitioners are now routinely testing women at the time of their annual exam in order to identify asymptomatic patients. Individuals with the highest risk are women between the ages of fifteen and twenty-five who have multiple sexual partners.

Pelvic Inflammatory Disease

Pelvic inflammatory disease (PID) is an infection in the upper part of the female reproductive system (see Figure 15–2). It has become a major health hazard for women, with victims numbering well over one million per year. Untreated PID can lead to **ectopic pregnancy** and sterility as a result of scarred and damaged fallopian tubes, the possibility of surgical **hysterectomy,** and, in some cases, death.

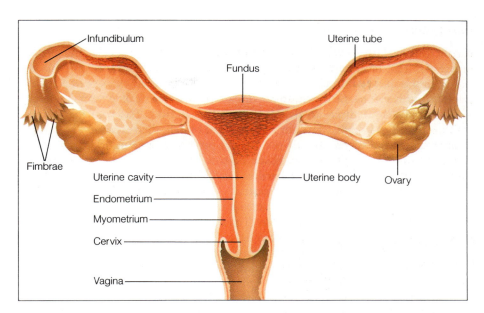

FIGURE 15–2 ■ **Uterus and Associated Female Reproductive Structures Showing Sites of Infection of PID.**
The figure has been sectioned to show internal structures.

Several organisms have been identified as potentially being responsible for PID, including *Neiserria gonorrhea*. Most PID, however, is caused by *Chlamydia*. In some cases, PID results from other organisms and more vigorous therapy is needed. Symptoms indicative of PID should never be ignored. Lower abdominal pain is the principal sign.

Because PID is most often a multimicrobial infection—that is, several organisms are causing the problem—multiple antibiotics are always used in the treatment. These include penicillin, tetracycline or doxycycline, and metronidazole (Flagyl).

Bacterial Vaginosis

Bacterial vaginosis is one of the most common vaginal inflammations and is frequently undetected by the patient. Sexual partners are sometimes asymptomatic carriers, although many experts do not consider bacterial vaginosis to be a sexually transmitted disease. It has been known in the past as *Haemophilus vaginalis* and gardnerella. Current opinion is that bacterial vaginosis is actually caused by at least four different bacterial organisms, all of which are normally present in the vagina. Diagnosis is made through the identification of so-called **clue cells** in a microscopic examination of vaginal mucous. Symptoms include a foul-smelling vaginal discharge. Generally, the patient has no other symptoms.

Treatment is with metronidazole (Flagyl). An alternative treatment with ampicillin is considerably less effective. Sexual partners are treated only if the female has recurrent infections.

■ *PROBLEM SITUATION* Your sexual partner informs you that she has bacterial vaginosis and has been treated and that you should also seek treatment. What would be your reaction? How might this information affect your relationship?

Chancroid

Chancroid is caused by a bacillus that produces a localized sore at the site of infection. The ulcerated sore usually has ragged edges, contains pus, bleeds easily, and is quite painful. The sore somewhat resembles the chancre of primary syphilis but is soft to the touch, so the disease is sometimes called "soft chancre."

Chancroid has a three- to five-day incubation period. The sore that subsequently develops usually starts out as a small red blotch, then enlarges and breaks open to form the **ulceration.** If not treated properly, large multiple sores can develop, leading to severe local tissue destruction, which is the most serious complication of the disease. The bacillus may also spread to the regional lymph nodes near the site of the initial infection.

Although some patients will heal without treatment, most will need antibiotics to arrest the progress of the disease. Tetracycline is the antibiotic of choice. Some strains of the chancroid bacillus have developed resistance to tetracycline, so erythromycin or other antibiotics must be used. Both males and females can be asymptomatic carriers of the bacillus, in some cases long after their sores have healed.

In 1985, an outbreak of chancroid occurred in Boston. In the nine months from January 8, 1985, to September 30, 1985, fifty-three cases (fourteen in females and thirty-nine in males) were diagnosed in the Boston area, compared to a total of two cases in the previous two years. This particular outbreak was traced to prostitute activity in a specific area of Boston. Nationwide, in 1983, there were 847 cases of chancroid, with 90 percent of the cases occurring in Florida, New York, Georgia, and California. In 1987, 4,998 cases were reported, most of them from New York, Florida, and Texas. In 1988, 5001 cases were reported.

Granuloma Inguinale

Granuloma inguinale is the least common of the sexually transmitted diseases caused by bacteria. The organisms, known as Donovan bodies, cause ulcerations on the skin of the groin area and on the genitals. The ulcerations are small, round, and filled with pus, and they spread progressively from the site of the infection. If the disease is not treated, regional lymph nodes may become involved and pain and fever may develop. In many untreated cases, the disease may result in death.

The incubation period for granuloma inguinale is about two to three months. Some cases have been reported to have much longer incubation periods. One characteristic of granuloma inguinale is a sour odor that is emitted from the sores after the disease has progressed for many months.

Lymphogranuloma Venereum

Lymphogranuloma venereum is a chlamydial infection of the lymph system in the genital region. The incubation period may be shorter than one week or as long as three weeks. Infection begins with a small, ulcerated sore at the site of contact. The sore disappears in a short period of time. Infection of the lymph system follows and is accompanied by swelling, tenderness, and pain in the groin area. In female patients, the swelling may occur in the area of the rectum. Systemic effects include headache, fever, chills, and arthritis-like pains in the joints.

Some patients show only mild symptoms of lymphogranuloma venereum, whereas others may be severely debilitated by the disease. A skin test, the Frei test, was used to diagnose the disease prior to 1974. Presently, diagnosis is accomplished through the use of a blood test and culture. Treatment is with tetracycline or other antibiotics. Occasionally, surgery is a necessary part of the treatment.

Viral Diseases

Acquired Immunodeficiency Syndrome (AIDS)

According to the National Center for Health Statistics, more than 99 percent of the American population has heard of AIDS. However, only two-thirds of those surveyed knew that AIDS can destroy the body's immune system and that a pregnant woman can give AIDS to her unborn baby. Only about one-fourth knew that AIDS can damage the brain.

Acquired immunodeficiency syndrome (AIDS) is caused by a virus known as HIV or HIV-1 (human immunodeficiency virus). Other names used in the past for the same virus are HTLVIII (Human T-lymphotropic virus type III) or LAV (lymphadenopathy-associated virus). The disease is transmitted primarily through the transfer of infected bodily fluids, particularly blood and semen, by high-risk sexual practices or through the use of infected needles. It can also be transmitted prenatally to a baby from an infected mother. Prior to the development of the test for checking donated blood for the presence of antibodies, some transmission occurred through blood transfusions.

AIDS became an obvious public-health issue in early 1981 with the identification of the disease among a group of gay men in New York. Recent evidence indicates that cases of AIDS occurred in the United States much earlier than

FAST FACTS

A prominent doctor has stated "there's no such thing as safe sex for someone contemplating sex with an HIV-positive person."

GUIDELINES TO YOUR GOOD HEALTH

To reduce the risk of getting or giving to others a sexually transmitted disease:

1. Avoid intimate contact with anyone having unexplained sores or rashes, especially in the genital area.
2. Avoid sexual contact with others if you believe or know that you have a sexually transmitted disease.
3. Refrain from engaging in casual sex.
4. Be sure to use a condom when engaging in sexual activity, including vaginal or anal intercourse and fellatio.
5. Avoid having multiple sexual partners.
6. Avoid sexual activity that involves the transfer of bodily fluids.
7. If you use hypodermic needles, use the sterile disposable type from a sealed package.
8. If you travel to any underdeveloped countries, take sterile needles and syringes with you in case you must be given any injections while traveling.

FAST FACTS

A 1988 report in the *Journal of the American Medical Association* stated that one in every sixty-one babies born in New York City is born with HIV antibodies.

FAST FACTS

The time period from infection with HIV until a diagnosis of AIDS averages about eight years, but from diagnosis to death averages only about eighteen months.

1981 but were not identified as such at the time. An article in *Newsweek* in November 1987 suggested that a teenager who died in St. Louis in 1969 actually died from AIDS.

The World Health Organization reported that AIDS cases worldwide increased 56 percent in 1987. More than 106,000 cases have been reported in the United States since 1979, and it has been estimated that the actual number may be more than twice that figure. Over 32,000 new cases were reported in the United States for the year 1988 alone.

The origin of AIDS has been a hotly debated issue. Many experts believe that it originated in Africa, possibly in Zaire, and was subsequently transmitted to Haiti, a country with close political and economic ties to Zaire. From there, it moved to the United States, transmitted by travelers vacationing in Haiti. We will probably never know for certain how the disease originated, but it's here now and we must deal with it.

In January 1988, it was reported that French scientists had identified another virus that can cause AIDS and have called it HIV-2. In contrast to HIV-1, the HIV-2 virus is not detected by currently used blood tests. As of 1989, this virus has been identified in only one patient in the United States. The patient was a West African who came to the United States in 1987 and in New Jersey in December of that year was discovered to be infected with HIV-2.

AIDS is currently more prevalent on the East and West Coasts and less prevalent in the middle American states. It is also more common in urban than in rural areas. Most cases occur in young to early-middle-aged adults. The disease is more common among men than women and, on the basis of a percentage of the population, more common among blacks and Hispanics than whites. As of May 1987, 37,000 teenagers have tested positive for HIV antibodies.

The U.S. Centers for Disease Control has considered the possible relationship between HIV infection and tuberculosis. A marked increase in tuberculosis cases was noted in New York City between 1984 and 1986, and further study showed an abnormally high concentration of these cases among those patients who tested positive for HIV infection. Much evidence has now been gathered to suggest a causal relationship between TB and AIDS in these cases.

The average incubation period for AIDS may range anywhere from six months to eight years or more before the patient becomes symptomatic. One study of transfusion-related AIDS cases showed an average incubation period of 8.23 years. The course of the disease may also be quite variable, but the average time from the onset of symptoms to death is about ten months.

TABLE 15–2 ■ Reported AIDS Cases in Areas of Highest Incidence

Year	New York City	California	Florida	Texas
1984	1,416	1,030	314	248
1985	2,178	1,979	551	485
1986	3,290	2,656	840	940
1987	3,182	4,872	1,627	1,681
1988*	6,061	5,867	2,827	2,235

*As of 8-31-89

SOURCE: U.S. Centers for Disease Control, USPHS

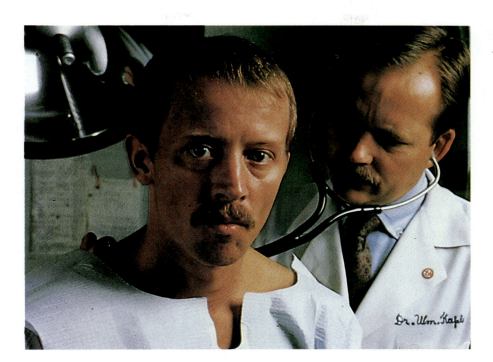

Evidence suggests that all HIV positive people will ultimately develop symptoms of their infection.

Symptoms may include persistent diarrhea, fever, drenching night sweats, fatigue, weight loss of fifteen pounds or more than 10 percent of body weight, and the presence of one or more opportunistic infections. Those individuals who exhibit signs and symptoms of the disease but do not have an opportunistic infection are said to have AIDS-related complex (ARC). Current evidence suggests that the disease ultimately leads to death in all patients.

Approximately 70 percent of those with AIDS are male homosexuals. Others who are commonly infected include intravenous drug users and **hemophiliacs.** Hemophiliacs acquired AIDS through transfusions of a substance used to control their hemophilia. This factor was obtained from the blood of large numbers of donors, many of whom carried the AIDS virus. Today, through the development of methods to test donated blood for the presence of antibodies to HIV, and more recently for the antigen itself, our blood supply is considerably safer.

AIDS is not a disease of gay men only. Anyone can get the disease, and, in countries where the disease has been around longer, there are as many heterosexuals with it as homosexuals. In Africa, for example, heterosexual spread is principally through the sexual activity of prostitutes. Heterosexual activity is now the principal way the disease is spread in Haiti. AIDS is well on its way to becoming another of the common STDs.

The AIDS virus virtually destroys the immune response of the patient by invading a specific cell of the immune system known as the **T lymphocyte.** This allows a variety of other organisms to infect the patient. The most common causes of death are Kaposi's sarcoma (a form of skin cancer) and *Pneumocystis carinii* pneumonia. Other commonly found opportunistic infections include *Candida albicans* infection, tuberculosis, cytomegalovirus, and a variety of other parasites. The virus also attacks the **B lymphocytes** and **monocytes,** reducing the immune response even further.

FAST FACTS

In New York City, AIDS is the leading cause of death for women ages twenty-five to thirty-four.

> **FAST FACTS**
>
> A study done by the National Center for Health Services Research and Health Care Technology Assessment estimated that the lifetime cost for the care of one AIDS patient is about $60,000.

Dementia—deterioration of a person's mental state—is also associated with AIDS. Until recently, it was thought to occur only in the later stages of the disease, but recent evidence shows that dementia often occurs in persons with early HIV infection and no other signs or symptoms of AIDS.

Recent evidence indicates that HIV can infect (in addition to the T lymphocytes and other cells of the immune system) cells of the brain, skin, bowel, and rectum. Research reported in February 1988 suggests that the virus can affect "a particular epithelial cell type, found in the rectum, that regulates the amount of fluid found in the bowel." This finding might, in part, explain why anal intercourse appears to be such a high-risk activity for transmission of HIV.

Many experts believe that a person who has been infected with HIV will eventually show symptoms of the disease to some degree. The time from exposure to the development of symptoms may be fifteen years or longer. The degree of infection may range from mild symptoms through a full-blown case of AIDS resulting in death. Opinions about the incidence of infection and the potential consequences for those exposed to the virus are at this point educated speculation. Only time and experience with AIDS will tell the true story.

Treatment. Until recently, there was no treatment, no vaccine, and no cure for AIDS or AIDS-related complex. Treatment was directed only at the opportunistic infections as they arose. There still is no cure and no vaccine. In 1987, however, Burroughs Wellcome Company was granted FDA approval to market a new drug named zidovudine under the brand name Retrovir. This drug, previously known as azidothymidine or AZT, is, at this writing, the only drug effective as a treatment for HIV infections. It is not a cure for AIDS. Company literature states that it "prolongs lives of certain AIDS and ARC patients," "reduces risk and severity of opportunistic infections," "improves immune status," and "helps patients feel better, resume more productive lives." On August 17, 1989, Louis Sullivan, Secretary of the Department of Health and Human Services, announced that AZT can halt the progress of AIDS when used in patients "who are only mildly infected." He added that "We are indeed entering the period when AIDS may become a treatable disease." Sullivan cautioned that "even those who are under AZT treatment remain capable of transmitting the disease." At an average wholesale price of $120 per hundred capsules and a dosage of two capsules every four hours around the clock, the monthly cost of Retrovir therapy is over $430. The price to the consumer generally approaches about $600 per month. The drug works by inhibiting replication of the virus.

A variety of other cures and treatments are available both in and outside of the United States; however, none thus far have proved to be effective. In 1988, a drug called peptide-T was approved for extended trials in humans. Limited trials have shown that the drug has no harmful effects and that it leads to "signs of improvement in AIDS symptoms, including improved sense of well-being, skin conditions, mental functioning, weight, and decreased diarrhea."

> **FAST FACTS**
>
> A new antiviral drug DDI (dideoxyinosine) was released in 1989 for use in AIDS patients unable to tolerate AZT.

Prevention. The way to reduce the risk of AIDS is to engage in safe sexual activity, in which the chance of transmission of the virus through bodily fluids is eliminated. We are no longer talking about risk *groups,* such as gay males or IV drug abusers. Our concerns are for risk *behaviors.* Any sexual or other intimate activity that allows for the exchange of bodily fluids places an uninfected person at risk.

Obviously, the best way to avoid contact with HIV is to abstain from sexual activity entirely. For those engaging in intimate relationships, safe-sex practices are a must. Sexual activities such as anal intercourse, vaginal intercourse, and oral sex are high-risk behaviors if practiced without the protection of a condom. We recommend that condoms be used in all relationships unless the partners have been monogamous with each other for at least five years and have been tested and are free of HIV antibodies.

A test has been available since March 1985 to check blood samples for HIV viral antibodies. A positive test means that there has been some prior exposure to the virus, which precipitated antibody production against it. This test is useful to test blood before it enters our country's blood supply to prevent accidental transmission of the virus to blood recipients. Its usefulness in testing people for the presence of the antibodies is not clear. A positive test does not indicate whether or not an individual will develop AIDS at some future time. It simply indicates a prior exposure to the virus. It does not mean that the person has the disease.

The ELISA test, the screening test in general use, sometimes indicates false positive results; that is, the test is positive but the tested blood is not infected. A more precise test, the Western Blot, is used for confirmation. In a recent study of blood donors in California, twenty-four of twenty-five tests on blood from female donors and seventy-five of seventy-six tests on blood from male donors were confirmed to be negative with the Western Blot, although all were positive with the ELISA. False positive tests with the ELISA are three times more common for women than for men.

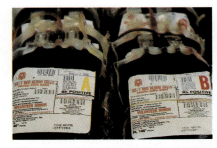

All units of donated blood are tested for the presence of HIV antibodies. Positive blood is discarded.

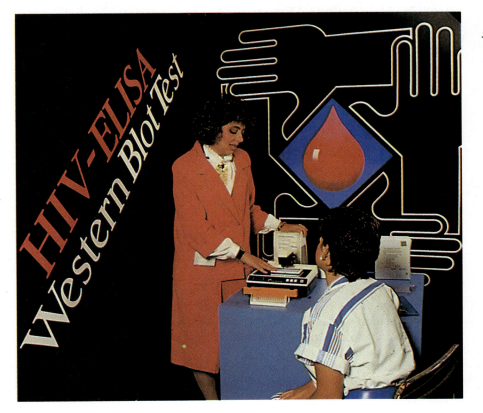

The ELISA is a general screening test for HIV antibodies. The Western Blot is used for confirmation of Positive ELISA test results.

> **FAST FACTS**
>
> In 1989, a 10-minute test known as SUDS became available for HIV antibody testing, affording results in a few minutes in your physician's office.

False negative tests are also possible, but these are usually related to situations in which the person tested has been exposed to the virus but the time from exposure to the test date has not been long enough for sufficient antibodies to build up in the person's blood. It is estimated that about one infected blood unit per 100,000 donations occurs as the result of this "window period."

There is currently a patchwork of laws regarding HIV antibody testing. In some states, test results may not be revealed to anyone other than the patient. In other states, results may be made known to certain individuals, such as the person's spouse. In still other states, reporting of the results is mandatory.

There is still a great deal of debate in the scientific community about AIDS, primarily because so much about it is still unknown. According to Dr. Peter H. Duesberg of the University of California at Berkeley, HIV may not be the sole cause of AIDS and, in fact, may not be a cause at all. According to a January 1988 news article, Dr. Duesberg believes that "the virus may be an opportunistic organism that found a willing host in the AIDS patient who became sick from something else." Many well-known figures in the scientific community agree with Dr. Duesberg, while many others disagree with him. We can only hope that science comes up with more information about this deadly disease and that a cure or effective prevention is discovered.

AIDS has led to many problems in addition to its obvious health consequences. A type of "AIDS hysteria" has surfaced in some areas and among some groups of people. This hysteria is based on fear and a lack of knowledge about the true nature of the disease. Discrimination against persons afflicted with AIDS has occurred in schools and in the workplace. Because AIDS has occurred to a great degree in the practicing gay male population, increased **homophobia** has led to discrimination against gay men and women. Much of the debate over AIDS has related to political and social issues as well as to public-health issues.

Herpes Simplex

Herpes simplex virus is known to cause both herpes I (HSVI) and herpes II (HSVII). Herpes I generally appears as cold sores around the mouth and lips, whereas herpes II is usually found in the genital area. Clinically, the two viruses are not distinguishable from one another, and treatment for both infections is the same. As a result of sexual practices such as oral sex, herpes I can be readily transmitted to the genital area and herpes II can be transmitted to the area of the mouth.

The herpes viruses are transmitted by direct contact with an infected individual. Within about two weeks after contact, the patient develops a series of blisters at the site of infection. Soon, the blisters break open, leaving painful sores that gradually heal and disappear.

The virus then migrates to the ganglia of the fifth cranial nerve, where it remains dormant (inactive), sometimes for only a short period of time and sometimes for the life of the patient. Approximately one-third of herpes patients develop subsequent outbreaks. In those patients in whom the disease recurs, the time interval between recurrences may be quite varied. Subsequent outbreaks can be triggered by a number of factors, including stress, other illnesses, excessive sun exposure, menstrual periods, and virtually any other event that can affect the patient's immune system.

It appears that the virus takes advantage of its host's weakened resistance and migrates back up the nerve pathways to the original site of infection to cause

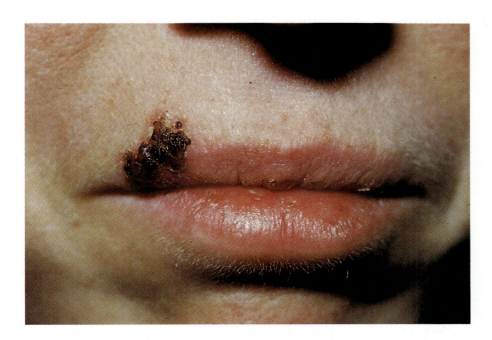

Herpes simplex infections often occur around the mouth and may be called cold sores, fever blisters, or sun blisters.

a repeat outbreak of the disease. For some patients, these subsequent outbreaks come as often as once or twice a month. For others, it may be several years between recurrences.

The disease is communicable throughout the period of active infection and for a few days before the blisters appear. During this entire time, the patient is said to be "shedding" virus. Evidence indicates that some people may come in contact with and be infected by herpes simplex virus without developing any visible symptoms. These individuals may still be able to transmit the disease to others.

There is presently no cure for herpes simplex virus infections. Prevention is through the avoidance of contact with an infected individual during the active stage of the disease and whenever viral shedding might occur. Treatment includes topical applications of ointments to reduce pain and discomfort and the use of the drug acyclovir.

Acyclovir is the only drug therapy currently approved by the FDA as a specific treatment for herpes. It comes in ointment form to be applied directly to the lesions and in capsule form. The ointment is not recommended for other than the initial outbreak and is not widely used except in specific situations, such as pregnancy. When taken by mouth, acyclovir shortens the course of the outbreak, reduces the risk of transmission by reducing viral shedding, and suppresses subsequent outbreaks. It may be used continuously as suppressive therapy in those patients who have very frequent recurrences, but it is recommended that it not be taken for longer than six months consecutively.

There is an association between genital herpes and increased risk of cancer of the cervix. Females with herpes simplex virus should get yearly **Pap smears.**

Herpes infections in the birth canal at the time of delivery present an extreme danger to the newborn. An infant acquiring herpes at birth will often develop a systemic form of the disease, which can be fatal. Babies at risk must be delivered by **Caesarean section.**

Hepatitis B

Hepatitis is any disease that causes an inflammation of the liver. Hepatitis B is one of a group of liver diseases caused by viruses.

Transmission of hepatitis B is similar to that of AIDS, through the use of contaminated needles and through contact with infected body fluids such as blood and semen. Sexual transmission, therefore, is not uncommon. Because the same types of sexual practices that can transmit the AIDS virus can also transmit the hepatitis B virus, it is not surprising that as many as 80 percent of practicing male homosexuals acquire hepatitis B at sometime during their lives.

The incubation period for hepatitis B is two to five months. The onset of symptoms, which are similar to those of hepatitis A, is gradual. Symptoms usually include nausea, lethargy, loss of appetite, and a yellowish skin color, usually first seen in the whites of the eyes. Cola-colored urine and white, clay-like stools may also occur.

Passive immunity to hepatitis B can be achieved through the use of a hepatitis B immune globulin (HBIG) specific for hepatitis B. HBIG is given in a two-shot series at a cost of approximately $150. To be effective, the injections must be started within ten days of exposure. Gamma globulin and immune serum globulin, used as passive immunity for hepatitis A, are ineffective for hepatitis B.

There is active immunity available for hepatitis B in the form of a three-shot series of hepatitis B vaccine. The second injection follows the first by a month and the third follows the second by five months. The vaccine is relatively expensive—about $150 wholesale for a three-shot vial. It is recommended for those at high risk, such as gay males, laboratory workers, dentists, dental hygienists, and any others who might come in contact with the body fluids of infected individuals. Before the vaccine is administered, the individual must have a blood test to see if there has been prior exposure and natural immunity already has developed.

Until 1986, all hepatitis B vaccine was made from the blood of a pool of blood donors who had active immunity to hepatitis B. Because of this, there was a fear that AIDS might be transmitted to persons receiving the vaccine, because the high-risk groups for both diseases are somewhat the same. There is no evidence to indicate that such transmission is possible. In July 1986, the FDA approved a new hepatitis B vaccine, manufactured through recombinant DNA techniques. The new vaccine should relieve all fears of incidental disease transmission through vaccination.

Human Papilloma Virus or HPV (Venereal Warts)

Venereal warts are viral in origin. They may appear anywhere in the genital region and may be found inside the urethra, vagina, or anus. Frequently, one sexual partner may have warts while the other is completely free of them. There is a direct association between venereal warts and cancer of the uterine cervix. Any female with a history of venereal warts should have an annual Pap smear.

Although there are no really effective techniques for the removal of venereal warts, some relief may be achieved through the application of podophyllin or trichloroacetic acid to chemically burn off the warts, or they may be removed with freezing, burning, or laser techniques. Only trained practitioners should attempt the removal of venereal warts, since great care must be taken to avoid damage to surrounding tissue. Internal warts require special treatment.

FAST FACTS

Venereal warts are three times more common than genital herpes, according to data from the Centers for Disease Control.

GUIDELINES TO YOUR GOOD HEALTH

The following are suggestions that, if followed, will help you maintain a strong immune system.

1. Eat a balanced diet containing adequate amounts of vitamins, minerals, and other nutrients.
2. Participate in a regular exercise program.
3. Get adequate sleep each night.
4. Develop a personal stress reduction program.
5. Maintain a proper body weight.
6. Do not use drugs known to adversely affect the immune system such as "poppers" or marijuana.
7. Do not consume excessive amounts of alcoholic beverages.
8. Do not use tobacco products.

Molluscum Contagiosum

Many individuals are susceptible to molluscum contagiosum, a viral skin disease sometimes known as pox virus. Most infected people are asymptomatic, but some complain of itching, tenderness, and pain where the lesions are present. Transmission is by direct contact.

The incubation period may range from one to six months. Molluscum appears as raised, smooth, shiny lesions with a slight **umbilication,** or depression, at the center. There may be a single lesion or as many as twenty. In some patients, hundreds may occur.

Treatment is with topical application of podophyllin, freezing with liquid nitrogen, or removal by surgery or laser.

■ Other Sexually Transmitted Diseases

Candida Albicans

Candida albicans, also known as *Monilia,* is a yeast that is found as part of the normal fauna and flora of the vagina as well as the throat and gastrointestinal tract. Generally, the yeast, being a fungus, is kept under control by the bacteria found in the same areas. However, certain factors can lead to a disruption of these normal controls, allowing the yeast to begin to grow unchecked. Some contributing factors include diabetes and the use of birth control pills or antibiotics. Yeast infections are not generally sexually transmitted, although males may act as asymptomatic carriers. Noncircumsized males may develop active infections.

Yeast grows well where it is warm and moist. Thus, in the summer, there is often a marked increase in vaginal yeast infections principally caused by the wearing of nylon bathing suits. Nylon reduces the evaporation of water, providing a very suitable environment for the growth of yeast. Bathing suits and underwear made of cotton, which is a more breathable fabric, are preferable.

FAST FACTS

A researcher from the University of Florida has suggested placing cotton underwear in a microwave for five minutes at high power to kill candida.

Symptoms of yeast infection include a whitish vaginal discharge, inflammation, and itching. In severe cases, there may be pain with intercourse because of swelling of the labia.

Yeast infections are treated with antifungal vaginal creams and suppositories. Generally, sexual partners of women with yeast infections do not have to be treated unless they develop symptoms.

Trichomonas Vaginalis

Trichomonas vaginalis is a protozoa that causes a **vaginitis** in the female. It can also cause a urethritis or prostatitis in the male, but the majority of male contacts will be asymptomatic. It is estimated that about 2.5 million women per year in the United States acquire the infection. *Trichomonas* is almost always sexually transmitted.

The incubation period may extend from four to twenty-eight days. Symptoms include a vaginal discharge that may range from frothy white to greenish or yellow. Vaginal soreness and itching and pain on intercourse may also occur. Many women, however, are asymptomatic. Treatment is with the drug metronidazole (Flagyl), except during the first trimester of pregnancy. Vaginal creams to relieve the symptoms may be safely used during that time.

Pubic Lice

There are three types of lice that are parasitic on humans—head lice, public lice, and body lice (see Figure 15–3). Body lice are the only ones known to carry any diseases and are, fortunately, the least common of the three types. In reality, body lice do not live on the body. They live in clothing and crawl on to the body only to feed.

Head lice are quite common, and outbreaks are frequently found among school children. Lice do not hop or fly but crawl from the clothing of one child to that of others. They may also be transmitted by direct contact and through the sharing of combs and hairbrushes.

Pubic lice are usually found in the pubic area but may seek out any short, course body hair, such as that of the armpits, eyebrows, and eyelashes. The lice are transmitted by direct contact and through fomites (inanimate objects such as carpets, bedding, and furniture).

The female louse is about the size of a pinhead (one to two millimeters in length). A louse has three pairs of curved claws that resemble those of a crab—hence the name "crab louse." Lice live on human blood and are easy to see on the body after they feed because of their deep red color. The main symptom is intense itching caused by irritation from the waste material produced by the lice and by a chemical in their saliva that is injected into the wound to prevent coagulation of the blood while they feed. Dark brown specks of the waste material can sometimes be seen on underwear and bedding.

When the female louse lays eggs, known as nits, she attaches them firmly near the base of the victim's hair follicles, a suitably warm environment for the eggs to hatch. The nits look very much like dandruff to the untrained eye with one exception; they do not come loose easily. After several days, the eggs hatch and the newly hatched nymphs begin their three- to four-week life cycle.

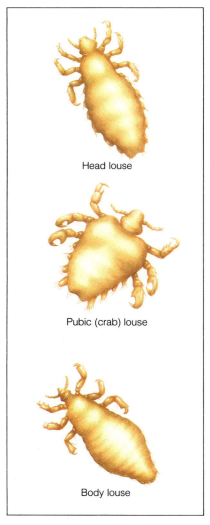

FIGURE 15–3 ■ **Head, Pubic and Body Lice.**

GUIDELINES TO YOUR GOOD HEALTH

The following will help you to reduce the risk of complications from a sexually transmitted disease:

1. If you have had an outbreak of herpes I or herpes II, maintain a strong immune system to help prevent recurrences.
2. If you are female and have had venereal warts, be sure to have a regular Pap smear.
3. If you are a female prone to vaginal yeast infections, wear cotton underwear and bathing suits rather than those made of nylon and be sure pantyhose have a cotton insert in the vaginal area.
4. Seek medical care at the first sign of any suspicious abnormality.
5. After being treated for a sexually transmitted disease, go back to your health-care practitioner for a follow-up visit to be sure the treatment was successful.
6. Seek medical care if you are informed by a sexual partner that he or she has a sexually transmitted disease.
7. Be open and honest in advising health-care personnel of your sexual contacts if you are diagnosed as having a sexually transmitted disease.

Treatment. Lice can be killed with lindane (Kwell), a prescription insecticide product, or a variety of over-the-counter preparations. Lindane comes in both shampoo and lotion forms and requires a prescription because it can be absorbed through the skin. Lindane should never be used on infants or pregnant women. Lice on the eyelashes cannot be safely treated with insecticides. Petroleum jelly can be applied to smother the arthropods.

Current research indicates that the over-the-counter preparations, which contain synthetic pyrethrins and are not absorbed through the skin, are just as effective as lindane when used properly. Natural pyrethrins are insecticidal agents produced in plants to prevent damage from insects. Treatment must be effective in killing the nits as well as the adult lice. Care must be taken to kill any lice present on bedding, carpeting, furniture, and so on, because lice can live off the body without feeding for up to ten days. Sprays are available for treating fomites. Clothing must be washed in hot water and detergent.

A severe **dermatitis** may develop as a result of an infestation from lice. Infections may also result from scratching. If either of these occur, they must also be evaluated and treated.

Individuals with pubic lice should be examined for other sexually transmitted diseases, since gonorrhea, syphilis, and trichomonas infections frequently coexist with lice infestations. Females between the ages of fifteen and nineteen and males over the age of twenty are the most common carriers of lice.

Scabies

Scabies is caused by a tiny itch mite so small that it can not be readily seen with the naked eye. The female mite burrows under the superficial layers of the skin to lay her eggs. Burrows can be as much as one and one-half inches in length.

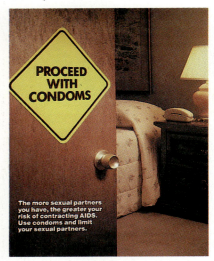

Condoms are helpful in preventing the transmission of a number of sexually transmitted diseases.

Infestations may take as long as two or three months to fully develop. Symptoms include intense itching, especially at night. Red, raised lesions (papules) or tracks caused by the burrows may be visible. The mite can sometimes be identified by scraping the skin surface of a papule and examining the material under a microscope.

Scabies is transmitted by intimate contact and through fomites, as the mite can live off the body for several days without feeding. Outbreaks often occur where large numbers of people live in close contact, such as in nursing homes, dormitories, and prisons.

Treatment is with lindane lotion. The over-the-counter preparations used for treating lice are generally not useful in treating scabies, because they are not absorbed through the skin. For pregnant women and infants, a prescription preparation known as Eurax is available. Fomites must also be treated in the same manner as with lice.

Prevention of Sexually Transmitted Disease

There are several things that can be done to prevent the spread of sexually transmitted diseases. One of the most obvious is abstaining from premarital and extramarital sex. Many of us choose just such a life-style either because of religious or moral beliefs or because of the fear of contracting a sexually transmitted disease.

The principal risk factor for acquiring STDs is having multiple sexual partners. Many studies have been done that demonstrate this to be extremely important in both homosexual and heterosexual populations. Be selective and limited in choosing sexual partners, and you will markedly reduce, although not completely eliminate, your risk.

When having a new or indiscriminate sex contact, men should wear a condom, because it is the most efficient method of birth control in terms of the prevention of STDs. If there is any chance of disease transmission, you should insist on the use of condoms. Condoms provide protection to both partners, but in heterosexual contacts, the female is afforded greater protection than the male.

Soap and water will sometimes eliminate some of the organisms responsible for STDs. Although it is not particularly effective in preventing sexually transmitted diseases, it is prudent for you to wash with soap and water after a new or casual sexual contact.

Both males and females should retain some urine in their bladders so that they can urinate after having sexual intercourse. You can often eliminate organisms that infect the urethra, such as gonorrhea and chlamydia, in this manner.

> ■ **PROBLEM SITUATION** You are about to have sexual intercourse with someone you do not know very well. What is the most important thing that you can do to protect yourself from getting a sexually transmitted disease? What do you say to your partner?

POSITIVE BEHAVIORS

I *Place a check mark in front of each behavior that you now practice.*

_____ 1. I do not engage in sexual activity with more than one partner. (ONE PARTNER)

_____ 2. I seek medical care whenever I have the symptoms of any sexually transmitted disease. (SYMPTOMS)

_____ 3. If I have a sexually transmitted disease, I freely give health officials the names and addresses of my sexual partners so that they can be treated. (FREELY GIVE)

_____ 4. If my partner informs me that he or she has a sexually transmitted disease, I seek medical care as soon as possible. (MEDICAL CARE)

_____ 5. If I become pregnant, I will obtain a blood test for syphilis. If someone I know becomes pregnant, I will encourage her to obtain the blood test. (PREGNANT)

_____ 6. If I acquire herpes simplex, I will do all that I can to maintain a strong immune system to prevent recurrences. (PREVENT RECURRENCES)

_____ 7. If I am considered at risk for hepatitis B, I will seek active immunization. (HEPATITIS B)

_____ 8. I will (or will require my partner to) use a condom when having a casual sexual contact. (USE A CONDOM)

II. *For each behavior that you DO NOT ENGAGE IN, write in the appropriate space below the KEY WORD(S) located in the parentheses at the end of the statement. Then indicate whether you intend to keep or change that behavior.*

Behaviors I Don't Engage In   KEEP/CHANGE

_____   _____/_____
_____   _____/_____
_____   _____/_____
_____   _____/_____
_____   _____/_____
_____   _____/_____
_____   _____/_____
_____   _____/_____

III. *For each of the preceding behaviors that you choose to KEEP, write a statement indicating why you are choosing to keep that behavior.*

I choose to keep behavior _____ because:
                           KEY WORD

For each of the preceding behaviors that you choose to CHANGE, write a statement indicating how you plan to implement that change.

I will change behavior _____ by:
                        KEY WORD

Now You Know

1. TRUE. There are more than twenty diseases that can be transmitted through sexual contact.
2. TRUE. The rates of most sexually transmitted diseases have been on the increase since the mid 1950s. Prevention is the best way to break the chain of infection.
3. TRUE. Evidence conclusively points to the fact that the more sexual partners you have, the greater the risk of acquiring a sexually transmitted disease.
4. FALSE. The only sexually transmitted disease for which there is an immunization is hepatitis B. There is no immunization or lasting immunity available against any of the other STDs.
5. FALSE. The victims of many of the sexually transmitted diseases show no symptoms, yet can transmit the disease to others. If you come in contact with someone with an STD, seek medical care even if you do not have symptoms.
6. TRUE. Syphilis and gonorrhea, as well as a number of other STDs, are caused by bacteria and are easily treated with appropriate antibiotics.
7. TRUE. The use of condoms is the most effective way of preventing the transmission of gonorrhea and several other STDs.
8. FALSE. Most organisms that cause vaginal infections in women can cause urethral infections in men. Men will often be asymptomatic carriers and be able to transmit the disease to other female partners without having any signs of the illness themselves.
9. FALSE. Anyone can get AIDS through sexual contact with an infected individual. You need not be gay nor male to be susceptible.
10. FALSE. After treatment, herpes simplex virus remains in the body in a dormant state. Any reduction in immune system capability can lead to a recurrence of the infection.

Summary

1. There are more than twenty diseases that can be transmitted sexually, and their incidence has been on the rise since the mid-1950s.
2. Factors that have led to the increase in sexually transmitted disease include the birth control pill, impulsive behavior, ignorance, denial, irresponsibility, lack of reporting, the high incidence of asymptomatic victims, and lack of vaccines.
3. Syphilis is caused by a bacteria and is characterized in its early stage by a single painless sore called a chancre. The disease is easily treated with appropriate antibiotics. Untreated syphilis can result in horrible disfigurement and death.
4. Gonorrhea is the most widespread of the reportable sexually transmitted diseases; almost a million cases are reported nationwide annually. It is caused by a bacteria and can be successfully treated with appropriate antibiotics. Untreated gonorrhea can lead to sterility.
5. A number of diseases, such as chlamydia and bacterial vaginosis, can lead to cervicitis or vaginitis in the female and urethritis in the male. Many victims of these diseases are asymptomatic but can pass their disease to sexual partners. In both sexes, serious complications can result from untreated cases.
6. Some less common but serious sexually transmitted diseases caused by bacteria include chancroid, granuloma inguinale, and lymphogranuloma venereum.
7. AIDS is a viral disease that leads to destruction of the body's immune system, resulting in death from some opportunistic infection. AIDS patients invariably die from their disease.
8. Herpes is caused by a virus transmitted through direct contact with an infected individual. There is no prevention, other than avoiding contact with infected persons, and no cure. Once a person becomes infected, the virus remains in his or her body for life and may cause recurrences at times when there is reduced immune capability.
9. Hepatitis B is the only sexually transmitted disease for which there is a vaccine. Hepatitis B immune globulin can be used for passive immunity.
10. Venereal warts are caused by viruses and are becoming more common. There is an association between venereal warts and cancer of the cervix.
11. *Candida albicans* is a yeast. It causes an infection that can be treated successfully with appropriate vaginal creams. The organism is normally present in the vagina and can cause symptoms when allowed to overgrow because of the use of birth control pills or antibiotics, the wearing of nylon bathings suits, and other factors.
12. Pubic lice are transmitted through direct contact and through fomites. They are easily treated with over-the-counter remedies and prescription medications.
13. Scabies is caused by a tiny mite and can be transmitted through direct contact and fomites. Treatment with the prescription medication lindane is usually successful.
14. A number of measures can be directed at preventing the transmission of STDs. These include avoiding indiscriminate sex contacts, using condoms, and reducing your number of sexual partners.

References

1. Benenson, Abram, ed. *Control of Communicable Diseases in Man*, 14th ed. Washington, D.C.: American Public Health Association, 1985.
2. The Blade-Citizen. "Drug Hailed as Step Toward Managing AIDS." Oceanside, CA: Aug. 18, 1989.
3. California State Department of Health. *A Manual for the Control of Communicable Diseases*. California State Department of Health, 1977.
4. Clark, Cheryl. "AIDS Virus is Reported in Bowel, Rectal Tissues." San Diego Union, San Diego, CA. Feb. 5, 1988.
5. Friedman, Gary D. *Primer of Epidemiology*, 2d ed. New York: McGraw-Hill, 1980.
6. Kerrins, Joseph, and George Jacobs. *What We Need to Know about AIDS Now!*, 2d ed. Woods Hole, Mass.: Cromlech Books, 1989.
7. Mausner, Judith S., and Anita K. Bahn. *Epidemiology: An Introductory Text*. Philadelphia: W. B. Saunders Co., 1974.
8. Shurkin, Joel N. "The AIDS Debate: Another View." Los Angeles Times, Los Angeles, CA. Jan. 18, 1988.
9. U. S. Department of Health and Human Services, Centers for Disease Control. "Summary of Notifiable Diseases, United States, 1985, 1986." *Morbidity and Mortality Weekly Report* 33 & 34, no. 54 (1986, 1987).
10. U. S. Department of Health and Human Services, Centers for Disease Control. "Annual Summary: 1980, 1981, 1982, 1983." *Morbidity and Mortality Weekly Report* 29–32, no. 54 (1981–1984).
11. Youmans, Guy P., Philip Y. Paterson, and Herbert M. Sommers. *The Biologic and Clinical Basis of Infectious Diseases*, 2d ed. Philadelphia: W. B. Saunders Co., 1980.

Suggested Readings

Brandt, A. *No Magic Bullet*. New York: Oxford University Press, 1987.

Kerrins, Joseph, and George W. Jacobs. *The AIDS File*, 2d ed. Woods Hole, Mass.: Cromlech Books, 1988.

Morbidity and Mortality Weekly Report, 1989 STD Treatment Guidelines. Washington, D.C.: U.S. Public Health Service, Centers for Disease Control, 1989.

Purtilo, David T. *A Survey of Human Diseases*. Menlo Park, Calif.: Addison-Wesley, 1978.

Wickett, W. H. *Herpes: Causes and Control*. New York: Pinnacle Books, 1982.

CHAPTER 16

Becoming Heart Smart

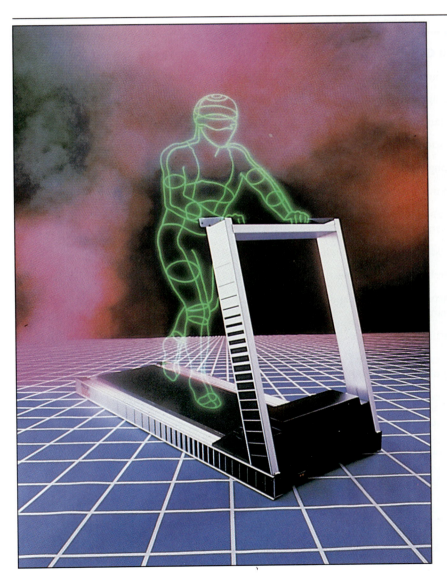

What Do You Know?

Are the following statements true or false?

1. Most deaths in the United States today are due to infectious diseases.
2. Most causes of death today are, at least to some degree, controllable.
3. It takes about an hour for blood to leave the heart, circulate through the body, and return to the heart.
4. A blood pressure of 150/100 would be considered high blood pressure.
5. High blood pressure with no known cause is called essential hypertension.
6. A diet high in saturated fat lowers the risk of cardiovascular disease.
7. High blood pressure has several early warning signs to alert you to seek medical care.
8. Cigarette smoking is the principal cause of premature death from cardiovascular disease.
9. Essential hypertension generally begins between the ages of forty and fifty.
10. It is best to maintain a high ratio of high-density lipoproteins.

Risk Factors and Their Relationship to Chronic Disease

At the turn of the century, infectious diseases were responsible for the majority of premature deaths in the United States. Through the development of immunizations and the discovery of the wide variety of antibiotics available to modern medical science, we have come a long way in conquering and treating these diseases. Infectious disease is no longer the threat it once was (with the exception of viral diseases such as AIDS).

TABLE 16–1 Years of Potential Life Lost (YPLL) Before Age 65[a]—United States, 1987

Cause of death	YPLL for Persons Dying in 1986	YPLL for Persons Dying in 1987	Cause-Specific Mortality Rate[b] 1987
All Causes (Total)	12,093,486	12,045,778	874.0
Unintentional injuries[c]	2,358,426	2,295,710	39.0
Malignant neoplasms	1,832,210	1,837,742	196.1
Heart diseases	1,557,041	1,494,227	313.4
Suicide/Homicide	1,360,508	1,289,223	21.2
Congenital anomalies	661,117	642,551	5.0
Prematurity[d]	428,796	422,813	2.7
Human immunodeficiency virus infection[e]	246,823	357,536	5.4
Sudden infant death syndrome	340,431	286,733	1.8
Cerebrovascular disease	246,131	246,479	61.3
Chronic liver disease and cirrhosis	231,558	228,145	10.7
Pneumonia/Influenza	175,386	166,775	28.8
Chronic obstructive pulmonary disease	128,590	123,260	32.2
Diabetes mellitus	121,117	119,155	15.6

[a]For details of calculation, see footnotes to Table V, *MMWR* 1988;37:45.

[b]Cause-specific mortality rates as reported by the National Center for Health Statistics (NCHS) are compiled from a 10 percent sample of all deaths.

[c]Equivalent to accidents and adverse effects.

[d]Category derived from disorders relating to short gestation and respiratory distress syndrome.

[e]1986 data is from CDC surveillance of acquired immunodeficiency disease cases. Data for 1987 is derived from death certificates coded to the *International Classification of Diseases, Ninth Revision* (ICD-9) codes 042-044 for HIV infection. These codes were introduced into the national vital statistics system by NCHS in 1987.

SOURCE: Morbidity and Mortality Weekly Report, Centers for Disease Control, Vol. 38/No.2.

Today the principal causes of death among the elderly include such chronic diseases as cardiovascular disease and cancer. In younger age groups, accidents, drug overdose, suicide, and homicide are among the threats to life (see Table 16–1). These causes of death are partially the result of life-style habits and are, at least to some degree, controllable.

For example, the primary risk factors associated with heart attack are diabetes, overweight, lack of exercise, smoking, and a family history of heart disease. Other risk factors include high stress levels and excessive amounts of saturated fat in the diet. The only factor over which you would have no control would be your family history. Certainly, weight, exercise, and smoking are factors over which direct control is possible. Even diabetes can be controlled somewhat. If you have a genetic predisposition for diabetes because of your family history, diet and exercise could delay the onset of the disease and could help control it should it develop.

Motor vehicle accidents are related to alcohol use, miles driven per year, seatbelt use and drug use. Drinking less than six drinks per week, wearing a seatbelt at least 75 percent of the time, and using drugs rarely or never can reduce your risk of being killed or seriously injured in an accident. The only factor in this area that you might not be able to control is miles driven per year if those miles were a necessary part of your employment.

Cancer risks can be substantially reduced through self-examination. Breast self exams and testicular self exams will be discussed in the next chapter. Annual pap smears for women and annual rectal examinations for everyone over forty years of age are essential. By not smoking and by reducing alcohol consumption, you will reduce the risk of several types of cancer as well as other diseases. Reducing exposure to the sun's harmful rays can all but eliminate the risk of skin cancer.

In this chapter and Chapter 17, we are concerned specifically with chronic diseases and the ways in which we can help to prevent problems associated with them. Table 16–2 indicates the most common causes of death for 20-year old males and females.

FAST FACTS

Heart disease is the third leading cause of "years of potential life lost" for people before the age of 65.

TABLE 16–2 ■ Chances of Dying per 100,000 People Within the Next Ten Years

Rank	White Females Aged 20 Cause of Death	
1	Motor vehicle accidents	145
2	Suicide	76
3	Nonmotor vehicle accidents	45
4	Homicide	42
5	Stroke	16
6	Leukemia	14
7	Pneumonia	11
8	Lymphosarcoma/Hodgkins	10
9	Cancer of the brain	8
10	Diabetes	8
11	Breast cancer	8
12	Circulatory defects	8
	All other causes	212
	All causes of death	603

TABLE 16–2 ■ **Chances of Dying per 100,000 People Within the Next Ten Years, continued**

White Males Aged 20

Rank	Cause of Death	
1	Motor vehicle accidents	563
2	Nonmotor vehicle accidents	289
3	Suicide	269
4	Homicide	146
5	Leukemia	20
6	Stroke	18
7	Lymphosarcoma/Hodgkins	17
8	Heart attack	17
9	Pneumonia	15
10	Cancer of the brain	11
11	Cirrhosis of the liver	11
12	Circulatory defects	11
	All other causes	<u>348</u>
	All causes of death	1,745

Black Females Aged 20

Rank	Cause of Death	
1	Homicide	270
2	Motor vehicle accidents	100
3	Nonmotor vehicle accidents	98
4	Suicide	59
5	Stroke	41
6	Cirrhosis of the liver	39
7	Pneumonia	28
8	Heart attack	17
9	Diabetes	16
10	Anemias	16
11	Complications of pregnancy	15
12	Leukemia	15
	All other causes	<u>575</u>
	All causes of death	1,289

Black Males Aged 20

Rank	Cause of Death	
1	Homicide	1,369
2	Motor vehicle accidents	500
3	Nonmotor vehicle accidents	449
4	Suicide	239
5	Cirrhosis of the liver	73
6	Stroke	48
7	Heart attack	47
8	Pneumonia	44
9	Alcoholism	31
10	Anemias	25
11	Rheumatic heart disease	20
12	Diabetes	18
	All other causes	<u>878</u>
	All causes of death	3,741

SOURCE: Centers for Disease Control Adult Health Risk Appraisal

Cardiovascular Disease

Some Physiology

To begin our discussion of **cardiovascular disease,** let us review some basic physiology related to circulation and the heart.

Each time your heart pumps, it pushes about 75 ml. (approximately 2½ oz.) of blood through your body. The entire trip—out from your heart, through the body, and back again—takes about one minute. The pumping action of the heart occurs in two phases, the contraction phase known as *systole* and the relaxation phase known as *diastole*.

Large arteries take the blood from the heart to the lungs and the rest of your body. As the blood moves further and further away, the arteries get smaller and smaller. The smaller arteries are called *arterioles*. These eventually reduce in size even more and become *capillaries*. Some capillaries are so narrow that blood cells have to pass through in single file.

It is in the capillaries that the exchange of gases and other substances takes place between the blood and the cells. Oxygen in the blood is transferred to the body cells, and, in turn, they give up their carbon dioxide and other waste materials for the blood to transport away for elimination from the body.

From the capillaries, the blood enters the venous system for the return trip back to the heart. The smaller veins are known as *venules*. Review the diagram of the circulatory system. (Figure 16–1.) Can you identify the only artery in the body that contains deoxygenated blood? How about the only vein that contains oxygenated blood?

Hypertension

What Is Blood Pressure? What causes high blood pressure and why should we be so concerned about it? Blood circulates in a closed system. In any closed system containing fluid, some pressure will be created. In the circulatory system, additional factors include the pumping action of the heart and the elasticity of the artery walls.

Your blood pressure is measured in millimeters of mercury similar to the way that barometric pressure is measured in inches of mercury. You might have your blood pressure taken and be told that it is 110/60 (that would be correctly expressed as 110/60 mm. Hg.). The upper number is called the *systolic* pressure, because it is the pressure in the arteries during systole. The lower number is the *diastolic* pressure, because it is the pressure in the arteries during diastole.

It is fairly easy to understand how systolic pressure is created in the arteries. When the heart contracts and forces blood out into the arterial system, that pumping action creates pressure. When the heart is at rest, what causes the diastolic pressure? The answer is **peripheral resistance.** Artery walls are lined with muscle tissue, which gives them a degree of elasticity. That elasticity creates pressure against the fluid in the arteries, even when the heart is at rest. The result is diastolic pressure.

What's Normal? Normal blood pressure varies from person to person. We can say that a particular sex and age group might have an "average" blood pressure, but we cannot define a "normal" pressure for any group. For example, it is generally accepted that the average blood pressure among the college-age

FAST FACTS

In urban-western cultures, blood pressure increases gradually with increasing age.

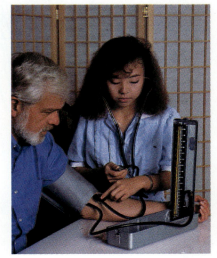

Each one of us should have his or her blood pressure checked on a regular basis. Any reading indicating the possibility of hypertension should be followed up by a thorough physical exam by a physician.

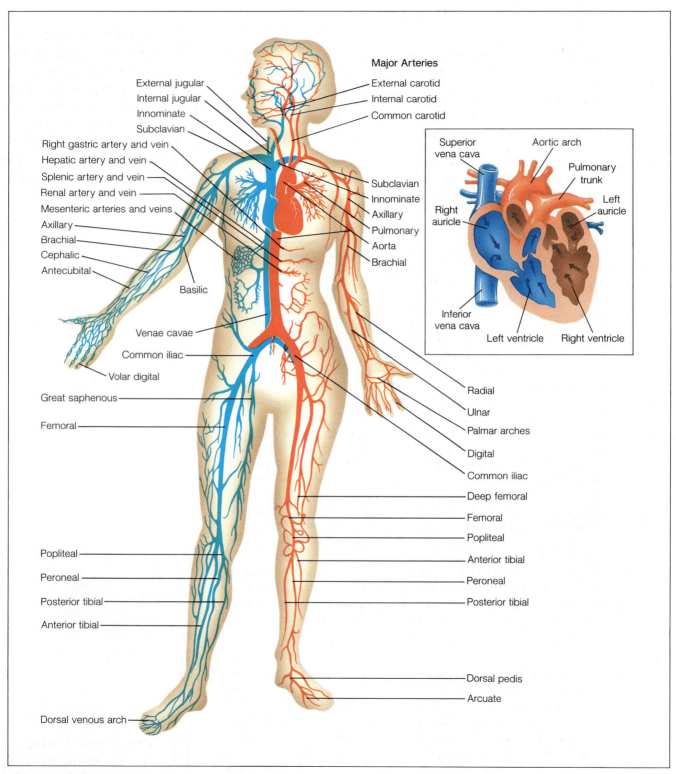

FIGURE 16–1 ■ The Circulatory System

population is about 120/80. That does not mean that you are abnormal if your blood pressure is either higher or lower than the average (as long as it isn't so high as to be considered dangerous).

Because pressure may vary greatly from person to person and still be considered within normal range, you should know your own normal blood pressure. Otherwise, you could not tell when pressure was abnormal, because you would have no normal values with which to make a comparison.

Let's assume, for example, that two students were traveling together in a car and had an accident. One student has a normal blood pressure of 120/80 and the other's is normal at 100/60. One of the first things that the paramedics would do on arrival at the accident would be to take the blood pressures of both victims. If both had a measurement of 100/60, would the paramedics be able to tell their condition without knowing the normal pressures of the two students?

What Is Hypertension? When a person's blood pressure is 140/90 or higher, **hypertension** (high blood pressure) is diagnosed. Although some medical practitioners believe that the diastolic pressure is more important than the systolic, most experts do not agree with that contention. It is true, however, that the diastolic pressure fluctuates less than the systolic in response to environmental factors such as stress and fear. Therefore, a change in diastolic pressure may be a more meaningful indicator that something is wrong. Of course, one reading of 140/90 does not mean that a person has hypertension. A few readings, several days apart and under low-stress conditions, should be made to confirm that true hypertension exists.

Twenty percent of Americans suffer from hypertension, making it the most common chronic disease in this country. Many people with hypertension are not even aware that they have it, because there are no early warning signs and no symptoms. For these reasons, it is sometimes known as the "silent killer." It is estimated that only about 30 percent of people with hypertension have it under control. Millions of others are not being treated for their hypertension or are receiving inadequate treatment.

In about 10 percent of patients diagnosed with high blood pressure, the problem can be traced to a specific organic cause, such as kidney disease or a brain tumor. In these cases, the hypertension, known as *secondary hypertension,* may be eradicated by correcting the underlying problem.

In the remaining 90 percent of hypertensive people, the high blood pressure can not be traced to any identifiable cause. This type of hypertension is known as *essential hypertension;* it is sometimes also called *primary hypertension, diastolic hypertension* or *idiopathic hypertension.* Does anyone in your family have essential hypertension?

Risk Factors. Although one of the risk factors for essential hypertension is a family history of the disease—something over which we have no control—there are things that we can do to help prevent the condition from developing. The two most important elements are diet and exercise. Aerobic exercise (see Chapter 6) is extremely important in maintaining cardiovascular fitness. Diet as it affects hypertension is important in two areas. The first and most significant is weight control. Failure to maintain low to average body weight places added burdens on the heart and the entire cardiovascular system. The second dietary factor is sodium intake. Americans generally consume far more salt than they need. The

---

FAST FACTS

Symptoms of hypotension (low blood pressure) are weakness, dizziness, and tiring easily. Most people with hypotension do not experience these symptoms and may actually have a greater life expectancy than people with "normal" average blood pressure.

FAST FACTS

Recent surveys have shown an increase in obesity among children of both sexes.

FAST FACTS

Smoking more than fifteen cigarettes per day is considered heavy smoking for women taking birth control pills. This presents a risk factor for cardiovascular disease.

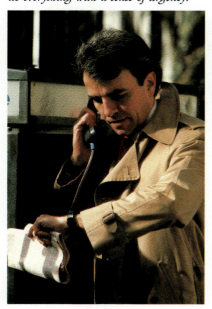

Type A individuals are competitive and do everything with a sense of urgency.

sodium in salt increases fluid retention and thereby increases blood pressure. It is essential that all of us, but especially those with a family history of hypertension, control our sodium intake. In addition to salt, sodium is found in many foods and food additives.

Another risk factor over which we have total control is smoking. Cigarette smoking is the principal cause of premature death from cardiovascular disease in this country. Some of the effects of smoking and nicotine were explored in Chapter 11.

Age, race, and sex are also risk factors. Black males tend to have the highest incidence of hypertension. Women have nearly double the rate of hypertension of men but seem to be less likely to develop long-term complications.

Type A or Type B. Two San Francisco cardiologists, Meyer Friedman and Ray Rosenman, studied the effects of stress on cardiovascular disease. Their first modest research study involved accountants during the tax season. They discovered that during the two weeks prior to April 15th (the tax filing deadline), the blood-cholesterol levels and blood-clotting rates of the accountants in their study rose significantly. During the months of May and June, after the tax season was over, the levels dropped back within normal range. Both blood-cholesterol level and clotting time are related to cardiovascular disease.

Friedman and Rosenman classified the individuals whom they studied as *Type A* and *Type B* personalities. Type A individuals tend to drive themselves very hard, are quite competitive and ambitious, do everything with a sense of urgency, and take on multiple tasks at the same time. Type B people are unhurried and noncompetitive, the reverse of Type A. Most of us are neither completely Type A nor Type B but somewhere in between. Some studies have shown that Type A people have a significantly higher incidence of cardiovascular disease. However, other studies suggest that Type A individuals have a better chance of surviving a heart attack than Type B individuals.

If you are a Type A person, you are not necessarily destined for an early death from cardiovascular disease. Other work by Friedman and Rosenman showed that Type A individuals can successfully alter those personality traits that place them at high risk.

At what age does essential hypertension begin? Although it varies greatly from person to person, on the average it begins between the ages of twenty and thirty. The complications generally begin to show much later in life, but we can do a great deal to prevent those complications with healthy life-style habits developed while we are still young.

Treatment. Hypertension should be treated with a combination of diet, exercise, drugs, and stress reduction. Proper diet is designed to reduce weight and limit salt intake. Exercise is necessary to maintain a healthy level of cardiovascular fitness. In many patients, hypertension could be controlled through diet and exercise alone. In the majority of patients, however, drugs are necessary. Once started, drug therapy will usually have to be continued for life.

The first line of defense in drug therapy is through the use of *diuretics*. Diuretics are drugs that remove fluid from the system, reducing the volume of blood and thereby reducing pressure inside the closed circulatory system. In individuals in whom the diuretics are not enough, *vasodilator* drugs are added to the regimen. These drugs relax the muscles in the artery walls, causing a subsequent reduction of pressure inside.

> ■ *PROBLEM SITUATION* Your father tells you that he has visited the family physician for a routine physical examination and has been told that he has high blood pressure. He feels fine, so he intends to do nothing about it until he experiences symptoms. What is your advice to your father? Why?

Arteriosclerosis

What happens if hypertension is not controlled? The arterial walls consist of three layers. The middle layer, or media, is a layer of muscle. If hypertension causes the pressure inside the arteries to remain constantly high, the muscles of the media are continuously challenged to push back against that pressure. This causes the muscles of the media to become big and hard. (*Arteriosclerosis* means "hardening of the arteries.") The enlarging of these muscles causes the opening in the artery (the lumen) to become smaller, restricting the flow of blood and leading to additional increase in pressure. Also, the hardening of the muscles causes the artery walls to lose some of their elasticity. (See Figure 16–2.)

In extreme cases, the lumen may become completely obstructed, reducing circulation to almost zero. The four parts of the body that are most susceptible to damage from this reduced circulation are the heart, brain, kidneys, and extremities. Lack of circulation to the extremities can result in tissue death and **gangrene,** necessitating amputation of a limb. This is generally a problem in the legs, not the arms. Kidney failure, resulting from lack of effective circulation to the kidneys, can lead to death.

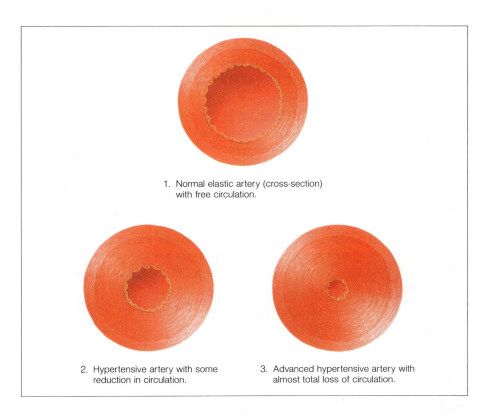

FIGURE 16–2 ■ **Hypertension in an Artery**

1. Normal elastic artery (cross-section) with free circulation.
2. Hypertensive artery with some reduction in circulation.
3. Advanced hypertensive artery with almost total loss of circulation.

Angina Pectoris. In the heart, a number of serious conditions may arise. One of the more common is *angina pectoris,* which literally translated into common terms means "pain in the chest." Angina results from a lack of circulation to cardiac muscle, which leads to inadequate oxygen supply at times of increased demand. Angina patients usually have an adequate oxygen supply during nonstressful times but not enough to meet extra needs at times of exertion, such as during physical activities, sex, or sometimes just walking up a flight of stairs. The resulting lack of oxygen causes severe pain.

Treatment for angina generally involves the use of a variety of drugs designed to dilate the coronary arteries, thereby increasing the blood and oxygen supply to the cardiac muscle. Some patients take their medication only when an angina attack occurs, whereas others may have to take the drugs on a regular basis to prevent attacks.

Heart Attack. If an artery transporting blood to the heart muscle becomes obstructed, the tissue it normally feeds will die from the inability to receive oxygen. This event is called a *myocardial infarction* (MI), or heart attack. The portion of the heart muscle that dies because of lack of oxygen ultimately forms scar tissue. The scarred area is called an infarct. (See Figure 16–3.)

The size of the obstructed artery will determine the size of the affected area and the victim's chances of survival. Some heart attacks destroy very small areas of heart muscle and may not even be felt by the victim; these are sometimes called "silent heart attacks." Others may be so massive as to kill the victim within a few minutes.

Congestive Heart Failure. Another result of arteriosclerosis may be *congestive heart failure* (CHF). In congestive heart failure, the ventricles (the lower chambers of the heart) may fail to pump adequately, causing blood to back up into the circulation of the victim's lungs. Fluid is then forced into the lungs and the victim has difficulty breathing, which may possibly lead to death.

Transient Ischemic Attack. Several complications in the brain may be caused by arteriosclerosis. A *transient ischemic attack* (TIA) is a temporary lack of oxygen to a portion of brain tissue. Symptoms vary, depending on the portion of brain not receiving adequate circulation, and may include temporary paralysis, slurred

GUIDELINES TO YOUR GOOD HEALTH

The following can help to reduce your risk of cardiovascular disease:

1. Reduce the amount of salt in your diet.
2. Maintain acceptable body weight.
3. Participate in aerobic exercise for at least twenty minutes every other day.
4. Do not use tobacco.
5. Set aside a few minutes each day for a quiet time to relax.
6. Reduce the level of saturated fat in your diet.
7. Check your blood pressure regularly.

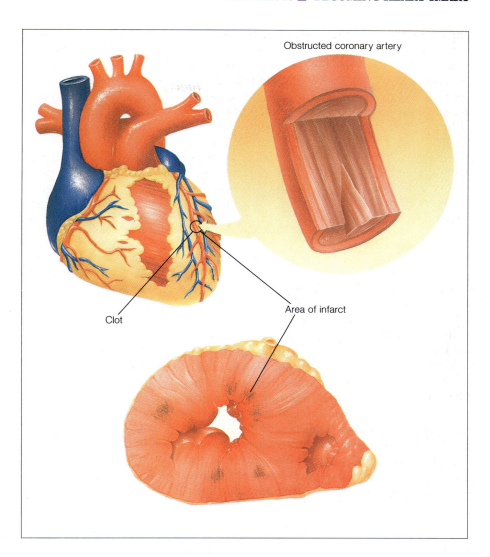

FIGURE 16–3 ■ **Myocardial Infarction**

speech, blurred vision, and loss of consciousness. TIAs normally last less than twenty-four hours.

Stroke. A *stroke,* also known as a cerebrovascular accident (CVA), can be caused by a variety of events, including the breaking of capillaries in the brain or the ballooning of a blood vessel that produces pressure on surrounding brain tissue. Often, complete obstruction of an artery as a result of arteriosclerosis is a cause. Strokes can cause permanent damage to brain tissue. Symptoms may resemble those of a transient ischemic attack but are not temporary. Long-term rehabilitation is frequently necessary to return a stroke victim to a fairly normal life. Strokes may also kill their victims.

■ *PROBLEM SITUATION* Your sister is several pounds overweight, doesn't exercise, and smokes twenty cigarettes a day. What can you do to encourage her to change these life-style factors?

GUIDELINES TO YOUR GOOD HEALTH

If you or someone you know exhibits the following signs or symptoms, which may suggest a heart attack, seek medical care immediately:

1. Pain or a squeezing sensation in the chest located directly below the breastbone.
2. Chest pain that radiates from the chest, usually to the left arm, neck, jaw, and back.
3. Nausea associated with the preceding symptoms.
4. Perspiration, fainting, lightheadedness, and shortness of breath.

Atherosclerosis

We have talked about how long-term untreated hypertension can cause arteriosclerosis and how that can subsequently lead to a variety of problems in the body. Another form of arteriosclerosis that can cause the same problems is atherosclerosis, a disease of fat metabolism.

In atherosclerosis, fatty deposits known as plaques are deposited along the inner lining, or **intima,** of the artery walls. These fatty deposits narrow the lumen of the artery, thereby reducing circulation and increasing pressure within the arteries. The accumulation of fatty deposits probably begins very early in life. Autopsies done on soldiers killed in the Vietnam War showed that many of them had well-developed atherosclerotic plaques even in their late teens and early twenties. Some scientists have theorized that this process may start even before birth. Figure 16–4 shows how plaque develops in atherosclerosis.

When fats are taken into the body and digested, they are combined with protein so that they can be transported from place to place. These fat-protein molecules are known as lipoproteins. Lipoproteins are classified in several dif-

FIGURE 16–4 ■ **Early and Late Atherosclerosis**

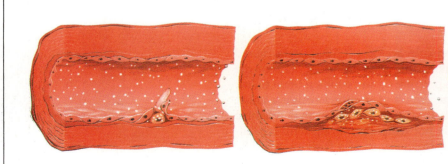

1. The beginning of the accumulation of atherosclerotic plaque on the intima of an artery wall.

2. The plaque increases in size and becomes incorporated in the artery wall.

3. The artery becomes extremely narrowed and clot formation becomes likely.

ferent ways, but for our discussion, we will use the classification system that separates them by density. In this system, they are identified as high-density (HDL), low-density (LDL), and very-low-density (VLDL) lipoproteins.

High-density lipoproteins are, in part, responsible for transporting excess fat to the liver, where it can be metabolized and removed from the body as waste. The low-density lipoproteins are responsible for moving excess fatty materials to areas of the body where they can be stored. In what ratio would you like to have your HDLs and LDLs? It is better to have a high ratio of HDLs to LDLs in order to reduce the accumulation of excess fat stores in the body. What can you do to effect changes in this ratio?

It is well documented that aerobic exercise increases HDL/LDL ratios. Therefore, a well-planned fitness program can help you reduce the storage of fat by

---

SELF-INVENTORY 16.1

Your Risk for Cardiovascular Disease

The following factors relate to your risk for cardiovascular disease. Respond to each statement by placing a check mark under the appropriate column to the right of the statement.

	Yes	No	Not Sure
1. Do you know your blood pressure?	___	___	___
2. Have you had your blood pressure checked within the last year?	___	___	___
3. Is your blood pressure within normal range?	___	___	___
4. Do you do aerobic exercise at least three times a week for at least 20 minutes each session?	___	___	___
5. Do you have a family history of cardiovascular disease?	___	___	___
6. Have you ever been told that you have hypertension?	___	___	___
7. Do you consume large amounts of salt (over 3,000 mg. per day) in your diet?	___	___	___
8. Do you smoke cigarettes?	___	___	___
9. Do you drink excessive amounts of alcohol (more than six drinks per week)?	___	___	___
10. Do you have a high-fat diet?	___	___	___
11. Do you have a high-calorie diet?	___	___	___
12. Are you a type A personality?	___	___	___

If you answered "Yes" to the first four questions and "No" to the others, you are at low risk for cardiovascular disease. Many of these questions relate to life-style factors over which you have control. Positive changes in these behaviors can significantly reduce your risk.

FAST FACTS

A three-ounce chocolate bar contains over 16 grams of saturated fat and 18 milligrams of cholesterol.

increasing the amount of HDLs, which subsequently increases the rate at which excess fat is removed from your body.

Diet, of course, is an important factor. Reducing the intake of **saturated fat** will reduce the quantity of low-density lipoproteins, thereby increasing the HDL/LDL ratio. Fat saturated with hydrogen is most abundant in animal products, dairy products, and vegetable fats that are solids at room temperature, such as coconut oil. See Chapter 4 for a discussion of saturated fat versus unsaturated fat in the diet.

Atherosclerosis can lead to the same complications as arteriosclerosis caused by high blood pressure. In addition, the two conditions often complicate each other, leading to the victim's even faster deterioration.

POSITIVE BEHAVIORS

I. *Place a check mark in front of each behavior that you now practice.*

_____ 1. I know my normal blood pressure reading. (BLOOD PRESSURE)
_____ 2. I maintain a low level of saturated fat in my diet. (SATURATED FAT)
_____ 3. I encourage my family members and friends to have their blood pressures checked regularly and to maintain healthy diets. (ENCOURAGE)
_____ 4. I avoid being overweight or obese. (OVERWEIGHT)
_____ 5. I participate in a regular program of aerobic exercise. (AEROBIC EXERCISE)
_____ 6. I control the amount of salt in my diet. (SALT)
_____ 7. I do not smoke cigarettes. (CIGARETTES)
_____ 8. If I am being treated by my physician with drugs for hypertension, I follow his or her instructions and take my medication regularly. (MEDICATION)

II. *For each behavior that you DO NOT ENGAGE IN, write in the appropriate space below the KEY WORD(S) located in the parentheses at the end of the statement. Then indicate whether you intend to keep or change that behavior.*

Behaviors I Don't Engage In   KEEP/CHANGE
_____   _____/_____
_____   _____/_____
_____   _____/_____
_____   _____/_____
_____   _____/_____
_____   _____/_____
_____   _____/_____
_____   _____/_____

III. *For each of the preceding behaviors that you choose to KEEP, write a statement indicating why you are choosing to keep that behavior.*

I choose to keep behavior _____ because:
                            KEY WORD

For each of the preceding behaviors that you choose to CHANGE, write a statement indicating how you plan to implement that change.

I will change behavior _____ by:
                        KEY WORD

Now You Know

1. FALSE. Most deaths in the United States today are caused by chronic diseases such as cancer and cardiovascular disease, illnesses over which we can exercise some degree of control through a healthy life-style.

2. TRUE. Deaths from motor vehicle accidents, homicide, drug overdose, and suicide are among the principal threats to life in younger age groups. Some control can be exercised over chronic diseases through positive changes in life-style habits.

3. FALSE. It takes only about one minute for blood to make the complete trip from the heart, through the body, and back to the heart.

4. TRUE. Any blood pressure reading above 140/90 would be considered hypertension and would require follow-up by a physician.

5. TRUE. High blood pressure with no known cause is called essential, primary, or diastolic hypertension.

6. FALSE. Too much saturated fat leads to the formation of excess cholesterol and to a poor HDL/LDL ratio. Fat in the diet should be monounsaturated or polyunsaturated, such as is found in canola, olive, safflower, or sunflower oils.

7. FALSE. There are no early warning signs of high blood pressure. For this reason, it has become known as "the silent killer."

8. TRUE. Although other factors, such as obesity and lack of exercise, contribute to death from cardiovascular disease, the leading factor is cigarette smoking.

9. FALSE. Essential hypertension generally begins during the third decade of life, between the ages of twenty and thirty.

10. TRUE. High-density lipoproteins contribute to the removal of excess fats from the body.

Summary

1. At the turn of the century, most deaths were due to infectious diseases. Today, chronic diseases, over which we have some degree of control, are responsible for the majority of deaths.

2. Diabetes, overweight, lack of exercise, and cigarette smoking are the primary risk factors associated with heart disease.

3. Normal blood pressure varies from person to person; however, a blood pressure above 140/90 should be investigated by a physician.

4. Systolic pressure is the top number of a blood pressure reading and is caused by the pumping action of the heart. Diastolic pressure is the bottom number and is the result of peripheral resistance.

5. Ninety percent of all hypertension in the United States is essential hypertension; that is, there is no identifiable cause.

6. Twenty percent of Americans suffer from hypertension, making it the most common chronic disease in this country.

7. There are drugs that can be used to treat hypertension. Diet and exercise are extremely important and may completely eliminate the need for drugs in some people.

8. Aerobic exercise, maintenance of normal body weight, not smoking, and stress reduction all help to reduce the risk of cardiovascular disease.

9. A heart attack may result from obstruction of the arteries that feed oxygenated blood to the heart muscle. This may result from long-term arteriosclerosis or atherosclerosis.

10. Atherosclerosis is a disease of fat metabolism and is aggravated by obesity, lack of exercise, and a diet high in saturated fats.

11. Both arteriosclerosis from hypertension and atherosclerosis may lead to heart attack, congestive heart failure, angina pectoris, stroke, and other cardiovascular problems.

References

1. Bahlmann, J., and H. Liebaw. *Stress and Hypertension*. New York: Doubleday and Co., 1986.
2. Dunkle, Ruth E., and James W. Schmidley. *Stroke and the Elderly*. New York: Springer Publishing Co., 1987.
3. Freis, E. D. *The Treatment of Hypertension*. Baltimore: University Park Press, 1978.
4. Jones, Kenneth L., Louis W. Shainberg, and Curtis O. Byer. *Disease*, 2d ed. San Francisco: Canfield Press, 1975.
5. Kaplan, Norman, and Jeremiah Stamler. *Prevention of Coronary Heart Disease*. Philadelphia: W. B. Saunders Co., 1983.
6. Kochar, Mahendr S., and Karen D. Woods. *Hypertension Control*. New York: Springer Publishing Co., 1985.
7. Martin, Anthony, and A. John Camm. *Heart Disease in the Elderly*. New York: John Wiley and Sons, 1984.
8. Purtilo, David T. *A Survey of Human Diseases*. Menlo Park, Calif.: Addison-Wesley, 1978.

Suggested Readings

American Heart Association. *Heartbook: A Guide To Prevention and Treatment of Cardiovascular Disease.* New York: Elsevier-Dutton, 1980.

American Heart Association. *1988 Heart Facts.* Dallas: American Heart Association, 1989.

Bennett, Cleaves M. *Control Your Blood Pressure Without Drugs.* Garden City, N.Y.: Doubleday and Co., 1984.

Caris, T. *Understanding Hypertension.* New York: Warner Books, 1986.

Kaplan, N. M. *Prevent Your Heart Attack.* New York: Pinnacle Books, 1987.

Purtilo, David T. *A Survey of Human Diseases.* Menlo Park, Calif.: Addison-Wesley, 1978.

CHAPTER 17

Dealing With Chronic Disease

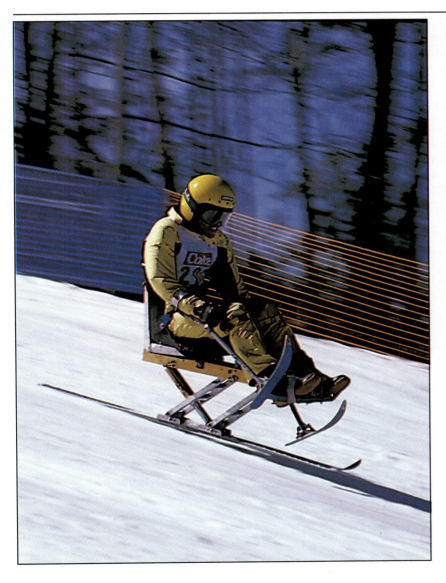

What Do You Know?

Are the following statements True or False?

1. A tumor or growth that is not cancerous is termed "benign."
2. Breast cancers occur only in women.
3. Lung cancers are easy to cure if discovered early.
4. Breast self examination is only a secondary means for discovering breast cancers.
5. The greatest risk for cancer of the testicles is among men ages fifteen to thirty-four.
6. Arthritis is a disease of only the elderly.
7. Arthritis can be prevented or cured by diet.
8. Type II diabetes can often be controlled through diet and exercise without the use of medication.
9. Epilepsy is a disease of children and is inherited.
10. Sickle-cell anemia does not affect only blacks.

Cancer

General Information about Cancer

Cancer, which is really a collection of diseases, is the second leading cause of death for all age groups in the United States and the leading cause of death among women forty to fifty-four years of age. Approximately one out of every four of us will develop some kind of cancer during our lifetime. Although cancer attacks older people more frequently than younger people, there are some forms of cancer that are far more prevalent among the young. During the past twenty to thirty years, case rates for cancer have been on the rise. There are many factors that account for this rise, including an increase in life expectancy (which allows more people to reach the age at which cancer is most prevalent), better diagnostic techniques, and the reduction in death rates from communicable disease.

The American Cancer Society reports that one out of every two cancer victims are saved today, compared to one out of four previously (see Figure 17–1). More lives could be saved with changes in life-style and the early diagnosis of cancer. Early diagnosis means that the malignancy must be detected before it has the opportunity to spread (see Table 17–1).

Terminology

A *tumor* is any swelling or enlargement in the body. Tumors are not necessarily made up of solid tissue nor are they necessarily cancerous. A *neoplasm* is a new growth of solid tissue and may be either *benign* (noncancerous) or *malignant* (cancerous).

Malignant tumors are characterized by disorderly and uncontrolled growth of cells. Benign tumors also involve abnormal cell growth, but they are sur-

FIGURE 17–1 ■ Cancer Incidence and Deaths by Site and Sex—1988 Estimates

SOURCE: "Cancer Facts and Figures—1988" American Cancer Society, New York, 1989.

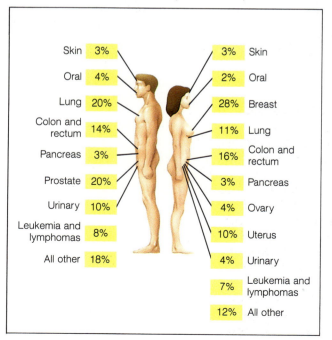

Cancer incidence by site and sex†

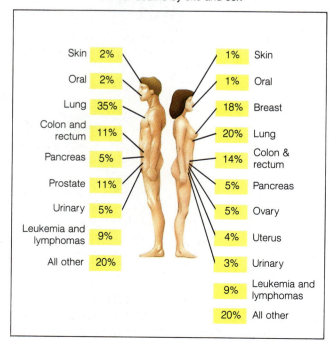

Cancer deaths by site and sex

†Excluding non-melanoma skin cancer and carcinoma in situ.

TABLE 17-1 ■ American Cancer Society Recommendations for Cancer Detection

Detection Procedure	Cancer	Who	When
Health counseling and cancer checkup	Thyroid, testes, prostate, ovary, lymph node, mouth, and skin	Everyone over age 20	Every 3 years between the ages of 20 and 40; yearly after age 40
Breast self-examination	Breast	All women over age 20	Every month
Breast physical examination	Breast	All women over age 20	Every 3 years for women age 40 and under; yearly thereafter
Mammography (breast X-ray)	Breast	All women over age 35	Baseline between the ages of 35 and 40; every 1 to 2 years between the ages of 40 and 49; yearly thereafter
Pelvic examination	Reproductive system cancers in women	All women over age 20	Every 3 years for women age 40 and under; yearly thereafter
Pap test (microscopic examination of cells)	Cervical	Women ages 20 to 65; younger women who are sexually active	After two negative exams 1 year apart, perform at least every 3 years[a]
Endometrial (uterine) tissue sample	Uterine	Women at high risk[b]	At menopause
Test for blood in stools	Colo-rectal	Everyone over age 50	Annually
Digital rectal examination	Rectal	Everyone over age 40	Annually
Sigmoidoscopy (examination of colon/rectum)	Colo-rectal	Everyone over age 50	After two negative exams 1 year apart, perform every 3 to 5 years

[a] The American College of Obstetrics and Gynecology recommends a *yearly* Pap test.
[b] High-risk women have histories of infertility, obesity, failure to ovulate, abnormal uterine bleeding, or estrogen therapy.
SOURCE: American Cancer Society.

rounded by a well-defined capsule that keeps them from invading surrounding tissue or spreading to other parts of the body. Benign tumors include growths such as **warts, cysts, polyps,** or **moles.** If you develop any of these benign growths, you should ask your physician about what course of action would be appropriate.

The spread of malignant cells to parts of the body distant from the site of the original tumor is called **metastasis,** and the new tumors are called *metastases*. They may occur when malignant cells leave the original tumor site and enter either the blood or **lymph system,** which transports them to other parts of the body where they begin to grow and set up secondary cancer sites. Once metastasis occurs, it becomes extremely difficult to successfully treat the victim's disease.

A *carcinoma* is a cancer in epithelial tissue such as skin or mucous membranes, whereas a *sarcoma* is a cancer in connective tissue such as bone, cartilage, or muscle. **Adenocarcinomas** arise from mucous glands found in epithelial tissue.

There are other specific cancers that we will discuss later, such as melanomas, lymphomas, and leukemias.

Benign versus Malignant Growths

No one is certain why certain cells begin to grow abnormally and uncontrollably. Theories point to changes in the DNA of the normal cell, possibly caused by such agents as radiation, chemicals, and viruses. Chance **mutations** might also play a role.

When abnormal growth does take place, it may be either benign or malignant. Benign tumors do not invade surrounding tissue, nor do they metastasize because of the capsule enclosing them. Generally, a person can have such growths removed surgically without any long-term effects. Rarely does a benign tumor kill its victim, although in a part of the body such as the brain, it might have that potential. Some benign tumors (moles, for example) can become malignant if they are subjected to certain types of excessive irritation.

The cells of a malignant tumor have a number of abnormalities that can be detected through microscopic examination. These include irregular size and shape, abnormal numbers of **chromosomes,** abnormal numbers of **nucleii,** ratio of nucleus to **cytoplasm,** and the way the cells take on stain for microscopic viewing. Malignant cells are capable of invading surrounding tissue and metastasizing to parts of the body far removed from the original site.

Risk Factors

Because the causes of cancer are still uncertain, we approach discussions of cancer prevention in terms of risk factors. Such risk factors include age, race, sex, hereditary influences, exposure to carcinogenic substances, socioeconomic factors, and occupational hazards.

Heredity. Most experts agree that there are some hereditary influences related to the risk of developing cancer. If you have immediate relatives with cancer, you are at a higher risk of developing cancer yourself. This is especially true of colon and breast cancers. It follows that if you have such a family history, you must be especially wary of the warning signs of cancer. You must also include self-examination, regular visits to your health-care professional, and proper diet in your life-style. Table 17–2 shows cancer's seven warning signs.

TABLE 17–2 ■ **Know Cancer's Seven Warning Signals**

1. Change in bowel or bladder habits.
2. A sore that does not heal.
3. Unusual bleeding or discharge.
4. Thickening or lump in breast or elsewhere.
5. Indigestion or difficulty in swallowing.
6. Obvious change in wart or mole.
7. Nagging cough or hoarseness.

If you have a warning signal, see your doctor.

SOURCE: American Cancer Society

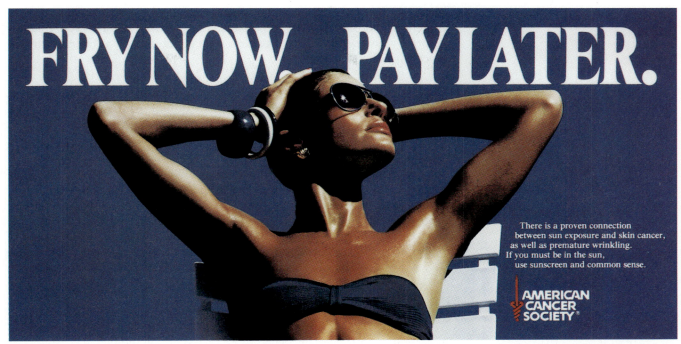

Evidence indicates that excessive exposure to ultraviolet radiation early in life leads to later development of skin cancer.

Age. Most cancers occur among older people, but some cancers—such as cancer of the kidney, acute leukemias, and a particular form of cancer of the eye known as **retinoblastoma**—are more often found among the young. Cancer of the colon and lung, in contrast, are generally found in older people. Cancer is the second leading cause of death among children between five and twelve years of age.

Carcinogenic Substances. Exposure to carcinogenic substances poses some degree of risk, depending on the nature of the substance and the degree of exposure. Many chemicals have been labeled **carcinogenic,** meaning that they have been determined to cause cancer in either humans or laboratory animals. One must be careful in evaluating the risk from these substances because, in some studies, exposure in the laboratory setting far exceeded normal exposure levels.

Some environmental hazards are also known to be carcinogenic. It is well documented that increased exposure to the ultraviolet radiation in sunlight substantially increases the risk of skin cancer. Pipe smokers may develop cancer of the lip and tongue from the heat of the pipe held in the mouth for long periods.

Other carcinogens include radiation from x-rays, numerous viruses, cigarette smoking, asbestos, certain drugs, several chemicals found in nature, and a variety of food additives.

Diet. A great deal has been written discussing the relation between diet and some forms of cancer. Links have been suggested between dietary factors and cancers of the colon, breast, stomach, bladder, prostate, and others. For example, cancers of the colon and rectum are less common among people who eat high-fiber diets, and cancers of the breast and colon seem to occur more frequently in those with high-fat diets. Booklets on the subject are available from the American Cancer Society.

Other Factors. Some cancers occur in both sexes but are more prevalent among members of one sex than those of the other. For example, cases of breast cancer among females outnumber cases in males two hundred to one. Lung cancer occurs more frequently in males than in females (but females seem to be working quite hard to catch up).

Other factors are socioeconomic and geographic. Breast cancer is found more often among the wealthy, whereas cancer of the cervix occurs more frequently among lower socioeconomic groups. This is primarily because women in lower socioeconomic groups tend to begin having sex earlier in life, are more likely to have multiple sex partners, and more frequently have untreated infections of the cervix. Cancer of the breast is quite prevalent in the United States but is rare in Japan (although Americans of Japanese decent have just as high an incidence as other Americans).

Cancer Cures

By definition, cancer is considered to be "cured" if the individual is cancer free for five years after treatment. Some cancers have very high cure rates whereas others have a poor **prognosis.** Skin cancers can be nearly 100 percent curable, but lung cancers are only about 5 to 10 percent curable.

There are two major factors that determine the cure rate of any particular type of cancer. They are the ease with which the cancer can be detected and the length of time the cancer remains localized before metastasis takes place. The easier a cancer is to discover and the longer it remains localized, the greater the chance of a successful cure. Skin cancers have a high cure rate because they

GUIDELINES TO YOUR GOOD HEALTH

The following will help you to reduce the risk of developing cancer:

1. Do not smoke cigarettes.
2. Avoid excessive exposure to ultraviolet radiation (i.e., sunlight, both natural and artificial).
3. Have all growths such as warts, moles, and cysts checked by your doctor.
4. If female, have a Pap smear as recommended by your physician.
5. Do breast self examination monthly.
6. If male, do testicular self examination monthly.
7. Encourage your friends and relatives over the age of 40 to have an annual rectal examination.
8. Encourage your female friends and relatives to have a baseline mammogram between the ages of 35 and 40 and subsequent mammograms as recommended by their physicians.

are easy to find and, for some types, never metastasize. Cancer of the ovary, on the other hand, has no early symptoms and is almost impossible to detect before metastasis takes place.

Signs and Symptoms

There is often no pain or other obvious symptom to enable early detection of cancer. There are, however, a variety of warning signs that, if they should occur for more than two weeks, may or may not indicate a problem and should be investigated by a physician. This is absolutely essential, since time is of the essence in diagnosing and treating cancer.

Cancer can be detected many different ways; but an absolute diagnosis can be confirmed only by **biopsy**. A biopsy involves the surgical removal of cells from the suspect tissue and subsequent examination under the microscope to detect malignant cells.

Types of Cancer

Skin Cancer. Although there are more than 300 types of cancer, about 90 percent of cancer cases are the result of the thirty most common types. Skin cancers outnumber all other types of cancer combined, reportedly numbering over 500,000 cases each year. The three major types of skin cancer are *squamous cell carcinoma* (occurring in the surface layers of epithelial tissue), *basal cell carcinoma* (found in the deeper layers of epithelial tissue), and **melanoma** (occurring in the pigment-forming cells of the skin). Of the three, melanoma affords the poorest **prognosis.**

Some individuals come from what are termed "melanoma-prone" families and, in some reported cases, have had literally hundreds of melanomas removed surgically during their lifetimes. The American Cancer Society has an audiovisual presentation specifically designed to educate melanoma-prone individuals.

FAST FACTS

A 1988 report in the *Journal of the American Medical Association* stated that "by 1990, one of every 1,000 Americans at 20 years of age will be able to claim to have beaten cancer."

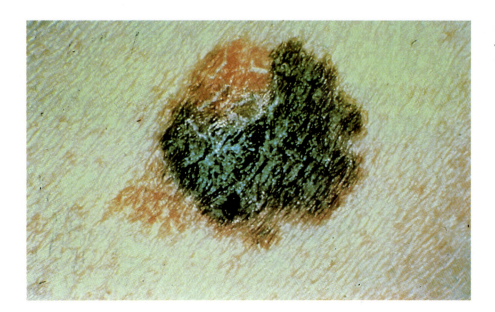

Malignant melanoma is the most aggressive of the skin cancers and affords a poor prognosis if not discovered early.

The principal risk factor for skin cancer is exposure to ultraviolet radiation, with sunlight being the number-one environmental source of exposure. The risk is greatest for fair-skinned individuals. Recent studies have shown that repeated exposure to sunlight is cumulative and that it may lead to the development of cancer many years after exposure has taken place. The incidence of skin cancer is significantly higher in sunbelt states than in other areas. It is extremely important to avoid prolonged exposure to sunlight (such as sunbathing) and to use an effective sunscreen when such exposure cannot be avoided.

The use of tanning beds to maintain a tan when weather doesn't permit going to the beach also poses a threat of skin cancer. The ultraviolet radiation emitted by tanning beds that causes you to tan is the same kind that places you at risk for skin cancer.

Signs of skin cancer may include any abnormal skin condition, especially a sore that appears not to heal or bleeds easily or a change in the size or color of a mole or other darkly pigmented spot.

> ■ **PROBLEM SITUATION** You have noticed that a sore on your leg doesn't seem to be healing normally. In fact, it bleeds easily when you touch it. Should you be concerned? What should you do?

Lung Cancer. The leading cause of cancer death overall is lung cancer. Nationwide, it is number one for both men and women. By the year 2000, as many women as men are expected to die annually from lung cancer. Case rates are also on the rise among black men.

The Surgeon General's report for 1979 stated, "Cigarette smoking is the single most important environmental factor contributing to premature mortality in the United States." The American Cancer Society indicates that at least 75 percent of all lung cancer deaths are directly related to smoking. No one, other than those working for the tobacco industry, would refute these statements. See Chapter 11 for a further discussion on the subject of smoking and health.

Lung cancer has an extremely poor prognosis. As indicated earlier, ninety to ninety-five out of every one hundred lung cancer victims will be dead within five years after treatment, even with the best modern medical care. Warning signs include coughing and possibly slight pain in the chest. These symptoms often go unnoticed, however, because smokers may have them even when no cancer is present. By the time severe symptoms (such as spitting up blood) occur, it is often too late for a cure or effective treatment. Generally, metastasis has already occurred to several other sites. Even X-ray diagnosis is difficult, because a cancerous lesion in the lung must be as large as 2 cm. in size before it can be detected.

Breast Cancer. Presently, breast cancer is the number-two cancer killer of U.S. women and the leading cause of death for women between the ages of 40 and 54. It is estimated that one out of ten women will develop breast cancer sometime during their lives and that one-third of those women will die from the disease.

The specific causes of breast cancer are not known, although some experts believe that diets high in fats play a role in the development of the disease. Hereditary factors also play a role. A study done in January 1988 reported that a group of women with breast cancer were found to have a particle in their

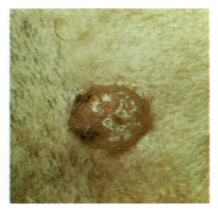

Basal cell carcinoma remains localized but can cause extensive tissue destruction.

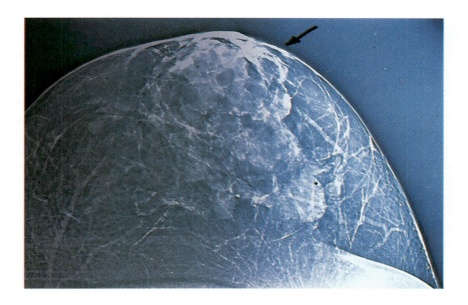

A mammogram is used to detect breast tumors too small to be felt by direct breast examination. This mammogram shows extensive cystic breast disease.

blood identified as a **retrovirus.** The particle was found in the blood of thirty-one of the thirty-two women studied. These findings have not been confirmed, and research is expected to continue over the next few years.

Women at greatest risk are those (1) over fifty years of age, (2) with a family history of breast cancer in a first-degree female relative (mother or sister) or maternal aunt, (3) with a history of previous malignancies, (4) with early onset of menstruation or late menopause, and (5) who have no children or had their first child after age 30. Radiation exposure is also considered to be a risk factor for breast cancer.

Most masses in the breast, whether benign or malignant, are detected by either the woman herself or her sex partner. A few masses are found by practitioners during routine annual examinations. Approximately 80 percent of breast masses are benign and are classified as either fibroadenomas or fibrocystic breast disease.

Fibroadenomas may be either single or multiple lumps and are more common among women during puberty or young adulthood. They have characteristic, well-defined boundaries and are usually mobile and not tender.

Fibrocystic change usually has its onset between the ages of 30 and 35 years. The problem appears to be hormonal. Fibrocystic lumps are generally well delineated, round, mobile, and tender.

Most malignant lumps occur in women between the ages of 40 and 80. These adenocarcinomas are irregular in shape and usually are not tender until the disease is well advanced. They may be fixed to the skin or underlying tissue, which causes a characteristic dimpling appearance. They are most commonly found in the upper outer quadrant of the breast. Early metastasis may occur through the regional lymph nodes.

Breast self examination (BSE) is extremely important for all women because, as mentioned previously, the majority of lumps are detected by the victim herself and because early detection is the key to successful treatment. It is important for women to begin BSE early so that they can become familiar with their normal breast configuration. Knowing what your breasts feel like when they

FIGURE 17–2 ■ **Breast Self-Examination.**

SOURCE: American Cancer Society.

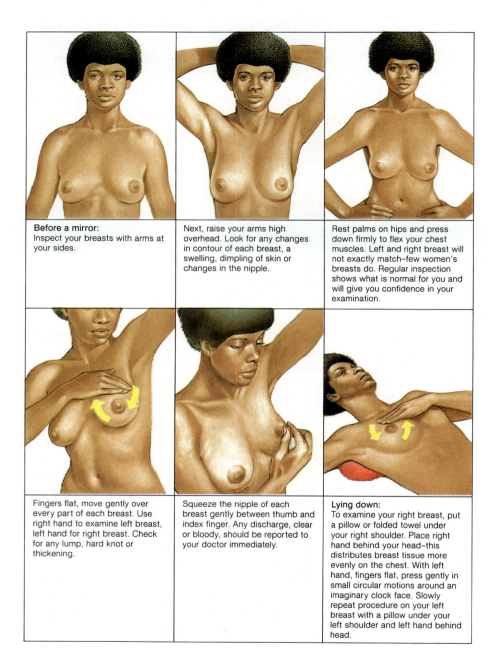

are normal will make it that much easier to detect abnormalities. Annual **mammograms**—special low-dose x-rays to detect breast tumors—are recommended for women over the age of 40. A *base-line mammogram,* which is important because it shows what the breast looks like when it is normal, is recommended for women age 35 to 40. Between the ages of 40 and 50, a mammogram should be done every one or two years. After age 50, annual mammograms are recommended.

Treatment for breast cancer includes surgery, radiation, and chemotherapy. A *lumpectomy* is a surgical procedure in which just the tumor is removed. A biopsy of the tumor is performed to determine if a lump is benign or malignant. *Mastectomies* (breast removal) range from subcutaneous mastectomy, in which some of the breast tissue underlying the skin is removed, to modified radical mastectomy, in which the entire breast is removed along with the regional lymph nodes from under the arm.

Radiation therapy involves irradiating the lymph nodes under the arm as well as surrounding tissue to prevent recurrence of cancer. Chemotherapeutic agents are used to reduce the incidence of metastasis resulting from surgery in which malignant cells may have spread into the bloodstream.

> *PROBLEM SITUATION* Your sister is 38 years old, has been doing breast self examinations regularly, and has not had any abnormal breast lumps. What should she do as a precautionary measure sometime during the next few years? Why?

Colorectal Cancer. The third most common form of cancer and the leading killer following lung cancer in both sexes is cancer of the colon and rectum. These cancers are almost always adenocarcinomas.

More than 60 percent of all colorectal cancers could be detected either through fingertip examination of the rectum or with the use of a **sigmoidoscope.** Annual rectal examinations are recommended for all people past the age of forty. Rectal bleeding, blood in the stool, and changes in bowel habits are early warning signs. Risk factors include a past history of **ulcerative colitis** or rectal polyps (benign growths in the rectum). **Hemorrhoids** are not a risk factor.

Much has been written about the possible relation between diet and colorectal cancer. Although it has been extremely difficult to establish a cause-and-effect relationship between the two, epidemiologic evidence strongly suggests that a high-fiber and low-fat diet tends to reduce risk. One theory suggests that high levels of fiber in the diet help speed the movement of waste materials out of the colon and rectum, thereby reducing the time that these materials remain in contact with the walls of these organs. This subsequently reduces chemical reactions that, in time, might cause malignant disease to develop.

Surgery is the principal treatment for colorectal cancer, although it is often used in combination with chemotherapy and radiation. A study published in 1986 indicated that surgery alone was more effective than surgery in combination with other therapies. Surgery involves a colostomy in only 15 percent of cases. Colostomy is a procedure in which all or part of the colon is removed and waste material empties into a bag on the abdominal wall.

Prostate Cancer. Generally occurring in men past the age of fifty, prostate cancer is an adenocarcinoma. This disease often goes undetected because of the mistaken diagnosis of benign enlargement of the prostate, a condition that occurs in a large percentage of older men. It is a cancer that is slow to metastasize, so early detection should enable a cure in most patients.

One of the symptoms of prostate cancer is difficulty in urination, also a symptom of benign prostate enlargement. Treatment is with surgery. Removal of the prostate gland leads to dry ejaculation during sexual intercourse. Early detection is possible through rectal examination of the prostate.

FAST FACTS

According to a recent study, depression does not necessarily make a person more susceptible to developing cancer although that belief has been held for some time.

Testicular Cancer. Cancer of the testes occurs most frequently in younger men between the ages of 15 and 34. Men with undescended or partially descended testicles are at greatest risk. The American Cancer Society indicates that the current five-year survival rate is 68 percent but could be much higher if these cancers were discovered earlier.

Because most cancers of the testes are discovered by men themselves, testicular self examination should be practiced on a regular basis to detect abnormal lumps (see Figure 17–3). The self examination takes less than three minutes of your time once a month. You should report any lumps to your physician immediately for further diagnosis. Not all lumps are cancerous, but none should be ignored. Treatment is usually surgical but may be combined with radiation and chemotherapy.

Cancer of the Uterine Cervix. Uterine cancers may affect either the uterine cervix or the endometrium (see Chapter 8). Cancers of the cervix are squamous cell carcinomas and occur at the junction of the squamous epithelium of the cervix and the columnar epithelium of the endometrium. Because their exact location is known, they are relatively easy to detect. Also, they remain localized

FIGURE 17–3 ■ **Testicular Self-Examination.**

SOURCE: American Cancer Society.

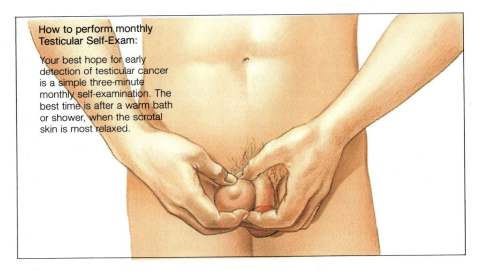

How to perform monthly Testicular Self-Exam:

Your best hope for early detection of testicular cancer is a simple three-minute monthly self-examination. The best time is after a warm bath or shower, when the scrotal skin is most relaxed.

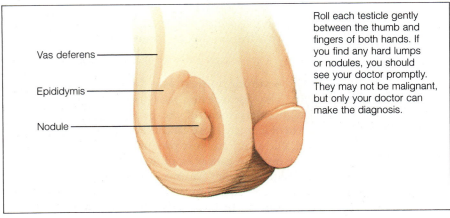

Roll each testicle gently between the thumb and fingers of both hands. If you find any hard lumps or nodules, you should see your doctor promptly. They may not be malignant, but only your doctor can make the diagnosis.

> **SELF-INVENTORY 17.1**
>
> ## How Can I Protect Myself from Cancer?
>
> Answer the following questions to identify your own personal risk of developing cancer.
>
> | | Yes | No |
> |---|---|---|
> | 1. Do you smoke? | | |
> | cigarettes | ___ | ___ |
> | pipes | ___ | ___ |
> | cigars | ___ | ___ |
> | 2. Do you use smokeless tobacco products? | | |
> | chewing tobacco | ___ | ___ |
> | snuff | ___ | ___ |
> | 3. Do you often work or play in the sun? | ___ | ___ |
> | 4. Are you taking high dose estrogens? | ___ | ___ |
> | 5. Do you work with or near industrial cancer-causing agents such as asbestos, nickel, uranium, chromates, petroleum, vinyl chloride? | ___ | ___ |
> | 6. Do you have x-rays taken frequently? | ___ | ___ |
> | 7. Do you eat many foods that are high in fats? | | |
> | fried foods | ___ | ___ |
> | whole milk/cheeses | ___ | ___ |
> | fatty meats | ___ | ___ |
> | potato chips | ___ | ___ |
> | 8. Do you have more than two drinks of alcoholic beverages per day? | ___ | ___ |
> | 9. Do you do breast self examinations regularly (females)? | ___ | ___ |
> | 10. Do you do testicular self examinations regularly (males)? | ___ | ___ |
> | 11. If over 40 years of age, do you have an annual rectal examination (males and females)? | ___ | ___ |
> | 12. If over 35 years of age, do you follow the recommendations for mammography (females)? | ___ | ___ |
>
> If you answer "yes" to any of questions 1 through 8 or "no" to any of questions 9 through 12, there is something you can do to protect yourself. Ways to reduce your risk of cancer are discussed in this chapter.
>
> SOURCE: Adapted from National Cancer Institute.

for as long as ten years, so early detection usually makes a complete cure highly probable.

Women at greatest risk are those over the age of 35 who have had early intercourse (prior to fifteen years of age), multiple sex partners, frequent childbearing, or frequent untreated infections of the cervix. Uterine cancer is most common among women in low socioeconomic groups.

The Papanicolau smear (or Pap smear) is the principal method of detecting cancer of the cervix. Because of this simple and inexpensive test, cancer of the cervix has declined substantially over the past forty years. If you are a sexually active woman, you should have a Pap smear done annually. Results are reported as a Roman numeral from I through V, with I being normal and V being confirmed malignancy. Results in categories II, III, or IV require follow-up examination.

Cancer of the Endometrium. Also an adenocarcinoma, cancer of the endometrium runs high among women who have had a late menopause, no children,

FAST FACTS

Arthritis is the most common of all chronic diseases, but it seldom causes death.

or long-term use of high-dose estrogens. Most diagnoses are made among women between the ages of 50 and 64.

Endometrial cancer is relatively easy to discover and remains localized for a long time, thus presenting a good prognosis. Unusual bleeding or discharge is a warning sign. The Pap smear is about 50 percent effective in detecting endometrial cancer.

Cancer of the Ovary. The poorest prognosis of the cancers of the female reproductive system is given for cancer of the ovary. It has no early warning signs and is usually discovered after it has spread. Pain is a symptom in later stages, but by then it is often too late for a successful cure.

Lymphoma and Leukemia. Cancers of the lymph system are called **lymphomas**. Hodgkin's disease, for example, is a form of lymph-node cancer. It can involve lymph nodes throughout the body.

Leukemias are cancers of the blood-forming tissues. Acute lymphocytic leukemias usually occur in children, whereas chronic lymphocytic leukemias and acute granulocytic leukemias usually occur in adults. Overall, there are nearly ten times as many cases of leukemia among adults as among children. The onset of chronic leukemias is much slower and life expectancy is much longer than for acute leukemias.

Early signs of leukemia may include fatigue, loss of weight, nose bleeds, bruising, and repeated infections. Blood tests and bone-marrow biopsies are used to diagnose the disease.

Chemotherapy has been more effective in treating leukemias and lymphomas than in treating any other types of cancer. Many different drugs are available and are used alone or in combinations.

■ Arthritis

Literally, *arthritis* means "inflammation of a joint." There are over one hundred types of arthritis, although some are far more common than others. Evidence indicates that nearly 97 percent of all adults over the age of sixty have enough arthritis to be detectable on x-ray. See arthritis warning signs on Table 17–3.

Some of the more common forms of arthritis are discussed in the following sections. Other types include bursitis, fibrositis, scleroderma, gonorrheal arthritis, infectious arthritis, psoriatic arthritis, and rheumatic fever.

Rheumatoid Arthritis

The most serious of the common forms of the disease is *rheumatoid arthritis*. Estimates are that it affects about one million people. Rheumatoid arthritis attacks the joints and various other organs of the body, causing increased pain and progressive damage with each successive attack. The disease can occur at all age levels but appears more often in middle life and is found three times more often in women than in men. Attacks may last as long as six to eight weeks.

The joints of the hands, arms, legs, hips, and feet are the most frequently affected. In addition to the swelling, redness, heat, and pain that may occur in

TABLE 17–3 ■ Arthritis Warning Signs
Persistent pain and stiffness on arising
Pain, tenderness, or swelling in one or more joints
Recurrence of these symptoms, especially when they involve more than one joint
Recurrent or persistent pain and stiffness in the neck, lower back, knees, and other joints

SOURCE: "Arthritis—The Basic Facts," Arthritis Foundation, 1978, p. 6.

the affected joints, rheumatoid arthritis may cause fever, lethargy, poor appetite, weight loss, and anemia.

The joints are surrounded by a protective membrane known as the *synovial membrane*. Lubrication and cushioning are provided through the synovial fluid within the joint, a lubricant so effective that humankind has never been able to match it. In attacks of rheumatoid arthritis, the synovial membrane is gradually eroded away, synovial fluid may be lost, and the joint becomes damaged. With each attack, more damage is done, sometimes leading to immobility and distortion of the joint. (See Figure 17–4.)

The cause of rheumatoid arthritis is unknown, although there appears to be some genetic influence. A genetic marker has been identified in the blood of rheumatoid arthritis patients, but the exact significance of this marker, as well as the factors that precipitate attacks of the disease, are still undetermined. Many experts believe that stress is an important factor in the initiation of the disease in susceptible individuals.

Treatment is directed at relieving pain and reducing inflammation. This is generally accomplished through the use of nonsteroidal anti-inflammatory drugs

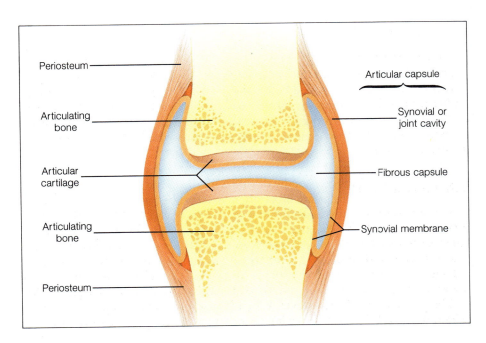

FIGURE 17–4 ■ Diagram of Joint.

GUIDELINES TO YOUR GOOD HEALTH

The following suggestions can help reduce your risk of developing arthritis or help you to avoid complications in treating arthritis.

1. Don't participate in activities that could potentially lead to joint damage.
2. Maintain body weight at a proper level.
3. If you develop arthritis, follow your physician's treatment instructions carefully.
4. Be aware that no relationship has been discovered between diet and arthritis.
5. Don't spend money or waste time on vitamin therapies, nonapproved drugs, gadgets and devices, or nontraditional medical practitioners.

(NSAIDs), the most well known of which is aspirin. Other NSAIDs include ibuprofen, indomethacin, and naproxen. Exercise is an important part of any therapy for arthritis and should be directed at keeping the affected joints mobile without causing further damage. Application of heat may also be helpful.

Juvenile Arthritis

According to the Arthritis Foundation, approximately 250,000 children in the United States have *juvenile arthritis*. More girls are affected than boys.

Symptoms resemble those of rheumatoid arthritis and may include skin rashes, inflammation of the eyes, retarded growth, and abnormal swelling of the lymph nodes. Without appropriate treatment, juvenile arthritis can be crippling.

Osteoarthritis

Osteoarthritis is often called the "wear and tear" disease. It is the most common form of arthritis, and it is said that if you live long enough, you will develop it to some degree. Symptoms include pain in and around the affected joints and loss of mobility of the joint. Most victims of osteoarthritis are over forty years of age, but it may occur in younger people as the result of an injury or overuse of a joint.

Osteoarthritis is a mild form of arthritis and rarely cripples its victims. Pain is moderate and the progress of the disease is gradual. The weight-bearing joints such as the knees and hips are most often affected, but the joints of the lower part of the spine may also become involved. Women tend to develop the disease earlier than men. One symptom particularly characteristic of osteoarthritis is the appearance of small bony protrusions at the end joints of the fingers. These are called Heberdon's nodes, and their appearance tends to be genetically determined.

Treatment of osteoarthritis includes nonsteroidal anti-inflammatory drugs, exercise, heat, and surgery, if necessary. Weight reduction is also important in overweight patients. If joints suffer considerable damage, joint-replacement surgery may be indicated. As with other forms of arthritis, there is no cure, but the progress of the disease can be slowed significantly reducing the risk of further joint damage.

Gout

Gout is a form of arthritis that is related to an inherited inability to control levels of a chemical known as uric acid. In gout, this chemical, which is normally found in the blood, occurs in excessive amounts. Approximately 1½ million people are affected by gout, which attacks men far more frequently than women. The excess uric acid forms solid crystals, which accumulate in the affected joints. These needle-like crystals cause extreme pain and severe inflammation. Gout may affect the joints of the ankle, foot, and knee, but the joint most often affected is that of the great toe.

Some experts think that diet may have an effect on gout because certain foods contain large amounts of purines—chemicals associated with increased uric-acid levels in the body. In general, however, it is believed that the uric acid taken in with food is not significant because most of the chemical appearing in the blood is formed by the body itself. Alcoholic beverages and diuretics can aggravate attacks.

Treatment is through the use of drugs that either prevent the formation of uric acid or cause it to be more rapidly metabolized and eliminated. Some victims of the disease may need to take medication for their entire lives to prevent attacks. Gout is the most effectively controlled form of arthritis.

Ankylosing Spondylitis

Ankylosing spondylitis, also known as Marie Strumpel disease, is arthritis of the spine. There is no known cause, although there seems to be a strong genetic influence. It affects the small joints of the spine and causes pain in the lower back and legs and stiffness of the spine. The hips and shoulders may also be affected, and inflammation of the eyes may occur.

The disease can begin as early as age sixteen but usually occurs between the ages of seventeen and twenty-five. It occurs more commonly among men. General symptoms include fatigue, weight loss, anorexia, and low-grade fever.

Systemic Lupus Erythematosus (SLE)

Systemic lupus erythematosus is a form of arthritis that principally affects women between twenty and forty years of age. It appears to be more common among dark-skinned races. The skin, joints, and internal organs may become inflamed as the result of periodic flare-ups of the disease. The cause is unknown, but current theories include the possibility of alterations in the immune system or infection by a virus or other unidentified organism. There does appear to be some hereditary influence because the rate of occurrence is approximately twenty times greater than normal among relatives of those already affected by the disease.

Symptoms of lupus may include skin rash, joint pain, fever, weight loss, anemia, and kidney failure. Loss of hair may accompany skin involvement of the scalp. Another characteristic sign is the formation of ulcers on the mucous membranes of the mouth. The disease is sometimes confused with rheumatoid arthritis but can be distinguished from it with appropriate laboratory tests.

A Few Final Thoughts

Victims of arthritis can become extremely frustrated over the inability to cure their illness. This frustration may lead to reliance on quackery and unproven remedies. The problem becomes even more serious when the patient passes up effective treatment to try some ineffective "cure." Victims of arthritis tend to be easy prey for charlatans.

> ■ **PROBLEM SITUATION** Your mother is complaining of pains in her joints, especially the joints of her arms and hands. A neighbor has suggested that she buy a copper bracelet and wear it on her wrist. What might be wrong with your mother? What should she do about it?

■ Diabetes Mellitus

In *diabetes mellitus,* the body is unable to properly metabolize carbohydrate as the result of the inadequate production of the hormone *insulin.* Protein and fat metabolism are also affected. Insulin is produced by the beta cells of the pancreas and is essential for both the metabolism of carbohydrate and its use by body cells as a source of energy.

The two principal types of diabetes are Type I (insulin-dependent or juvenile-onset diabetes) and Type II (noninsulin-dependent or mature-onset diabetes). (See Table 17–4.) Type I diabetes generally occurs in persons under the age of thirty-five. Onset is rapid as compared to Type II diabetes. The Type I diabetic is unable to produce insulin in any appreciable amount. Most Type I diabetics appear to be undernourished at the onset of the disease.

Approximately 100,000 cases of juvenile-onset diabetes are diagnosed in the United States each year. Type I diabetics must take injections of insulin to control their disease. Diet and exercise are also important control measures, as they are for Type II diabetics.

Type II diabetes generally occurs after the age of thirty-five and has a slower onset. Approximately 80 percent of all diabetics have this type. The Type II diabetic either is able to produce insulin but not in a quantity sufficient to meet

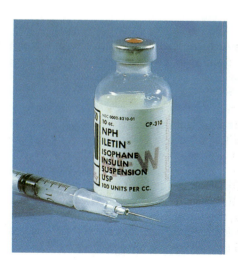

Type I diabetics must use insulin to control their disease.

TABLE 17-4 ■ A Comparison of the Essential Features of Type I and Type II Diabetes

Feature	Type I	Type II
Other names	Juvenile, growth-onset	Adult-onset, maturity-onset
Age of onset	Usually under 35	Usually over 35
Type of onset	Abrupt (days to weeks)	Usually gradual (weeks to months)
Nutritional status at onset	Usually undernourished	Usually obese
Symptoms	Excessive thirst, excessive appetite, and increased urination	Frequently none
Naturally produced insulin	Negligible to absent	Present; may be in excess but relatively ineffective because of obesity
Associated fat abnormalities	High levels of cholesterol	Cholesterol and triglycerides frequently elevated and related to obesity
Insulin	Needed for all patients	Necessary in only 20 to 30 percent of patients
Medication taken by mouth	Rarely effective	Effective
Diet	Mandatory, along with insulin for control of blood-glucose level	Diet alone frequently sufficient to control blood-glucose level

Adapted from Eli Lilly and Company, *Diabetes Mellitus*, (Indianapolis: Eli Lilly and Company, 1980).

all of his or her metabolic needs, produces chemically incorrect insulin, or has an improper balance between insulin and *glucagon,* a chemical that normally opposes insulin in the body. Obesity is clearly related to the onset of Type II diabetes. Although most diabetes in older persons is of this type and is very mild, the complications of Type II diabetes can be more severe in this age group.

There appear to be hereditary patterns associated with diabetes, especially Type II, but these patterns are not well understood. It is clear, however, that you must avoid becoming obese if you have a family history of diabetes.

Many people with diabetes are unaware that they have it. It is estimated that as many as five million Americans, or 40 percent of all diabetics, are undiagnosed. The average Type II diabetic has the disease for six years before it is detected. Symptoms include increased urination, thirst, and hunger; disturbances in vision; irritability; numbness or tingling in the feet; and fatigue. The disease affects twice as many women as men in the over-fifty age group.

> **FAST FACTS**
>
> A California company is developing a nasal spray for the administration of insulin to diabetics.

Type II diabetes can often be controlled by diet and exercise alone. Diet is designed to meet the metabolic needs of the patient while keeping weight at normal levels. Carbohydrate intake must be carefully regulated as well. Exercise is important because it aids in the body's use of glucose through the burning of calories. Several drugs can be taken orally, if necessary. These medications induce the secretion of needed insulin and enable it to more effectively perform its normal functions of carbohydrate metabolism.

A diabetic's blood-sugar level must be carefully controlled so that he or she can avoid the complications of the disease. A variety of home testing methods are presently available, including color test strips and electronic measuring machines.

Failure to control blood-sugar levels can result in damage to the circulatory system, which may lead to heart attacks, strokes, kidney failure, and gangrene in the extremities. In patients with both diabetes and atherosclerosis, the diabetes may increase the rate of progression of their atherosclerosis. Diabetic retinopathy, an eye disease resulting from inadequately controlled diabetes, is the leading cause of blindness in the United States.

> **PROBLEM SITUATION** Your mother and grandmother are both Type II diabetics. They have told you that you must not eat sugar because it will cause you to also become a diabetic. Are they correct? What should you do to reduce your risk of Type II diabetes in the future?

Other Chronic Diseases

Chronic Obstructive Pulmonary Disease

The term *chronic obstructive pulmonary disease* (COPD) applies to chronic bronchitis, emphysema, and asthma. Fifty thousand deaths per year in the United States are directly related to COPD, with more than half of them being caused by emphysema. Nearly three-fourths of the deaths are among white males.

Chronic bronchitis is the term given to chronic and recurrent productive cough. To be defined as such, it must continue for at least three months per year in two successive years. The condition is characterized by excessive mucous production and often occurs along with emphysema. Smoking is the leading cause of chronic bronchitis. It occurs about equally in men and women.

Emphysema is characterized by abnormal enlargement of the air spaces in the lungs, resulting in destruction of the walls of the alveoli. Often the bronchial tubes are obstructed either partially or completely, thereby reducing lung capacity. A barrel-chested appearance, resulting from many years of labored breathing, is a later sign of emphysema. Although there is one form of emphysema that is hereditary, the majority of cases result from smoking. Emphysema occurs more frequently among men than women.

Asthma is a disease in which the bronchial tubes and trachea show an oversensitive response to stimuli such as allergens, stress, pollens, cigarette smoke, perfumes, and so on. In an acute asthmatic attack, the airways constrict and become so narrowed that the patient has great difficulty in breathing. The victim wheezes and has a feeling of tightness in the chest. Often there is excessive

> **FAST FACTS**
>
> Approximately one-third of all asthmatics are under seventeen years of age.

secretion of abnormally sticky mucous, which causes further obstruction. Although asthma is not caused by cigarette smoking, smoke can seriously aggravate the condition and can lead to acute attacks in susceptible individuals.

Epilepsy

Epilepsy is a disorder of the brain characterized by seizures. In reality, it is not a single disease and may result from head injury, tumors, drug overdose, exposure to poisons such as lead, diseases such as **encephalitis** from measles, or other causes. Epilepsy afflicts approximately two million Americans.

Epilepsy is not a well-understood disease. Attacks happen when abnormal electrical disturbances occur in the brain. Often, these abnormalities temporarily block normal electrical transmission in the brain. The result is a seizure, the nature of which depends on the type of disturbance and its location in the brain.

The most common and the most violent type of epileptic seizure is the *tonic-clonic* (previously known as *grand mal*) seizure. The victim's muscles become spastic (the tonic phase), followed by violent shaking, sometimes of the entire body (the clonic phase). Unconsciousness ensues. After a short period of time, the victim usually awakens confused, disoriented, and extremely tired.

Another type of seizure is the *absence* form (previously known as *petit mal*). This type of epilepsy occurs most often in children, primarily from ages six to fourteen, and is often mistaken by teachers and parents as daydreaming. A child with absence seizures may have as many as fifty to one hundred seizures per day.

A third type of seizure is the *psychomotor*, or partial, seizure. In this type of seizure, the victim may exhibit repetitive, purposeless movements, may drool, or may simply stare as in an absence seizure.

Some people with epilepsy experience a warning, or *aura*, prior to a seizure. The aura may come as a funny taste, a sound, or a visual disturbance. Epilepsy can often be controlled with medication. Many drugs are available by prescription for the control of specific types of seizures.

■ Genetic Disorders

Sickle-Cell Anemia

Sickle-cell anemia is a genetic disease that affects individuals whose ancestors come from areas of the world where malaria was prevalent. Although it affects mostly blacks in the United States, it is not a disease of blacks only. In some parts of the world, its victims are mostly white. Its relationship to malaria has been studied extensively. Individuals who carry the gene for sickle-cell anemia appear to be protected by it against dying of malaria.

Sickle-cell anemia affects the **hemoglobin** of the red blood cells. During a sickle-cell crisis, the red blood cells lose their normal round shape and begin to clog the smaller blood vessels, sometimes causing severe pain. Some victims are affected very seriously, whereas others may have only mild symptoms. Many victims of the disease require frequent blood transfusions.

A blood test is available to detect carriers of the sickle-cell gene. Carriers are said to have sickle-cell trait. They do not have the disease. If two carriers meet and mate, however, they have a one-in-four chance of producing a baby with the disease itself.

FAST FACTS

The word *epilepsy* comes from the Greek word for "seized." In early days, people with epilepsy were thought to be seized by demons.

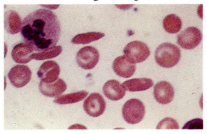

In a sickle cell crisis, red blood cells lose their normal round shape and clog small blood vessels, causing severe pain.

Amniocentesis and other screening techniques are also available to determine whether or not an unborn baby is affected by the disease. Unfortunately, the test does not indicate the degree to which the fetus might be affected.

Cystic Fibrosis

Cystic fibrosis is a genetic disease of the exocrine glands that affects mostly whites of northern European decent. It primarily affects the lungs by clogging them with abnormally thick mucous. Individuals with cystic fibrosis require regular and vigorous physical therapy to keep their lungs clear. Digestion is faulty because of a deficiency of pancreatic enzymes, and there is an excessive loss of salt in the sweat. The life expectancy of cystic fibrosis victims is varied, but most do not live past their teenage years.

There is no prenatal diagnosis through amniocentesis, nor is there a carrier blood test for cystic fibrosis. The only way for two people to know that they are carriers is to have a child be born with the disease.

An August, 1989 newspaper article reported that researchers at the Hospital for Sick Children in Toronto, Canada have isolated the gene that is responsible for cystic fibrosis. This discovery could potentially lead to the development of a treatment for this disease. Dr. Robert Beall of the Cystic Fibrosis Foundation stated that this discovery was "the most exciting event since the disease was first described in the medical literature 50 years ago".

Tay-Sachs Disease

Tay-Sachs disease, an inborn defect of lipid metabolism, primarily affects Ashkenazi Jews, people of central European Jewish decent. One in twenty-seven people in this population carries the gene. In the general population, the disease is found in about one in 150 people. Tay-Sachs is a horrible disease in which the child is born apparently normal but, during the next three to four years, develops progressive loss of vision, paralysis, and dementia and wastes away to die an agonizing death. There is both a carrier detection test and prenatal diagnosis through amniocentesis available for Tay-Sachs.

Phenylketonuria (PKU)

Phenylalanine is a common amino acid found in many foods. In children born with phenylketonuria, the body is unable to metabolize phenylalanine properly, and it builds up in the blood, causing brain damage. The disease is controlled through a diet low in phenylalanine-containing foods. Current information indicates that children with PKU should remain on this special diet until they are teenagers. Every state in the United States requires a blood test for PKU for all newborn babies.

POSITIVE BEHAVIORS

I. *Place a check mark in front of each behavior that you now practice.*

___ 1. I use an effective sunscreen when I participate in outdoor activities. (SUNSCREEN)
___ 2. I do not smoke cigarettes. (CIGARETTES)
___ 3. I do breast self examinations regularly and/or I encourage my female friends and relatives to do so. (BREAST SELF EXAM)
___ 4. I have an annual Pap smear and/or I encourage my female friends and relatives to do so. (PAP SMEAR)
___ 5. I do testicular self examinations and/or I encourage my male friends and relatives to do so. (TESTICULAR SELF EXAM)
___ 6. If I found any abnormal growth or lump on my body, I would seek medical evaluation as soon as possible. (MEDICAL EVALUATION)
___ 7. If I belong to a high-risk group for a genetic disease, I will obtain genetic screening or amniocentesis if available when planning to have a child. (GENETIC SCREENING)

II. *For each behavior that you DO NOT ENGAGE IN, write in the appropriate space below the KEY WORD(S) located in the parentheses at the end of the statement. Then indicate whether you intend to keep or change that behavior.*

Behaviors I Don't Engage In   KEEP/CHANGE
_____   _____/_____
_____   _____/_____
_____   _____/_____
_____   _____/_____
_____   _____/_____
_____   _____/_____
_____   _____/_____

III. *For each of the preceding behaviors that you choose to KEEP, write a statement indicating why you are choosing to keep that behavior.*

I choose to keep behavior _____ because:
                          KEY WORD

For each of the preceding behaviors that you choose to CHANGE, write a statement indicating how you plan to implement that change.

I will change behavior _____ by:
                        KEY WORD

Now You Know

1. TRUE. A noncancerous growth is termed "benign" and a cancerous growth is termed "malignant."
2. FALSE. Breast cancers occur in men as well as in women but much more infrequently. However, in a man, a breast cancer may be more aggressive and harder to cure.
3. FALSE. Lung cancers are difficult to cure. Only about 5 to 10 percent of patients live more than five years after treatment.
4. FALSE. Breast self examination is the most important tool for diagnosis of breast cancers because the vast majority of breast lumps are discovered by such examinations.
5. TRUE. The greatest risk for cancer of the testicles is among younger men; therefore, testicular self examination should be done regularly by all men past the age of puberty.
6. FALSE. Approximately 250,000 children in the United States are afflicted with juvenile arthritis, and rheumatoid arthritis can strike at any age.
7. FALSE. There is as yet no scientific evidence to substantiate claims that changes in diet or the use of vitamin supplements has an effect on the prevention or treatment of any form of arthritis.
8. TRUE. Many Type II diabetics can control their disease through a diet designed to maintain proper body weight and reduce sugar intake and through exercise, which helps the body use glucose properly.
9. FALSE. Epilepsy can occur at any age and may be caused by any event that leads to brain damage resulting in seizures.
10. TRUE. Sickle-cell anemia affects groups of people whose ancestors come from areas of the world where malaria has been a prevalent disease.

Summary

1. A tumor is any swelling or enlargement. A neoplasm is a tumor consisting of solid tissue. Malignant neoplasms grow in a disorderly and uncontrolled manner and are cancerous.
2. Risk factors for cancer include age, sex, exposure to carcinogenic substances, diet, socioeconomic factors, and geographic factors.
3. Cancer is considered to be "cured" if the person who has the disease lives for five or more years after treatment.
4. Skin cancer cases outnumber all other types of cancer combined. The principal risk factor is exposure to ultraviolet radiation. The most serious type of skin cancer is malignant melanoma.
5. Lung cancer is the number-one cancer killer overall. Only five to ten out of every one hundred patients treated will survive more than five years. The principal risk factor is cigarette smoking.
6. Breast cancer can be detected in most cases by the woman herself when she does a breast self examination. In addition to BSE each month, every woman should have a baseline mammogram when she is between the ages of thirty-five and forty.
7. Young men ages fifteen to thirty-four are at highest risk for testicular cancer and should do testicular self examinations regularly.
8. Annual Pap smears for the detection of cancer of the uterine cervix are essential for all sexually active women.
9. There are more than one hundred types of arthritis, some of which can cause serious debilitation and death. Over 97 percent of adults over the age of sixty will develop enough arthritis to be detectable on x-ray.
10. Type I diabetes usually affects people under the age of thirty-five and Type II diabetes usually affects people over the age of thirty-five. Type I diabetics must use insulin. In many cases, Type II diabetics can control their disease through diet and exercise.
11. Chronic obstructive pulmonary disease consists of asthma, emphysema, and chronic bronchitis. Cigarette smoking is the principal causative factor of emphysema and chronic bronchitis. Asthma may be aggravated by cigarette smoke.
12. The three major types of seizures in epilepsy are tonic-clonic, abscence, and psychomotor.
13. Genetic diseases include sickle-cell anemia and Tay-Sachs disease, for which there are carrier detection tests and prenatal diagnosis.
14. Carriers of the gene for cystic fibrosis find out that they are carriers only by having a child with the disease.
15. Phenylketonuria is caused by an inability to metabolize the amino acid phenylalanine. It is controlled through diet.

References

1. Arthritis Foundation. "Arthritis: The Basic Facts." Atlanta: Arthritis Foundation, 1978.
2. Blade-Citizen. "Scientists Isolate Cystic Fibrosis Gene." Oceanside, CA: Aug. 24, 1989.
3. Dennis, Betty. "Diabetes Therapy, Part 2: Insulin Therapy and Complications of Diabetes." Chapel Hill, N.C.: Health Sciences Consortium, 1981.
4. Dolger, Henry, and Bernard Seeman. *How to Live with Diabetes*. Pyramid Books, 1965.
5. Jones, Kenneth L., Louis W., Shainberg, and Curtis O. Byer. *Disease*, 2d ed. San Francisco: Canfield Press, 1975.
6. National Cancer Institute, Department of Health and Human Services. *Cancer Treatment Reports*. Washington, D.C. (January 1984): 68.
7. Office of Cancer Communications. *The Breast Cancer Digest*. Washington, D.C.: U.S. Department of Health and Human Services, NIH Publication no. 80-1691, 1980.
8. Purtilo, David T. *A Survey of Human Diseases*. Menlo Park, Calif.: Addison-Wesley, 1978.
9. Raasch, Ralph H. "Diabetes Therapy, Part 1: Pathophysiology, Glucose Tests, and Dietary and Oral Hypoglycemic Treatment." Chapel Hill, N.C.: Health Sciences Consortium, 1981.
10. Shimkin, Michael B. *Science and Cancer*. Washington, D.C.: U.S. Department of Health and Human Services, NIH Publication no. 80-568, 1980.
11. Stanbury, John B., James B. Wyngaarden, and Donald S. Frederickson. *The Metabolic Basis of Inherited Disease*, 2d ed. New York: McGraw-Hill, 1966.
12. Stern, Charles A., and Ralph M. Grawunder. *Senior Citizens Health Education Project*. San Diego: San Diego State University, 1978.
13. Young, Patrick. *Asthma and Allergies: An Optimistic Future*. Washington, D.C.: U.S. Department of Health and Human Services NIH Publication no. 80-388, 1980.

Suggested Readings

American Cancer Society. *Cancer Facts and Figures—1988*. New York: American Cancer Society, 1989.

Beattie, Edward J., Jr., and Stuart D. Cowan. *Toward the Conquest of Cancer*. New York: Crown Publishers, 1980.

Eli Lilly and Co. *Diabetes Mellitus*. Indianapolis: Eli Lilly and Co., 1980.

Gershwin, E., and E. Klingelhofer. *Asthma—Stop Suffering, Start Living*. Reading, Mass.: Addison-Wesley, 1986.

National Institutes of Health. *Cancer Treatment Reports*. Washington, D.C.: U.S. Government Printing Office, 1984.

Purtilo, David T. *A Survey of Human Diseases*. Menlo Park, Calif.: Addison-Wesley, 1978.

Rosenbaum, E. H. *Can You Prevent Cancer?* St. Louis: C. V. Mosby Co., 1983.

Young, Patrick. *Asthma and Allergies: An Optimistic Future*. Washington, D.C.: U.S. Department of Health and Human Services, NIH Publication no. 80-388, 1980.

SECTION VI

Taking Control of Your Health

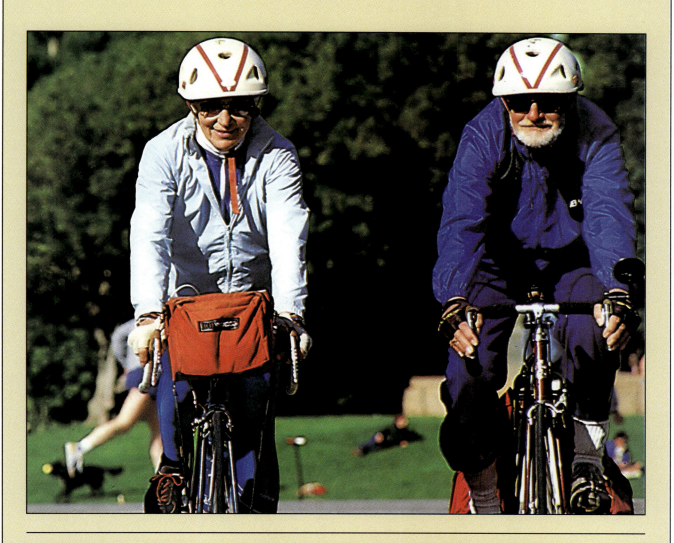

Chapter 18: Consumer Health
Consumer Protection Agencies
The Power of Advertising
Consumer Protection Skills
Accuracy of Health Information
Health Care
Health Insurance
Over-the-Counter Drugs and the Consumer

Understanding Your Prescription
Generic Drugs
Drug Laws

Chapter 19: Occupational and Environmental Risks
Sources of Toxic Waste and the Chemical Industry

The Hazardous Materials in Our Environment
The Nature and Extent of the Problem
Toxic Substances: Who Is at Risk?
DBCP: A Case Study
Community Health Protection
Accidental Injury: The Number-One Health Problem

CHAPTER 18

Consumer Health

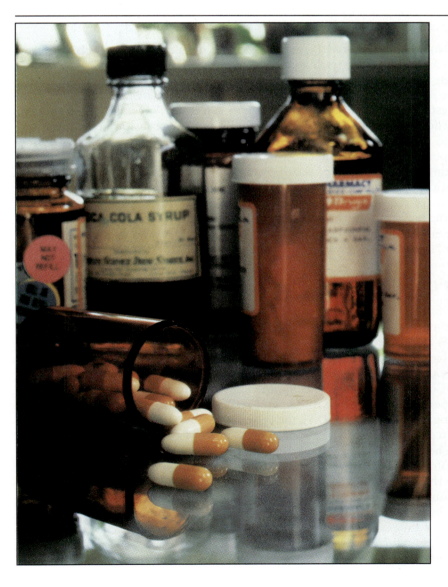

////////

What Do You Know?

Are the following statements true or false?

1. The Consumer Bill of Rights gave consumers the right to voice their complaints about unsafe and unsanitary working conditions.
2. Puffery is an advertising technique frequently used to sell products.
3. When buying a product, the salesperson's verbal promises are legally binding.
4. If you have a consumer complaint, you should first try to resolve it with the person with whom you did business.
5. The Office of Consumer Affairs is the primary federal agency responsible for the safety of health products.
6. Any time that elective surgery is recommended, you should get a second opinion.
7. With traditional health insurance, the individual has the freedom to choose any physician or hospital in the world to provide his or her health care.
8. A major disadvantage about the health care provided by health maintenance organizations is that there is a high deductible that the individual must pay before insurance coverage begins.
9. Drug prescriptions are written in Latin to discourage the average consumer from reading them.
10. Generic drugs are always as good as their brand-name counterparts.

If one were to assign a date to the birth of the modern consumer protection movement, it would have to be March 15, 1962, when President John F. Kennedy sent a message to Congress. The four goals he outlined have become known as the Consumer Bill of Rights. The Rights include the following:

1. The right to safety—to be protected against the marketing of goods that are hazardous to health or life.
2. The right to be informed—to be protected against fraudulent, deceitful, or grossly misleading information, advertising, labeling, or other practices and to be given the facts a consumer needs to make an informed choice.
3. The right to choose—to be assured, whenever possible, of access to a variety of products and services at competitive prices or, in those industries in which competition is not workable and government regulation is substituted, to be assured of satisfactory quality and service at fair prices.
4. The right to be heard—to be assured that consumer interests will receive full and sympathetic consideration in the formulation of government policy and fair and expeditious treatment in its administrative tribunals.

No president had ever before devoted such detailed attention to the problems of consumers or put forth such detailed goals for Congress to meet in dealing with these problems. President Kennedy's leadership served to encourage the states to enact consumer protection measures of their own and inspired them to establish their own enforcement agencies. Kennedy's message also stimulated the development of more effective self-policing systems by businesses and awakened the mass media to their responsibility for serving consumers' needs. Most important of all was the effect on consumers themselves. The message gave them a stronger sense of their power, an increased awareness of their rights, and a strengthened determination to act on their own behalf. Consumers became aware of the need to prepare and educate themselves to deal more effectively in the marketplace. The need for consumer protection led to the emergence of the emphasis on the "let the seller beware" *(caveat vendor)* concept rather than the "let the buyer beware" *(caveat emptor)* concept.

Consumer Protection Agencies

To further ensure the rights of consumers, the Consumer Protection and Environmental Health Service was established in 1968 under the auspices of the U.S. Department of Health, Education, and Welfare (presently the Department of Health and Human Services). Shortly after 1968, this agency split into two separate agencies: the Environmental Protection Agency (EPA) and the Office of Consumer Affairs. Presently, there are four major federal agencies whose responsibilities deal with consumer protection. These agencies are the Food and Drug Administration (FDA), the Federal Trade Commission (FTC), the United States Postal Service (USPS), and the Office of Consumer Affairs.

The Food and Drug Administration is an agency of the U.S. Department of Health and Human Services. The FDA is the primary federal agency responsible for the safety and efficacy of health products. This agency is responsible for consumer protection in the areas of falsely represented or worthless drugs; medical devices; cosmetics; food contaminants; and the safety and effectiveness of new drugs. The Food, Drug, and Cosmetic Act, which was established in 1938, is still considered today to be the primary federal legislation providing consumer protection in the United States.

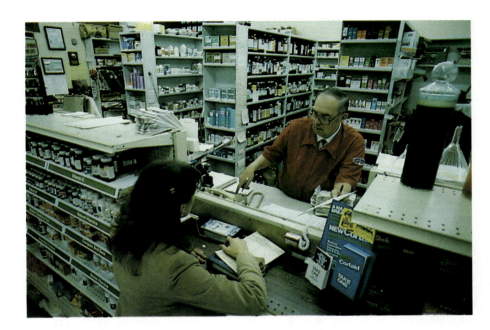

Ask your pharmacist; he or she is there to help you.

The Federal Trade Commission provides consumer safeguards against deceptive claims in advertising. Before the FTC can take legal action, however, fraud must be evident.

The United States Postal Service attempts to protect the consumer from fraud and quackery conducted through the U.S. mail. Mail fraud is a scheme to get money or anything of value from an individual by offering a product, service, or investment opportunity that does not live up to its claims. Prosecutors must prove that the claims were intentionally misrepresented and that the mails were used in some way to carry out the scheme.

The Office of Consumer Affairs was established in 1971 as part of the Executive Office of the President of the United States. In 1976, the office became part of the Department of Health, Education, and Welfare (presently the Department of Health and Human Services). The Office of Consumer Affairs conducts investigations, conferences, and surveys on consumer problems. This office also encourages and coordinates research and consumer education programs.

■ The Power of Advertising

In the American economy, producers of goods and sellers of services are all busy contending for the consumer's dollar. They want consumers to buy from them, not from their competitors. To achieve this end, each manufacturer and merchant uses all available means of persuasion. The volume and variety of advertising is tremendous. It is found in magazines and newspapers and can be seen and heard on television and radio. It seems that wherever there is an available space, such as on matchbook covers and milk cartons, there is some form of advertising. But what does an advertisement really tell you? When looking at a commercial or reading an advertisement, what is being sold? Are we being asked to buy a product or an image?

All people want to live happy and healthy lives and to be loved and well-liked by friends and family members. If at all possible, people also want to be

FAST FACTS

The average American is exposed to 1,500 advertising messages a day.

able to afford the good things in life. Advertisements are directed toward assuring us that we can have it all—if only we buy what they are selling. Obviously, no one automatically becomes popular and irresistible by buying an advertised perfume or cologne. Drinking a specific brand of beer will not enhance one's sex appeal. And I guarantee you that serving a particular type of potato chip will not turn a boring party into a gala event! If we are to be wise consumers, we have to pay attention not only to the obvious messages that advertising conveys but to the hidden messages as well—those messages that appeal to our psychological self. Consumers must be able to separate fact from fiction if they are to make intelligent decisions about whether or not to buy a product or use a service.

> ■ *PROBLEM SITUATION* You read an advertisement in a magazine telling about a revolutionary new cream that prevents the facial skin from wrinkling with age. All you have to do is apply the cream twice a day for three months, and your facial skin becomes immune to the wrinkling process. This cream can only be purchased by mail order, and the company's name and address are listed on the advertisement. How would you analyze this advertisement? If you were interested in buying this cream, what questions should you ask yourself? What sources could you contact to obtain further information?

Many advertisements do not supply the information needed to make an intelligent decision. Empty words are used instead of facts. This advertising technique, known as **puffery,** is frequently used to sell products. The purpose of puffery is to magnify or exaggerate the characteristics or value of a product, thereby making it more desirable to the consumer. Puffery, however, does not provide specific facts about the product. Therefore, since no false information is being directly stated, it is not an illegal advertising technique. Examples of puffery include the following:

- Coke is it.
- Bayer works wonders.
- Ajax cleans like a white tornado.
- Try the clean makeup—Covergirl.

As you can see, nothing substantial is being said about these products. It is up to the consumer to interpret the message that is being conveyed and then to decide whether or not to buy the product. The ultimate goal of puffery is persuasion. Can you think of an advertisement that uses puffery as the primary communication technique?

Advertisements and commercials are not the only techniques used to try to get the consumer to buy certain products. Effective packaging, using bright colors, attractive shapes, and catchy names, has a considerable influence on consumer buying. From the manufacturer's point of view, successful packaging produces "brand identity." The consumer immediately knows and recognizes the product when it is seen on the shelf. The liquid cleaner whose label shows a bald-headed man wearing one earring with arms crossed over his chest is immediately identifiable. Some products have such strong brand identities that

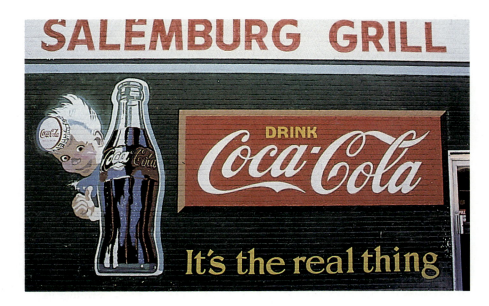

Advertisers know what they are trying to say—but do we know?

even children who have not yet learned to read can recognize them. Just ask any child which cereal has the tiger on the box. Other techniques, such as sales, coupons, rebates, and money-back guarantees, are used to encourage consumers to buy certain products.

If you are a smart shopper, there are many good and legitimate deals to be had; however, part of smart shopping is knowing when you are being "ripped off." To avoid being taken advantage of, consumers should follow these principles:

1. Be suspicious of offers that are "too good to be true." In the world of business, nobody gives away something for nothing.

2. Be suspicious of salespeople who offer special deals if you "act now." Important purchases must be carefully considered. Don't feel pressured to buy. You may regret it later.

3. Shop around to compare quality and prices. Wise shoppers look for quality as well as price. The low-priced product may not be the best buy.

4. Determine whether a sale price is actually a good price. Don't assume that the word "sale" means "best value." Some businesses overprice their merchandise, so when there is a sale and the prices are lowered, the consumer may be paying what other stores regularly charge. Some sale!

5. Inquire about whether the quoted price of an item includes such extras as delivery charges or installation or if those services will involve an additional charge.

6. Don't rely on verbal promises or arrangements. They are not legally binding. Get everything in writing and have the person who made the promises sign and date the agreement.

7. Determine whether the product comes with a guarantee. A guarantee is a statement given to the purchaser by the seller at the time of sale that states what will be done if the product fails to perform as expected. The buyer should ask: (1) What is guaranteed? (2) What is it guaranteed against? (3) For how long is it guaranteed? (4) What will the seller or manufacturer do? (5) What do I have to do? (6) What are the conditions of the guarantee?

8. If there is a contract to sign, take your time reading everything. If there are any blank spaces in the contract that the salesperson says will be filled in later, DO NOT SIGN. If you don't understand the contract and any questions asked still remain unanswered, DO NOT SIGN.

9. Investigate the reliability of unfamiliar businesses by checking with friends and local consumer agencies.

10. Remember, a bargain is only a bargain if the product is something that you need or want and it is at a price you are willing to pay.

11. Don't be afraid to ask questions. That is your right!

■ Consumer Protection Skills

Have you ever bought a product just because of the way it was advertised? Did the advertisement say that the product was highly effective and extremely reliable? Did you rush right out to the nearest store and buy the product? When you got home and tried the product, did it live up to its claims, or were you disappointed? How many times have you thrown part or all of a product in the garbage because it just did not do what the advertisement said it would do? With each product that you have thrown away, you have also thrown away valuable money. And what's almost as infuriating is that the product continues to be falsely advertised and others are also throwing away their money buying it. By saying and doing nothing about this deception, you are allowing advertisers and manufacturers to make profits from your losses. What can you do about inaccurate or misleading advertising?

> ■ *PROBLEM SITUATION* You have just bought a hand and body soap that claims to be "milder and less irritating" than other soaps. The word "hypoallergenic" even appears on the package. Shortly after washing your hands, you develop a slight itching rash that lasts for several minutes. What would be your reaction? What would you do with the soap?

If you buy a product and find that it does not measure up to the promises made for it, complain to the advertiser, to the medium in which you saw the advertisement, and to your local consumer protection agency. If the advertisement is on national television, complain to the Federal Trade Commission. It might sound like an overwhelming task, and you may even say to yourself, "Why bother?" The reason you should bother is that you need to let the proper organizations know about your problem. Not only is this the fastest way to get your complaint resolved, but it also gives the manufacturer a chance to keep you as a satisfied customer and gain new customers by making improvements. If you know the correct steps to follow, registering your complaint will be easy. The following points are important if you want to ensure success:

1. Assess whether you have a legitimate complaint. Only when you have followed the directions and used the product in a safe, competent manner and then there has been failure or dissatisfaction are you eligible for reimbursement or damages.

2. Always remain coolheaded. Don't become overly emotional. Wisely plot your strategy, and you'll be more likely to win in the end.

SELF-INVENTORY 18.1

What Kind of Shopper Are You?

Place a check mark in the column that most accurately describes your attitudes and behaviors regarding shopping.

	True	False	Sometimes
1. I love to go shopping.	___	___	___
2. I am usually one of the first in line when the doors open for a store-wide sale.	___	___	___
3. I am an impulse shopper.	___	___	___
4. When a new product comes out in the stores, I usually buy it.	___	___	___
5. I am a sucker for a good value.	___	___	___
6. I like to spend time window shopping.	___	___	___
7. I have difficulty saying "no" to a good sales pitch.	___	___	___
8. I buy brand-name products because they are better than generic.	___	___	___
9. If I am dissatisfied with a product, I usually throw the item away rather than return it.	___	___	___
10. I don't have the time to shop around for the best buy.	___	___	___
11. I go into a store, buy what I need, and then leave.	___	___	___
12. I feel that shopping is a bother.	___	___	___
13. I often overpay for products and services.	___	___	___
14. I read labels and compare products for their quality before looking at the price.	___	___	___
15. I will not sacrifice quality for price.	___	___	___
16. If I am dissatisfied with a product, I return it and ask for a refund.	___	___	___
17. I will not buy a product if I have any doubts about it.	___	___	___
18. If I have a complaint about a product or service, I ask to speak to the person in charge.	___	___	___
19. I feel that I am a wise consumer and do not let people in the marketplace take advantage of me.	___	___	___

Scoring:

If you answered "Yes" to questions 1 through 7, you are what every salesperson hopes for. You probably have a house full of items that you never use. You need to learn how to become a wise consumer and not give in to all your buying desires.

If you answered "Yes" to questions 8 through 13, you are probably spending more money than you need to and not taking the time to determine if you are buying quality merchandise. You need to learn how smart consumer skills can save you money without having to sacrifice quality.

If you answered "Yes" to questions 14 through 19, you are a wise consumer. Keep up the good work!

3. Be persistent. Don't give up if you initially experience failure.

4. Learn about the organizational structure of the company to which you are complaining. If you don't get satisfaction at one level, go up to the next. This shows your willingness to keep on going until you reach the president of the company.

5. Learn to increase the vehemence of your letters gradually rather than openly attacking the company. By coolly accelerating the intensity of your complaint, you can have maximal psychological impact on those to whom you are complaining.

6. Have sufficient evidence to substantiate your claim. You should (1) report your complaint promptly, (2) state the problem as clearly as possible, (3) describe the product in question fully, (4) state how the company can rectify the problem, and (5) include photocopies of any supportive evidence. (Figure 18–1 illustrates what the U.S. Office of Consumer Affairs recommends as the format to follow when writing a letter of complaint.)

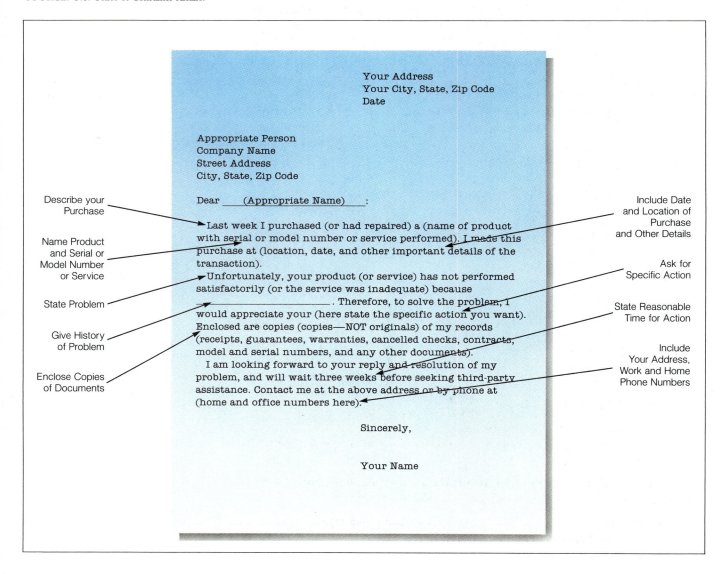

FIGURE 18–1 ■ **How to Write a Letter of Complaint**

SOURCE: U.S. Office of Consumer Affairs.

If you get no positive results, begin writing to support agencies such as the Better Business Bureau (BBB), and send copies of your letter to the company along with a statement of what you are doing. By involving other agencies that can affect the company you are complaining to, you increase the impact of your complaint. Because companies fear adverse publicity, a letter to a newspaper or "action line" may also help you to get results. If all else fails, you may consider suing in small claims court.

The Wheeler-Lea Amendment, which was passed in 1938, is that portion of the Federal Trade Commission Act that deals with truth in advertising. This act empowers the FTC to establish certain kinds of regulations governing advertising content and to take action against advertisers whose messages it deems harmful to the consumer. There is nothing in the Wheeler-Lea Amendment to prevent advertisers from using puffery, as long as they don't deceive the consumer in the process. To sustain high standards of truth and accuracy in national advertising, a self-regulatory system was established within the advertising industry in 1971. The National Advertising Division (NAD) of the Better Business Bureau investigates questionable advertisements and negotiates settlements. The NAD systematically monitors radio, television, and print advertising. A consumer who wishes to file a complaint about an advertisement may do so in the following way:

1. Prepare a written statement citing the "where, when, and what" of the advertisement. If the advertisement is in print, enclose an original copy.
2. Send the complaint to the National Advertising Division in New York City.
3. Send a copy of your correspondence to your congressional representative.

Wise consumers should follow the advice of consumer advocate David Horowitz when he says, "Fight Back!"

Accuracy of Health Information

Because advertisements are designed to sell, how can consumers be assured that the information being conveyed is nonbiased and accurate? Here are some questions to help the consumer determine whether sources of health information are accurate and reliable.

1. What is the purpose of the material? Is it produced to sell products, make money, or present factual information in order to make a professional contribution?
2. Is it presented in an educational or scientific manner, or does it use exaggerated claims and make misleading and inaccurate statements?
3. Is the author qualified in terms of educational background and professional experience?
4. Are the data based on appropriate research findings and the experiences of experts in the health field or on the opinions of a few individuals?
5. Is the research acceptable to medical, dental, public health, and other reputable authorities and organizations?
6. What evidence exists to support or refute conflicting claims about health information?

Very simply stated, when trying to analyze the accuracy and reliability of health information, you need to ask yourself:

- Who says so?
- How does that person know?
- How did he or she find out?
- Is anything missing?
- Does it all make sense?

GUIDELINES TO YOUR GOOD HEALTH

You should contact your primary-care physician if you experience the following:

1. A symptom or condition is too severe to be endured.
2. An apparently minor symptom persists for a few days with no easily identifiable cause.
3. Symptoms return repeatedly for no apparent reason.
4. There is doubt about the condition.

Health Care

When was the last time you bought something expensive? Did it take you a long time to save up enough money to buy it? While you were saving up the money, did you check to see which stores sold what you wanted and how much each was charging? Did you look for advertisements and cut out the ones from places that offered the best deal? Did you ask questions that helped you to eliminate certain stores from your list? Did you narrow down your selection to two or three sources and then decide where you would buy the item? If all of the preceding questions sound familiar and you have gone through this decision-making process, then ask yourself the following question: Did you spend as much time and effort in the investigation and selection of your primary-care physician? If the answer is "no," are you placing more value on material possessions than you are on your health and life? Medical care is the most vital consumer service that any of us will ever buy. Yet we are often ignorant of the medical background and fee scales of available physicians and generally have no idea about how to find the physician most suitable for our needs.

The first step toward proper health care is to choose the right primary-care physician. Your primary-care physician is the one on whom you will depend for routine medical treatment and also the one who will refer you to a specialist or admit you to a hospital should that ever become necessary. It is important that you choose a physician when you are healthy, before you need one. This gives you the opportunity to decide what you want and to evaluate whether the physician meets your criteria. It also gives the physician a chance to get to know you and to become familiar with your medical history. It is recommended that you choose a family practitioner or a general internist as your primary-care physician. Never bypass your primary-care physician by referring yourself to a specialist. Specialists usually are not familiar with your total health picture and tend to see health problems in terms of their own area of expertise. Your primary-care physician will refer you to a specialist when necessary. (Refer to Table 18–1 for a list of medical specialties and subspecialties.)

When selecting a physician, it is helpful to inquire about the physician's credentials. Credentials may be ascertained by contacting the physician's office, by consulting medical societies and hospitals with which the physician is affiliated, or by looking in reference books such as *The Directory of Medical Specialties* or *The American Medical Directory*. It is a good idea to select a physician who is either "board certified" (has completed the qualifying requirements and has

FAST FACTS

Only 13 percent of the nation's physicians are women.

TABLE 18–1 ■ Medical Specialties and Subspecialties

Specialty/Subspecialty	Description
Allergy:	A subspecialty of internal medicine concerned with the diagnosis and treatment of allergic reactions.
Anesthesiology:	Administration of drugs to prevent pain or to induce unconsciousness during surgical operations or diagnostic procedures.
Cardiology:	A subspecialty of internal medicine concerned with the diagnosis and treatment of the heart and blood vessels.
Dermatology:	Diagnosis and treatment of skin disorders.
Endocrinology:	A subspecialty of internal medicine concerned with the diagnosis and treatment of glandular disorders.
Family Practice:	General medical care for patients and their families.
Gastroenterology:	A subspecialty of internal medicine concerned with the diagnosis and treatment of the digestive tract.
Hematology	Diagnosis and treatment of blood disorders.
Internal Medicine:	Diagnosis and nonsurgical treatment of internal organs of the body.
Neonatal Medicine:	A subspecialty of pediatrics concerned with the diagnosis and treatment of disorders of newborn infants.
Nephrology:	Diagnosis and treatment of kidney disorders.
Neurology:	Diagnosis and nonsurgical treatment of disorders of the brain, spinal cord, and nerves.
Nuclear Medicine:	Use of radioactive substances for the diagnosis and treatment of disease.
Obstetrics/Gynecology:	Care of pregnant women and the diagnosis and treatment of disorders of the female reproductive system.
Oncology:	Diagnosis and treatment of cancerous tumors.
Ophthalmology:	Medical and surgical care of the eye, including the prescription of corrective lenses.
Orthopedics:	Treatment of diseases, fractures, and deformities of the bones and joints, and diseases of the muscles.
Otolaryngology:	Diagnosis and treatment of ear, nose, and throat disorders.
Pathology:	Examination of organs, tissues, body fluids, and excrement to detect disease.
Pediatrics:	The medical care of children through adolescence.
Physiatry:	Treatment and rehabilitation of physical handicaps.
Plastic Surgery:	Correction or repair of body or facial structures through surgery.
Preventive Medicine:	Prevention of disease through good health practices, immunization, and environmental control.
Proctology:	Diagnosis and treatment of disorders of the lower digestive tract.
Psychiatry:	Diagnosis and treatment of mental and emotional disorders.
Pulmonary Medicine:	A subspecialty of internal medicine concerned with diseases of the lungs.
Radiology:	Use of radiation for the diagnosis and treatment of disease.
Rheumatology:	A subspecialty of internal medicine concerned with arthritis and related disorders.
Thoracic Surgery:	Surgical treatment of the lungs, heart, and large blood vessels within the chest cavity.
Urology:	Diagnosis and treatment of disorders of the urinary tract in both males and females, and the genital organs in the male.

passed the board examination in a given specialty, thereby becoming a "diplomate" of that board) or "board eligible" (has completed the qualifying requirements but has not yet passed the board examination). Most physicians also belong to one or more professional societies. The criteria for membership in these groups vary and are not a guarantee of a physician's skill. However, initials such as A.C.S. (American College of Surgeons) appearing after a physician's name give some indication of the physician's medical training. If the physician has met additional criteria, he or she may be elected a "fellow" of the society and permitted to use that designation. For example, the initials F.A.C.S. appearing after a physician's name indicate a Fellow of the American College of Surgeons. Some societies require their members to complete a minimum number of hours of ongoing training annually to keep up with new medical developments.

Try to select a physician who is affiliated with a good hospital that is connected with a medical school. If the hospital has a formal program for training medical students and resident doctors, affiliated physicians can keep up with the latest medical advances. Also, if you are in need of hospitalization, you can be admitted to that hospital because your physician has privileges there.

Besides inquiring about a physician's credentials and medical affiliations, you should also consider the following information before making your selection:

1. Is the physician's office conveniently located?
2. Are the office hours ones that work with your schedule?
3. What is the charge for a routine visit?
4. Can major bills be paid in installments?
5. Will medical insurance cover any costs?
6. Who covers for the physician when he or she is not available?
7. How does the physician feel about referring patients to specialists?

If you are satisfied with the answers, your next step is to make an appointment for a routine examination. Only after a personal visit will you be able to judge whether the physician is the right one for you. A thorough health examination is the best situation in which to evaluate a new physician. If you are pleased with the way you were treated and believe that the doctor met your personal and professional criteria, you have been successful in finding yourself a primary-care physician. If, however, you are dissatisfied, keep searching until you find the kind of bedside manner you are looking for.

GUIDELINES TO YOUR GOOD HEALTH

When compiling a list of physicians to choose from, names can be obtained from the following sources:

- The department of medicine at a nearby medical school
- A local accredited hospital
- Another local health-care professional
- The county medical society
- Your previous physician
- Relatives, friends, and co-workers

A successful doctor-patient relationship involves communication. As the patient, you have every right to ask questions and receive direct and honest answers from your physician. But, as the patient, you also have the obligation to be open and honest with your physician when you have a medical problem. In order to receive the proper diagnosis and treatment, you must disclose any information that could be contributing to your problem. In a doctor-patient relationship, the doctor is required to keep in confidence anything that you reveal.

> ■ *PROBLEM SITUATION* You are new in town and need to choose a primary-care physician. Describe your ideal physician. Is it a male or a female? How old? What does he or she look like? What sort of demeanor will he or she have? What will the office look like?

One of the most difficult decisions that arises in a doctor-patient relationship occurs when the doctor advises the patient to have elective, or nonemergency, surgery. Any surgical procedure involves two inherent risks: the surgical procedure itself, and the anesthetic being used. It is estimated that 10 to 20 percent of the 21 million operations performed annually are not necessary. Some of the more commonly overprescribed operations are hysterectomies, tonsillectomies, gall bladder and prostate gland removal, and back and knee surgery. Before agreeing to any elective surgery, you should know the answers to these questions:

1. What does the doctor say is the matter with you?
2. What is the operating procedure for the surgery that is being recommended?
3. Who does your doctor recommend to perform the surgery? (Primary-care physicians usually are not surgeons.)
4. What are the benefits of having the surgery?
5. What are the risks of having the surgery, and how likely are they to occur?
6. How long would the recovery period be and what is involved?
7. What are the costs of the surgery?
8. What costs will your medical insurance cover?
9. What will happen if you don't have the surgery?
10. Are there other ways to treat your condition that could be tried first?

When thinking about elective surgery, one way you can help yourself to reach a decision is to seek the advice of another qualified physician. This advice is called a *second opinion*. Any time that elective surgery is recommended, you should get a second opinion. Most medical insurance plans will pay for it, and some even insist on it as a precondition to paying for the surgery. A second opinion should not be used to delay or avoid having an emergency operation. With emergency surgery, any delay could be life-threatening, so second opinions are seldom possible for this kind of surgery.

Some people do not feel comfortable about letting their doctor know that they are getting a second opinion. Not only is this practice sound, but it is one that every conscientious doctor will recommend. By informing your physician that you are getting another opinion, your medical records can be sent to the second doctor. In this way, you may be able to avoid the time, costs, and discomfort of having to repeat tests. When you ask questions, receive thorough information, and have the opinions of two qualified doctors, you increase your chances of making the decision that is right for you.

Health Insurance

Health insurance is a necessity for everyone, especially because of the constant and enormous rise in health-care costs. Buying health insurance is no easy task. There are hundreds of companies to buy from, offering thousands of combinations of coverage. Millions of Americans are fortunate to be covered by group health insurance plans through their jobs; however, millions of other Americans are without any coverage whatsoever. And even those who are insured usually have far less insurance than is necessary to ensure that they will not become bankrupt because of health-care bills.

Additional insurance is equally necessary for the millions of Americans over 65 years of age who are covered by Medicare, because the program provides only partial coverage. Medicare today is paying only 38 percent of the total health bill for persons age 65 and older. Of the 28 million Americans over the age of 65, 83 percent have at least one policy to supplement the inadequate coverage of Medicare.

Most individuals have little understanding of what protection they may or may not have through their health insurance until they need to use it. It then comes as an overwhelming shock when these individuals discover the sizable amount of out-of-pocket money that must be paid. If you are among those who do have health insurance, do you know what kind of coverage yours provides?

There are three general categories of health insurance plans—traditional health insurance, health maintenance organizations, and public health insurance. Traditional health insurance—also referred to as private, prepaid health insurance—can be obtained through private insurance companies such as Blue Cross/Blue Shield. With this type of health insurance, the system that provides the health care is separate from the system that pays for the care. This is why health insurance companies are called third-party payers. These companies guarantee to reimburse health-care providers for their services within specified guidelines, but they do nothing to help provide health care or to assure the quality of that care.

Health maintenance organizations, commonly referred to as HMOs, are organizations that provide comprehensive health care. They are owned and operated by a variety of different organizations. The HMO that provides your health care also pays for it, so the organization that you choose has a vested interest in assuring the quality of that care.

Public health insurance programs are sponsored by the government at the federal, state, and local level. Programs such as Medicare and Medicaid are examples of public health insurance. Medicare is a federal insurance program. It provides health insurance benefits for persons 65 years of age or older and to certain disabled younger persons under the age of 65. Medicaid is a federal-state partnership assistance program that provides health-care services for public assistance recipients, the aged, the blind, the disabled, and members of single-parent families with dependent children.

Let's examine the benefits offered by traditional health insurance plans as compared to those offered by health maintenance organizations to help determine which type of plan best suits your individual health-care needs.

Traditional Health Insurance

With traditional health insurance, you can be covered by either a group or an individual policy. Group coverage usually is less expensive and provides better

---

FAST FACTS

It is estimated that 30 to 40 million people in the United States have no health insurance.

FAST FACTS

The Better Business Bureau states that individuals can assess the value of health insurance policies by comparing the amount of money a company pays out in claims to the amount received in premiums. For group policies, a minimum of $75 should be returned for every $100 collected and for individual policies a minimum of $60 should be returned.

coverage, because your employer pays for part of it and also handles some of the administrative details. If you are eligible for a group policy, be sure to find out what type of coverage you have so that you can determine if you need to purchase supplemental insurance. Also find out if you can convert your group coverage to an individual policy should you leave your place of employment. The individual coverage will probably cost more, but it is better than leaving yourself with no coverage at all. If your new place of employment offers group health insurance, you can then cancel your individual coverage.

With traditional health insurance, an individual has the freedom to choose any physician or hospital in the world to provide his or her health care. Most traditional health insurance provides coverage for the following types of benefits: hospital and medical, surgical, major medical, and disability. Hospital, medical, and surgical benefits are present in one form or another in most health insurance policies. Sometimes major medical and disability benefits are not a part of health insurance coverage. They may have to be purchased separately. Always check to determine what the provisions are in your specific policy.

Major medical is designed to supplement your basic health benefits by providing protection against the high costs of prolonged illnesses or serious accidents. Most group insurance policies include major medical coverage. If it is not included, however, it is wise to buy this type of coverage. Major medical insurance is generally not very expensive because you are insuring against a highly unlikely event and the policies usually have a high deductible. (More about deductibles will be mentioned in this section.) Once your medical bills rise above the deductible, major medical will cover a substantial percentage of your costs.

Disability benefits offer protection from loss of income resulting from illness or accident. It is important to check how your policy defines "disability." If your policy defines it as "the inability to perform duties pertaining to any occupation," you would have to be unable to do ANY type of work in order to collect money. If, however, your policy defines it as "the inability to perform duties pertaining to the individual's type of occupation," you would be able to collect.

Many of these benefits have cost-sharing stipulations that divide up the costs between the insurance company and the individual. There is tremendous variety in these, so it is extremely important for an individual to understand the provisions of his or her specific coverage. Most plans have a **deductible.** This is a fixed sum of money that the insured individual must pay each year before the insurance coverage becomes effective. For example, if your deductible is $100 per year, you would have to pay the first $100 of your medical bills before your insurance would cover any costs. When the next year rolls around, you must again pay $100 toward your medical bills before your insurance coverage begins taking care of any costs.

Another cost-sharing stipulation found in many health insurance policies is the **copayment.** A copayment is the amount of money that the insured individual pays toward each medical charge before the insurance company assumes the remaining charges. For example, if an office visit to your physician costs $50, your copayment might be $10 and your insurance company would pay the remaining $40. If you purchased a prescription drug, however, your copayment might be only $2. Copayments vary according to the type of medical service received.

The third type of cost-sharing is called **coinsurance.** Coinsurance divides the medical expenses proportionately between the insurance company and the in-

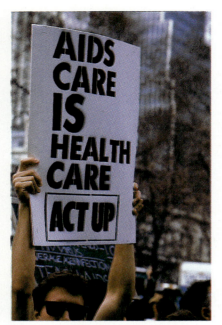

With the advent of AIDS, health insurance has become a must in our society.

FAST FACTS

Consumers should be wary of insurance policies covering cancer, diabetes, and other specified diseases. The policies have uncommon restrictions and limitations that are frequently hidden.

dividual. The individual pays a specific percentage of the charge rather than a specific dollar amount. Usually the insurance company assumes 80 percent of the cost and the individual assumes the other 20 percent. For example, if an individual's medical bill is $7,500, he or she is responsible for paying 20 percent of the bill, or, in this case, $1,500. Having to pay this amount can still be a financial burden to many people.

In addition to deductibles, copayments, and coinsurance, most traditional health insurance will cover the cost for physicians' services and surgery based on a schedule of "usual and customary" fees. What is considered to be "usual and customary" is determined and defined by the insurance company. For each service or procedure, the insurance company sets a predetermined amount that it will pay for that service or procedure. This fee is usually determined by the amount that a sampling of physicians charge for the same service or procedure. If your medical bill is higher than what is deemed usual and customary by your insurance company's standards, you are responsible for paying the difference.

Another fact that should not be overlooked is that most insurance companies pay for medical care only when an individual is ill. What this means is that you, as the patient, need to be diagnosed as having a disease or medical condition if you want your insurance company to pay the bill. The physician, however, is ethically expected to diagnose only what is supported by the examination. The conflict arises when the physician is asked to fill out your insurance form, because what she or he writes down determines who pays the bill. Unfortunately, preventive health care is rarely covered by traditional health insurance. Let's say, for example, that while you are undergoing a routine health examination, your physician notices that you have not had an immunization against tetanus in the past ten years. It would be a good preventive measure to get a tetanus booster at this time. If you do, however, traditional health insurance will not cover it. Your insurance company would pay for the injection only if you had a puncture wound or laceration.

Most traditional health insurance policies will not cover an individual for any illness or condition that exists, or had existed in the past, at the time the policy is purchased. Denial of this type of coverage is called a **preexisting condition clause.** Insurance companies include this clause to help keep their costs down. Exclusion of coverage for preexisting conditions creates a gap in an individual's health-care coverage. It is probably those very conditions that are the most costly to the individual. Some policies have preexisting condition clauses that last for a specified period of time. Others have clauses that last for as long as the policy remains in effect. If you have a preexisting health condition and you are buying individual health insurance, buy a policy that has a limited preexisting condition clause. At least once the specified period is over, coverage will begin.

Health Maintenance Organizations (HMOs)

Health maintenance organizations have existed for more than fifty years. The HMO concept began on the West Coast. Kaiser Foundation Health Plan, the nation's largest HMO, currently has more than four million members. As more people learn about HMOs, the quality of care they provide, and the potential savings they offer over traditional health insurance, the number and popularity of HMOs will continue to increase. HMOs offer an important alternative to traditional health insurance. They provide a complete range of health-care services to their members in exchange for a regular (usually monthly) fee. Unlike traditional health insurance, an HMO has no deductibles, seldom requires any coinsurance, and provides preventive health care. Many HMOs offer membership only to individuals of particular groups, such as employees of a university or members of a union. Other HMOs can be joined on an individual basis. In all cases, the benefits of the membership remain the same: comprehensive health care for a single regular fee. If you become a member through your employer, a large part of the membership fee, or even the entire amount, is paid by your employer. No matter how much medical care is needed, your membership fee will not increase. Rates for a given year may go up because of inflation, but an HMO cannot raise just your membership fee for any reason. Also, your membership cannot be canceled as long as you pay your fee and remain a member of the enrolling group.

When you enroll in an HMO, you agree to obtain your health care through the physicians and other health-care personnel associated with that HMO. When you need medical care, you usually go to a neighborhood HMO facility. Assembled under one roof are primary-care physicians, specialists, laboratory and X-ray facilities, and even a pharmacy. During your first visit, you will be asked to choose a primary-care physician. This physician will be responsible for most of your medical care while you are a member of that particular HMO. Should you become unhappy or dissatisfied with your original selection, you are free to select a different primary-care physician at any time. HMOs have a designated service area, which is a specific geographical area in which its members must live. If you live outside of this area, you cannot become a member of that HMO.

As is the case with traditional health insurance, HMOs offer hospital, medical, and surgical benefits. The main difference, however, is that HMOs offer more comprehensive coverage. Disability insurance is not a part of HMO coverage. All physician services, including checkups, preventive medical care, and referrals made by your primary-care physician to a specialist, are covered. One of the most significant HMO benefits is the coverage of prescription drugs. Usually there is a copayment ranging from $1 to $5, depending on the plan.

HMOs also provide out-of-area coverage. This means that if you need emergency or medical care anywhere in the world (or if you are more than a certain distance away from an HMO facility), the HMO will pay for a large portion of the medical expenses until you are able to return to your HMO facility. Usually the member is responsible for a 20 percent coinsurance payment. If you do obtain medical care outside of your HMO's service area, get as much written documentation as possible from the attending physician, including a statement of the diagnosis and treatment. Also make sure to get a copy of your bill. Your HMO may require this information before it will provide any coverage.

Although HMOs offer comprehensive and quality health care at a reasonable price, you may encounter some disadvantages. For one thing, you are required to choose a physician from those in the HMO. This means severing ties with the physician you used before joining the HMO. If you have developed a valued doctor-patient relationship and think that your physician is qualified and competent to attend to your medical needs, you may be hesitant to start seeing another physician. If this is the case, you may be lucky enough to find that your physician is affiliated with the HMO. You can then continue seeing that physician and also obtain the more comprehensive coverage offered by the HMO. Another possible disadvantage is that many people feel frustrated by long waits

FAST FACTS

The Health Maintenance Organization Act of 1973 requires all employers with 25 or more employees to offer workers an opportunity to join a qualified HMO if one exists in the area.

for appointments and crowded waiting rooms. You may have to make an appointment for a routine checkup or some other preventive care well in advance. For health problems needing prompt attention, however, you usually get an immediate appointment.

Remember that although HMOs generally provide quality and comprehensive health care, it is unrealistic to say that once you join an HMO, you will experience the epitome of health care. No person or organization is perfect, and if you are expecting perfection, you are bound to be disappointed. Before selecting any health insurance plan, you must consider your own specific health-care needs and carefully examine the specific costs, benefits, coverage, exclusions, and limitations of each plan.

■ Over-the-Counter Drugs and the Consumer

Many of us have been ill sometime during the past year. We all have experienced everyday colds, upset stomachs, allergies, pain, and many other common medical problems. Because of the high cost of medical care, the lack of physicians in remote areas, or the simple fact that our illness is minor, we sometimes need to diagnose and treat ourselves. Our first task is to determine what illness we have. Our second is to decide what, if anything, to do about it. And our third, if we determine it to be necessary, is to choose a medication or other treatment. We generally face that task with little knowledge about **over-the-counter (OTC) drugs,** their effects, the appropriateness of their use in the situation, and nondrug alternatives.

Once you have diagnosed your own medical problem and have determined that it is something you can deal with yourself, you have to choose the proper medication, if any, to treat the illness or injury. This is no easy task. It has been estimated that there are more than 500,000 different over-the-counter drug products in this country containing approximately 10,000 different active ingredients. When you walk into a pharmacy, you may be overwhelmed by the vast number of products for the same problem, each advertising its advantages over all the others. What do you choose for your cold—Dristan, Sinex, Contac, Sine-Aid, Nyquil, or some other product? Do you trust the advertising to be honest? Can you ask the pharmacist's advice? Are there books you can buy to help you make those choices?

First, let's consider possible reference books that you might consider for your home library. In choosing a resource, you must take care that the book you buy isn't biased and isn't trying to sell you something. The three books that we have found to be the most useful are *The Handbook of Nonprescription Drugs,* available from the American Pharmaceutical Association; *The PDR (Physician's Desk Reference) for Nonprescription Drugs,* available from the Medical Economics Company; and *About Your Medicines,* available from the United States Pharmacopeial Convention. These books may also be available at your local public library.

Analgesics

First, a note of caution about advertising, because so many of the drug ads we see on television are for **analgesics** (pain relievers). Most drug advertisements contain exaggerations of the truth. The consumer has to sort out fact from fiction. Have you seen the television ads that suggest that extra-strength Tylenol

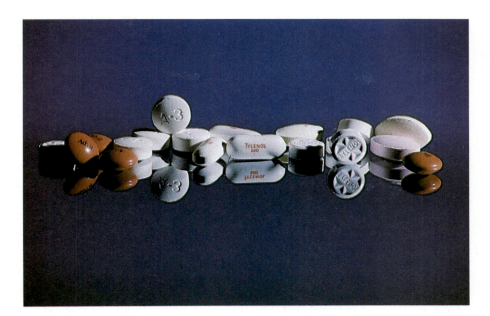

For those people who cannot tolerate aspirin, there are many substitutes available under assorted brand and generic names.

is stronger than regular-strength aspirin or regular-strength Excedrin? Of course that's true. An extra-strength dose (500 mg.) of any drug is stronger than a regular-strength dose (325 mg.) of any drug. Is extra-strength Tylenol a better pain reliever than extra strength aspirin? The answer is a resounding no! Is it better at reducing fever? Again no! How about inflammation? Aspirin is **anti-inflammatory** but Tylenol is not. Are there times when Tylenol is a better choice than aspirin? Yes, in pregnant women (aspirin is **contraindicated** in pregnancy) and in persons who suffer from the gastric distress sometimes caused by aspirin, a salicylate. That problem occurs in approximately 2 percent of the population. Aspirin and other salicylates also should not be given to children or teenagers who have or are recovering from viral illness such as the flu or chicken pox because of the risk of *Reye's Syndrome,* an often fatal illness.

While we are on the subject of aspirin and acetaminophen (the generic name for Tylenol), let's examine other pain relievers available without a prescription. Recently, the Food and Drug Administration allowed a change in the status of the drug ibuprofen. It is now possible to buy ibuprofen in a 200 mg. strength without a prescription under the brand names Advil, Nuprin, Medipren, and others. It is also manufactured in 300 mg., 400 mg., 600 mg., and 800 mg. strengths under the brand names Motrin, Rufen, Morpen, and others and requires a prescription in those strengths. Ibuprofen is a nonsteroidal anti-inflammatory drug (NSAID) and, other than aspirin, is the only drug in this class available without a prescription. Not only are these drugs able to relieve pain but, as their name indicates, they have anti-inflammatory properties as well.

There are a number of aspirin, acetaminophen, and other salicylate combination products on the market. Are combination products more effective than single drugs? Recent studies have suggested that single drugs are just as effective as combination products and they have fewer long-term side effects. One drug often found in combination products that you should avoid is *phenacetin*. Phenacetin has been linked to kidney damage with long-term use.

FAST FACTS

Aspirin can deteriorate. If it has a furry look or a vinegar-like odor, it should be discarded.

How about **buffered aspirin?** Is it safer or more effective than plain aspirin? The buffering in a buffered aspirin tablet is not nearly enough to counteract the acidity of the aspirin. If you are one of those people who can't tolerate aspirin by itself, it would be better to buy an antacid product such as Mylanta or Maalox and simply take a dose of the antacid with each dose of aspirin. It would be far more effective and probably less expensive than buying a buffered aspirin product.

> ■ *PROBLEM SITUATION* You have an inflammation in your ankle from a running injury. Should you purchase aspirin, acetaminophen, or a combination product to relieve your pain? Why?

Cold and Allergy Preparations

Are you ready to take a look at another category of drug products? Let's examine cold and allergy preparations. Most confusion in this area lies in choosing the right product. You could buy a product like Dristan, which advertises its ability to treat all twelve symptoms of a cold at once. But how often do you have all twelve symptoms at once? Rarely, if ever.

Combination cold and allergy preparations generally consist of an **antihistamine,** a **decongestant,** an analgesic, and possibly caffeine. An antihistamine's purpose is to dry up excessive secretions, like the runniness of your nose. A principal side effect of antihistamines is drowsiness. Decongestants reduce stuffiness and include drugs such as pseudoephedrine (Sudafed), phenylpropano-

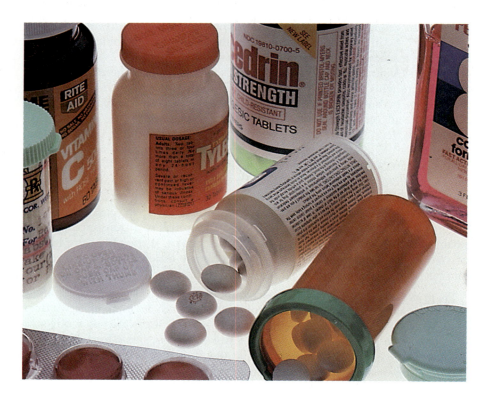

Many prescription and over-the-counter medications are available to treat colds and allergies.

GUIDELINES TO YOUR GOOD HEALTH

Don't take any medication until you ask your physician or pharmacist the following questions:

1. Do I really need this medication?
2. What is the medication for? How will it help me?
3. What are the unwanted side effects of this medication? If they occur, what should I do? Which side effects should be reported?
4. Are there any other medicines that should not be taken while this medicine is being taken?
5. How should I take this medicine?
6. Can I stop taking the medication early if the symptoms disappear?
7. How soon should I expect results?
8. Can I drink alcohol while taking this medication?
9. Are there any foods I should avoid while taking this medication?
10. Can a generic drug be prescribed rather than a brand-name drug so that I can save money?
11. What should I do if I accidentally miss a dose?
12. Is it safe to operate machinery or drive while taking this medication?
13. Should the prescription be refilled, and if so, under what circumstances?

lamine, and phenylephrine. Since these drugs mimic the actions of the sympathetic nervous system (they are **sympathomimetics**), they tend to cause stimulation and wakefulness as side effects. Some people become very restless when using them. Analgesics relieve headache and the other aches and pains often associated with colds and allergies. The most frequently used analgesics are aspirin and acetaminophen. Caffeine is included in many products because of its ability to constrict cerebral blood vessels, thereby reducing headache. It is usually considerably more expensive to buy a combination product than to buy the various ingredients separately. We recommend having as part of your home medicine chest a generic antihistamine such as chlorpheniramine, a generic decongestant such as pseudoephedrine, and a bottle of aspirin or acetaminophen. Then, when a medical problem arises, take only what you specifically need to treat the problem: an antihistamine for a runny nose, a decongestant for stuffiness, and an analgesic for the aches and pains. That would be the safest and least expensive alternative.

When treating the cough often associated with colds and allergies, the same precautions apply as with the tablet and capsule preparations. Many products are combinations of ingredients, usually an **expectorant** to loosen mucous, a cough suppressant, an antihistamine, and a decongestant. Again, use only what is needed, both for safety and economy.

■ *PROBLEM SITUATION* Your sinuses are congested from an allergy. You also have a slight headache from the congestion. What over-the-counter products should you use to relieve your symptoms? Why?

> **FAST FACTS**
>
> More than 50 percent of the people in the United States will receive at least one prescription drug this year, with the average being seven per person.

■ Understanding Your Prescription

Many people think that prescriptions are written in Latin or possibly in some kind of code that the average person is unable to read. This is not true. Prescriptions are written in English. Prescription writing does, sometimes, use a type of special shorthand that the average lay person might not understand (see Table 18–2).

Consider the following prescription:

Rx Tetracycline 250mg. #40
Sig: i po qid × 10 days

The prescriber is requesting that the pharmacist dispense 40 capsules of the antibiotic tetracycline in the 250 milligram strength. The directions to be typed on the label follow the word "sig." They are one capsule (i) by mouth (po) four times daily (qid) for ten days.

Another example:

Rx Sulamyd Ophth. Drops 15ml
Sig: ii gtts os tid and hs

The medication is Sulamyd eye (ophthalmic) drops in the 15 milliliter container. The directions are two (ii) drops (gtts) in the left eye (os) three times daily (tid) and at bedtime (hs). Using the abbreviations in Table 18–2, you should now be able to read and interpret the instructions on your own prescriptions.

Most states require that a prescription contain certain elements. These generally include the name and address of the prescriber; the name and address of the patient; the date; the name, strength, and quantity of the drug; and the prescriber's signature. Refill instructions may be included on the original prescription or may be given later by telephone. Some states have specific requirements regarding the use of generic drugs (to be discussed later in this chapter).

Most prescriptions do not have to be in writing. The exception to this is for the Schedule II controlled substances. Federal laws require that these medications be prescribed on a special triplicate (three-part) prescription blank.

■ Generic Drugs

If you were to discover a new drug that you thought might be effective in treating a disease such as herpes or AIDS, what is the first thing you would do? You would patent the drug to prevent someone else from stealing your discovery. Then you would begin scientifically conducted research studies to find out if the drug was effective and safe.

It could take as long as ten to twelve years and cost many millions of dollars to conduct all the necessary research on a new drug before you could get it to the marketplace. A new drug patent is good for only seventeen years, leaving the developer and manufacturer of the new drug with possibly five to seven years to recover all of its research investment. This explains, at least in part, why new drugs are sometimes so expensive. After the patent expires, other manufacturers, who have little or no research investment, can manufacture the drug at a much lower cost and therefore supply it to the public at a cheaper price.

Sometime during the discovery, development, and marketing of a new drug, it will be given three names: a chemical name, a **generic name,** and a **brand**

TABLE 18-2 ■ **Commonly Used Abbreviations in Prescription Writing**

Symbols	Latin Word	English
Ad	Ad	To, up to
Ad lib	Ad libitum	At pleasure
aa	Ana	Of each
a	Ante	Before
a.c.	Ante cibos	Before meals
aq	Aqua	Water
b.i.d.	Bis in die	Twice a day
caps = capsul	Capsule	A capsule
c	Cum	With
dexter	Dexter	Right
d	Dies, dosis	A day, a dose
et	Et	And
gr.	Granum	Grain
gtt	Gutta	A drop
h	Hora	Hour
hor. som., h.s.	Hora Somni	At bedtime
inj.	Injectio	Injection
Noct	Nox notis	Night
non	Non	Not
non. rep.	Non repetatur	Do not repeat
Ocul.	Oculus	The eye
o.d.	Oculus dexter	Right eye
o.s.	Oculus sinister	Left eye
o.u.	Oculo Uterque	Both eyes, in each eye
omn. hor.	Omni hora	Every hour
P.O.	Per os	By mouth
Placebo	Placebo	To please, satisfy
p.c.	Post cibos	After meals
p.r.n.	Pro re nata	As needed
q.i.d.	Quater in die	Four times daily
Rx	Receipe	Take (thou)
ss	Semis, semi	Half
s., sig.	Signa, signatur	Label
s	Sine	Without
Stat.	Statum	Immediately
t.i.d.	Ter in die	Three times daily
tab	Tabella	Tablet
ut. dict.	Ut. Dictum	As directed

name. The generic name is the common name. "Aspirin" is a generic name. The chemical name is usually long and complicated and is rarely used other than by researchers. One example of a relatively simple chemical name is that of aspirin—acetylsalicylic acid.

Manufacturers give their products brand names. Bayer, St. Joseph, and Empirin are examples of brand names for aspirin. Generally, brand names are designed to direct consumers to that particular brand of product and advertising revolves around brand-name selection. Such names are often catchy and easy to remember for the consumer—for example, Sleep-Eze (obviously a sleeping

Although the names are different, many products contain the same ingredients.

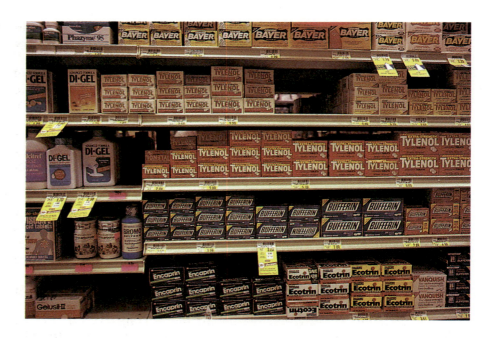

pill), Nyquil (to provide you with a tranquil night), and Herpecin (to relieve the symptoms of herpes cold sores).

Unique and clever brand names are also used when drug companies advertise prescription medications to prescribers. A commonly prescribed drug for the symptoms of menopause is conjugated estrogen (generic name). The original developer of this drug named it Premarin (brand name) because it was first taken from PREgnant MARe urINe. Get it?

Once the patent on a drug expires, other manufacturers will begin manufacturing the same drug either under their own brand name or under the generic name. Prices may vary greatly from one manufacturer to another. What is the consumer to do? Is it important to ask for a more expensive brand, or are the less expensive, generically named brands just as good?

Consumer advocates would have us believe that all brands of a drug are the same and that there are no quality differences between a more expensive brand and the less expensive generic drug. This is not entirely true. The economic factors that come into play in the manufacturing of any product also must be considered in drug manufacturing.

We usually apply the old saying, "You get what you pay for," when we buy most products. Basically, what we mean is that the more something costs, the better the quality. Of course, you can often find the better-quality product at a lower price by shopping around. It is true, however, that a purchaser would expect longer wear, less shrinkage, and fewer problems with a $30 shirt than with a $10 shirt. Likewise, you would expect better-quality sound from a $1,000 stereo receiver than from a $200 receiver.

These same principles apply to drugs. You should expect better quality from more expensive products. It is true that drugs' contents must be labeled and that you should expect each and every bottle to have the same amount of active ingredient if it is labeled as such. For example, if you had ten different brands of aspirin and they were all labeled "aspirin, 5 grains," you would expect them all to have the same effect in relieving your headache. This, however, is not always the case.

Does this mean that generic drugs are not as good as brand names and shouldn't be used? Not at all. There are many instances when less expensive generic drugs are the best choice and other times when they are not. For example, a patient on thyroid medication should not switch from brand to brand because of significant bioavailability differences between brands. The same holds true for certain heart and high blood pressure medications. However, most antibiotics, antihistamines, muscle relaxants, and pain relievers are available in quality generic products.

The key to the effectiveness of a drug is what is known as its **bioavailability**—that is, how available is the drug to the body for its intended purpose once it is taken. Many factors come into play in determining bioavailability. Binders used to hold tablets together, fillers to take up space, coatings on tablets, preservatives, flavoring agents, and many other additives can have an effect on the bioavailability, and therefore the effectiveness, of a drug.

Drugs are tested to determine whether or not they contain the labeled amount of active ingredient, and in the majority of cases they do. But they can not be tested in people to see if they are all equally effective. In addition, bioavailability testing is expensive and is not done routinely on an ongoing basis. Recently, the Food and Drug Administration has begun to require drug companies to have their products meet certain bioavailability standards.

The problem for the consumer is the difficulty in knowing when to ask for brand names and when to ask for generic drugs. It is very important that as a consumer, you establish a relationship with a pharmacist similar to that which you would establish with your physician, dentist, or other health-care practitioner. Then you can feel comfortable in asking for advice and consultation from your pharmacist. He or she knows best when a generic drug is appropriate and when a brand name should be chosen.

> ■ *PROBLEM SITUATION* You have been given a prescription by your physician. She suggests that it might be quite expensive. What options are available to you?

FAST FACTS

Generic drugs are estimated to be 30 to 50 percent cheaper than brand-name drugs.

■ Drug Laws

Federal and state laws governing prescription writing and dispensing directly affect the consumer in terms of his or her ability to obtain prescription medications when they are needed. Let's take a look at some of the factors considered by the Food and Drug Administration when it decides whether a new drug should be available over the counter or on a prescription-only basis.

The first concern is the nature of the illness for which the drug is used and the degree to which the patient can diagnose the problem without medical advice. For instance, the average person could most likely diagnose his or her own cold, allergy, headache, or stomachache. Therefore, most medications for these problems are available without a prescription. However, a prescription is required for medications for diabetes, high blood pressure, and syphilis because these conditions could not be readily self diagnosed.

The second consideration in determining the status of a drug is related to the ability to safely use the medication by simply following directions on the package. Some antihistamine drugs for allergies such as diphenhydramine hydrochloride (Benadryl) and chlorpheniramine maleate (Chlortrimeton) are available over the counter, whereas others such as clemastine fumarate (Tavist) require a prescription. This is because some of them are safe to take using the package directions and information. For others, special precautions and information need to be given to the patient, and therefore they require a prescription.

Lastly, the method of administration is considered. If a drug was to be taken by mouth, it would be expected that everyone would know how to administer it. But if it was to be given by injection, some special knowledge would be necessary. One such drug is vitamin B_{12}, which can be purchased over the counter in orally administered tablets but which requires a prescription in injectable form. The injection has the same pharmacological action as the tablets and is no more dangerous to use, but it requires the patient to know how to give herself or himself an injection, a technique requiring some special training. The only injectable drug available today without a prescription is insulin, needed by diabetics. These patients are trained in injection technique by their physicians and are able to administer their own insulin.

Legend Drugs

To distinguish prescription medications from those available without a prescription, the FDA requires manufacturers of prescription drugs to imprint on the package the statement, "CAUTION: Federal law prohibits dispensing without prescription." This statement is known as the *federal legend;* therefore, prescription drugs are sometimes called "legend" drugs.

Legend drugs do not all require a written prescription. With a few exceptions, prescribers can telephone prescriptions to the pharmacist. In most states, anyone from the prescriber's staff may make the call on the doctor's behalf, but usually only the pharmacist may take the call.

All legend drugs require the prescriber's approval for refills. That approval can be given on the original prescription or later by phone. In most states, pharmacists are permitted to give emergency supplies of medications if the prescriber is unavailable to grant permission for refills.

Controlled Substances

Some drugs, because of their potential for abuse, come under special laws and are generally known as **controlled substances.** The controlled substance laws, first introduced in 1965 and later amended as the Comprehensive Drug Abuse Prevention and Control Act of 1970, have been further amended a number of times and place specific additional restrictions on those drugs that people use recreationally. Under these laws, drugs are divided into categories known as *schedules.* There are five schedules of drugs, with abuse potential decreasing as the schedule number increases (refer to Table 18–3).

Schedule I drugs are those that are considered to have no known medical use in the United States (other than for research) and have a high abuse potential.

TABLE 18-3 ■ **Legal Classification of Controlled Substances**

Schedule	Drug Examples	Abuse Potential	Medical Use
I	Heroin, LSD, PCP, peyote	High	None recognized Only legal use is for research
II	Cocaine, amphetamine, codeine, secobarbital	High	Some medical use Written prescription required Prescription cannot be refilled
III	Tylenol with codeine, aspirin with codeine	Moderate	Medically used Prescription required (telephone prescription is all right) May be refilled up to 5 times in 6 months
IV	Valium, Librium, Darvon, phenobarbital	Low	Medically used Prescription required (telephone prescription is all right) May be refilled up to 5 times in 6 months
V	Cough syrups containing codeine, lomotil	Low	Medically used Prescription required (telephone prescription is all right) May be refilled up to 5 times in 6 months

These include heroin, PCP, and LSD, among others (see Chapter 13).

Schedule II drugs have the highest abuse potential of the legal drugs. This category includes cocaine, most barbiturates, most amphetamines, and most opiates. Prescriptions for drugs in this schedule must be written on special triplicate prescription forms. The prescriber retains one copy of the form and gives two to the patient to take to the pharmacist. The pharmacist keeps one for the files and sends the triplicate copy to the state drug enforcement agency. Prescriptions for schedule II drugs are valid for only seven days from the date written, must be entirely in the prescriber's handwriting, and cannot be refilled.

Drugs in *schedule III* have less abuse potential than those in schedule II and include such products as Tylenol with codeine. Valium, Librium, and Darvon are in *schedule IV*. The principal group of drugs in *schedule V* are the cough syrups containing codeine. The main prescription limitation on drugs in schedules III, IV, and V relates to refilling of prescriptions. Refills are limited to five times or six months, whichever comes first. It's important to note that drugs are placed in these schedules based on their abuse potential. How dangerous they might be or how serious their side effects might be are not considered.

Federal law requires that the package of a controlled drug bear the letter "C" containing a Roman numeral to indicate which schedule it is in. Many states require that pharmacists keep prescriptions for these drugs in separate files, and periodic inventories of scheduled drugs are required.

■ ***PROBLEM SITUATION*** Your relative has cancer and is being given morphine, a schedule II drug, for pain. He is almost out of medication. What must you do to obtain more medication for him?

POSITIVE BEHAVIORS

I. *Place a check mark in front of each behavior that you now practice.*

_____ 1. I shop around to compare quality and prices. (SHOP)

_____ 2. If I am dissatisfied with a health product or service, I take positive action to rectify the problem. (ACTION)

_____ 3. I ask my physician questions about fees, diagnoses, and treatments. (ASK QUESTIONS)

_____ 4. I critically analyze advertisements that promote health products and services. (ANALYZE)

_____ 5. I actively support social changes that will ensure safe and effective health products and services. (ACTIVELY SUPPORT)

_____ 6. I get routine checkups and laboratory tests as preventive health-care measures. (PREVENTIVE)

_____ 7. I have selected a primary-care physician who is responsible for most of my health care. (PRIMARY PHYSICIAN)

_____ 8. I know what kind of coverage my health insurance provides. (INSURANCE)

_____ 9. When I am ill and choose to treat myself, I am careful to take only those medications that are designed to treat my specific symptoms. (SPECIFIC SYMPTOMS)

_____ 10. I take all my prescriptions to the same pharmacist and seek advice on any questions I might have regarding my medications. (ADVICE)

II. *For each behavior that you DO NOT ENGAGE IN, write in the appropriate space below the KEY WORD(S) located in the parentheses at the end of the statement. Then put a check mark in the appropriate column to indicate whether you are going to keep or change that behavior.*

Behaviors I Don't Engage In   KEEP/CHANGE

_____/_____
_____/_____
_____/_____
_____/_____
_____/_____
_____/_____
_____/_____
_____/_____
_____/_____

III. *For each of the preceding behaviors that you choose to KEEP, write a statement indicating why you are choosing to keep that behavior.*

I choose to keep behavior _____ because:
                              KEY WORD

For each of the preceding behaviors that you choose to CHANGE, write a statement indicating how you plan to implement that change.

I will change behavior _____ by:
                          KEY WORD

Now You Know

1. FALSE. The Consumer Bill of Rights gave consumers the right to safety, the right to be informed, the right to choose, and the right to be heard.
2. TRUE. Puffery is the primary communication technique found in advertisements.
3. FALSE. Verbal promises or arrangements are not legally binding.
4. TRUE. Many problems are often caused by errors or misunderstandings. The problem can frequently be corrected at the level at which it originated.
5. FALSE. The Food and Drug Administration is the primary federal agency responsible for the safety of health products.
6. TRUE. Getting a second opinion can help you to avoid unnecessary surgery.
7. TRUE. The individual has the freedom to choose any physician or hospital to provide his or her health care.
8. FALSE. One of the advantages of health maintenance organizations is that they have no deductibles.
9. FALSE. Drug prescriptions are written in English, although some special abbreviations are used in them. The wise consumer should learn how to read and interpret prescriptions.
10. FALSE. In most cases, generic drugs will work just as well as brand-name equivalents. There are a few situations, however, in which that is not the case. Be sure to discuss each prescription with your pharmacist so that you can make an informed choice.

Summary

1. The Consumer Bill of Rights guarantees the consumer the right to safety, the right to be informed, the right to choose, and the right to be heard.
2. The four major federal agencies whose responsibilities deal with consumer protection are the Food and Drug Administration, the Federal Trade Commission, the United States Postal Service, and the Office of Consumer Affairs.
3. Puffery is the primary advertising technique used to sell products. Its purpose is to magnify the characteristics or value of a product, thereby making it more desirable to the consumer.
4. It is the consumer's right to expect quality products and services at fair prices. If there is consumer dissatisfaction, it is up to the consumer to initiate the proper actions to resolve any problems.
5. Medical care is the most vital consumer service that anyone will ever buy. The first step toward proper health care is choosing the right primary-care physician.
6. When selecting a primary-care physician, names can be obtained from such sources as an accredited hospital, the county medical society, and relatives, friends, and co-workers.
7. A large percentage of operations performed annually are not necessary. When elective surgery is recommended by a physician, obtain the advice of another qualified physician. Seeking a second opinion, however, should not be used to delay or avoid having emergency surgery.
8. The three categories of health insurance plans are traditional health insurance, health maintenance organizations, and public health insurance.
9. Both traditional health insurance and HMOs are prepaid medical plans. Unlike traditional health insurance, however, an HMO has no deductibles, seldom requires any coinsurance, and provides preventive health care.
10. Most health insurance coverage includes hospital, medical, and surgical benefits. Major medical and disability insurance can be purchased separately to supplement the basic health benefits.
11. It has been estimated that there are more than 500,000 over-the-counter drug products in the United States containing approximately 10,000 different active ingredients.
12. Drugs are usually sold over-the-counter if they are for problems that the average person could self-diagnose, they can be taken safely by following the package directions, and they are administered in ways other than by injection.
13. Drugs that have a potential for abuse are termed controlled substances and are placed in categories, or schedules, based on the degree of abuse potential. Schedule I consists of drugs that have a high abuse potential and are of no known medical value in the United States. Drugs in schedules II through V can be obtained by prescription and have decreasing abuse potential.
14. Drugs in schedule II require a triplicate prescription and cannot be refilled. Other controlled substances can be refilled a maximum of five times or within six months, whichever comes first. The prescriber's permission is needed for refills.
15. Generic drugs are usually just as effective as their brand-name equivalents. There are some exceptions. An individual should always consult with the pharmacist regarding each prescription.

References

1. *About Your Medicines.* Rockville, Maryland: The United States Pharmacopeial Convention, Inc., 1987.
2. Barofsky, Ivan. (Editor) *Medication Compliance: A Behavioral Management Approach.* Charles B. Slack, Inc., Thorofare, N.J.: 1977.
3. Bennett, William I., Stephen E. Goldfinger, and G. Timothy Johnson. *Your Good Health.* Cambridge, Mass.: Harvard University Press, 1987.
4. *Consumer's Resource Handbook.* Washington, D.C.: U.S. Office of Consumer Affairs, 1984.
5. Cornacchia, Harold J., and Stephen Barrett. *Consumer Health: A Guide to Intelligent Decisions,* 4th ed. St. Louis: Times Mirror/Mosby College Publishing, 1989.
6. Corry, James M. *Consumer Health: Facts, Skills and Decisions.* Belmont, Calif.: Wadsworth Publishing Co., 1983.
7. Govoni, Laura E., and Janice E. Hayes. *Drugs and Nursing Implications,* 3d ed. New York: Appleton-Century-Crofts, 1978.
8. *Handbook of Nonprescription Drugs.* Washington, D.C.: American Pharmaceutical Association, latest ed.
9. Hensel, Bruce. *Smart Medicine.* New York: G. P. Putnam's Sons, 1989.
10. Morris, Mary. *The Truth about Your Diet.* Chicago: William Mulvey Inc., 1988.
11. *Physicians' Desk Reference for Nonprescription Drugs.* Oradell, N.J.: Medical Economics Co., 1989.
12. Price, James H., Nicholas Galli, and Suzanne Slenker. *Consumer Health: Contemporary Issues and Choices.* Dubuque, Iowa: William C. Brown Publishers, 1985.
13. Rosenfeld, Isadore. *Modern Prevention: The New Medicine.* New York: Bantam Books, 1987.
14. Rosenfeld, Isadore. *Symptoms.* New York: Simon and Schuster, 1989.
15. Smith, Wesley J. *The Doctor Book.* Los Angeles: Price Stern Sloan, Inc., 1987.
16. *The American Medical Association Family Medical Guide.* New York: Random House, 1987.
17. Vickery, Donald M., and James F. Fries. *Taking Care of Yourself: A Consumer's Guide to Medical Care,* 3d ed. Reading, Mass.: Addison-Wesley, 1986.
18. Weast, Robert C. (Editor) *". . . take as Directed.* Cleveland: Chemical Rubber Co., 1967.
19. "What Insurance Do You Need?" *Consumer Reports.* Vol. 54, No. 6 (June 1989): 375–378.

Suggested Readings

Consumer Reports. New York: Consumers Union, current issues.

FDA Consumer. Washington D.C.: U.S. Department of Health and Human Services, current issues.

Harvard Medical School Health Letter. Boston: Harvard Medical School, current issues.

National Council Against Health Fraud (NCAHF) Newsletter. Loma Linda, Calif.: National Council Against Health Fraud, Inc., current issues.

Rosenfeld, Isadore. *Second Opinion,* 2d ed. New York: Bantam Books, 1987.

Rosenfeld, Isadore. *Symptoms.* New York: Simon and Schuster, 1989.

Taintor, Jerry F., and Mary Jane Taintor. *The Oral Report: The Consumer's Common Sense Guide to Better Dental Care.* New York: Ballantine Books, 1989.

The New Medicine Show, 6th ed. New York: Consumers Union, 1989.

Vickery, Donald M., and James F. Fries. *Taking Care of Yourself: A Consumer's Guide to Medical Care,* 3d ed. Reading, Mass.: Addison-Wesley, 1986.

CHAPTER 19

Occupational and Environmental Risks

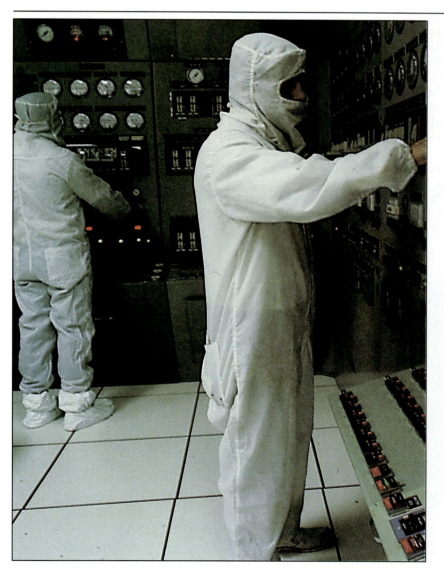

What Do You Know?

Are the following statements true or false?

1. Most serious occupational health problems are related to blue-collar jobs in construction, factories, ship yards, steel mills, and mines.
2. If a material is used in industry or available as a consumer item, you can assume that it is safe to breathe or touch.
3. Health problems related to toxic exposure in the workplace or environment are easy to identify because they occur immediately after exposure.
4. Once a toxic waste site is identified, it is usually very difficult to clean up.
5. Most occupational health problems are difficult to treat and cure.
6. The rapidly expanded production of organic chemicals from the petrochemical industry has brought limitless benefits to society without incurring any related costs.
7. Occupational and environmental health problems are usually manifest as lung problems. Other body organs and systems are rarely harmed by chemicals and ionizing radiation.
8. Common household products contain hazardous materials and generate hazardous waste when disposed of.
9. The unleashed power of the atom may determine the fate of the earth.
10. The country with the highest number of deaths caused by fires and burns is Canada.

Oozing liquid in every color of the rainbow seeped into the basements and backyards of the residents of a quiet and content neighborhood near Niagara Falls, New York. Children were sent home from the 99th Street Elementary School with nausea, headaches, runny noses, and watering eyes. Pets developed tumors and lost their fur. Located in the center of this community was Love Canal, a sixteen-acre landfill into which tons of chemicals known to cause cancer, birth defects, and myriad other health effects had been dumped.

Residents of the neighborhood dealt with their ailments individually, never guessing that the landfill and Hooker Chemical, the company dumping its chemical wastes into Love Canal, were to blame. It was not until residents, primarily housewives, began talking about their individual problems that their suspicions were aroused. The local homeowners association then conducted a survey in the community, asking residents about their health problems. The survey revealed the increased occurrence of miscarriages, birth defects, asthma, and urinary-tract diseases.

Initial assumptions that government agencies would "take care" of the disastrous problems plaguing the community were soon replaced by a realization of the harsh reality that the residents themselves would have to fight to protect their families. At first local, state, and federal agencies denied that there was any danger to the residents' health. Even when they finally acknowledged the hazard, they were slow to act.

Is Love Canal a unique and horrible aberration? Unfortunately not. Love Canal was the first of what was to become a decade of discoveries of toxic chemical pollution and its consequences. There are more than 24,000 hazardous waste sites throughout the United States, of which over 900 are considered to pose an imminent and serious threat to the public's health. Despite the fact that more than $8.5 billion has been invested by Congress to remedy the problem, only thirteen sites had been cleaned up with support from the Federal Superfund as of mid-1987.

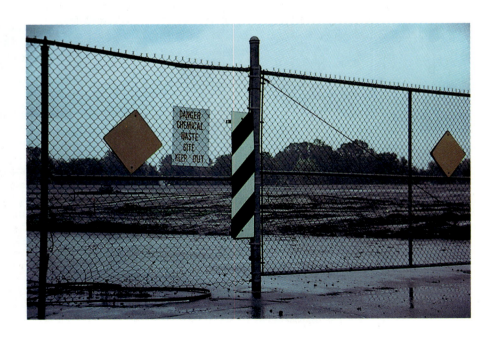

The experience at Love Canal should put us all on guard to the potential dangers of chemical and other wastes.

Sources of Toxic Waste and the Chemical Industry

Plastic trash and grocery bags, insecticides, computers, televisions, styrofoam cups and fast-food containers, synthetic fabrics and paint—this seemingly benign list of common products belies the danger inherent in the expansion of the petrochemical industry, which has made all of these products an integral part of our lives. Manufacture of such products has caused untold occupational illness, environmental damage, and public health problems, either in their production or through the disposal of the resulting toxic wastes.

Even though hazardous waste problems have received an enormous amount of attention by the media and through legislation and regulation, toxic chemicals are still at the core of the majority of toxics issues. Hazardous chemicals have caused problems both when they are used and when they are accidentally released. The worst, and probably best known, catastrophe occurred in Bhopal, India, claiming the lives of over 2,500 people and injuring more than 20,000 when a pesticide manufacturing plant released methyl isocyanate, an extremely toxic gas, into a residential area.

The Hazardous Materials in Our Environment

If you consider the sheer number of toxic chemicals used today, you may have a clear perspective of the inherent difficulty in regulating them. Approximately 60,000 substances are thought to have some toxic effects, which range in severity from skin irritations to death.

Most hazardous substances are organic (carbon-containing) chemicals. Nearly 225 billion pounds of synthetic organic chemicals were produced in 1985. Organic chemicals provide a host of products that we have come to rely on, such as synthetic fabrics like rayon and nylon, which can be produced much more inexpensively than products using natural fibers like cotton and wool. Although organic chemicals have provided an economic boon to many industries, they also have produced most of the environmental contamination and occupational illnesses. Ninety percent of the 165 potential human **carcinogens** are organic compounds, and most of the priority pollutants listed by the Clean Water Act are organic.

Certain synthetic organic chemicals, like the pesticide DDT, do not break down easily in nature and persist for long periods of time. As they enter living systems (plants or marine and animal life at various levels), they **bioaccumulate.** Thus, initially small amounts emitted into the air and water or entering the food chain may be found in amounts multiplied many-fold in human tissues, because humans are at the top of the food chain.

Household Hazardous Waste

The proliferation of chemicals also extends to products that we use everyday in our homes to clean, kill insects, and fix our cars. Public-interest groups have identified and recognized *household hazardous waste* as a danger. Cities and counties across the country have established local programs to deal with this problem.

Consumers often do not acknowledge household toxics as being dangerous to use or hazardous to dispose of. Potentially toxic products that are prominently

Safe disposal of common household wastes is an urgent problem.

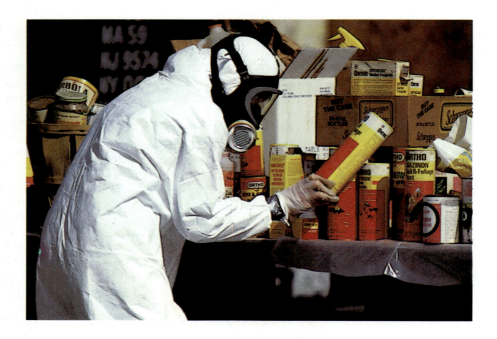

displayed on grocery store shelves include window cleaner, drain opener, furniture polish, toilet-bowl cleaner, and pesticides. Many of these materials can cause eye, skin, or respiratory tract irritation as well as headaches, nausea, and dizziness—all symptoms that may be experienced after a product's use but that may not be traced back to the product. Long-term illnesses such as heart disease, cancer, or birth defects may also be related to prolonged use of common household products.

Individuals can make a difference in the fight to reduce production and exposure to toxic chemicals right in their own homes. Safe substitutes can be used that reduce the risk of exposure and that are considerably less expensive (refer to Table 19–1 for specific alternative products).

FAST FACTS

The Environmental Protection Agency lists about 48,000 commercially produced chemicals. Less than 500 of these have been tested for their reproductive, mutogenic, or cancer-causing properties, and only about 1,000 were tested for their acute effects. Almost nothing is known about the toxic effects of 38,000 of these chemicals.

There Are Large Information Gaps

Generally, little is known about toxic materials. The National Academy of Sciences estimates that fewer than 2 percent of these chemicals have been adequately tested for human toxicity. This means that we know very little about the short- and long-term health effects that may occur if workers or others are exposed to these materials. We have learned a great deal about some toxic materials, such as asbestos or vinyl chloride, but only at the expense of people who have had prolonged exposure to them, which has often resulted in death or very serious or unusual illness.

Information is also sorely lacking about the environmental effects of these substances on marine and animal life, plants, water, and air. Further, it is not possible to estimate the extent of human and environmental exposure to toxics, because adequate data does not exist. Questions about the levels of contamination of our drinking water and the air we breathe outside and inside our homes or workplaces—as well as the impact such contamination will have on us during our lifetimes—remain largely unanswered today.

TABLE 19–1 ■ Alternatives to Household Toxics

Product	Health Effects	Nontoxic Alternatives
Aerosols	Eye and throat irritation; headaches; heart problems; lung cancer; birth defects	Use nonaerosol products in spray bottles (e.g., pump sprays).
Air fresheners	Skin eruptions; damage to nervous system, liver, kidneys, and lungs	Leave opened box of baking soda in room or refrigerator. Set out a small saucer of pure vanilla or vinegar in an open dish. Simmer cloves and cinnamon in boiling water.
All-purpose cleaners	Irritation of eyes and respiratory tract	Mix ½ cup vinegar with 1 quart water for a surface cleaner. Dissolve baking soda in water for a general cleaner. Or mix ½ cup borax, ½ tsp. liquid soap, and 2 tsp. trisodium phosphate or TSP (a mineral available in hardware stores) in 2 gallons of water.
Bleach	Respiratory-tract irritation	Use dry bleach or borax, which is a good greasecutter.
Disinfectants	Skin eruptions; damage to nervous system, liver, kidneys, lungs	½ cup borax to 1 gallon hot water.
Drain cleaners	Skin and eye irritation; asthma attacks; severe tissue damage	Use a drain strainer regularly and once a month pour ½ gallon boiling water down drain. If clogs occur, use a plunger, wait 15 minutes and then flush thoroughly with boiling water. Use a metal snake to unclog drain.
Oven cleaners	Dermatitis; asthma; severe tissue damage	Sprinkle on water followed by layers of baking soda. Rub gently with fine steel wool. Sprinkle salt on spills while they are warm, then scrub. Prevent spill cleanups by using oven liners.
Glass cleaners	Irritation of eyes and respiratory tract; skin irritation; nausea; headaches	Wash windows with ¼ to ½ cup white vinegar to 1 quart warm water, rub dry with newspapers.
Oil-based paint	Irritation of eyes and respiratory tract; skin eruptions; difficulty in breathing; liver and heart damage; cancer; birth defects and convulsions	Use latex and water-based paints, which are also available in enamels and stains.
Paint remover	Skin eruptions; damage to liver, kidneys, nervous system, and lungs; heart attacks	Mix 1 pound TSP with 1 gallon hot water, brush on, leave 30 minutes, remove paint with a scraper; this is probably most effective on water-based paints. Use an alkali-type paint remover or a heat gun and scraper. Be sure to protect yourself from fumes by using a mask.
Paint thinner	Nausea; vomiting; headaches; damage to liver, kidneys, and nervous system	Do not use oil-based paints that require a paint thinner.
Auto cleaning products	Damage to central nervous system, kidneys; ether penetrates intact skin	No alternative. Follow instructions and keep containers tightly capped.
Antifreeze and brake fluid	Damage to kidneys, metabolic symptoms; facial paralysis; eye irritation; rapid breathing	No alternatives. Follow instructions.

SOURCE: San Diego Environmental Health Coalition—The World Is Full of Toxic Waste. Your Home Shouldn't Be. 1989.

Hazardous Wastes

Currently, the manufacture of many common products requires the use of hazardous materials and generates hazardous wastes. At the end of World War II, the United States was generating 1 billion pounds of hazardous wastes per year. Estimates now put the annual amount of hazardous wastes at over 266 million tons.

According to the Congressional Budget Office, in 1983 chemical and allied products accounted for about 48 percent of total industrial waste, metal-related industries for 28 percent, petroleum and coal products industries for 12 percent, and all other industries for 13 percent (see Figure 19–1).

The most important health and environmental problems related to hazardous wastes are associated with disposal of these wastes. For many years, hazardous wastes were disposed of on the land, under the assumption that they would degrade into harmless products or would be contained in a landfill. These assumptions turned out to be erroneous. In almost all cases, wastes put into landfills are not contained but leak out into groundwater or are moved by environmental forces to other locations. These organic chemical substances either do not degrade or degrade into other hazardous materials.

The Nature and Extent of the Problem

To understand the effects of occupational and environmental factors on health, it is necessary to ask several basic questions:

1. What is an occupational or environmental health problem?
2. How do we recognize it? Who diagnoses it?
3. What are the substances and conditions that are associated with this problem?
4. Who is at risk of acquiring this health problem?

Once these basic issues are defined, it is possible to develop approaches to the prevention and control of the specific occupational or environmental health problem.

FIGURE 19–1 ■ **Distribution of Industrial Hazardous Waste Generation, by Major Industrial Group, 1983 (latest available data).**

SOURCE: *State of the Environment: A View toward the Nineties* Conservation Foundation, Washington, D.C., 1987.

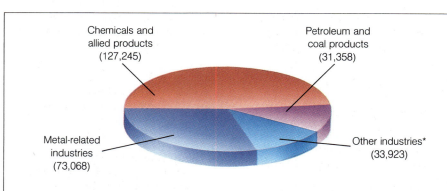

*Includes rubber and plastic products, miscellaneous manufacturing, motor freight transportation, wood preserving, drum reconditioning industries, nonelectrical machinery, transportation equipment, and electric and electronic machinery.

Human Health Effects

Examples of health effects related to occupational or environmental exposure include many types of damage to organs and impairment of physiological functions. Probably one of the best-known manifestations of occupational disease is the decreased lung function that results from breathing certain dusts and fibers. Coal miners have long been known to suffer from pneumoconiosis, or black lung disease. This condition leaves the miners' lungs permanently scarred and their respiratory function drastically reduced. Since the early part of this decade, inhaled asbestos has been known to cause a scarring of the lungs called asbestosis. Asbestos can also cause cancer, the highest risk being associated with lung cancer.

The lungs are a major route for hazardous substances to enter the body. When the particles are small, the substance is initially in direct contact with the lungs. By means of minute blood vessels, the lungs also may serve to transport harmful materials to various other parts of the body, such as the liver, kidneys, heart, and nervous system. Thus, a toxic substance's effect may be on the nervous system, causing weakness or convulsions, or on the reproductive system, resulting in a miscarriage or birth defect. Every organ and system in the body can potentially be affected by workplace or environmental toxins. The National Institute of Occupational Safety and Health (NIOSH) last developed a list of the ten most important occupationally related diseases in 1982. (See Table 19–2.) These diseases were ranked on the basis of three criteria: frequency of occurrence, severity of health impact, and availability of preventive measures.

TABLE 19–2 ■ **The Ten Leading Work-related Diseases and Injuries—United States, 1982**

1. Occupational lung diseases: asbestosis, byssinosis, silicosis, coal workers' pneumoconiosis, lung cancer, occupational asthma
2. Musculoskeletal injuries: disorders of the back, trunk, upper extremity, neck, lower extremity; traumatically induced Raynaud's phenomenon
3. Occupational cancers (other than lung): leukemia; mesothelioma; cancers of the bladder, nose, and liver
4. Amputations, fractures, eye loss, lacerations, and traumatic deaths
5. Cardiovascular diseases: hypertension, coronary artery disease, acute myocardial infarction
6. Disorders of reproduction: infertility, spontaneous abortion, teratogenesis
7. Neurotoxic disorders: peripheral neuropathy, toxic encephalitis, psychoses, extreme personality changes (exposure-related)
8. Noise-induced loss of hearing
9. Dermatologic conditions: dermatoses, burns (scaldings), chemical burns, contusions (abrasions)
10. Psychologic disorders: neuroses, personality disorders, alcoholism, drug dependency

SOURCE: *Morbidity and Mortality Weekly Reports*. 32 (January 21, 1983).

> **FAST FACTS**
>
> In 1989, 60 percent of Americans lived in cities that violated Environmental Protection Agency clean air standards.

Although occupational skin problems are the most frequently reported conditions, because they are generally not life threatening (unlike lung diseases), they are not ranked number one.

A wide range of health problems can be caused or aggravated by workplace exposures. Certain solvents can cause heart arrhythmias (irregular heartbeats), which can precipitate heart failure and trigger a heart attack. Certain solvents can cause **neurological** problems, such as tremors, weakness, or even paralysis. Exposure to lead can cause convulsions in children and mercury can make people seem crazy. In fact, the character of the Mad Hatter in *Alice in Wonderland* is based on the experiences of hat makers who used mercury in the felting process. Many of them went "mad" because of their exposure to toxic levels of mercury. Increasing numbers of chemicals and physical agents or emissions, such as ionizing radiation, have been linked to an increased occurrence of cancer (see Table 19–3).

Environmental Health Effects

Workplace and environmental **toxins** have affected the broader environment. In 1962, Rachel Carson issued a powerful warning in her book, *Silent Spring*, describing the consequences of pesticide use on our environment. One of the most dramatic examples was DDT, a pesticide used extensively until the 1960s and finally banned in 1973. It was recognized that this organic substance did not break down in the environment but actually had the capacity to bioconcentrate in nature. Pelicans, for example, were threatened with extinction because their eggs' shells became extremely fragile as a result of DDT exposure. The survival of the species was in doubt, but the banning of DDT reduced the threat of extinction. Only recently, decades later, have we begun to see a resurgence of the pelican population.

Recently, scientists have documented that the **ozone** level in the atmosphere is diminishing as a consequence of the use of chemicals called **chlorofluorocarbons (CFCs)** in refrigeration, plastics, and other products. If this trend continues, the lower levels of atmospheric ozone will increase the levels of ultraviolet (UV) light coming to earth. This is likely to result in an increased incidence of skin cancer, impaired human immune systems, and retarded plant growth. Recently, government and industry have initiated measures to reduce the production of CFCs.

The extensive use of hydrocarbons for fuels is related to an increase in carbon dioxide levels in the atmosphere. Higher levels of atmospheric carbon dioxide act to retain heat, causing a *greenhouse effect*. It is believed that global temperatures will slowly rise and ultimately endanger our delicate ecosystem. Figure 19–2 shows the ten cities with the highest averages of days per year in violation of ozone standards.

Another environmental problem exists with the phenomenon of **acid rain.** Sulfur dioxide and nitrogen oxides are released into the atmosphere, some by natural means but most by human means, especially from the burning of fossil fuels. Sulfur dioxide and nitrogen oxide gases are transformed to acids by chemical reactions with sunlight. These acid molecules remain suspended in the clouds and are eventually brought back to Earth by precipitation in the form of rain or snow. Extremely high levels of acid then accumulate in lakes and streams, which endanger fish and other aquatic life. Many trees absorb the acids through their root systems and leaves, causing forests to die.

> **FAST FACTS**
>
> In the world's rainforests, which help maintain the oxygen-carbon dioxide balance and prevent escalation of the greenhouse effect, an area the size of a football field is being destroyed every second.

TABLE 19–3 ■ Confirmed and Suspected Occupational Carcinogens by Target Organ

Target Organ/Tissue	Occupational Carcinogen Confirmed	Occupational Carcinogen Suspected
Bone		Beryllium
Brain	Vinyl chloride	
Gastroenteric tract	Asbestos	
Hematopoietic tissue (leukemia)	Benzene Styrene butadiene and other rubber manufacture substances	
Kidney	Coke oven emissions	Lead
Larynx	Asbestos, chromium	
Liver	Vinyl chloride	Aldrin Carbon tetrachloride Chloroform DDT Dieldrin Heptachlor PCBs Trichloroethylene
Lung	Arsenic Asbestos Bis (chloromethyl) ether Chloromethyl methyl ether Chromates Coke oven emissions Mustard gas Nickel Soots and tars Uranium Vinyl chloride	Beryllium Cadmium Chloroprene Lead
Lymphatic Tissue		Arsenic Benzene
Nasal Cavity	Chromium, isopropyl oil, nickel, wood dusts	
Pancreas		Benzidine PCBs
Pleural Cavity	Asbestos	
Prostate		Cadmium
Scrotum	Soots and tars	
Skin	Arsenic Coke oven emissions Cutting oils Soots and tars	Chloroprene
Urinary Bladder	4-Aminobiphenyl Benzidine B-Naphthylamine	Auramine 4-Nitrodiphenyl Magenta

SOURCE: M. Key, ed., *Occupational Diseases: A Guide to Their Recognition* (Washington, D.C.: Government Printing Office, 1977).

FIGURE 19–2 ■ **Ten Leading United States Cities in Violation of Federal Smog Standards**

SOURCE: Environmental Protection Agency

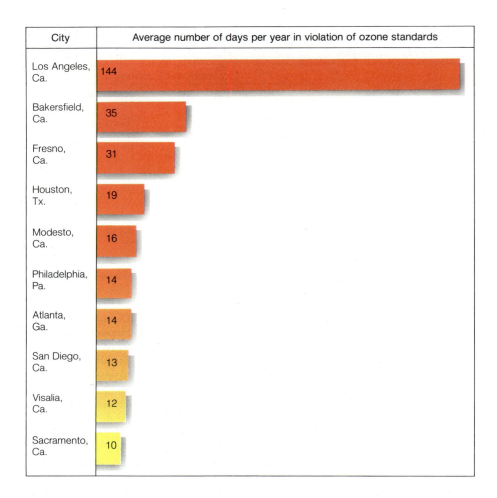

The Threat of Nuclear War—The Last Epidemic

The effects of many substances present in our workplaces and communities have the potential to dramatically affect the health of human beings and other living things. However, the disastrous consequences of the diminishing ozone layer and the greenhouse effect pale when compared with the potential danger of nuclear annihilation introduced by the development of the atomic bomb.

In the summer of 1945, during the second World War, the United States dropped an atomic bomb on Hiroshima and, several days later, another one on Nagasaki. The resulting nuclear holocaust heralded the start of a new era. Atomic weapons were incredibly destructive compared to previous warfare techniques. In Hiroshima, over 100,000 people died at once of direct trauma from the shock wave and severe burns from the extreme heat (at the epicenter, the heat was comparable to that of the fireball of the sun). Those near the epicenter were vaporized. Others succumbed later to radiation sickness and disease.

Today, we have single weapons that each can kill more than one million people. The world's nuclear arsenals have destructive power equivalent to over one million Hiroshimas. Albert Einstein, commenting on the implications of

CHAPTER 19 ■ OCCUPATIONAL AND ENVIRONMENTAL RISKS 483

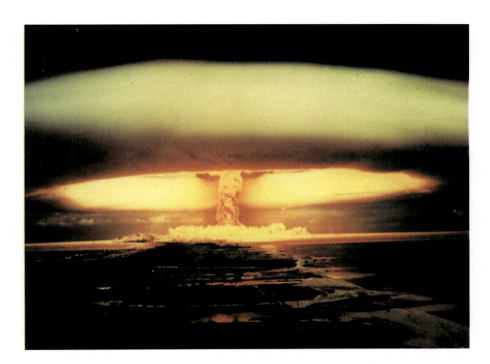

Caution: Nuclear arms can be harmful to your health.

nuclear weapons said, "The unleashed power of the atom has changed everything except our way of thinking, and thus we drift toward unparalleled catastrophe. We shall require a substantially new manner of thinking if mankind is to survive."

In 1983, Carl Sagan and Paul Ehrlich, along with a team of scientists, went on to describe still more devastating scenarios involving nuclear weapons. They reported on new scientific findings that suggested a phenomenon called *nuclear winter*. This would be the result of the multiple effects of toxic fumes and smoke, dust particles, levels of ionizing radiation, and a depleted ozone level in the stratosphere. The scenario involves a nuclear explosion (perhaps involving as little as 10 percent of the current arsenal) followed by the occurrence of massive fires in forests and urban industrial areas. The fires would liberate large volumes of fumes and dust that would float upward and block out most of the sunlight. This would cause a dramatic temperature drop to freezing levels, preventing normal photosynthesis from occurring for months to perhaps years in most of the northern hemisphere and undoubtedly affecting the southern hemisphere as well. These effects, combined synergistically with increased levels of radiation and diminished ozone levels, would so severely disrupt agriculture and delicate ecosystems that life on this planet might cease. As Carl Sagan states:

Health impacts can range from a single organism, an individual—you and I—to effects involving entire ecosystems and the survival of life on our planet.

■ **PROBLEM SITUATION** You have recently seen a TV show about nuclear war. The vivid portrayal of death, disease, and destruction was frightening. The images continue to haunt you. You are trying to forget the entire issue, but you can't put it out of your mind. What should you do?

FAST FACTS

United States weapons plants release radioactive particles in the air and dump huge quantities of potentially cancer-causing waste into water supplies according to C.D.C. research. Up to 20,000 children in eastern Washington may have been exposed to radioactive iodine from the milk of cows who grazed in contaminated pastureland.

SECTION VI ■ TAKING CONTROL OF YOUR HEALTH

GUIDELINES TO YOUR GOOD HEALTH

By following these single guidelines, you will be able to avoid and minimize injury from common hazardous substances:

1. When using a toxic material in your home, always read and follow the directions. Use only as much of the product as instructed.
2. When possible, use a nontoxic product or the least toxic product available.
3. Avoid using aerosol sprays. Avoid breathing fumes of aerosol mists. Use pump sprays instead of pressurized cans.
4. At work or in your home, make sure that you use appropriate protective clothing or equipment if you are exposed to potential toxics in the air or on surfaces.
5. Keep a list in your home and workplace of emergency and informational numbers to guide you in the appropriate use and disposal of hazardous materials.

■ Toxic Substances: Who Is at Risk?

Individuals from many segments of the population may be exposed to hazardous substances. Workers in various trades and professions, members of their families, and residents of communities where water, air, soil, and food contain hazardous substances are all placed at increased risk of developing toxic-related health problems. In order to effectively prevent exposure to hazardous substances and materials, it is necessary to determine what jobs and settings represent an actual or potential threat to health.

Workers

In the past, it was generally understood that blue-collar workers such as miners, construction workers, and factory and millworkers had dangerous jobs that could entail serious injuries resulting from falls, burns, and acute mechanical trauma (fracture or amputation), as well as damage to specific organs, like the dust-related lung diseases discussed earlier. Only within the last few decades has it been recognized that white-collar workers such as office workers or health practitioners (see Table 19–4) and high tech employees such as those in the electronics industry can also be exposed to health hazards.

Neighbors and Communities

Exposure to hazardous materials is not limited to workers only. The potential of workplace exposures to become community environmental problems has been dramatically demonstrated, as at Love Canal, with ever increasing frequency. A classic example of such a situation was the poisoning of Minamata Bay, Japan, where members of the community were exposed to mercury that had been discharged from a local plant directly into the bay. First the fish died, and then the cats who ate the fish "went crazy." Several years later, adults developed severe weakness and tremors, and subsequently, two hundred infants were born with

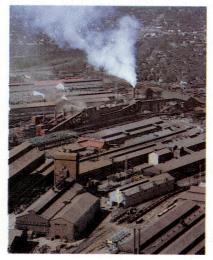

Toxic substances may travel beyond the boundaries of individual plants into surrounding neighborhoods and communities.

TABLE 19–4 ■ Examples of Possible Exposures Related to Various Occupations

Occupation	Potential Exposures
1. Agriculture (Migrant workers' wives work in fields while pregnant and sustain work as long as able)	Multitude of substances and conditions, including physical and biologic. Excessive work hours; intermittent and prolonged heavy work. Chemicals, especially pesticides, herbicides, insecticides, solvents, dusts, fumes, gases, heat and high humidity, infections (bacterial, viral, rickettsial), and vibration.

2. Cleaning personnel
  a. Launderers
  b. Dry cleaners
	
	Contaminated clothing, detergents, enzymes, soaps, heat, humidity.
	Contaminated clothing, heat, perchloroethylene, Stoddard solvent, naphtha, benzene, trichloroethylene, and others.

3. Clerical personnel	Carbon tetrachloride and various other cleaners, physical stresses, poor illumination, ergonomic deficiencies.
4. Domestic workers (homes, hotels, motels, office buildings)	Alkalies, bleaches, detergents, heat, cold (physiologic factors), shift work, at times hard work and various solvents in cleaning agents.
5. Electronics assemblers	Antimony, epoxy resins, lead, methyl ethyl ketone, methylene chloride, tin, trichloroethylene, and visual stresses and strain.
6. Hairdressers and cosmetologists	Acetone, aerosol propellents (freons), benzyl alcohol, ethyl alcohol, hair dyes, hair spray resins (polyvinylpyrrolidone), halogenated hydrocarbons, and other solvents of a wide variety.

7. Hospital/health personnel
  a. Registered nurses, aides, orderlies, physicians, students, patients
  b. Dental hygienists
  c. Laboratory workers (clinical and research)
	
	Alcohol anesthetic gases, ethylene oxide, infectious diseases (bacterial and viral), puncture wounds, and x-ray radiation.
	Anesthetic gases, infectious diseases (bacterial and viral), mercury, puncture wounds, ultrasonic noise, vibration, and x-ray radiation.
	Infectious diseases (bacterial and viral); puncture wounds; wide variety of toxic chemicals, including carcinogens, mutagens, and teratogens; and x-ray radiation. Many workers are subject to shift rotation.

8. Opticians and lens grinders	Coal tar, pitch, volatiles, hydrocarbons, iron oxide, other polishing and grinding dusts and solvents.
9. Photographic processors	Bromides, caustics, iodides, iron salts, mercuric chloride, pyrogallic acid, and silver nitrate.
10. Plastic fabricators	Acids, acrylonitrile, alkalies, hexamethylenetetramine, peroxide, phenol formaldehydes, styrene, urea formaldehydes, vinyl chloride, and vinylidene chloride. High heat and humidity.
11. Printing operatives	Benzene, carbon tetrachloride, ink mists, lead, methanol, methylene chloride, microwave, 2-nitropropane, pigments, trace metals, toluene, and various solvents, including trichloroethylene. Ultraviolet, microwave, and other radiation sources. Noise and vibration.
12. Sign painters and letterers	Epichlorohydrin, lead chromate pigments, lead oxide, toluene, trace metals, and xylene. A wide diversity of other chemicals as solvents and strippers.

13. Textile and related operatives
  a. Textile operatives
  b. Sewers and stitchers
	
	Asbestos, dyes, flame retardants, formaldehyde, heat, noise, raw cotton dust, synthetic fiber dusts.
	Asbestos, cotton and synthetic fiber dusts, flame retardants, formaldehyde, noise, and organic solvents.

(continued next page)

TABLE 19–4 ■ **Examples of Possible Exposures Related to Various Occupations,** continued

Occupation	Potential Exposures
c. Upholsterers (Some specific chemicals encountered in the preceding occupations are benzene, carbon disulfide, chloroprene, perchloroethylene, styrene, toluene, and trichloroethylene)	Same as above.

14. Transportation
   a. Bus, taxi, truck, and other vehicle drivers
   b. Airlines
	Carbon monoxide, polynuclear aromatics, lead, and other combustion products of gasoline and jet fuels; circadian dysfunctions; heat; physical stresses; shift changes; and vibration (ultrasonic, noise, and hypersonic).

SOURCE: Adapted from American College of Obstetrics and Gynecology, *Guidelines on Pregnancy and Work.* Rockville, MD: NIOSH, 1977.

FAST FACTS

Between 5,000 and 20,000 lung-cancer deaths per year are caused by radon, a gas that has been found to be present in many homes in the United States.

a severe cerebral palsy-like disease. Mercury in the mother's blood stream had crossed the placenta and entered the developing fetus. The mercury concentrated in the fetal brain, destroying many of the brain cells and leaving the surviving infant with severe mental and physical retardation.

In recent years, the release of pesticides containing methyl isocyanate in Bhopal, India, the worldwide radioactive contamination associated with the Chernobyl nuclear plant explosion in the Soviet Union, and the malfunction of the Challenger launching in the United States have all exemplified the dangers and risks to human health and well-being associated with high technology. No longer are the main threats to health associated with visible black smoke from factory stacks and steel mills or the dust and obvious dangers that exist in the mines. New technologies and recently developed materials have created new risks and have exposed different working populations to toxic-related health problems.

Not only have the new chemicals created new at-risk populations, but the time span over which the effects of these toxic exposures last has also been dramatically expanded. In recent decades, we have seen the focus of attention shift from acute effects (poisonings, sore throats, lung damage) to chronic diseases like cancer and obstructive lung problems (bronchitis, emphysema). The increasing recognition that chemically induced genetic changes may not appear for several generations and that chemicals persist in the environment for decades and longer makes it difficult to foresee the impact of many of these toxic materials (for example, DDT, PCBs, and radioactive materials) on future generations.

■ DBCP: A Case Study

What Is an Occupational Disease? Who Is at Risk?

A toxin in the workplace can eventually find its way to nearby residents of the plant as well as to distant citizens via air, water, and food contamination. The experience of a group of workers in a chemical plant in the Central Valley of

California illustrates the problems of exposure to a new breed of chemicals and such a chemical's various health effects on diverse populations. Dibromochloropropane (DBCP), as the following case study shows, contaminated land and water in both the immediate area of the plant, because of storage in nearby lagoons, and throughout the state of California, because of its extensive use in agriculture. Eventually, ground water and thousands of wells were contaminated, as were California crops.

Sterility Is an Occupational Hazard

The DBCP case study involves a group of employees who worked in a plant's agricultural chemical division making pesticides. The employees of this company worked and lived in a small town. They socialized together and were well acquainted with each others' families. In the mid-1970s, they noticed that individuals who had worked in the agricultural chemical division of the plant for a period of time were not having children. These employees were mostly young male workers who were married and trying to have children. They asked the company whether anything at work could be related to their problem. A company representative said that there were many chemicals in production and that none was known to have an effect on fertility.

Finally, after several years of wondering and worrying, seven of the men went to a physician, who tested their ability to produce sperm. The results were shocking. All seven had zero sperm production. The men reported this information to the company and the union. Within a day, the regulatory agency charged with protecting worker health, the Occupational Safety and Health Administration (OSHA), found information that one of the chemicals that was currently being produced in their unit (DBCP) had been studied and reported on in the scientific literature in 1961. The report described that in addition to damage to the liver and kidneys, this chemical caused serious damage to sperm-forming tissue in several species of male animals. Unfortunately, this information, so critical to the protection of the workers, had not been transmitted to the workers, who were working daily with this toxic pesticide. Although the study was originally reported in 1961, the episode described here occurred in 1977. For sixteen years, workers had been exposed to DBCP daily and had worked without skin or lung protection, because no one had ever warned them of the dangers of the chemical or informed them of measures to take to prevent exposure to the hazardous substance.

Environmental Exposures Occur via Air, Drinking Water, and Food

In the months that followed, it was revealed that workers in other plants in the United States and other parts of the world (Israel) had been similarly affected. Because of the serious, work-related health effects of DBCP, production was temporarily stopped.

As work proceeded to determine how extensive the consequences of DBCP exposure had been, it was discovered that large amounts of the material had been stored on-site in lagoons, causing substantial contamination of soil and ground water in the area. It soon became known that DBCP was used extensively in agriculture throughout the state of California and that most of the crops

Do the fruits and vegetables you eat contain pesticide residue?

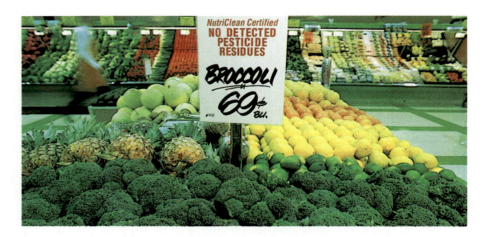

coming out of California contained DBCP residues. Further review of the literature also identified DBCP as an animal carcinogen and a suspected human carcinogen. In 1979, the Environmental Protection Agency, the federal agency charged with protecting community health, banned DBCP's further use on crops.

In 1987, ten years after the "discovery" of DBCP's toxicity, the water from thousands of wells in California was found to be unsafe to drink because of high levels of DBCP. It is estimated that the half-life of DBCP in the soil (the amount of time it will take for half of it to disappear) is 141 years! Although DBCP can no longer be used on crops in the United States, OSHA ended the moratorium on the chemical's production in the late 1970s and permits it to be produced for export for agricultural use abroad. This banned chemical then returns to the United States on imported food products for our consumption. What does the DBCP experience teach us about the nature of hazardous materials, their harmful health effects, and the actions that can be taken to prevent and control future exposures?

Who Diagnoses Occupational Health Problems?

It is extremely important to note who originally diagnosed the DBCP related health problems. It was not a company doctor, it was not the individual worker's physicians, and it was not a company official. The problem was identified by the workers themselves. This is not an unusual event. Very frequently when work-related problems surface, it is the employees themselves who make the diagnosis. Remember this if you suspect that a health problem you have may be related to your work setting. Talk to others around you and see if they share your problems. In evaluating whether the health condition is related to work, consider whether it seems to go away on the weekends or when you take a vacation.

> ■ **PROBLEM SITUATION** You suspect that a sore throat and cough you have had for some time may be related to exposure to a toxic substance in your workplace. What should you do to check out the possibility of this connection?

What Are the Health Problems?

In the case of the DBCP exposure, the immediate at-risk group was clearly the workers in the Agricultural Chemical Division and their families. In the past, reproductive problems such as infertility, miscarriages, and birth defects were considered to be related only to maternal exposures. In recent years, however, the DBCP episode and research done on the reproductive outcomes of the wives of men who were working in operating rooms, as well as previous information on lead exposures, have emphasized the impact of toxic exposures on the reproductive outcomes of *both* women and men.

The DBCP experiences also raised consciousness concerning the wide range of health effects that can result from occupational and environmental exposures. It is now recognized that effects can be quite subtle and less visible than traumatic injuries or the obvious consequences of chronic lung disease that coal miners and asbestos workers experienced. It is said that workers exposed to some of the newer chemicals produced by the petrochemical industry (pesticides like DBCP) are "silent canaries." In the past, coal miners brought caged canaries into the mines with them. The canaries were slightly more sensitive to the toxic gases in the mines than the men who worked there. When the toxic gases started accumulating in the mines and the canary fell over, the miners knew this was the warning for them to leave. Today, workers are functioning like canaries—dying or falling sick or losing important functions such as reproductive capacity when they are exposed to the newer chemicals we know little about. They are warning the rest of us that the materials they are working with may endanger us as the toxics appear in our drinking water, in the air we breathe, or in the products we eat or use.

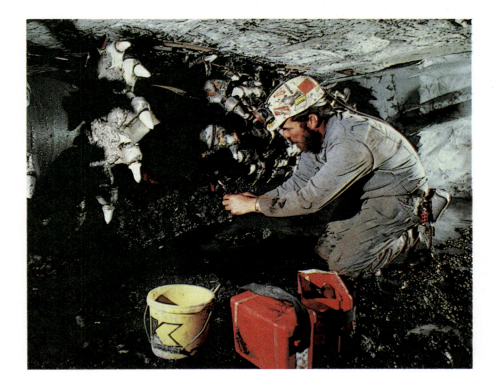

This coal miner probably knows the health dangers he faces, but we don't always know when we may be exposed to similar toxic substances such as asbestos from brake linings.

Could the DBCP-Related Sterility Have Been Prevented?

Was the DBCP incident inevitable? It should be apparent that if the workers had been warned about the materials that they worked with, they might have been able to take precautions that would have eliminated or minimized their exposures. Several years after the incident, the California legislature passed a *Worker Right-to-Know Law,* which has now become implemented on a national basis as the *Hazard Communication Law.* This regulation requires producers of hazardous materials and employers who use these materials to make available in the workplace specific information about the health effects of these substances (i.e. what to do in the event of accidents, spills, or unanticipated emissions). Paralleling this type of protective legislation, many communities, counties, and states have implemented *community* right-to-know programs to assure that citizens in neighborhoods can also be fully informed about the nature and location of hazardous materials near their homes, schools, and parks. It is hoped that with more information available to workers and communities, tragic situations such as Love Canal and pesticide-related sterility will not occur.

The DBCP episode demonstrated that a given hazardous material can affect many community members. Usually its impact is on the workers first, since they usually have the larger and more prolonged exposure to the substance. However, family members are frequently affected, indirectly when their childbearing capacity is affected (in the case of reproductive toxins), or more directly when children are harmed by toxins that parents bring home from the workplace on soiled clothing or via breast milk in the case of nursing mothers. An example of this phenomenon is the children who have developed lead poisoning as a result of lead dust brought into the home on their parents' work clothes. The DBCP situation demonstrates how consumers of food contaminated with pesticide or community members who drink water from contaminated wells or neighbors who live within airborne spread of the pesticide may be exposed to the material. Thus, workplace toxins may expose individuals who are not present on the workplace site.

The creation of a Hazard Evaluation Service and Information System (HESIS) was another measure implemented in the wake of the DBCP experience. It provides free information about workplace toxins to all employers, employees, and health practitioners who can call hazardous-materials experts by telephone. The latter make available the most recent information on substances to the people who need to know. Programs of this nature, available and used nationwide, may prevent many of the problems that have been encountered in the past. There is usually very little that can be done once people have developed occupational and environmental diseases. The primary emphasis must be on prevention.

The Right to Know

One of the major points in this discussion is that workers and individual consumers often are not informed about the health and environmental effects of exposure to toxic chemicals. Sometimes, as we discussed earlier in the chapter, there is little information about a substance, even though it is allowed to be widely used. Disclosure of information about known and suspected toxic effects from exposure to hazardous materials is a controversial issue, just as labeling of cigarette packages was controversial for many years. Many consumer products are inadequately labeled with regards to the actual ingredients they contain and the effects of exposure to these ingredients.

Because workers are usually the first group to be exposed to hazardous materials, many state governments, and recently the federal government, have enacted worker right-to-know or hazard communication standard laws. These statutes require that information is provided to workers about the specific chemicals they are exposed to and the potential health effects. This "right to know" has also been extended to community residents who want information about local industries that use hazardous chemicals or generate toxic waste. In this way, firefighters can obtain information about the contents of a chemical or manufacturing warehouse and thus be prepared to combat a fire properly. Similarly, land-use planners can better determine appropriate zoning for industrial facilities in relation to residential or high-density areas.

Community Health Protection

Given the industrial or agricultural nature of most areas of the United States, individuals throughout the country can expect to encounter problems with hazardous materials and wastes in one way or another. It is important for them to be able to have access to information that can assist them in resolving their problems. The following is a list of suggested organizations, government agencies, or types of groups that concerned individuals can use as a resource:

Local/Regional
- Poison Control Center
- American Lung Association
- Public-interest consumer/environmental/toxics groups
- County Health Department
- County/Regional Air Quality Board
- County/Regional Water Quality Board
- Department of Agriculture
- County District Attorney (for enforcement)

State
- Department of Health Services
- State Water Resources Control Board
- State Air Resources Board
- Food and Agriculture Department
- State Attorney General's Office

Federal/National
- Consumer Product Safety Commission
- Environmental Protection Agency

One lesson from the DBCP and Love Canal examples is that each of us has to be attentive to the actual and potential health problems in our workplaces, our homes, and our communities. Although government and industry are supposed to be responsible for assuring healthful and safe environments in our neighborhoods and on the job, protection has all too often been lacking or inadequate. This suggests the necessity of a multi-leveled prevention and control approach.

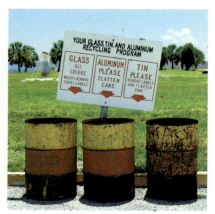

You can play an important part in the prevention and control of environmental damage. Recycle!

Individuals themselves must be knowledgeable about actual and potential hazards in their workplaces, schools, homes, and communities. When groups of people complain about particular types of health problems that are new or occur in unusual numbers, these concerns should be heeded and investigated. Individuals can play a critical role by practicing safe work and play habits, learning about potential health hazards, and personally attempting to limit the use of toxic materials (for example, eliminating the use of styrofoam cups, selecting safe alternatives to household toxics, disposing of toxic materials safely, and so on).

However, many elements of ensuring occupational and environmental health lie outside the realm of the efforts of individuals (except as responsible citizens). This is when the efforts of government, industry, unions, public-interest groups, and scientists must combine to deal with the substantive changes that are necessary to contain the current threat that toxic materials and wastes pose to human and environmental health.

Where Do We Go from Here?

Are we to be saddled with the health and environmental hazards associated with toxic chemical use if we want to maintain our current standard of living? Can we enjoy technological benefits without sacrificing our future? These questions are central to the discussion of hazardous waste and materials "management." Recent evidence indicates that the flurry of laws and regulations that have been passed during the preceding decade have addressed only the tip of the iceberg. The overriding theme of these laws has been the assumption that these wastes and materials are a permanent part of industrial America and therefore must be handled "as safely as possible" to maintain an "acceptable" amount of environmental degradation, damage to human health, or both.

This approach has resulted in little reduction of air and water pollution. In fact, according to Barry Commoner in a June 15, 1987, *New Yorker* article, "For all the air pollutants other than lead, the average annual rate of decline in emissions was 1.52 percent between 1975 and 1981 but only 1.16 percent between 1981 and 1982. Indeed, since 1982 the long-term, if gradual, decline in air pollutant emissions has come to a halt. Between 1982 and 1985, there was an average annual increase of 0.87 percent in these emissions." Pollutants that have been banned—such as in lead in gasoline, DDT, and PCBs—have shown a marked decrease in the environment. Environmentalists and government officials are beginning to heed this evidence by promoting not merely waste management but "toxics use reduction" (see Table 19–5.)

The reduced use of toxics eliminates worker and community exposure to toxic chemicals (via the waste-site and the home) through innovation, by using different (less toxic or hazardous) products to meet social needs, and by changing production processes to eliminate the use of toxics. Some industries have begun to convert manufacturing processes that were previously dependent on toxic chemicals to cleaner, safer systems. A good example is Cleo Wrap, the world's largest producer of gift wrap in Tennessee. This company converted from the use of organic solvent–based printing inks to water-based inks. This allowed them to replace the organic solvents used in the cleaning process with water-based cleaning solutions and soaps. The change persuaded Cleo Wrap's suppliers to develop a full range of water-based ink colors that did not previously exist and that can now be distributed to others.

TABLE 19–5 ■ **Preferred Techniques for Reducing Toxics Hazards at Their Source and Hazardous Waste Management Techniques**

Toxics Reduction Techniques	Description
Toxics Use Reduction	Reducing or eliminating the manufacture and use of toxic and hazardous chemicals so as to reduce risks to human health and the environment.
Reduction in or ban on production	Reducing or banning the production of hazardous chemicals, including bans on specified uses.
Input substitution	Using safer substitutes for raw materials or other hazardous chemicals.
Waste Reduction: At the Source	Reducing or avoiding the generation of wastes, including releases of toxic and hazardous pollutants to all media (air, water, and land), so as to reduce risks to human health and the environment.
Process changes	Altering manufacturing practices to reduce or eliminate wastes.
Operational changes	Improving "housekeeping" practices to reduce or eliminate wastes.
In-process recycling	On-site recycling in which wastes are conveyed in a closed loop back into the manufacturing process.
Treatment Techniques:	The following treatment techniques are not source reduction techniques and should only be utilized after all reduction efforts have been exhausted. All of these methods leave hazardous waste residuals and/or involve air and/or water releases.
On-site treatment	Physical treatment, chemical treatment, biological treatment, thermal treatment
Off-site recycling/resources recovery	Leaves hazardous waste residual for disposal
Off-site treatment	Physical treatment, chemical treatment, biological treatment, thermal treatment
Residual repositories	Solid residuals from recycling and treatment, disposed with ground and air cover. A form of land disposal.

SOURCE: Adapted from *A Community Perspective of Hazardous Waste Planning: A Handbook*. Toxics Coordinating Project and the Environmental Health Coalition, (San Diego, Calif.: 1987).

> **FAST FACTS**
>
> CFC emissions account for about 15 percent of the greenhouse effect.

Another example of source reduction is the current attempt to halt the depletion of the ozone layer by reducing CFC production. In the spring of 1988, the U.S. Senate ratified an international treaty limiting the use of the chemicals that destroy the ozone layer. E. I. DuPont de Nemours and Company, the major producer of CFCs, announced the discontinuation of their manufacture. In a commentary (*Los Angeles Times,* April 3, 1988), biophysicist Donella H. Meadows from Dartmouth College describes this teamwork:

The world's scientists, with their international networks that transcend politics, spotted the problem, learned a tremendous amount of atmospheric chemistry in a short time, and steadily supplied crucial information to the political process.

Citizen activists and environmental organizations in many countries mobilized pressure and educated politicians. Some of the organizations that deserve special mention are the Natural Resources Defense Fund, the World Resources Institute, Friends of the Earth U.K., and the Institute for European Environmental Policy.

National governments, in particular those of the United States, Canada, the Scandinavian countries, and eventually West Germany, led the way in the negotiations.

Major corporations that manufacture CFCs played a generally constructive role.

Finally, and most important, the United Nations Environmental Programme and its director, Tolba, provided skillful, untiring leadership in calling meetings and keeping the discussions going.

It's easy to poke fun at environmentalists or argue that the United Nations is worthless or say that national governments are hopelessly self-seeking or believe nothing good about big corporations. But every one of those actors was essential to the ozone agreement. Given the changing news about ozone and other global environmental problems, we'll probably need them all again.

At the same time that problems with hazardous materials are escalating, progress is evident as individual consumers are selecting safe substitutes for hazardous chemicals and recycling waste materials. Many communities and institutions such as schools and hospitals are beginning to make informed choices in the purchase of paints, pesticides, food supplies, and packaging. For instance, the use of styrofoam cups is being eliminated by certain food chains and schools. The use of paper and wood products that **biodegrade** are being substituted in many situations. As Congressman Albert Gore, in the forward to *Hazardous Waste in America,* states succinctly:

It is as if our civilization has lost a sense of its future. We are so busily engaged in making miracle products for our present enjoyment from substances deposited in the earth over a million years, we don't stop to consider the environmental burden we are placing on future generations. We have pillaged the past and pawned the future, telescoping time for the benefit of a fleeting present. Only when the consequences begin to manifest themselves in our own generation do we demand that changes be made.

■ Accidental Injury: The Number-One Health Problem

Depending on how you look at it, the biggest personal, public, and environmental health problem today may well be accidental injuries. In terms of sheer numbers, in 1987, there were 8.8 million disabling injuries and 94,000 deaths from accidents in the United States. Put another way, eight million people who are alive today can expect to die from accidents. Table 19–6 breaks these figures down into four classifications—motor-vehicle, work, home, and public accidents. Notice that the direct costs of accidents totaled more than $133 billion. As you might expect, half of these accidents involved motor vehicles.

TABLE 19–6 ■ Accident Facts, 1988

Category	Deaths	Death Rate per 100,000 Population	Disabling Injuries	Cost[b]
All Classes[a]	96,000	39.1	9,100,000	$143.4 billion
Motor-Vehicle	49,000	19.9	1,800,000	70.2 billion
Work	10,600	4.3	1,800,000	47.1 billion
Home	22,500	9.2	3,400,000	17.4 billion
Public	18,000	7.3	2,300,000	10.9 billion

[a]The totals for the four separate classes may be more than for the category "all classes" because some accidents are included in more than one category and numbers have been rounded off.

[b]Costs include lost wages, medical expenses, insurance costs, property damage, fire loss, and indirect loss from work accidents.

SOURCE: *Accident Facts* (Chicago: National Safety Council, 1989).

Accidents are the fourth leading cause of death in the United States, but that statistic belies the true extent of the problem because so many accidental deaths occur at a young age. From the ages of one through thirty-seven, as many people die from accidents as from all other causes combined! In the fifteen- to twenty-four-year-old age group, 55 percent of all deaths are due to accidents. If you add the categories of homicide and suicide to accidents, 82 percent of deaths in this age group can be attributed to violent means.

Using the measure of *years of potential life lost* (YPLL), accidents become the nation's number-one public health problem. YPLL is usually calculated by subtracting the age at which a person died from sixty-five. Since accident victims are usually young, they would be expected to live many more years than those who died of chronic diseases such as cancer or heart disease. (See Table 16–1 for a comparison of YPLL factors.)

Analyzing Accidents

Accidents result because of a combination of direct and indirect factors. A common way of analyzing the elements of an accident is by using the **epidemiological** triangle, which considers host, agent, and environmental factors (see Figure 19–3). Environmental factors include all conditions in the environment that make unintentional injury more likely, such as weather, lighting, or surface conditions. The agent refers to lethal characteristics of the instrument of injury. Any hard object that a person collides with, causing bodily harm, is considered to be an agent. If you were to fall off your motorcycle and hit your head on the ground, the concrete pavement would be the agent. We are most concerned with the host, or human, factor when considering the prevention of accidental injury and death. Human factors such as age, sex, skill level, alcohol and drug consumption, and even socioeconomic status influence the likelihood of an accident occurring.

People who are likely to have more than their share of accidents are called **accident prone.** The *80:20 theory* states that during a specific period of time, such as one year, 20 percent of the population will experience 80 percent of all accidents. Accident proneness may be short-term, as, for example, when temporary conditions such as acute stress, physical disability, alcohol or drug use,

FIGURE 19–3 ■ **Epidemiology of Accidents**

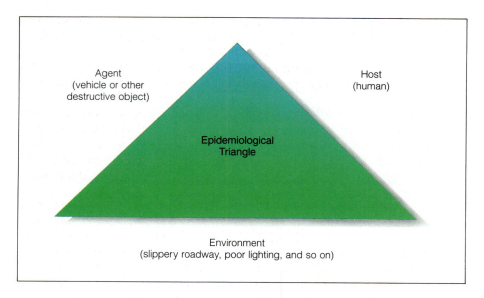

fatigue, or overwhelming emotions exist. Long-term accident proneness is associated with more enduring human characteristics, such as aggressive personality traits, physical impairment, ignorance, misperceptions of unsafe conditions, or improper attitudes.

The possibility of an accident occurring is always present as long as people take risks. All of us engage in risk-taking behaviors at one time or another as a means of stretching our limits and adding greater adventure to our lives. In order to have a safe and meaningful adventure, we need to minimize the possibility of an accident occurring while engaging in risk-taking behaviors. To do so, we must be able to accurately judge how safe an experience is by becoming thoroughly knowledgeable about the activity and by participating within the limits of our skills.

Motor-Vehicle Accidents

If there were one action that a typical college student between the ages of eighteen and twenty-five could take to prolong his or her life, it would be to wear a safety belt at all times when driving or riding in a car. The second most important action would be to never ride in a vehicle driven by someone who has been drinking alcohol. If you were to follow these two simple rules, your chances of living a long life would be greatly enhanced.

Although most motor-vehicle accidents occur in urban areas, almost two-thirds of all auto deaths happen in rural areas. The reason for this is that speed increases drastically on the open road. As a matter of fact, speed and reckless driving are the two most common reasons cited for fatal accidents. Alcohol is a factor in just 20 percent of all injury crashes, but it is a factor in 50 percent of all fatal crashes and 60 percent of all single-vehicle fatalities.

Consider the case of Bruce Kimball, the 1984 Olympic silver medalist in diving, who, in 1988, lost control of his car after he had been drinking and ran into a crowd of teenagers, killing two and injuring a third. He took two young lives, damaged another, and possibly ruined his own chances for a fruitful life. It is clearly inexcusable and irresponsible to operate a motor vehicle when you have had more than one ounce of alcohol to drink. That means that anything more than one twelve-ounce can of beer is too much for a driver to consume.

FAST FACTS

Even when blood alcohol content has returned to zero, driving skills can be impaired the morning after intoxication.

Even though the legal limit for driving under the influence of alcohol is a blood alcohol content (BAC) of 0.10, in most states, the chance of having an accident is greatly increased with as low a level as 0.03 BAC.

Some traffic accidents are inevitable, but injuries resulting from car crashes can be prevented to a great extent. The most important action you can take is to always use a passenger restraint—either a lap belt, lap/shoulder harness, or passive air bag (which is not yet available as standard equipment on most cars). Because ejection is the most frequent cause of motor-vehicle deaths, it is essential for us to have and use restraints. As of July 1, 1987, thirty-one states have legislated mandatory safety belt use and all fifty states have mandatory child safety seat laws. Nevertheless, a study done in December 1987 found that actual use of safety belts was just 42 percent.

Eighty percent of all motorcycle deaths occur among fifteen to thirty-four year olds, and the group with the highest risk is the eighteen to twenty-four year olds. Based on miles driven, death rates are fifteen times higher for motorcycles than for cars. What can you do to help cut down motorcycle fatalities? Wear a good helmet at all times! It is estimated that states that have enacted helmet laws have reduced motorcycle deaths by 30 to 40 percent. What's your opinion about legislation governing such personal actions as the wearing of motorcycle helmets and automobile safety belts?

Nonmotor-Vehicle Accidents

If you were to analyze the deaths resulting from nonmotor-vehicle accidents, you would notice that different age groups are particularly susceptible within each accident category. Drowning victims, for example, are most likely to be children between the ages of one to three and young people in the fifteen to twenty-four-year-old age range. Most drownings involve swimming beyond one's ability or the use of alcohol. Almost half of those who drown are found to have been under the influence of alcohol. Infants and small children are at greatest risk of accidental poisonings and burns from fires.

Older Americans are the victims of more than half of the deaths from accidental falls, mostly occurring over rugs or on stairs or wet floors. As people get older, they lose some of their general strength and their bones become more brittle. A common scenario is for an older person to fall and break a hip, become hospitalized, and develop pneumonia in the hospital, ultimately leading to death. This person's death certificate may list pneumonia as cause of death, but was the fall actually the more important causative factor?

> ■ *PROBLEM SITUATION* Your grandparents have recently moved into a new apartment, and you are concerned about their safety because you consider them to be frail and susceptible to accidental falls. Using the three epidemiological categories of host, agent, and environment to guide your analysis, what would you recommend doing to make their new living situation as safe as possible?

Fires

You may not have realized that the United States has a higher incidence of deaths from fires than any other industrialized nation in the world, more than twice the number occurring in Canada, the country that is second in fire-related

---

FAST FACTS

An average accident costs safety-belt users $534, compared to $1,583 for motorists not using restraints.

FAST FACTS

More than 25,000 accident victims die each year because they don't get proper emergency care on time.

Fires can be costly to life and property. Try to make your home as fireproof as possible.

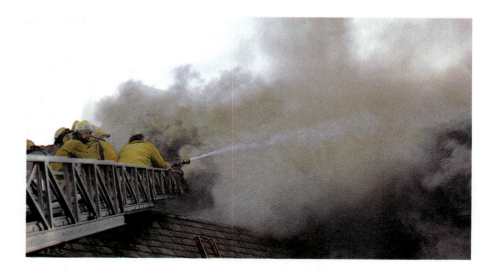

deaths. Most household fires (where three-fourths of all fire and burn deaths take place) are caused by faulty or incorrectly used heating equipment. However, fires that cause injury and death are most commonly the result of cigarettes and other smoking materials. Frequently, cigarettes are left smoldering on furniture upholstery or mattresses and ignite at night when people are asleep.

Besides not smoking and using safe electrical appliances, there are a number of precautions that you can take so that fires won't cause personal injury or death. First of all, every household should be equipped with smoke detectors. These are relatively inexpensive, costing between $10 and $50. There should be at least one on every floor in the house and one placed near each bedroom. It is recommended that the batteries be changed twice a year to insure that they are working. A good time to remember to change them is when you change your clock to and from daylight savings time.

GUIDELINES TO YOUR GOOD HEALTH

If you encounter a house fire that requires you to use a fire extinguisher, be sure to follow these steps:

1. Break the seal and remove the pin on the handle *before* nearing the fire.
2. Make sure that the fire extinguisher works by giving the handle a quick squeeze.
3. Approach the fire low to the ground to avoid inhaling smoke.
4. Aim the spray from the extinguisher at the base of the fire, holding the extinguisher in an upright position.
5. Move the extinguisher in a sweeping motion across the flames, starting at the bottom.
6. Back away from the fire when the extinguisher is emptied. Do not turn your back on the fire.

A second precaution to take to prevent fire-related injuries is to plan an escape route to use in the event that a fire should break out in your home. If you have never done so, draw a rough floor plan of your home and decide which routes of escape you would use if a fire occurred at various places in the house. It would also be a good idea to conduct a practice fire drill from time to time.

Finally, you should have an all-purpose fire extinguisher readily available, preferably a dry chemical extinguisher that is triple rated for use with class A, B, and C fires. Class A fires involve ordinary solids, such as wood, paper, or textiles; class B fires are caused by flammable liquids; and class C fires are electrical fires. Be sure that you know how to properly operate the fire extinguisher, place it where it will be easily accessible, and be sure that it is maintained in good working order. During a fire is no time to learn how to use a fire extinguisher or to find out whether it will work.

POSITIVE BEHAVIORS

I. *Place a check mark in front of each behavior that you now practice.*

_____ 1. I do not use toxic household products when nontoxic alternatives are available. (TOXICS)

_____ 2. I recycle all of my aluminum cans, glass bottles, and other reusable containers. (RECYCLE)

_____ 3. I keep myself well-informed about threats that exist in my environment and what I can do to control them. (INFORMED)

_____ 4. I never drink and drive, nor do I ride in a vehicle that is operated by someone who has been consuming alcohol. (DRINKING/DRIVING)

_____ 5. I always wear a safety belt while driving in a car or truck. (SAFETY BELT)

_____ 6. I see to it that there are functional smoke detectors placed in appropriate locations in my house or apartment. (SMOKE DETECTORS)

II. *For each behavior that you DO NOT ENGAGE IN, write the KEY WORD(s) located in the parentheses at the end of the statement in the columns below. Then put a check mark in the appropriate column to indicate whether you are going to keep or change that behavior.*

Behaviors I Don't Engage In   KEEP/CHANGE
_____   _____/_____
_____   _____/_____
_____   _____/_____
_____   _____/_____
_____   _____/_____
_____   _____/_____

III. *For each of the preceding behaviors that you choose to KEEP, write a statement indicating why you are choosing to keep that behavior.*

I choose to keep behavior _____ because:
                              KEY WORD

For each of the preceding behaviors that you choose to CHANGE, write a statement indicating how you plan to implement that change.

I will change behavior _____ by:
                         KEY WORD

Now You Know

1. FALSE. New technologies and recently developed materials have created new risks and have exposed different occupations to toxic-related health problems. Smoke-stack industries have been replaced by "clean" industries such as electronics, health-care services, and research and development laboratories as some of the more toxic places to work.

2. FALSE. There exists an information gap about the environmental effects of industrial materials. Data on long-term or chronic effects are particularly incomplete.

3. FALSE. It is increasingly being recognized that health problems caused by chemicals are taking decades and even generations to appear, especially when genetic changes are induced.

4. TRUE. It is usually very difficult to clean up a toxic waste site because of technical, financial, and political barriers. Only a very small number of the more than 24,000 hazardous waste sites in this country have been cleaned up.

5. TRUE. Most occupational health problems are not easily treated, reversible, or curable. This is why prevention, by minimizing exposure to toxics in the community, is so important.

6. FALSE. Although the petrochemical industry has provided many useful products, its proliferation has caused untold occupational illness, environmental damage to air and water sources and the ozone layer, and public-health problems related to the production of chemicals or disposal of the resulting toxic wastes.

7. FALSE. Although the lungs are a major route for substances to enter the body, harmful materials can and do reach all organs of the body.

8. TRUE. There is a substantial list of toxics used as common household products. A big problem is that most consumers don't recognize these products or their wastes as being dangerous. Many household products reach the market without having been adequately safety-tested.

9. TRUE. The threat of nuclear war, whether intentional or by accident, is considered by many (including such prestigious groups as the American Public Health Association and Physicians for Social Responsibility) to be the major environmental issue of our day. Even a small part of the world's nuclear arsenal, detonated for a brief period of time, would plunge us into a nuclear winter that would probably result in the end of life on our planet. According to Albert Einstein, "the unleased power of the atom has changed everything except our way of thinking."

10. FALSE. Canada is second to the United States, which has twice as many fire-related deaths.

Summary

1. Toxic exposures in the community can be associated with a wide range of acute and chronic health effects.

2. There are hazardous waste sites all over the United States. More than 900 are considered to pose an imminent and serious threat to the public's health.

3. Toxic chemicals represent a serious health problem in their production, use, storage, transportation, and disposal. Incidents like the one in Bhopal, India, involving the release of a toxic gas, or in Minimata, Japan, where many members of the community were poisoned by mercury that had been discharged from a local plant, are testimony to the international dimensions of the problem.

4. The health consequences of occupational and environmental exposure to toxics may involve every organ system.

5. Some chemicals, especially certain organic compounds like pesticides, do not break down easily in nature and persist for long periods of time. As they enter living systems (plants, animals, and sea life), they bioaccumulate and end up concentrated manyfold in human tissues.

6. For the majority of chemicals in commerce, data about their full range of effects on human health are inadequate.

7. The continued production and proliferation of nuclear weapons may lead to the "last epidemic" our civilization will experience if, by design or accident, a small percentage of the current arsenal is detonated. The resulting nuclear winter may end all life on this planet.

8. Today, hazardous materials or conditions influence the health of not only blue-collar workers but also workers in high tech, "clean" industries such as electronics, health care, and research laboratories.

9. Hazardous materials do not stay inside the factory gates. It is necessary for community members, health practitioners, and land-use planners to know what materials are being produced and used in their communities.

10. Substituting safe alternatives for household toxics is something individuals can do to reduce the burden of toxic materials in our communities.

11. When using the measurement of years of potential life lost, accidents are the number-one public health problem.

12. The three epidemiological factors considered in accident analysis are the environment, the agent, and the host.

13. The action that is most important to survival for those in the eighteen- to thirty-five-year-old age group is the use of safety belts when riding in a car, followed by not riding in a vehicle in which the driver has been consuming alcohol.

References

1. *A Community Perspective of Hazardous Waste Planning: A Handbook.* San Diego, Calif.: Toxic Coordinating Project and the Environmental Health Coalition, 1987.
2. Baker, Susan, et al. *The Injury Fact Book.* Lexington, Mass.: Lexington Books, 1984.
3. Bever, David L. *Safety: A Personal Focus.* St. Louis: The C. V. Mosby Co., 1987.
4. Brodeur, Paul. *Expendable Americans.* New York: Viking/Compass, 1974.
5. Brown, Michael. *Laying Waste: The Poisoning of America by Toxic Chemicals.* New York: Washington Square Press, 1981.
6. Brown, Michael. *The Toxic Cloud.* New York: Harper and Row, 1987.
7. Carson, Rachel. *Silent Spring.* Greenwich, Conn.: Fawcett Publications, 1962.
8. Chavkin, Wendy, ed. *Double Exposure: Women's Health Hazards on the Job and at Home.* New York: Monthly Review Press, 1984.
9. Committee on Trauma Research. *Injury in America: A Continuing Public Health Problem.* Washington, D.C.: National Academy Press, 1985.
10. Dadd, Debra L. *Non-Toxic and Natural.* New York: Jeremy P. Tarcher, Inc., 1984.
11. Ehrlich, Paul, Carl Sagan, et al. *The Cold and the Dark: The World after Nuclear War.* New York: W. W. Norton, 1984.
12. Epstein, Samuel S. *The Politics of Cancer.* San Francisco: Sierra Club Books, 1978.
13. Epstein, Samuel S., Lester O. Brown, and C. Pope. *Hazardous Waste in America.* San Francisco: Sierra Club Books, 1982.
14. Freudenberg, Nicholas. *Not in Our Backyards: Community Action for Health and the Environment.* New York: Monthly Review Press, 1984.
15. Gibbs, Lois M. *Love Canal.* Albany: State University of New York Press, 1982.
16. Heifetz, Ruth. "Women, Lead and Reproductive Hazards: Defining a New Risk," in *Dying for Work: Workers' Safety and Health in Twentieth Century America.* Bloomington: Indiana University Press, 1987.
17. "Leading Working Related Diseases and Injuries." *United States Morbidity and Mortality Weekly Reports* 32 (1983): 24–26.
18. Legator, Marvin S., ed. *The Health Detective's Handbook: A Guide to the Investigation of Environmental Health Hazards by Nonprofessionals.* Baltimore, Md.: Johns Hopkins University Press, 1985.
19. Postel, Sandra. "Controlling Toxic Chemicals," in Lester O. Brown, ed., *State of the World, 1988.* New York: W. W. Norton, 1988.
20. Robertson, Leon S. *Injuries: Causes, Control Strategies and Public Policy.* Lexington, Mass.: Lexington Books, 1983.
21. Sarokin, David J., et al. *Cutting Chemical Wastes.* New York: Inform Inc., 1985.
22. Sinclair, Upton. *The Jungle.* New York: Doubleday, Page and Co., 1906.
23. Solomon, Frederic, and Robert Q. Marston. *The Medical Implications of Nuclear War.* Washington, D.C.: National Academy Press, 1986.
24. *State of the Environment: A View Toward the Nineties.* Washington, D.C.: The Conservation Foundation, 1987.
25. Terkel, Studs. *Working.* New York: Ballantine Books, 1985.
26. Waller, Julian. *Injury Control: A Guide to the Causes and Prevention of Trauma.* Lexington, Mass.: Lexington Books, 1985.
27. Weir, David, and Mark Shapiro. *Circle of Poison: Pesticides and People in a Hungry World.* San Francisco: Institute for Food and Development Policy, 1981.
28. Whorton, M. D. "Male Occupational Reproductive Hazards." *Western Journal of Medicine* 137 (1982): 521–524.

This chapter written by Ruth Heifetz, M.D., Department of Community Medicine, University of California at San Diego and Diane Takvorian, M.S.W., Executive Director, San Diego Environmental Health Coalition.

Suggested Readings

Accident Facts. Chicago: National Safety Council, 1989.

Berry, Thomas. *The Dream of Earth.* San Francisco: Sierra Club Books, 1988.

Brown, Michael. *Laying Waste: The Poisoning of America by Toxic Chemicals.* New York: Washington Square Press, 1981.

Chavkin, Wendy, ed. *Double Exposure: Women's Health Hazards on the Job and at Home.* New York: Monthly Review Press, 1984.

Ehrlich, Paul. *The Machinery of Nature.* New York: Simon and Schuster, 1987.

Seymour, John, and Herbert Girardet. *Blueprint for a Green Planet.* Englewood Cliffs, N.J.: Prentice-Hall, 1987.

State of the Environment: A View Toward the Nineties. Washington, D.C.: The Conservation Foundation, 1987.

Waller, Julian. *Injury Control: A Guide to the Causes and Prevention of Trauma.* New York: Lexington Books, 1984.

SECTION VII

The Final Transition

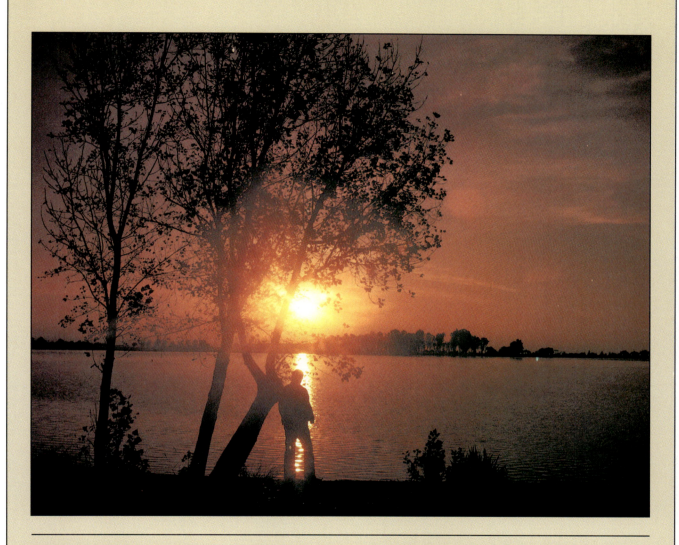

Chapter 20: Maturing Gracefully
Aging versus Being Old
The Process of Aging
Theories of Aging
Ageism
Overcoming the Stereotypes of Aging
Physiological Changes of Aging
Alzheimer's Disease and Aging
Sexuality and Aging
Successful Retirement
Caregiving: Taking Care of an Elderly Parent

Chapter 21: The Ultimate Loss
The Role of Death in Life
Concepts of Death and Dying
Fears of Death and Dying
The Process of Dying
Dying with Dignity
Funerals
Handling Grief

CHAPTER 20

Maturing Gracefully

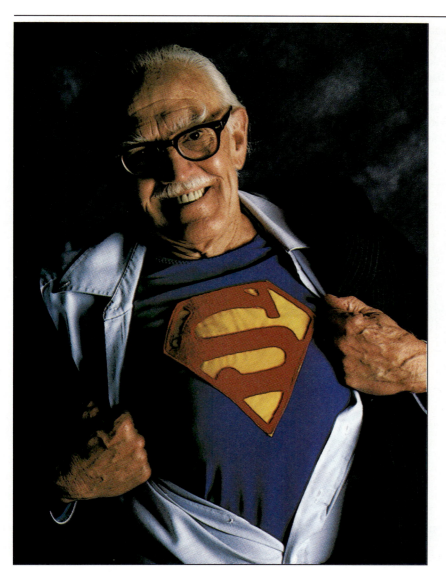

What Do You Know?

Are the following statements true or false?

1. Men tend to live several years longer than women.
2. Ageism is a form of discrimination against the elderly.
3. Senility is an inevitable consequence of growing old.
4. Intelligence declines with age.
5. People who are in excellent physical health throughout their lives will not show signs of aging as they grow older.
6. One of the earliest visible signs of aging is the appearance of wrinkles.
7. Osteoporosis is an age-related disorder characterized by decreased bone mass.
8. There is no cure for Alzheimer's disease.
9. The major barrier to sexual intimacy among the elderly is usually the male's inability to maintain an erection.
10. It is almost always a female child who cares for an aging parent.

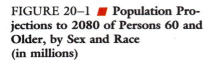

FAST FACTS

The United States has more residents over the age of sixty-five than it has teenagers.

Aging versus Being Old

Old age is not a disease. **Aging** is a physiologic process that continues from birth to death. People grow older each day. According to the U.S. Bureau of the Census (1987), there are 29 million Americans, 12 percent of the U.S. population, who are sixty-five years of age and over. By the year 2000, 45 million Americans will be in this age group. Population projections show that by the year 2000, individuals over the age of sixty will compose 17 percent of the total U.S. population, and by the year 2050, this age group will make up almost 25 percent. (See Figure 20–1.) In 1970, the average life expectancy for males in the United States was 67.1 years and for females it was 74.7 years. By 1986, it had risen to 71.3 years for males and 78.3 years for females.

A person's overall attitude toward life will determine how he or she approaches growing older. Each stage of life has its changes, and with each stage, some things are lost but other things are gained. In our society, when a person reaches the age of sixty-five, he or she is considered "old." By this definition, "old" is based on chronological status, or the year in which an individual was born. This criteria is too simplistic and limiting. It is more useful and appropriate to think of aging as having three facets: biological, psychological, and social.

Biological age is based on the physical changes that occur as a person becomes older. The biological age indicates the number of years a person will be likely to survive. This prediction is based on factors such as heredity, life-style, and environmental conditions. Looking at this concept of biological age, if a man who celebrates his sixty-fifth birthday has a projected life span of about ninety

FIGURE 20–1 ■ **Population Projections to 2080 of Persons 60 and Older, by Sex and Race (in millions)**

SOURCE: The 1989 Information Please Almanac.

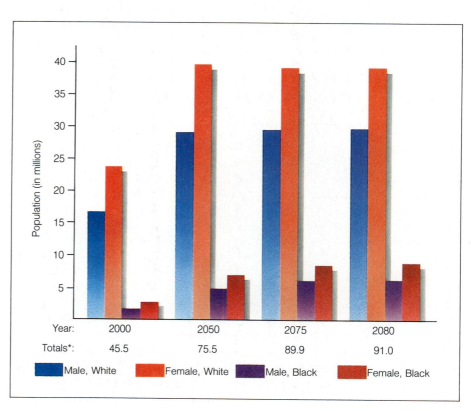

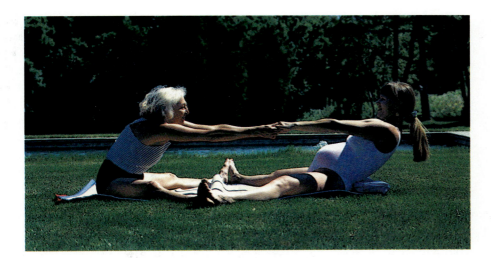

Think young, act young, feel young!

years, he would not be considered biologically old at age sixty-five. **Psychological age** is based on how a person thinks and feels as he or she becomes older. If a sixty-five year old man perceives himself as being forty, his psychological age is less than his chronological age. **Social age** is based on how a person behaves as he or she becomes older. Psychological age is usually a good indicator of social age. If a sixty-five year old woman feels young, her social age is going to reflect the behaviors of an individual younger than sixty-five. Being "old," therefore, is a combination of several factors. How a person looks, feels, and acts are very important in the aging process. So next time you celebrate someone's seventieth birthday, remember, that person may really be seventy years young!

■ The Process of Aging

To understand the process of aging, we must first examine the properties of a human cell, for it is in our cells that aging begins. The cell is the smallest unit that has all the properties associated with life. It reproduces itself through a splitting process called division. The one cell divides to make two cells, the two divide to make four, and so on, until the billions of cells that make up an adult are produced. When a cell divides, each new cell receives an equal amount of chemical components needed to carry on reproduction. Cells are made up of organic molecules. These molecules consist of sugars, fats, proteins, and nucleic acids. Each plays a special role in the life of a cell.

We need to look more closely at the nucleic acids to understand the aging process. Nucleic acids are found in the nucleus of each cell. There are two main types of nucleic acids: **deoxyribonucleic acid**, or **DNA**, and **ribonucleic acid**, or **RNA**. The DNA controls all of the characteristics of living things. DNA governs the chemical processes in the cell by producing RNA. RNA directs the formation of proteins. The proteins govern the cell's metabolism, form much of the cell's structure, and help regulate cell division.

FAST FACTS

In the years between 1980 and 2000, the numbers of people over age 80 will nearly double—from 5.2 million to 10.1 million.

■ **PROBLEM SITUATION** Suppose that an elderly male, who is a family friend, asked you to guess his age. How would you respond?

> **FAST FACTS**
>
> The longest human life span reliably recorded is 114 years of age.

Theories of Aging

In 1961, Dr. Leonard Hayflick discovered that human cells growing in a culture could divide only a limited number of times before they all aged and died. The cells could undergo about fifty divisions before dying. Dr. Hayflick calculated, on the basis of fifty divisions by cultured embryonic human cells, that a human's life span should be about 110 to 120 years. That is how long it would take for that many cell divisions to occur in the body. When Dr. Hayflick examined the cell cultures as they aged, he found that even though there were many cells still capable of dividing, these cells showed specific structural and functional changes. He concluded that when enough of these changes occur in vital organ cells, such as those in the heart, the whole body dies, even though there may be cells still capable of living. This theory of aging is known as the *genetic limit theory*.

A number of theories have been proposed to explain how Hayflick's genetic limit is expressed in the cells of our bodies. All of the theories assume that aging represents a loss of control over various bodily processes and that this loss occurs at the cellular level in the DNA. Let's look at the various theories of aging.

The Error Hypothesis

The *error hypothesis* proposes that aging is caused by defects or errors in DNA and RNA duplication. These errors can result from attacks on the DNA by polluting chemicals present in the air we breathe and in the food we eat. Unrepaired damage to the DNA of a cell can cause that cell to produce errors in RNA and protein formation. Once an error is made in RNA or protein, it continues to result in faulty duplication. This cumulative increase of errors is responsible for aging. Attempts are being made to modify the course of "error-induced" aging.

The Free Radical Theory

During the process of metabolism, certain molecules, called free radicals, are produced. They can also be produced by accident if oxygen combines with the cellular molecules. Free radicals have a strong tendency to link to other molecules. The result is that uncontrolled free radicals can cause accumulated damage to the membranes surrounding cells and to the cellular molecules of RNA and DNA. This process is known as *free-radical aging*. Scientists are trying to find ways of protecting the cells from free-radical damage. One attack on free-radical aging is the use of chemicals called antioxidants. An antioxidant inhibits reactions promoted by oxygen. If you have heard vitamin E being promoted as an "anti-aging" vitamin, it is because vitamin E is a natural antioxidant. It is speculated that vitamin E may defuse free radicals, thus helping to slow the aging process. So far, however, there is no conclusive evidence demonstrating that additional amounts of vitamin E can prolong life.

The Cross-linkage Theory

The *cross-linkage theory* proposes that aging is due to the formation of chemical bridges, or cross-linkages, between protein molecules. When these cross-linkages form between protein molecules, they cannot be undone by the cell's normal repair mechanisms. These cross-linkages adversely affect the protein structures in the body. Cross-linkages are also formed between DNA molecules. Such cross-linkages not only prevent DNA from participating in cell division, but they also interfere with the production of RNA. Cross-linkages in protein and DNA can be caused by chemicals that are normally present in cells as a result of metabolism and by environmental pollutants, such as tobacco smoke. The number of cross-linkages found in the human body increases with age. Research is being conducted to determine if there is any effective way to dissolve these cross-linkages.

The Brain Hypothesis

The *brain hypothesis* proposes that aging is due to a decline in the body's ability to maintain homeostasis. **Homeostasis** is the ability to keep bodily processes in a state of equilibrium or balance. Many symptoms of aging are caused by a breakdown in the control of hormone production. Because the hypothalamus is the center of control over bodily homeostasis and is responsible for triggering the release of hormones, it is theorized that the hypothalamus malfunctions with aging. Experiments are being conducted to determine if administration of certain drugs can correct hypothalamic breakdown.

The Autoimmune Theory

The *autoimmune theory* proposes that the body's immune system malfunctions with age. The major components of the immune system are two types of white blood cells—B cells and T cells. The main function of the B cells is to produce antibodies, which destroy disease-producing organisms. The main function of the T cells is to attack and destroy cells that are foreign to the body. The aging process seems to cause the B and T cells to behave abnormally, attacking not only disease organisms and cells but also the body's own normal, healthy cells. This destruction of the body by its own protective immune system is called **autoimmunity**. Scientists are trying to find methods that may rejuvenate the immune system, thereby preventing the development of autoimmune aging. There is also evidence indicating that restricting one's diet by eating less, but maintaining an adequate and well-balanced diet, may slow the rate of autoimmune aging. More research needs to be done in this area.

■ Ageism

When you are in a room with an elderly person, do you feel uncomfortable? Do you avoid having to converse with this person? Have you accepted the stereotype that elderly people are dull and forgetful and are incapable of engaging in worthwhile conversation? Or, if you do talk with this person, do you expect him or her to be opinionated or argumentative and to ramble on with old ideas? If you have responded "yes" to any or all of these questions, you may be contributing to ageism. **Ageism** is a form of discrimination on the basis of age. In regard to the elderly, it refers to prejudice against the elderly solely because of their age.

Many young people, because of misconceptions and ignorance, fear growing old. They have grown up in a nuclear family surrounded only by parents and siblings. These youngsters may have limited contact with their grandparents and with other elderly people. All they know is the media-projected image of

FAST FACTS

Special-interest groups, such as the Gray Panthers and the American Association of Retired Persons (AARP), have become increasingly effective in combatting ageism and improving the quality of life for the elderly.

Age is no barrier to learning.

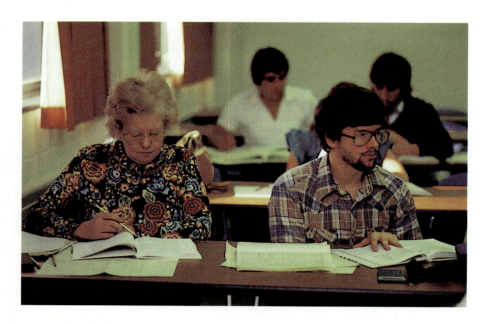

old age. When television depicts the elderly as being senile, withdrawn, sickly, sexless, and constipated, it is no wonder that young people fear growing old. Instead of viewing old age as an achievement and a natural stage of life with its own merits, wisdom, and beauty, our society all too often ignores, rejects, and isolates the elderly.

Society has perpetuated negative stereotypes about aging and being old. What we believe about being old can become self-fulfilling prophecies. If we treat the elderly as bumbling incompetents who are unable to think clearly and intelligently, they may begin to believe it themselves. It is easy to patronize the elderly by talking down to them or by not allowing them to perform tasks that they are perfectly capable of doing. This kind of behavior is demeaning. We cannot accept stereotypical portraits of the elderly that portray them as crabby, helpless, ineffectual, and nonproductive people.

If we believe that the elderly can't function in society, can't maintain their own health, and can't handle their own affairs, we are fueling the fires of ageism. And, ironically, we will all become victims of our own prejudice, because the obstacles we place in the paths of the elderly today will be there some day for us to overcome.

> ■ *PROBLEM SITUATION* Suppose you are shopping in a grocery store. An elderly woman, whom you have never seen before, starts talking to you as if she knows you well. What would you do? Would you continue the conversation with her, or would you walk away?

■ Overcoming the Stereotypes of Aging

People assume that the aging process inevitably brings with it mental incompetence, physical incapacitation, and social isolation. Labeling all elderly people as poor, sick, and lonely is a great injustice. Many are financially secure and in

SELF-INVENTORY 20.1

What Are Your Attitudes Regarding the Elderly?

Place a check mark in the column that most accurately describes your feelings about the elderly.

SA = Strongly Agree
A = Agree
NO = No Opinion
D = Disagree
SD = Strongly Disagree

	SA	A	NO	D	SD
1. I feel that most elderly people are forgetful.					
2. I feel that elderly people are incapable of making important decisions.					
3. I feel that television accurately portrays how elderly people look and behave.					
4. I feel angry when I think about how the elderly are treated in our society.					
5. I would feel comfortable leaving a child in the care of an elderly person.					
6. I feel that elderly people should be allowed to continue working until they no longer wish to do so.					
7. I feel that most elderly people belong in nursing homes.					
8. I feel that most elderly people are too old to enjoy sex.					
9. I enjoy interacting with elderly people.					
10. I don't feel that people over the age of 65 should be allowed to drive.					
11. I feel that young people can benefit from the wisdom of the elderly.					
12. I get bored spending time with an elderly person.					
13. I feel that more government money should be spent on health care, food programs, and housing for the elderly.					
14. I feel that elderly people are no longer productive members of society.					
15. I feel that adult children should have the responsibility of taking care of elderly parents.					

Scoring: If you answered "Strongly Agree" or "Agree" to questions 4, 5, 6, 9, 11, 13, and 15 and "Strongly Disagree" or "Disagree" to questions 1, 2, 3, 7, 8, 10, 12, and 14, you have a positive attitude regarding the elderly.

If you answered "Strongly Disagree" or "Disagree" to questions 4, 5, 6, 9, 11, 13, and 15 and "Strongly Agree" or "Agree" to questions 1, 2, 3, 7, 8, 10, 12, and 14 you have a negative attitude regarding the elderly.

Why do you think you feel the way you do about the elderly?

What suggestions do you have for getting to know an elderly individual and finding out what he or she is really like?

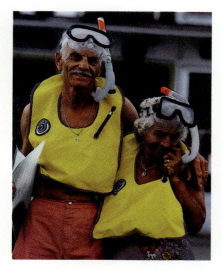

Many older people are discovering various leisure-time activities that help them stay alert and healthy.

good health. They have numerous friends and have maintained close family ties. Changes may occur, but those people who are interested and involved in life work around whatever declines they experience. These people don't sit and wait; they plan and anticipate. Healthy older people are happy, alert, and active. A person's enthusiasm, creativity, and motivation do not dwindle with age. With stimulation and new challenges, most older individuals remain involved in life and continue to function at a high level.

The aging years can bring opportunities for growth and activities that are exciting and meaningful. As stereotypes break down, the elderly are increasingly recognized as having profound capabilities. They are concerned with factors that will help them continue to lead healthy and productive lives. They are participating in exercise programs, eating nutritious foods, moving to less stressful environments, and fighting the negative stereotypes of old age. Even the political clout of the elderly is growing, and they are actively lobbying in their own behalf. Although there is no remedy for aging itself, a lot can be done about how we age. It takes longer to become old today than ever before. Most elderly persons are likely to stay healthy and active well into their seventies and even their eighties. Today's elderly "are not just getting older, they're getting better!"

Many people believe that senility is an inevitable consequence of growing old. **Senility** is usually characterized by physiological degeneration in the brain. It is true that there are degenerative diseases of the brain that afflict old people, but there are also degenerative diseases of the brain that afflict people of all ages. In many instances, the signs of senility do not result from brain damage. Senility may actually be a behavior resulting from such factors as environmental conditions, overmedication with drugs, malnutrition, anemia, certain viral infections, anxiety, loneliness, or depression. If properly identified, the behavior may be fully reversible. Unfortunately, in our society, the word "senile" has become a catch-all phrase used to refer to any elderly person who responds too slowly or who is forgetful. It's interesting how forgetfulness in a younger person is considered to be indicative of an overly busy schedule. In an elderly person, however, that same forgetfulness is indicative of senility. The indiscriminate use of the senility label, based on the assumption that senility is inevitable at a certain age and that nothing can be done about it, is one of the most harmful elements of ageism.

Another myth about growing old is that intelligence declines with age. This is certainly not the case. With good health and a stimulating environment, intelligence changes little with age. It is difficult to find a meaningful decline in mental functioning in the general population before age sixty. The most rapid decline takes place between the late sixties and early seventies. Only after eighty do mental abilities fall below the average mental performance of younger people.

There are a number of steps a person can take to keep the mind alert. First, one should remain socially involved. Studies have shown that elderly people who frequently interact with family and friends fare better mentally than those who isolate themselves. Second, a person should keep his or her mind stimulated, perhaps by enrolling in adult education classes. Elderly people have enrolled in and successfully completed courses in subjects such as real estate, photography, computers, politics, and auto mechanics, just to mention a few. Third, an elderly person should continue to get physical exercise. Good physical health has a positive effect on a person's mental health. And fourth, one should be flexible.

Being open to new experiences also keeps the mind open. It should be understood that elderly people are able to assimilate, process, and act on new information. Although they may require more time to think about the information before drawing conclusions, their answers are no less accurate. Learning and growth does not stop with age. We must not allow the elderly to fall prey to this myth of declining mental abilities.

When people get old, we assume that they must live with a relative or be put in a nursing home because they cannot take care of themselves. Right? Wrong! The fact is that about 10 percent of the elderly find it necessary to live with their immediate family, and of those who do, most are likely to be in their eighties. Only about 4 percent of the elderly in our society are institutionalized. Institutionalized, in this case, means residing in full-care nursing homes or wards for the chronically ill of hospitals. It may surprise you to learn that the overwhelming majority of older people continue to live in their own homes and care for themselves. (See Figure 20–2.) Although many suffer from one or more common medical problem, such as diabetes, hypertension, or arthritis, most manage exceptionally well. For those elderly who suffer from physical or mental disabilities that restrict their mobility, services are available that offer in-home assistance. This assistance still allows the elderly person to be in control of his or her life and to function, for the most part, independently. This sense of independence gives the elderly individual a feeling of self-worth and accomplishment.

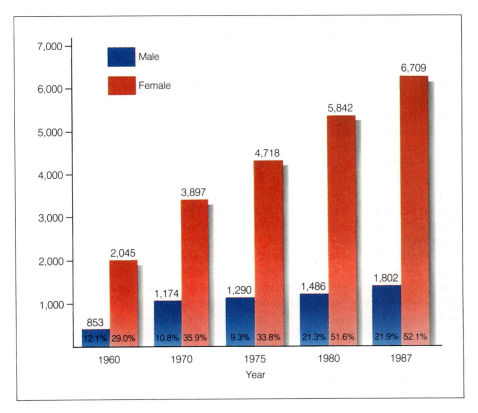

FIGURE 20–2 ■ **Persons 65 Years and Older Living Alone, by Sex (numbers in thousands)**

SOURCE: The 1989 Information Please Almanac.

The time has come for us to re-establish the dignity of the elderly. We must eliminate the negative stereotypes that are cruel, demeaning, and discrediting. Old age should not be a tragedy or a period of quiet despair and desolation. The elderly should not be ignored or kept out of sight. They are a group of people worthy of high regard. We need to value what they have accomplished and appreciate what they can continue to do. They have spent a lifetime "paying their dues" to society. It's about time that they reap some of the rewards. After all, their basic needs are no different than those of any other age group. We all want to love and be loved and to live happy, healthy, and meaningful lives. Is that too much to ask?

Physiological Changes of Aging

Aging begins at birth. From the day we are born, the body changes. Up until the teenage years, rapid growth takes place. By about the age of twenty-five, the body reaches its peak of physiological strength and skills. Then, at an extremely slow pace, we begin to experience a tapering off. Usually after age fifty, many individuals begin to notice changes indicative of greater age. Persons who eat a well-balanced diet, exercise regularly, maintain good health, and have a positive attitude about life are likely to feel the effects of aging more slowly than others. Eventually, however, all people will show signs of aging.

Wrinkles

One of the earliest visible signs of aging is noticed in the skin. Wrinkles appear. Less efficient functioning of oil glands, loss of the skin's elasticity, and loss of the underlying layer of fat cause wrinkling skin. Wrinkles are more pronounced where the fat loss has been the greatest and where there has been prolonged exposure to the sun, such as the face, neck, and hands. Skin cells nestle in **collagen**, a cushiony protein that gives fullness to our bodies. During childhood and youth, the protein aligns itself in fibers bunched together and parallel to each other. This arrangement is what gives the skin resilience and elasticity. Remembering the cross-linkage theory of aging, you should understand why the skin loses its elasticity as we age. The formation of cross-linkages between protein molecules lessens the strength of the collagen. One of the latest innovations in cosmetic surgery is a procedure in which cow-skin collagen, purified and ground up, is injected under the facial skin. This is supposed to puff up the face in the right places. It seems to work for about a year, but after that, the results begin to fade. The cost is several hundred dollars for each collagen treatment, which just proves what some people will do because of vanity.

As people grow older, they need to be more careful about protecting their skin from the sun. The more hours spent in the sun, the more melanin the cells secrete and the darker the skin becomes. **Melanocytes** are cells located in the skin and hair roots that manufacture the dark pigment, **melanin**. Melanin determines an individual's skin and hair color. As a person ages, a lot of his or her melanocytes die, leaving fewer to protect the skin. Without this protection, the skin burns rather than tans. Cells that are not protected by abundant melanin go crazy when bombarded by ultraviolet light. Their chromosomes break into fragments as the cells divide. This process can lead to the development of skin cancer. Ultraviolet light also tends to harden, thicken, and dry out the skin's outer layer, which is called the **epidermis**. Remember, wrinkling is inevitable. If you avoid the sun, however, the process is considerably slowed.

FAST FACTS

The sense of taste decreases with age. At age 30, each tiny elevation on the tongue has 245 taste buds. By age 70, each has only 88.

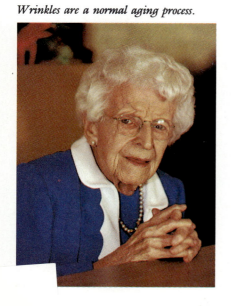

Wrinkles are a normal aging process.

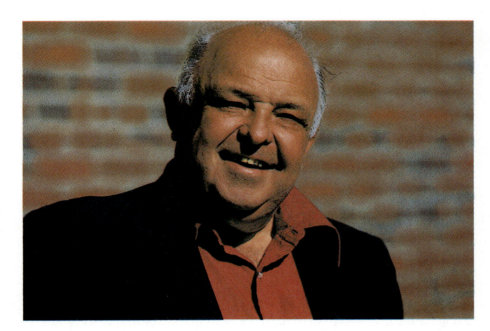

Gray hair and baldness do not detract from an older man's appearance.

Changes in Hair

Another change that occurs with aging is that hair becomes grayer, finer, and scantier. Hair turns gray because of a decline in the density and activity of melanocytes. Genes dictate the abundance of these cells. Blacks have more melanocytes, for example, than whites. Brunettes have more melanocytes than blondes. As a rule, beginning around the age of thirty, 10 to 20 percent of the hair's melanocytes either die or become inactive with each successive decade. Stress has nothing to do with how quickly one's hair turns gray. That's just another myth that needs dispelling.

Have you ever wondered why it is primarily the hair on our heads that turns gray? Since hair grows faster on the head than anywhere else on the body, the melanocytes located in the roots of head hair work harder, thereby shortening their lifespan. The melanocytes located in the roots of body hair do not work as hard and thus survive longer.

Like graying, balding is another sign of aging whose primary effect is on one's vanity. Men bald more frequently than women because genes for baldness are dominant in males but recessive in females. The actual balding process involves the death of hair follicles over many parts of the body. In men, however, hair in the ears, in the nose, and on the back becomes more prevalent with age. Before scalp hair falls out, beginning above the temples and continuing to the top of the head in the sequence termed male-pattern baldness, it gradually becomes finer. This process is influenced by a decrease in androgens that many (but not all) males experience as they get older. Although virtually all men experience some hair loss, not all become bald. At a certain point the process can stop. Whether this occurs depends mostly on heredity.

Changes in Vision

Most elderly people experience some loss of vision. Changes in vision usually occur gradually. Elderly people may have trouble with glare, have difficulty

> **FAST FACTS**
>
> Visual sensitivity to contrast may aid in the early detection of cataracts or glaucoma.

seeing objects close to them, or lose much of their peripheral vision. The extent to which these changes occur varies from one individual to another.

Cataracts are an eye condition endemic to the aging population. A cataract is a white cloudiness that covers the eye's lens, causing objects to appear blurred. The only remedy is surgical removal. Once the cataract is removed, use of convex glasses, a contact lens, or a permanently implanted intraocular lens imitates the eye's natural lens so that the individual can see clearly again.

Glaucoma is another eye problem occurring in the elderly. It is caused by a buildup of fluid within the eye because of the blocking off of passages through which the fluid normally drains. If left untreated, the high pressure eventually causes blindness. In chronic glaucoma, the draining mechanism tends to clog slowly. The victim may be aware of decreasing peripheral vision or the appearance of haloes around lights. If the condition is discovered early enough, symptoms and progression can be effectively treated with eye drops that relieve the pressure. Some physicians use laser treatment to open the clogged drainage canal. Other treatments are being used experimentally to determine their rates of effectiveness and safety.

Even though cataracts and glaucoma occur frequently in old age, they are not normal changes of old age. They need to be identified and treated promptly. Fortunately, many visual difficulties occurring in the elderly can be improved significantly by using adequate lighting, corrective lenses, magnifying glasses, and large-print reading materials. Elderly people usually have functional eyesight throughout most of their lifetime.

Changes in Hearing

Everyone loses some hearing with age. As a result, the older you are, the harder it becomes to hear high-frequency sounds. In many older people, hearing loss never becomes severe enough to cause problems, whereas in others, the loss may be incapacitating. Permanent hearing loss, or **presbycusis**, results from a gradual physical deterioration of structures in the inner ear. It is not known whether this loss is due to aging per se or to general wear and tear on ears by noise pollution. A person with a moderate degree of hearing loss may find communication difficult. Hearing aids are usually of value only when they are carefully adjusted to the particular hearing deficit. A poorly selected or poorly adjusted hearing aid may only increase noise and do nothing to enhance clarity.

When speaking to an elderly person with a hearing deficit, it is helpful to speak slowly and clearly. Get as close to the person as comfort will allow, and look directly at the person when speaking. Try to eliminate background noises. Don't engage in rapid-fire conversation. This may cause the person to become hesitant in responding. After speaking, allow the individual time for reflection before answering. Give explanations and instructions carefully and repeat them if necessary. Presbycusis can also amplify loud noises, so be aware of the noise level when listening to the stereo or watching television with an elderly person. It is important to understand what a person might be feeling if his or her hearing is deficient. The less an elderly person can hear, the more likely the person is to avoid communication. We must be alert and sensitive to possible hearing problems. A parent or grandparent who is gradually losing his or her hearing may become depressed and withdrawn. We must not allow a loved one to slip into quiet isolation.

> ■ *PROBLEM SITUATION* You have noticed that your father is not hearing as well as he used to. When you try to discuss it with him, he gets angry and says, "I can hear fine; you just need to stop mumbling." Would you pretend to go along with what he says to keep the peace, or would you pursue the issue anyway, knowing that he will become angrier?

Changes in Bones

As people age, their bones do not change in length but do change in chemical composition. Aging bones gradually lose their calcium, become weakened, and fracture easily. This can be caused by hormonal changes, lack of exercise, and inadequate consumption of calcium. **Osteoporosis** is an age-related disorder characterized by decreased bone mass and increased susceptibility to fractures. It affects all bones but typically the spine, wrist, and hip. Osteoporosis affects as many as 15 to 20 million individuals in the United States, including one out of every four women over the age of sixty. Sex, race, nutrition, exercise, and overall health influence bone mass. Bone mass is approximately 30 percent higher in men than in women and approximately 10 percent higher in blacks than in whites. Women are at higher risk than men because they have less bone mass than men and because for several years following menopause, the rate of bone-mass decline is accelerated. Factors suggesting a woman's susceptibility to osteoporosis include the following:

- Family history
- Early menopause
- Never having borne a child
- Sedentary life-style
- Underweight or petite build
- Fair complexion
- Smoking

Dietary precautions taken early enough in life can be protective against osteoporosis. Two nutrients are especially recommended: calcium and vitamin D. A female between the ages of eleven and twenty-four should consume 1,200 mg. of calcium each day. A female twenty-five years of age or older should consume 800 mg. of calcium each day. The major sources of calcium in the American diet are milk and dairy products. Each eight-ounce glass of milk contains 275–300 mg. of calcium. Skim or low fat milk is preferred to minimize fat intake. Many dark green vegetables are also good sources of calcium. For those unable to obtain 800–1,200 mg of calcium by diet, supplementation with calcium tablets is recommended. When trying to build up the body's calcium, avoid using nicotine, coffee, alcohol, large amounts of protein, and phosphorous (commonly found in sodas), because they are responsible for calcium depletion. Normal levels of vitamin D are required for optimal calcium absorption. The recommended vitamin D intake is 5 μg each day for adults. Persons who do not receive adequate daily sunlight exposure, such as those confined to home, are at special risk for vitamin D deficiency. If sun exposure is inadequate, vitamin D supplements can be taken. However, because vitamin D can be toxic at high doses, an elderly person should consult with a physician to determine what amount of vitamin D supplement may be needed. It is important to know that calcium alone can only prevent *further* bone reduction and must be combined with exercise, ideally before menopause, to prevent bone loss and build up a reserve of bone mass.

> **FAST FACTS**
>
> Activity influences how efficiently the body uses calcium. With immobilization or extended bed rest, calcium absorption decreases and urinary excretion increases.

It is important to know that calcium alone can only prevent *further* bone reduction and must be combined with exercise, ideally before menopause, to prevent bone loss and build up a reserve of bone mass.

Exercise can decrease the likelihood of falls, strengthen muscles, increase bone mass, and improve balance and agility. Participate in exercises that use the muscles connected to the body's larger bones. Weight-bearing exercise, such as walking, running, swimming, and bicycling, may reduce bone loss and increase bone mass. The optimal types and amounts of physical activities that will prevent osteoporosis, however, have not been established. If an elderly person is suffering from an osteoporotic spine, she (or he) should not subject her body to the trauma of toe touches and sit-ups. She must avoid activities that further stress the weakened vertebrae. She needs to lie straight, sit straight, and stand straight with the aid of low pillows, straight-backed chairs, and good standing posture. She must avoid back flexion, twisting, reaching, and lifting. Sudden forceful movements, such as picking up heavy objects or opening windows, are especially dangerous for the elderly. An exercise program consisting of posture correction and strengthening exercises for spine extension should be prescribed. Exercise at all ages is extremely important. If you, your parents, or your grandparents are not getting the proper type or amount of exercise, what are you waiting for? Call them up and get started today. It's never too late!

Physicians must emphasize measures that retard or halt the progress of osteoporosis before irreversible structural defects occur. Protective measures, such as increased calcium consumption, engaging in weight-bearing exercises, and appropriate use of estrogen replacement therapy, have been highly successful in the prevention and management of osteoporosis. Estrogen replacement seems to be the most successful, however, when started a few years before the onset of menopause. Since there are still unanswered questions about the relative safety of using estrogen, physicians may prefer to use this therapy only for patients who have a particularly high risk of osteoporosis.

Alzheimer's Disease and Aging

Alzheimer's disease is a form of dementia that mainly affects the elderly. **Dementia** refers to deteriorating mental functions, such as intelligence, memory, and behavior controls. More than fifty conditions are known to cause dementia. Alzheimer's disease, also known as primary degenerative dementia or senile dementia of the Alzheimer's type, is the most common cause of dementia. It accounts for about 50 percent of dementia cases. It is estimated that two million Americans are afflicted by Alzheimer's disease, a neurologic disease in which certain brain cells degenerate. This degeneration disrupts the brain's ability to make acetylcholine, a chemical transmitter that carries messages between brain cells. Without enough acetylcholine, the brain deteriorates. It is a gradual, progressive, irreversible, and incurable disease. There is no existing diagnostic test for Alzheimer's disease, so if the signs of dementia appear, all potential causes must be examined and ruled out to avoid making a false diagnosis. It is important to distinguish Alzheimer's disease from other forms of dementia that can be treated.

The cause of Alzheimer's disease is not known. Although the disease is not inherited, the risk of Alzheimer's is highest among those with relatives afflicted by it. Numerous factors have been identified as possible causes of the disease. They include viral infections, inadequate diet, a deficiency of certain brain chemicals, environmental toxins, and increased concentrations of aluminum in the

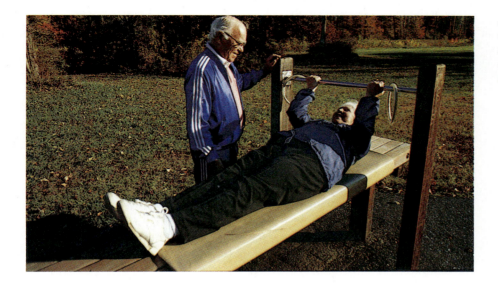

Seniors should exercise regularly. It is uplifting for the healthy, alert older person and can also be an important part of establishing a daily routine for the Alzheimer's victim.

brain. The first noticeable symptom of Alzheimer's disease is usually absent-mindedness. This is soon accompanied by a decline in reasoning, concentration, and judgment. The rate at which deterioration occurs varies. But as the disease progresses, the disease's victims become more confused and disoriented. They may develop a peculiar speech pattern called *intrusion*. This is when words or phrases from earlier conversations are repeated out of context.

In the final stages of Alzheimer's disease, afflicted individuals are helpless and dependent. Complete assistance is required in feeding, bathing, and dressing. There is loss of control over all body functions. At this point, such individuals cannot be left alone, even for a few minutes. They may wander off and get lost or may seriously injure themselves. There is total loss of recognition of potential dangers, such as knives, fire, or poisons. The hardship on the family is inconceivable. There is little left for the family to do but provide minute-to-minute custodial care. Individuals with Alzheimer's disease may continue to survive for a long period, but eventually they die from pneumonia or some other infection.

What can we do if a loved one is afflicted by Alzheimer's disease? How can we, as caregivers, improve the quality of the victim's life? The following suggestions may be helpful:

1. Get as much information as possible from the physician about the disease. Find out how far it has progressed in the individual. Determine what the individual's specific abilities and limitations are so that you can realistically approach the situation.
2. Provide a comfortable and stimulating environment for the individual. Intellectual stimulation and social contact are extremely important.
3. Keep the surroundings simple and uncluttered. Leave the individual's possessions where he or she is accustomed to seeing them. Provide familiar objects to help the individual feel less bewildered.
4. Establish a daily routine. Because Alzheimer's victims forget quickly, frequently repeated explanations are important and reassuring.
5. Let the individual do the tasks he or she can still manage to do. This reinforces self-worth.
6. Keep the person in the "here and now." Remind him or her of the day and time. Talk about yourself and other family members present in the house.

The majority of families work very hard to care for the ill family member. The task is emotionally and physically exhausting, and many relatives become overwhelmed with caregiving tasks. If you have a parent or grandparent with Alzheimer's disease, volunteer to stay with him or her so that another family member can take a break for a few hours. Providing alternatives that give the family some rest, such as day treatment, in-home help, or acute care hospitalization, can also allow the family to continue caring for the person without becoming exhausted. Self-help groups are an important resource for families. The Alzheimer's Disease and Related Disorders Association, whose national headquarters is located in Chicago, sponsors support groups in many communities throughout the United States. Current research is trying to find out more about the possible causes of Alzheimer's disease, and various treatments are being used with Alzheimer's patients to determine the effectiveness of each treatment. We hope that someday a cure will be found for this unmerciful disease.

■ Sexuality and Aging

Different people have different sexual desires, but there is normally no physical reason that healthy older individuals should not remain sexually active well into old age. The major barrier to sexual intimacy among the elderly usually lies in their own reluctance to be active. Attitudinal problems commonly include the male's fear of impotence, the woman's conviction that sex in old age is shameful or wrong, and other emotional stresses like those that interfere with sexual functions at any age. It is true that sexual ability and functioning decline through the years, but the elderly are just as capable of giving and receiving sexual satisfaction as people in their twenties or thirties. Elderly individuals need to understand the physical and psychological changes that they are undergoing. Ignorance and fear are powerful obstacles that can stand in the way of love, pleasure, and shared intimacy.

What changes can be expected by elderly men and women in regard to their sexual desires and abilities? Both men and women experience a "change of life" in middle age. In women, this period of time is called *menopause*. In men, this period of time is referred to as the *climacteric*.

When a woman is in her mid to late forties, her body's production of sex hormones slows down. Her menstrual cycle becomes irregular, and this may continue for a year or two before she completely stops menstruating. The cessation of menstruation is known as **menopause**. A woman is not considered to be postmenopausal until she has not had a menstrual period for one year. Many women sail through the menopausal years without any discomfort. Others experience symptoms such as headaches, insomnia, irritability, weight gain, and "hot flashes." Hot flashes are occasional warm, flushed feelings around the head and neck. These symptoms result from the hormonal imbalances occurring during this time. The woman also experiences vaginal changes, such as decreased vaginal lubrication, thinning of the vaginal walls, and less elasticity of the vagina. The lack of lubrication can be remedied by using a water-soluble lubricant (such as K-Y jelly) during sexual intercourse. If menopausal symptoms become a problem, estrogen replacement therapy is available. This is a controversial treatment, so a woman should evaluate the potential benefits and risks with her physician before making a decision about whether to try the treatment.

Even though a man's androgen and sperm production gradually decrease with age, there is no distinct physical menopause for men as there is for women. A small percentage of older men do experience notable declines in testosterone production. These men experience what has been termed male **climacteric**. It is characterized by chronic fatigue, depression, and lack of interest in sex. Some of the changes in a man's sexual ability and functioning may include a less firm erection, a longer time required to get an erection, a less intense orgasm, a smaller amount of semen ejaculated, and a rapid loss of erection after ejaculation. Both men and women may be alarmed by these changes. The man may feel sexually inadequate, and the woman may feel that she has failed as a lover. For these reasons, it is extremely important for sexual expectations to be realistic. Sex is more relaxed for the elderly than it is for youth. The incredible surges of sexual passion and the frequent desire for sex have long since disappeared. Yet physical and sexual intimacy with a loved one, no matter how altered from that of younger days, is comforting and renewing at any age and should be encouraged.

Successful Retirement

Gerontologists consider retirement and the death of a mate to be the two most traumatic events of later life. Perhaps the most difficult part of retirement is the abruptness of change and the lack of preparation for it. Many individuals fear that with retirement comes reduced income, loss of social participation, fewer experiences for self-expression, and less respect from others. The word "retirement" may, in itself, trigger negative feelings because it suggests a withdrawal and detachment from life. The key to successful retirement and use of leisure is to view this phase as a continuation of life rather than as an end to it. There are many people who have no problem with the prospect of retirement and who look forward to this period in life with enthusiastic anticipation.

There are many needs that must be accounted for in order for people to enjoy their later years. The Institute of Gerontology of the University of Iowa has compiled the following list of needs and drives.

1. The need to render some socially useful service.
2. The need to be considered a part of the community.
3. The need to enjoy normal companionships.
4. The need for recognition as an individual.
5. The need for opportunity for self-expression and a sense of achievement.
6. The need for health protection and care.
7. The need for suitable mental stimulation.
8. The need for suitable living arrangements and family relationships.
9. The need for spiritual satisfaction.

Although this list was specifically written with the elderly in mind, it hardly differs from the needs of people of all ages.

Caregiving: Taking Care of an Elderly Parent

From a life-span perspective, one can appreciate and come to understand the intricate relationship between rearing a child and caring for a parent. During the early part of the life span, parents provide food, shelter, clothing, love, and guidance for the child. These things are essential for the child's survival, development, and eventual independence. During child rearing, there is an im-

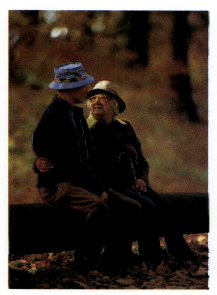

It's never too late to keep on loving.

FAST FACTS

Social Security is the only source of retirement income for nearly half (46 percent) of all aged persons and couples, and the median annual income is $6,270.

balance in the exchange of help in favor of the child. If parents care sufficiently for the child, they will meet whatever obstacles occur and make whatever sacrifices are needed to carry out the responsibilities of child rearing. Through all this, the child develops the basic attachment bond that provides a foundation for all later relationships. When the child is in young adulthood and the parents are in middle age, they are relatively independent from each other and there is greater mutual exchange of help. In the later part of the parents' life span, when the child has grown to middle age, the exchange of help may shift more in favor of the elderly parents. The process has been reversed. At this stage of life, caring for one or both parents is essential for their maintenance and continued survival in view of their decreasing growth and increasing dependence.

As America's population ages, the need for long-term care and caregivers increases. Traditionally, elderly parents were cared for by their children, and today, children are still essential as care providers to help satisfy the needs of their elderly parents. As elderly people grow older, lose friends, and become more dependent, they become more involved with their children. Ties with children may be the only remaining attachments they have, so children become even more important for assistance. Many sons and daughters make the mistake of assuming that their parents want or expect them to provide round-the-clock care. People value their independence more as they age, and having to move in with a son or daughter may be perceived as the final surrender of control over their lives. Elderly people dread being a burden to their children. They want their children to care about them, not for them. They want to live close to them, not with them.

The question of who cares for an aging parent rarely comes down to who should, who can, or who wants to. It is almost always the female in the family. Nearly seven out of every ten primary caregivers are female, and they spend an

FAST FACTS

In the years between 1980 and 2000, the numbers of people over age 80 will nearly double—from 5.2 million to 10.1 million.

GUIDELINES TO YOUR GOOD HEALTH

If you are taking care of an elderly parent and you notice any of the following warning signals, it is time to seek assistance from other family members or caregiving agencies.

1. No matter what you do, it isn't enough.
2. Your parent's condition is worsening, regardless of all your efforts.
3. You no longer have any time or any place just for yourself.
4. Other relationships in your life are falling apart because of the caregiving pressures.
5. Your caregiving duties are interfering too greatly with your other responsibilities, such as family and work.
6. You are doing everything by yourself, but you still feel guilty that you are not doing enough.
7. You can no longer find healthy ways of coping, so you engage in self-destructive behaviors, such as overeating or undereating, excessive use of alcohol, and so on.
8. You no longer feel good about yourself; you have lost your identity as a person.
9. You have become mentally or physically abusive to your elderly parent.

average of sixteen hours a week providing care. Female caregivers usually perform the household duties and tend to their parent's personal care, such as bathing, dressing, and so on. Male primary caregivers spend about five hours a week providing care, and many rely heavily on their wives or outside help. When males help out with caregiving, they tend to take on responsibilities such as managing finances or making home repairs.

Why is it that men do not share more of the caregiving responsibilities? One reason is that many older men are likely to be care recipients rather than caregivers. Another is that men are socialized differently. But the most surprising reason is that women themselves sometimes discourage men from helping out. Many men do care about helping their aging parent, but as children, they were much less involved in domestic matters than their sisters were. So when it comes to cooking, cleaning, feeding, bathing, and dressing, many men feel awkward and incompetent. As men share more of the child rearing duties (as today's younger fathers are doing), they will acquire more caregiving skills, which will make them more likely to step in when a parent needs help. Today's family is shrinking in size. Aging parents have raised fewer children, and the number of adult children available to provide caregiving for their parents will soon be smaller than in previous times. So, like it or not, men will have to share more of the caregiving responsibilities in the future simply because there will be fewer women around.

> ■ *PROBLEM SITUATION*   Do you think that it is your responsibility to personally take care of an aging parent? If you were faced with the decision of having to put your parent in a nursing home or having him or her live with you, what would you do? What factors would need to be considered before making your decision?

Caregivers need relief. Support services should be available all through the caregiving process and not just when the caregiver is about to drop from exhaustion. We need agencies to create programs that will share or relieve the caregiver's burden. Group sessions—either self-help groups or groups with trained leaders—can provide a setting in which caregivers can share their problems and concerns, develop skills for problem solving and coping, and provide mutual support. Changes must also occur in the workplace. Programs should be initiated that offer adult day care for the elderly parent while the caregiver is at work. Seminars could be conducted to discuss caregiving issues, and support groups consisting of fellow employees could be established. The Family and Medical Leave Act (HR 925), if passed, would give workers up to eighteen weeks of unpaid, job-guaranteed leave over a two-year period for the care of a dependent parent or a seriously ill child.

The children who are now adults are in the best position to truly individualize the care needed to fit their elderly parents' particular circumstances. They are also probably the best determiners of what type and degree of supplemental help or services should be provided. Regardless of the effectiveness of the help they provide, the adult children may not have the financial resources and skills to adequately take care of their parents. They may not be able to provide intermittent or continuous long-term care for those elderly parents who have become quite dependent. Assistance from other family members and service providers should be available to the primary caregiver as the elderly parents' needs become greater.

When you love somebody, you are more apt to undertake wearisome "labors of love" that offer little compensation. The following anecdote, recalled by Elaine Brody, associate director of research at the Philadelphia Geriatric Center, sums it all up:

> As the discharge procedure began for the 75-year-old hospital patient, several staff members wandered over to pay their respects because they knew he still needed assistance. When they asked who would look after him, he said, "Don't worry, Mom will take care of me." The gathering broke into laughter, thinking him a witty character. The next day a 92-year-old woman hobbled in, asked for her son, and took him away.

POSITIVE BEHAVIORS

I. *Place a check mark in front of each behavior that you now practice.*

_____ 1. I have conversations with elderly people. (CONVERSATIONS)

_____ 2. I am respectful to elderly people. (RESPECTFUL)

_____ 3. I am tolerant when an elderly person is driving in front of me. (TOLERANT)

_____ 4. I don't label the elderly by using negative stereotypes. (LABEL)

_____ 5. I initiate visits with elderly relatives or friends whenever possible. (INITIATE VISITS)

_____ 6. I protect my skin from the sun. (PROTECT SKIN)

_____ 7. I get adequate daily amounts of calcium through diet, supplements, or both. (CALCIUM)

_____ 8. I do weight-bearing exercise at least three times a week for a minimum of twenty minutes each time. (EXERCISE)

_____ 9. I get my eyes examined at least every two years. (EYES)

_____ 10. My present life-style is laying a good foundation for healthy aging. (GOOD FOUNDATION)

II. *For each behavior that you DO NOT ENGAGE IN, write the KEY WORD(S) located in the parentheses at the end of the statement in the column below. Then put a check mark in the appropriate column to indicate whether you are going to keep or change that behavior.*

Behaviors I Don't Engage In   KEEP/CHANGE
                                     _____/_____
                                     _____/_____
                                     _____/_____
                                     _____/_____
                                     _____/_____
                                     _____/_____
                                     _____/_____
                                     _____/_____
                                     _____/_____
                                     _____/_____

III. *For each of the preceding behaviors that you choose to KEEP, write a statement indicating why you are choosing to keep that behavior.*

I choose to keep behavior _____ because:
                            KEY WORD

For each of the preceding behaviors that you choose to CHANGE, write a statement indicating how you plan to implement that change.

I will change behavior _____ by:
                         KEY WORD

Now You Know

1. FALSE. Women are biologically tougher. Their system deteriorates more slowly, making them less susceptible to degenerative diseases.
2. TRUE. It is discrimination against the elderly solely because of their age.
3. FALSE. Only a small percentage of the elderly are senile, which results from physiological degeneration in the brain.
4. FALSE. Intelligence changes little with age.
5. FALSE. Persons who take care of themselves are likely to feel the effects of aging more slowly than others; however, eventually all people will show signs of aging.
6. TRUE. Less efficient functioning of oil glands, loss of the skin's elasticity, and loss of the underlying layer of fat cause wrinkling of skin.
7. TRUE. Osteoporosis is more prevalent in the elderly population, especially among women.
8. TRUE. Presently, research is being conducted to try to find a cure for Alzheimer's disease.
9. FALSE. The major barrier to sexual intimacy is usually the couple's own reluctance to be sexually active.
10. TRUE. Nearly seven out of every ten primary caregivers are female.

Summary

1. Aging is a physiologic process that continues from birth to death. It consists of biological, psychological, and social dimensions.
2. There are 29 million Americans who are sixty-five years of age and over. By the year 2000, there will be 45 million Americans in this age group.
3. It is in our cells that aging begins. All the theories of aging assume that aging represents a loss of control over various bodily processes and that this loss occurs at the cellular level in the DNA.
4. There are five basic theories of aging. The error hypothesis theory of aging proposes that aging is caused by defects in DNA and RNA duplication. The free-radical theory of aging proposes that uncontrolled molecules cause accumulated damage to RNA and DNA molecules. The cross-linkage theory of aging proposes that chemical bridges form between protein molecules and DNA molecules. These cross-linkages interfere with the normal functioning of protein and DNA. The brain hypothesis theory says that aging is due to a decline in the body's ability to maintain homeostasis. The autoimmune theory of aging proposes that the body's immune system malfunctions with age.
5. Ageism is a form of discrimination against the elderly solely on the basis of their age. Society has perpetuated negative stereotypes about aging and being old.
6. Senility is a condition that is caused by physiological degeneration in the brain. It is not an inevitable consequence of growing old. Senility may actually be a behavior resulting from factors such as environmental conditions, overmedication with drugs, anemia, certain viral infections, anxiety, loneliness, or depression. If properly identified, the behavior may be fully reversible.
7. Intelligence does not decline appreciably with age. The most rapid decline takes place between the late sixties and early seventies. Only after age eighty do mental abilities fall below the average mental performance of younger people.
8. The overwhelming majority of elderly people live in their own homes and care for themselves. Only about 4 percent of the elderly in our society are institutionalized.
9. Wrinkles are one of the earliest visible signs of aging. They are more pronounced where the fat loss has been the greatest and where there has been prolonged exposure to sun, such as the face, neck, and hands.
10. As a person grows older, his or her skin becomes more susceptible to burning instead of tanning. The ultraviolet light from the sun tends to harden, thicken, and dry out the skin's outer layer.
11. Graying and balding are other signs of aging. They are both inherited traits, and living a stressful life does not precipitate premature graying or balding.
12. Most elderly people experience some loss of vision; however, they usually have functional eyesight throughout most of their lifetime.
13. Permanent hearing loss, or presbycusis, results from a gradual deterioration of structures in the inner ear. Everyone loses some hearing with age.
14. Osteoporosis is a bone disorder characterized by decreased bone mass and increased susceptibility to fractures. It affects all bones but typically the spine, wrist, and hip. It affects as many as 15 to 20 million individuals in the United States.
15. Alzheimer's disease is a neurologic disease in which certain brain cells degenerate. It is the most common cause of dementia. Dementia refers to deteriorating mental functions. In the final stage of the disease, the individual is helpless and dependent and has lost control over all bodily functions. The cause of Alzheimer's disease is not known, and at the present time it is incurable.

16. Even though it is true that sexual ability and functioning decline with age, there is normally no physical reason why healthy older individuals should not remain sexually active well into old age.

17. Retirement has the potential for being a traumatic event of later life. The key to successful retirement is to view this phase as a continuation of life rather than as an end to it.

18. Children are the primary caregivers to help satisfy the needs of their elderly parents. Caregivers must be aware of when they are approaching unhealthy levels of stress and exhaustion. That is the time to seek assistance from other family members or caregiving agencies. More support services are needed to share or relieve the caregiver's burden.

References

1. Anderson-Ellis, Eugenia, and Marsha Dryan. *Aging Parents and You*. New York: Master Media Ltd., 1988.
2. Aronson, Miriam K. *Understanding Alzheimer's Disease*. New York: Charles Scribner's Sons, 1988.
3. Belsky, Janet K. *Here Tomorrow*. Baltimore: The Johns Hopkins University Press, 1988.
4. Cooper, Kenneth H. *Preventing Osteoporosis*. New York: Bantam Books, 1989.
5. Kart, Cary S., Eileen K. Metress, and Seamus P. Metress. *Aging, Health and Society*. Boston: Jones and Bartlett, 1988.
6. Kenney, Richard A. *Physiology of Aging: A Synopsis*. 2d ed. Chicago: Year Book Medical Publishers, 1989.
7. *Memory and Aging*. Chicago: Alzheimer's Disease and Related Disorders Association, Inc., 1987.
8. McIlwain, Harris H., Debra Fulghum Bruce, et al. *Osteoporosis: Prevention, Management, Treatment*. New York: John Wiley and Sons, 1988.
9. Osterkamp, Lynn. "Family Caregivers: America's Primary Long-Term Care Resource." *Aging* 358 (1988): 2–6.
10. Rhodes, Colbert. *An Introduction to Gerontology*. Springfield, Ill: Charles C. Thomas, 1988.
11. Sommers, Tish, and Laurie Shields. *Women Take Care*. Gainesville, Florida: Triad Publishing Co., 1987.
12. *The 1989 Information Please Almanac*, 42nd ed. New York: Houghton Mifflin, 1988.

Suggested Readings

Anderson-Ellis, Eugenia, and Marsha Dryan. *Aging Parents and You*. New York: Master Media Ltd., 1988.
Aronson, Miriam K. *Understanding Alzheimer's Disease*. New York: Charles Scribner's Sons, 1988.
Cooper, Kenneth H. *Preventing Osteoporosis*. New York: Bantam Books, 1989.
Dychtwald, Ken, and Joe Flower. *Age Wave*. Los Angeles: Jeremy P. Tarcher, Inc., 1989.
Kart, Cary S., Eileen K. Metress, and Seamus P. Metress. *Aging, Health and Society*. Boston: Jones and Bartlett Publishers, 1988.
Wise, David A. *The Economics of Aging*. Chicago: The University of Chicago Press, 1989.

CHAPTER 21

Ultimate Loss

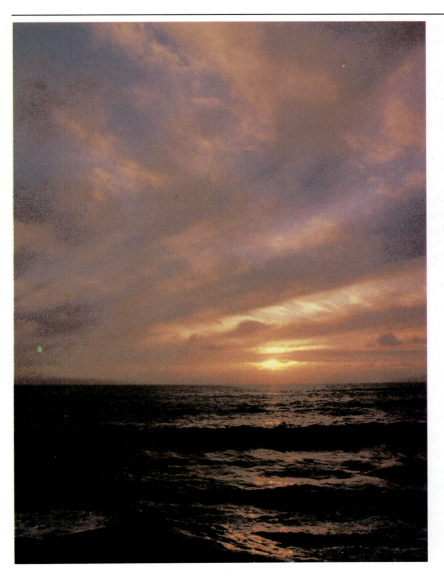

What Do You Know?

Are the following statements true or false?

1. No one has ever been pronounced legally dead and come back to life.
2. Fears of death and dying are first initiated when infants and young children experience separation anxiety when their parents leave them alone.
3. Grieving the loss of a loved one is usually made easier when the dying trajectory is prolonged and a period of anticipatory grief precedes the actual death.
4. A living will, stating that you do not wish to have doctors take heroic lifesaving measures in certain instances such as irreversible coma, is a legally binding document that physicians are bound to follow.
5. The term *euthanasia* refers to allowing patients to die by "pulling the plug" as well as to take direct steps to end their lives.
6. A hospice is a hospital where people go to die.
7. When purchasing funeral goods and services, it is best to buy a package that includes everything.
8. Grief, bereavement, and mourning are synonymous terms for the loss of a loved one.
9. Common reactions of acute grief include distorted perception, loss of appetite, bodily disturbances, restlessness, and disorganization.
10. When people are dying, they invariably go through a series of stages from denial to acceptance.

This is not meant to be morbid or frightening, but some day YOU WILL DIE. So will we and so will everyone else you know. Death is a certainty; we just don't know when, where, or how it will happen. It is the natural way of things that people are born, live their lives, and then die. The knowledge that we will die one day gives meaning to our lives. In fact, even before death arrives, its presence is felt in our lives. It affects everything we do and the levels of wellness that we attain.

Besides understanding death as it affects our health and wellness, there are many other reasons for studying death and dying. In a recent survey of why college students had enrolled in a course on death education, the following reasons were given most frequently:

- the recent death of a friend or relative
- a terminally ill parent or grandparent
- thoughts of suicide, either by oneself or a friend
- fears about one's own death
- preparation for the dying process, including knowledge about funerals, wills, how to talk to dying people, and so on
- an interest in helping others by teaching death education or working with dying patients, such as in a hospice
- an opinion that the topic seemed interesting and different.

The Role of Death in Life

To see that death plays a big part in our everyday lives, we need only look at the newspapers and books we read every day, the movies, plays, and television programs we watch, the songs we listen to, and so on. One of the major differences between the human species and other animals is that we anticipate potential death and personal extinction. Death, therefore, gives an added dimension or meaning to our lives. It is the idea of a finite life that causes us to organize and to plan how we will make use of the limited time we have on earth.

The concept of death's occurrence is difficult to handle for two reasons. First, death occurs too soon. There almost always are unmet goals to achieve or unfulfilled pleasures to experience. We may want to keep on living in order to reach life's goals and have pleasure whether life expectancy is forty years, as it was a few centuries ago, almost eighty years, as it is in the United States today, or more than one hundred years, as it may be in the twenty-first century. The second reason we find death difficult to handle is that we don't know what is beyond life. It represents for us the ultimate fear of the unknown.

To look at death on a personal level, here are some pertinent questions for you to think about and answer:

- When would you like to die?
- Would you like to know how much longer you have to live? Do you think the answer will be the same in forty or fifty years from now, if you're still alive then?
- What are your beliefs about an afterlife?
- When do you think about your own dying?
- How do you think you will die? What would you like the circumstances of your dying to be like?
- Would you want to outlive your mate/spouse?

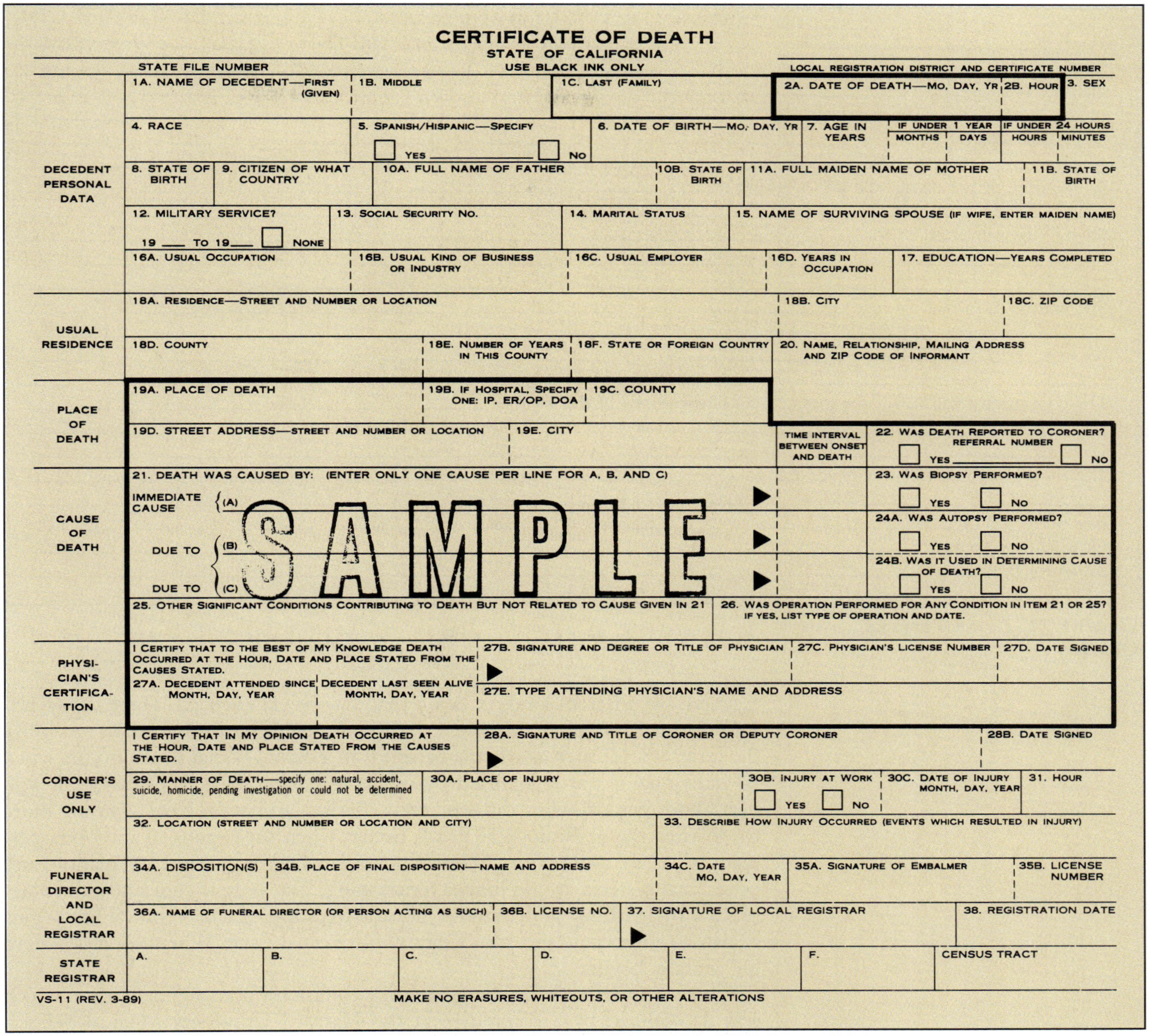

FIGURE 21–1 ■ Example of a Death Certificate

■ What will your death certificate look like? Your obituary? (See Figures 21–1 and 21–2.)

Another interesting question that you might want to ponder is, When does the process of dying begin? Is it at birth? Is it directly linked to aging? When does the aging process start? When is the dying process felt? When is it recognized? Does life end when the doctor says it does, or do we realize it ourselves? When do we accept that we are dying? As we get imminently close to death, when do we recognize and accept that nothing more can or should be done?

_____, age _____ died yesterday
from _____. She was a
member of _____
_____.
She is survived by _____
_____
At the time of her death, she was working on _____
_____
She will be remembered for _____
_____
_____
She will be mourned by _____
_____
because _____
_____
The community will suffer the loss of her contributions in the areas of _____
_____
She always wanted, but was never able to _____
_____
The body will be _____
Flowers may be sent _____
In lieu of flowers _____

FIGURE 21–2 ■ **A Personal Obituary**

There are different kinds of death that may be experienced. There is **psychological death**, which occurs when a person is unable to distinguish or recognize the outer world, such as when a person is in a coma. **Social death** occurs when an individual is not recognized by others as having existed. Occasionally you hear about parents who "disown" their children and never have anything more to do with them. **Biological death** occurs when the organs of the body permanently cease to function. **Clinical death** is when respiration, circulation, and other vital systems are no longer functioning. Not only is clinical death sometimes a tricky thing to determine, but the question of when clinical life begins is also an important and sometimes controversial issue. When do you believe life actually begins?

What about **legal death**, however? The commonly accepted definition, which was determined by a committee at the Harvard University Medical School, establishes the four criteria for a person to be considered dead as (1) unreceptivity and unresponsivity, (2) no movements or breathing, (3) no reflexes, and (4) a flat electroencephalogram, or EEG (the tracing of a device that measures brain waves). The last criterion—having no measurable brain waves—is the most definitive evidence that someone is truly dead.

■ Concepts of Death and Dying

Since none of us is aware of actually having been legally dead, for all intents and purposes, death is a thought or conceptualization. We can intellectualize about it and have all sorts of feelings connected with it, but our concept of death changes as we mature and develop or as we find ourselves in different situations. There is no simple explanation of why we think and feel the way we do about dying. In order to get a little more in touch with how you conceptualize death, try completing the following sentences. (Don't hesitate to give more than one response.)

- Death is _____.
- Death is like _____.
- Death means _____.
- When I think of a dying person, the scenario that comes to mind is _____.

One major thought about death is that it always involves loss—either the loss of our "self" or of a significant other. It involves being unable to experience this earthly world and the sensory satisfactions that make life worth living. It means that we can no longer exert control over our environment, nor can we complete projects that we've begun. Death is the end of our bodies (or other *things*)—which leads to the spiritual question of what (if anything) is left.

Perhaps now is a good time to ask that popular question, "Is there life after death?" (Or should we use the title of Raymond Moody's best selling book and ask if there's *Life After Life*?) The answer is . . . nobody knows. An impressive number of people have been considered dead and have returned to life, but none of them have actually had a verifiable flat brain wave for more than five minutes. Nevertheless, thousands of people have had what can be called *near-death experiences* and were revived. The amazing thing about these experiences is how similar the reports of what happened during them have been. A notable reaction of people who have had such experiences has been that they found it difficult, if not impossible, to describe in ordinary language what they went through. It may not surprise you, therefore, to learn that most people are not anxious to tell about their near-death experiences, as they're afraid that others won't believe what they find hard to put into words in the first place. In studies that asked people who had had near-death experiences to describe what occurred, the following events and feelings were most frequently reported:

- being pulled through a dark tunnel
- being surrounded by a beam of indescribably bright light accompanied by feelings of warmth and love
- detachment from one's body and the outer world
- meeting friends or relatives, some of whom they never met or heard of in their lifetime
- a feeling of peace, joy, and harmony
- a new view of spirituality or revelation and purpose in life.

These people also overwhelmingly agreed that they didn't want to come back to their earthly bodies. Although they were glad to still be alive, they had no great fear of death.

Fears of Death and Dying

Almost all of us harbor some fears about death to a greater or lesser degree. Let's look at how these fears develop, what forms they take, how people handle them, and the benefits of overcoming them.

FAST FACTS

An estimated 20 percent of adults in the United States have had a near-death experience.

Some fears and accompanying denial may be said to be inborn, because even infants react to isolation and separation. Yet how this fear manifests itself and whether it becomes so severe that it interferes with normal functioning is *learned*. Some of the fear stems from the anxiety of being separated from our parents as infants and young children. In a more direct way, children learn to fear death and dying by the way their parents react to it and the way they respond to their children's questions. If parents avoid the topic of death and exclude their children from all discussions and activities involved with death, their children are likely to be uncomfortable with death, too. If, on the other hand, death is talked about naturally and honestly in the household, the children are more likely to develop a healthier attitude about death.

How did your attitudes about death and dying evolve? Your responses to these more specific questions may give you some insights into the development of your death attitudes.

1. What was your first involvement with death?
   - Who died?
   - What were the reactions of the adults present?
   - What were your feelings and reactions?
2. How was death dealt with in your family? Openly? With a sense of secrecy or embarassment?
3. What has influenced your attitudes toward death the most?
   - Specific books?
   - Religious upbringing?
   - TV and movies?
   - Friends and family?

Another way for you to examine your attitudes about death and dying is to complete a validated death attitude instrument, such as Self-Inventory 21.1.

Why do people fear death as they do? One category of fears is associated with the *cessation of being*. Some people fear dying because of what will happen to those who depend on them when they are gone. They may be afraid that time will run out and they will not be able to complete important tasks or achieve certain goals in life. They may fear a loss of pleasure or the ability to think. Finally, associated with the cessation of being is the basic realization of the death of the self (*I will die*).

A second category of fears involves the fear of the *event of dying*. It may involve the physical pain that people think they will experience while dying. The following statement made by Don Robinson, a leading educator, before his death in 1980 addresses this point about the presence of physical pain while dying:

> Perhaps there is some built-in physiological reaction that numbs the emotions in the presence of imminent death or the recognized threat of death, something similar to the physiological numbing of pain that is so intense that the overload converts unbearable pain into unfeelable pain.
>
> This resumed numbing of the emotions coupled with the urge to absorb the most pleasure from the limited time remaining results in one's final days being among the most pleasurable. I somehow feel freed from responsibility. My anxieties fall away. I am carefree. This is ever so much more important than my illness, regardless of what may be the connection between them.

People also fear the helplessness and indignity that may come with being weak and incapacitated—a kind of psychological suffering. Also associated with the process of dying is the fear of growing old and infirm.

The last category of common reasons for fearing death has to do with the fears of what may occur *after death*. The most obvious fear related to this concern is that we may encounter some sort of hell or retribution after we die, especially if we have feelings of guilt about some actual or self-perceived wrongdoing. Many people fear their bodies decaying and being eaten by worms. The basic fear in this category, however, is a fear of the unknown—what is on the "other side" or what the future holds in store.

Fears of death and dying can also focus on others. Not only may we be concerned about our own suffering while going through the dying process, but we may also fear that those we love will be enduring pain and suffering. We may fear being abandoned as those we love die. This is common among children, who fear losing their parents, or among the elderly as they see their friends and relatives die off.

Fears of death are not necessarily bad, as long as the level of fear is not so intense that it interferes with our ability to function normally. A certain amount of fear of death is natural and may serve to motivate us to engage in fulfilling behaviors.

With regard to the death-related fear of oblivion, people do all sorts of things to overcome the fact that they will never return to this earth in this time and form. Some common actions include the following:

- Erecting monuments to themselves.
- Having children who will carry on the family name.
- Prolonging physical existence through mummification, transplantation of organs, or freezing of the body (called **cryogenics**). In the future we may see attempts made at **cloning** (genetically making an exact replica of a person) in order to gain immortality.
- Doing good deeds or otherwise working to gain fame and remembrance.

What other ways can you think of that people may use to try to overcome oblivion or seek immortality?

If we are able to overcome intense fears of death and accept that we will inevitably die, the positive consequences that result include the following:

- the tendency to act with honesty, courage, and strength
- the ability to make decisions boldly and with conviction, overcoming timidity
- the ability to be spontaneous in life and act naturally, to eliminate the fear of failure, and to achieve freedom in actions
- discovery of the focal point in our lives and the meaning in it.

Those who have faced a terminal illness and have been able to accept this fate usually begin to live every moment to the fullest. They become fully appreciative of the smallest and most mundane aspects of living, even everyday household chores and "dreary" weather conditions. In fact, a nationwide self-help group for terminally ill people and their families calls itself *Make Today Count* to signify that it encourages people to live every day to the fullest.

■ The Process of Dying

What comes to mind when you think of a dying person? In what environment do people usually spend their last hours? At home? In a hospital? Who's there with them? Loved ones? Doctors or nurses? What is their physical, spiritual, and mental-emotional state? Are they sedated or aware? In a coma or unconscious?

FIGURE 21–3 ■ **The Dying Trajectory**

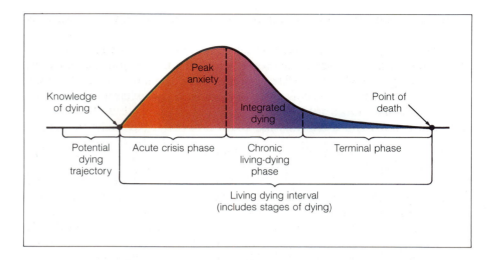

Basically, there are four ways to die: natural death, accidental death, suicide, and homicide. Dying may be considered passive (such as in the case of someone who dies from a chronic illness like cancer) or active (such as when someone's actions are responsible for causing his or her death). Cultural aspects, including religious rites, influence the way people go through the dying process. People usually die in a manner that is consistent with the way they live.

The pattern that people follow in moving through the dying process is called a **dying trajectory** (see Figure 21–3). Considering the advanced state of modern medical technology and the fact that most Americans die from chronic diseases, the typical dying trajectory lasts for a relatively long period. The actual dying trajectory begins at the moment a disease is diagnosed as being terminal. The time from that moment until the person actually dies is called the **living-dying interval**. It is during this interval that people need the most help in coping with the final stages of life and in experiencing death with dignity.

The most important work to date describing common reactions during this living-dying interval has been the pioneering research done by psychiatrist Elisabeth Kübler-Ross. According to Kübler-Ross, terminal patients and their loved ones experience one or more of the five following stages in coping with the impending or actual loss of life:

1. *Denial* is most often the initial response. People defend themselves against the pain of tragic loss by denying that the loss will or has occurred. Denial may take the form of continuing on with normal behavior as if the dying person were in good health or visiting clinic after clinic in an effort to find a cure for the terminal disease. Some people never get out of this stage and continue to deny the loss. However, individuals may move on and deal with their other emotional reactions.

2. Once someone has faced the reality that death and loss are inevitable, *anger* may be allowed to vent itself. It is natural to feel and express anger at the frustration of not being able to prevent the loss of a human life. Yet, it is important to recognize the anger and manifest it in a healthy manner rather than directing it at an innocent bystander. In a hospital setting, nurses, for example, are sometimes singled out as the target of a person's anger simply because they are accessible.

3. Although not one of the most common or important psychological stages of dying, *bargaining* of one sort or another sometimes occurs. It usually takes the form of an individual promising to behave properly if only good health is restored.

4. *Depression* can stem from many situations, and dying is a common cause. Depression is a normal and perhaps even desirable reaction to death; if, however, it lingers long enough to interfere with leading a full and fruitful life, overt steps (such as consulting a professional counselor) must be taken to relieve it.

5. Ideally, if the previous stages have been successfully dealt with, *acceptance* will be achieved and the reality of the loss will be integrated into one's life.

In addition to these five stages, there is always *hope* that things will get better or that meaning will be found in the loss.

As helpful as Kübler-Ross' theory of the stages of dying is in understanding emotional reactions to death and other losses, it is not without its faults. First, not everyone goes through these stages in a sequential order; rather, people usually vacillate from one stage to another. Some people may immediately become depressed and may never achieve acceptance. Furthermore, reactions other than the five identified by Kübler-Ross have been identified. Any of a wide array of defense mechanisms may be implemented as a way of handling dying. Nevertheless, Kübler-Ross' work has led the way in helping us understand many of our psychological reactions to death or loss.

Some influences on the quality of the living-dying interval and the grieving process that follows death include the suddenness of the dying trajectory and whether or not the trajectory follows an expected path. An expected and slow

---

SELF-INVENTORY 21.1

Hardt Death Attitude Scale

The following items are not intended to test your knowledge. There are no right or wrong answers.

Directions: Read each item carefully. Place a check mark next to each item with which you AGREE. Make no marks next to items with which you DISAGREE.

1. _____ The thought of death is a glorious thought.
2. _____ When I think of death, I am most satisfied.
3. _____ Thoughts of death are wonderful thoughts.
4. _____ The thought of death is very pleasant.
5. _____ The thought of death is comforting.
6. _____ I find it fairly easy to think of death.
7. _____ The thought of death isn't so bad.
8. _____ I do not mind thinking of death.
9. _____ I can accept the thought of death.
10. _____ To think of death is common.
11. _____ I don't fear thoughts of death, but I don't like them either.
12. _____ Thinking about death is overvalued by many.
13. _____ Thinking of death is not fundamental to me.
14. _____ I find it difficult to think of death.
15. _____ I regret the thought of death.
16. _____ The thought of death is an awful thought.
17. _____ The thought of death is dreadful.
18. _____ The thought of death is traumatic.
19. _____ I hate the sound of the word "death."
20. _____ The thought of death is outrageous.

Scoring and Interpretation

To score, add up the numerical values next to each item you checked and divide the sum by the number of items checked. This numerical value will fall on a statement or between two statements. If it falls between two statements, round off the average to the nearest whole number. The statement corresponding to that number represents your current attitude towards death.

SOURCE: Dale V. Hardt, "Development of an Investigating Instrument to Measure Attitudes toward Death," *Journal of School Health* 45 (February 1975): 96–99.

GUIDELINES TO YOUR GOOD HEALTH

Because all of us at some time in our lives will probably have the opportunity to visit and speak with a friend or relative who is dying, here are some helpful suggestions to follow.

1. You can feel awkward when speaking to a dying person, but if you are uncomfortable about knowing what to say or how to act, rely on the principle that honesty is the best policy. Say that you are unsure about what to say, and you'll get a response of appreciation and assurance.
2. The most important thing that you can give a dying person is the reassurance of physical touch. Simply sitting quietly and holding hands or exchanging hugs is all that is necessary.
3. Small talk is a good way to pass the time and may lead to other, more personal matters if the person wants to talk about deeper matters of the heart.

---

dying trajectory gives everyone time to tie up most unfinished business, both financial/physical and emotional/spiritual. It also allows loved ones to undergo a period of anticipatory grief, thus lessening the intensity of grief at the moment of death. However, a dying trajectory that is slower than expected can emotionally drain everyone. This lingering trajectory is an especially trying situation when the dying person is so weak and in such pain that there is virtually no real quality of life left.

In contrast, a death that occurs unexpectedly and suddenly, such as from a motor-vehicle accident, is a tremendous shock and doesn't allow anyone time to take care of unfinished business or to do preparatory grieving. Some dying trajectories are sudden but expected, such as those of deaths occurring during war or occurring as a risk of high-risk jobs or adventurous activities.

The typical dying trajectory—one that is expected and relatively slow—often presents some difficult moral decisions, such as if and when to tell a person that a condition is terminal. If you had terminal cancer, would you like to be told? When? By whom? In what manner? The key concept in approaching this decision is that people should be told as much as they want to know. Most people want to know if they're dying, but they don't necessarily want to know all the minute details. Although telling someone that he or she is dying is one of the hardest things you'd ever have to do, the dying person is usually grateful that somebody is being honest and open.

Speaking freely and openly with a dying person can be of tremendous comfort, because it will help alleviate his or her fear of being deserted and prevent the isolation that frequently accompanies the dying process. It's unfortunate, but once people are stuck with the label of "dying," friends come to see them less often and they may be treated as outcasts. One person with cancer told about being at a party with friends when he noticed that the host had served everyone drinks in regular glasses except for him; his drink was served in a disposable plastic cup. Informing dying individuals of their terminal illness also allows them to put their affairs in order. It allows them to come to a spiritual resolution about the meaning of life and death for themselves.

FAST FACTS

Recent research indicates that families with children who have cystic fibrosis (with limited longevity) appear to be much like other families for long periods of time rather than homes of chronic sorrow.

When talking to a dying person about his or her condition, the important thing is not to lie! This only leads to a situation of mutual pretense wherein the dying person senses the discomfort of the other person—whether it be a doctor, nurse, or family member—and therefore also avoids the topic of death. Mutual pretense of this sort obviously should be avoided, but we must recognize that doctors and nurses are human, too, and they may need help in talking to dying patients. Nevertheless, as time gets closer to actual death, most people know instinctively that they are dying. At that point, all that needs to be done is to provide them with a comfortable setting and a good listener with whom they can freely discuss their dying.

Dying with Dignity

If we can die in familiar surroundings with those whom we love around us, free from pain but aware and alert, we will have accomplished a good and dignified death. The aim is to die peacefully and painlessly at the appropriate time.

One way to accomplish this is to let your wishes be known beforehand. By filling out a **living will**, which is a signed statement declaring when a person would want life-sustaining procedures withheld or withdrawn, you can give physicians some guidelines to follow in making decisions about the use of life-support systems. (See Figure 21–4 for an example of a living will which includes a Durable Power of Attorney form if one wishes to use it.) Although living wills aren't legally binding on physicians, they do give them some directions to go by. Most states now have some sort of right-to-die laws, under which patients and their families can legally demand that life-support systems be withdrawn and that the patient be allowed to die in a natural way.

If a person is on a life-support machine such as a respirator and the "plug is pulled," this act of withdrawing lifesaving procedures is considered to be **passive euthanasia**. This is opposed to **active euthanasia**, or mercy killing, which is an overt act leading directly to death. Although some people advocate active euthanasia in certain cases, the controversy today usually centers around withholding heroic measures and allowing people with no hope of recovery to die. Legally, it is more difficult to "pull the plug" than to hook a patient up to a life-support system to begin with.

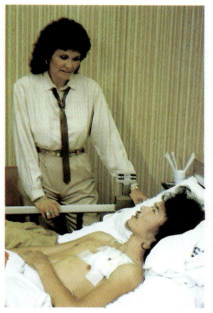

Hospices provide tender loving care to both those who are dying and to their families.

> ■ **PROBLEM SITUATION** Your grandmother is seventy-five years old and has excruciating pain from arthritis that can only be somewhat controlled with drugs. Though frail, she has remained alert and responsive. She has now developed pneumonia in the hospital and has been put on a respirator to help her breathing. If she were to lapse into a coma, would you ask that the respirator be disconnected? If she were still conscious and asked to be taken off the respirator and allowed to die, would you be in favor of asking the doctor to pull the plug? If you answered "yes" and the doctor refused, what might you do?

Formal programs exist that have been established specifically to meet the needs of dying patients and their families. The most notable of these is the hospice movement, which is not a new concept but has just recently been instituted on a large scale in the United States. **Hospice** is a humanistic program

FIGURE 21-4 ■ A Living Will

created to care for dying patients and their families. Analgesic drugs may be administered to free the patient from intense pain yet keep him or her alert enough to have meaningful relationships with family members and others. No intravenous feeding is provided, nor are heroic measures taken to prolong life unnecessarily.

The ideal is usually to provide the necessary support so that the patient can live his or her last days at home. Support is available to help with the patient's personal needs, to give the family a break from having to stay at home to take care of the patient, and to provide emotional support. Some hospices have built inpatient facilities for those families that can no longer give patients adequate care at home. Most hospices are staffed largely by volunteers, so the cost of these programs is minimal and services are very humane.

Funerals

Once upon a time, when someone died, the body was disposed of by members of the family or clan. Then the task was given to others, whose job it was to take the dead body away and take care of its disposal. These *undertakers,* as they were then called, were the forerunners of today's *funeral directors* (who sometimes also call themselves *grief counselors,* although they usually do not have any special credentials or degree in counseling). Funeral directors still look after the disposal of the body, but they also plan the memorial services for the deceased and handle other special arrangements for the survivors, such as shipment of the body if it is to be transported to another part of the country.

Funerals and memorial services, whatever form they may take, serve several practical functions. One such function is to mark the passage from one state of being or life to another. Just as we engage in rituals to mark other passages, such as marriage, graduation from school, and birth, so too do we have rituals acknowledging the passing away of another human being. Memorial services may be formal or religious in nature, or they may simply be gatherings of loved ones who meet to share memories of the deceased. Whatever form a memorial service takes, it should be a meaningful event for the bereaved, because it is a way of acknowledging the loss and helps with the grieving process. The memorial service is a declaration of the status of the deceased in society and shows that the social system remains after the loss of one of its members.

How the body is disposed of is, of course, a matter of personal preference. You can be buried in the ground, called **interment**. You can be **cremated**, whereby your body is burned in an extremely hot furnace until only ashes and unburnable bone fragments are left. Or you can be "buried" at sea. Cremation is becoming more and more popular because it is much less costly than ground burial and because burial land is scarce in some areas. The ashes, or *cremains,*

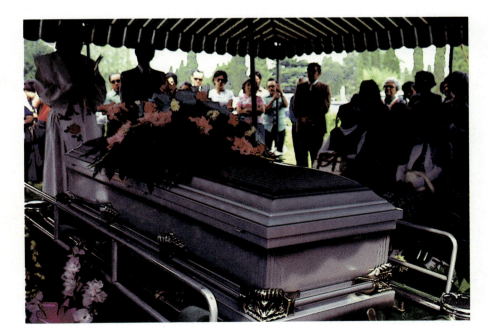

Funerals serve an important emotional and social function in all cultural groups.

as they are called, can then be kept in an urn, can be disposed of in the ground, or can be scattered at sea or over a wilderness area.

Most of you will at one time in your lives be responsible for making funeral arrangements for a family member or other loved one. For many, it will be the biggest single expenditure of money next to purchasing a home or car. Nevertheless, it is extremely difficult to be a good consumer when it comes to funerals. In her classic muckraking book, *The American Way of Death,* Jessica Mitford has pointed out several reasons why this is so.

1. Most people are totally ignorant about what to expect when they step into a mortuary or funeral home. This is due in part to their fear of anything having to do with death.

2. Decisions about a funeral must be made immediately, leaving no time to shop around.

3. Consumer decisions about funerals are made at a time of great emotional stress, and sometimes there are feelings of guilt that not enough was done for the deceased. This leads to the tendency to want to "get the best" or that "nothing is too good" for the dead person. Of course, whatever is done is for the survivors, since the deceased is no longer here on earth.

All of this leads to consumers of funeral services and products being easy prey for sales gimmicks. Sentiment is a boon to the funeral industry, making it easier to sell various funeral artifacts such as caskets and flowers. It must be noted, of course, that the funeral industry is profit oriented, just like any other business in our free-enterprise system. It should be expected that similar marketing and sales strategies will be used within the limits of good taste and sensitivity to people's emotional needs.

To save considerable money when making funeral purchases, make the funeral simple and personally meaningful. Buy only what is absolutely necessary. This can best be accomplished by purchasing each item separately instead of buying a package in which everything is included. That way you can avoid such things as embalming, which is usually not necessary unless the body is to be transported a long distance or kept for a long time before it's disposed of. Cremation, as opposed to earth burial, is much less expensive and should definitely be considered as a means of body disposal.

Another money-saving approach is to join a memorial society early in life; then funeral arrangements can be made ahead of time, even though they won't be needed for many years to come. A memorial society (there's one in just about every city in the United States and Canada) is a group that you need join only once in a lifetime for a nominal fee, usually about $25 to $50. The society contracts with local funeral homes to have them provide services for its members at a much lower cost than for people not affiliated with a memorial society. Although most cemeteries and mortuaries have pre-need agreements that you can purchase, they are still usually not as economical as memorial societies.

> ■ *PROBLEM SITUATION* After reading the portion of this chapter dealing with funerals, you decide to join a memorial society. You are asked to stipulate how you want your body disposed of. What will you say? While you're at it, what kind of memorial service would you want? What would you like said about you?

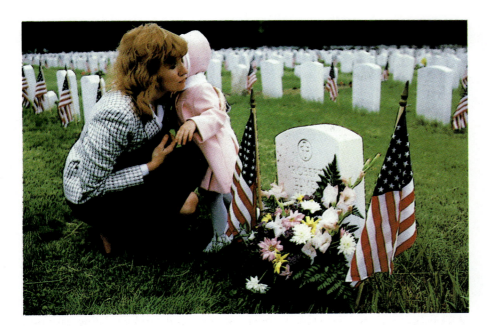

We all must grieve in our own way the loss of loved ones.

◼ Handling Grief

Dealing with the death of a loved one is like dealing with any other loss, but in most cases it is much more intense. In his book, *Loneliness and Love,* psychologist Clark Moustakis said, "All love leads to suffering," meaning that all relationships eventually end in parting or separation. The actual loss is termed **bereavement**. **Grief** is the emotional pain that accompanies the loss, and the expression of that grief or sorrow is called **mourning**.

In his book, *Death, Grief, and Caring Relationships,* **thanatologist** Richard Kalish identified four tasks that are necessary for optimal grieving:

1. Acceptance of the reality of death and loss.
2. Acceptance that grieving is painful.
3. Adjustment to a new environment with the absence of the lost loved one.
4. Establishment of new relationships.

The grieving process should enable survivors to gain a better understanding of the loss, stabilize and bolster their self-esteem, and utilize their social-support system. Grievers should be allowed a full expression of their feelings. The appropriate expression of these feelings of sorrow, anger, guilt, and despair is crying. These tears are part of the healing process, and crying should be encouraged for both men and women, as well as boys and girls.

One way of protecting ourselves against the loneliness that may follow the loss of a loved one is through the nurturing of intimate relationships. The first step is to establish an intimate knowledge of ourselves through such practices as contemplation or meditation, psychotherapy, journal writing, or some other

FAST FACTS

In our society, females are expected to express grief openly, whereas males are expected to inhibit such feelings in public.

> **FAST FACTS**
>
> The death rate of widowed and divorced parents of Israeli soldiers who were killed in action was significantly higher than that of parents who were still married, indicating that spouse support lessens grief-related stress.

kind of free writing such as poetry. Second is the development of a new intimate relationship with another person. This is not easily done, because it means that we are once more vulnerable to loss or separation and subsequent suffering. Nevertheless, a meaningful life necessitates taking such risks. Finally, we should similarly relate to other friends and acquaintances in an open and somewhat intimate way.

When death comes about with little or no warning, there isn't time to grieve in small doses or get used to the loss. Such a sudden dying trajectory leads to an unsettling *acute grief syndrome*. Symptoms of acute grief may affect a person's physical well-being, thought processes, emotional stature, or behaviors. Some of these manifestations include the following:

- Bodily disturbances such as tightness in the throat, weakness, sighing, and dryness in the mouth
- Distorted image of or preoccupation with the deceased
- Confusion and disorganization
- Guilt
- Hostile reactions or anger
- Social withdrawal and lack of interest in other people and activities
- Depression
- Loss of appetite
- Sleep disturbances
- Aimlessness or a restless searching for nothing in particular

The typical grief pattern is first to experience some sort of shock (in which case a doctor's attention may occasionally be required), then to go through general despair and depression, and finally to recover and to reestablish normal thinking and activities. From a therapeutic standpoint, the first twenty-four hours is a period of *resuscitation* from the initial shock, when most social support is needed. The next six months is seen as a time for *rehabilitation* in order to overcome some of the sleeplessness, disorganization, depression, guilt, anger, and other negative emotions. Finally, after six months comes a time for *renewal* and reestablishment of one's normal life-style.

As you can see, the grieving process is not an easy one. Reactions such as poor eating habits, irregular sleep patterns, a decrease in the social-support system, an increased dependency on alcohol, tobacco, tranquilizers, and other drugs, and other negative health-related behaviors can contribute to an increase in the morbidity and mortality rates of survivors. Widows and widowers are the most vulnerable, but parents, siblings, and children are also adversely affected. Widows are particularly at risk during the first six months of bereavement. Studies done by British psychiatrist C. M. Parkes and others found that there is a significant increase in heart disease among widowers during that first six-month period, supporting the old adage that you can, indeed, die of a "broken heart."

> **FAST FACTS**
>
> It has been found that people who don't grieve properly are more apt to become dependent on drugs (including alcohol), display antagonism toward others, and have shorter life spans.

> ■ **PROBLEM SITUATION** Your friend's brother has just died in a car accident, leading to a state of acute grief. How would you advise your friend about what to expect during the grieving process, and what could you do to help lessen the pain of bereavement?

POSITIVE BEHAVIORS

I. *Place a check mark in front of each behavior that you now practice.*

_____ 1. I do not mind facing personal questions related to my death and dying. (QUESTIONS)

_____ 2. I recognize that I have certain fears about death and dying, but they do not interfere with my quality of living. (FEARS)

_____ 3. I do not unnecessarily waste energy and resources trying to seek immortality. (IMMORTALITY)

_____ 4. Although I hope and expect to live a long, healthy, and happy life, I am ready to die at any time. (READY)

_____ 5. If someone I knew were dying of a terminal disease, I would feel comfortable in visiting that person and talking about dying if he or she wanted to. (TERMINAL)

_____ 6. I have thought about how I would like my body disposed of when I die and have communicated those wishes to a close friend or relative. (WHEN I DIE)

_____ 7. When I lose someone significant in my life, whether because of death or some other cause of separation, I usually recognize my emotions and allow them to be acted out in a natural way. (GRIEVING)

II. *For each behavior that you DO NOT ENGAGE IN, write the KEY WORD(S) located in the parentheses at the end of the statement in the column below. Then put a check mark in the appropriate column to indicate whether you are going to keep or change that behavior.*

Behaviors I Don't Engage In   KEEP/CHANGE

_____ _____/_____
_____ _____/_____
_____ _____/_____
_____ _____/_____
_____ _____/_____
_____ _____/_____
_____ _____/_____

III. *For each of the preceding behaviors that you choose to KEEP, write a statement indicating why you are choosing to keep that behavior.*

I choose to keep behavior _____ because:
                                       KEY WORD

For each of the preceding behaviors that you choose to CHANGE, write a statement indicating how you plan to implement that change.

I will change behavior _____ by:
                            KEY WORD

Now You Know

1. TRUE. Many people have had near-death experiences during which their respiration or heartbeat temporarily ceased, but the legal definition of death includes a flat brain wave (EEG), and no one with a flat EEG for more than five minutes has ever recovered consciousness.
2. TRUE. Our attitudes about the phenomenon of death are shaped as we react to our first, even temporary, separations.
3. TRUE. Anticipatory grief, which is the part of the grieving process that takes place before the actual moment of death, occurs when people have an extended terminal illness.
4. FALSE. A living will, though not a legally binding document, gives guidance to families and doctors in making medical decisions.
5. TRUE. Euthanasia is the broad term for the causing of a gentle or easy death to ease suffering. Active euthanasia is an overt action of mercy killing, but passive euthanasia is simply allowing nature to take its course and making no heroic efforts to keep a dying person alive.
6. FALSE. Actually, a hospice is a program that mainly helps dying people and their families in their homes, although many hospices do have facilities to provide inpatient supportive care.
7. FALSE. Keep funeral costs to a minimum by buying only goods and services that are needed. Embalming of the body, for example, is usually not required.
8. FALSE. Bereavement is the loss itself, grief is the emotional reaction to loss, and mourning is the expression of those emotions.
9. TRUE. When these and other adverse reactions to acute grieving are severe, professional counseling services are helpful.
10. FALSE. Although there are common stages involved in the dying process, not everyone experiences the same emotional reactions in the same sequences.

Summary

1. Everyone born will also die, making death an integral part of living.
2. Individuals who have had a near-death experience have almost universally reported that it was a positive yet indescribable experience.
3. All people have some fears related to dying. Sometimes these fears are so great that they interfere with optimal functioning.
4. Overcoming the fear of death and dying has beneficial consequences, such as bringing honesty, boldness, spontaneity, and meaning to one's life.
5. The dying process—beginning with the recognition that one has a terminal illness and ending in death—is called the dying trajectory. The length and expectancy of this trajectory, as well as the quality of life one has during this living-dying interval, varies.
6. Death with dignity means dying in familiar surroundings with loved ones on hand, free from pain but alert and without unnecessary, heroic measures taken to prolong life when little or no quality remains.
7. It is difficult to be a good consumer of funeral services because decisions must be made immediately and because the consumer is in an intensely emotional condition.
8. It is important for us to work through all of the phases of grieving for the loss of our loved ones in order to accept their death and adjust to a new environment without them.

Suggested Readings

Grollman, Earl. *Living When a Loved One Has Died*. Boston: Beacon Press, 1987.

Myers, Edward. *When Parents Die: A Guide for Adults*. New York: Viking Penguin, 1987.

Rando, Therese A. *Grieving: How to Go on Living When Someone You Love Dies*. New York: Lexington Books, 1988.

Ring, Kenneth. *Heading Toward Omega: In Search of the Meaning of the Near-Death Experience*. Fairfield, N.J.: Wm. Morrow and Co., 1985.

Rosenthal, Ted. *How Could I Not Be Among You?* New York: Persea Books Inc., 1987.

Veatch, Robert M. *Death, Dying, and the Biological Revolution*. New Haven, Conn.: Yale University Press, 1989.

Viorst, Judith. *Necessary Losses*. New York: Ballantine Books, 1986.

References

1. Becker, Ernest. *The Denial of Death*. New York: The Free Press, 1973.
2. "Don Robinson, Former PDK Editor, Dies in Santa Barbara." *News, Notes and Quotes* 25 (1980): 2.
3. Fowles, John. *The Aristos*. Boston: Little, Brown and Co., 1964.
4. Hardt, Dale V. "Investigation of the Improvement of Attitudes Toward Death." *Journal of School Health* 46 (1976): 269.
5. Kalish, Richard A. *Death, Grief, and Caring Relationships*. Monterey, Calif.: Brooks/Cole, 1985.
6. Kastenbaum, Robert. *Death, Society, and Human Experience*. St. Louis: C. V. Mosby Co., 1981.
7. Kastenbaum, Robert, and Ruth Aisenberg. *The Psychology of Death*. New York: Springer Publishing Co., 1976.
8. Kübler-Ross, Elisabeth. *On Death and Dying*. New York: Macmillan, 1969.
9. Moody, Raymond. *Life After Life*. New York: Bantam Books, 1975.
10. Moustakas, Clark E. *Loneliness and Love*. Englewood Cliffs, N.J.: Prentice-Hall, 1972.
11. Parkes, C. M., B. Benjamin, and R. G. Fitzgerald. "Broken Heart: A Statistical Study of Increased Mortality Among Widowers." *British Medical Journal* 1 (1969): 740.
12. Rodabough, Tillman. "Alternatives to the Stages Model of the Dying Process." *Death Education* 4 (1980): 1.

APPENDIX A

First Aid

We recommend that everyone complete both a course in first aid and a course in cardiopulmonary resuscitation. The written information that follows will serve as a guide but can not substitute for hands-on training.

Burns and Scalds

Minor Burns without Blisters (first-degree burns). Place burned extremity into cold water or cover burned part with a towel soaked in cold water until the pain stops (at least fifteen minutes).

Burns with Blisters (second-degree burns). Same as above. Do NOT break the blisters. Call your doctor for advice on how to cover the burn. ANY burn on the face, hands, feet, or genitals and any large burn should be seen by a physician.

Deep Burns (third-degree burns). Call 911 or an emergency ambulance. Do NOT apply cold water or any medication. Keep victim warm with a clean sheet and then a blanket until help arrives. Remove smoldering, wet, or chemically contaminated clothing. First, second and third degree burns are illustrated in Figure A–1.

Electrical Burns. Disconnect electrical power. Do NOT touch victim with bare hands. Pull victim away from power source with wood or a thick, dry cloth. ALL electrical burns need to be seen by a physician. Be prepared to do mouth-to-mouth resuscitation or CPR if necessary.

Convulsions

Protect the victim from injury. Move furniture and other objects away from the individual. Lay the victim on his or her side with the head lower than the hips. Put nothing in the mouth. Call 911 or an emergency ambulance.

Eye Injuries

Do NOT press on an injured eye. Do NOT apply medication. Any injured or painful eye should be seen by a physician. Consult a physician before removing a foreign body from the eye. Gently bandage the painful eye shut until you can get medical help. If a chemical is splashed in the eye, gently flush with water; continue this for at least fifteen minutes. If only one eye is affected by the chemical, be sure to hold the victim's head so that the chemical does not wash into the other eye (see Fig. A–2).

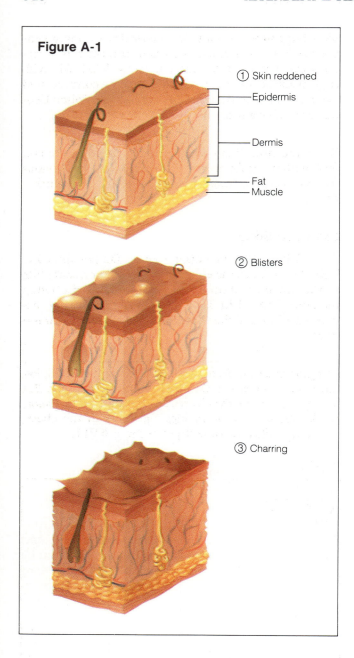

Figure A-1
① Skin reddened — Epidermis, Dermis, Fat, Muscle
② Blisters
③ Charring

Fainting

Keep the person in a flat position, raise the legs, and turn the head to the side. Do NOT give the person anything by mouth. Call your doctor.

Fractures

If an injured part is very painful, swollen, or deformed or if motion causes pain, suspect a fracture (see Fig. A–3). A fractured part should not be moved until it has been splinted. Call a physician or ambulance. Treat the victim for shock if necessary. Do NOT move a victim who may have a neck or back injury, as this may cause paralysis. Wait for help to arrive. Fractures are classified in Figure A–4.

Sprains

Apply a cold compress and elevate the injured arm or leg. If you suspect a fracture (see preceding section), call your doctor.

Head Injuries

Seek immediate medical assistance for any of the following:

- Unconsciousness or drowsiness
- Convulsions
- Inability to move any body part
- Oozing of blood or watery fluid from the ears or nose
- Severe or persistent headache
- Head injury in any child less than one year old

If there are no symptoms, you may let the victim sleep. However, awaken the victim every one to two hours and make sure that he or she can recognize you.

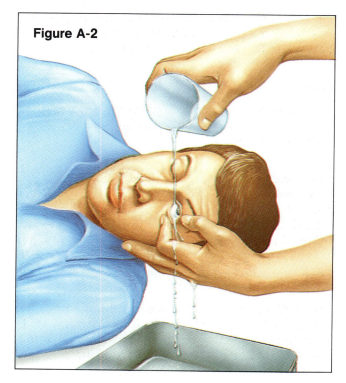

Figure A-2

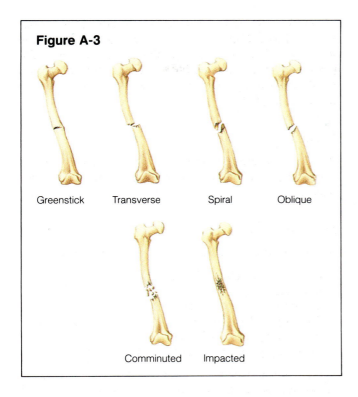

Figure A-3

Greenstick Transverse Spiral Oblique

Comminuted Impacted

Nosebleeds

With the victim sitting, squeeze the nostrils together between your thumb and index finger for at least five minutes. If bleeding persists, call a doctor.

Poisons

If a victim is unconscious, becoming drowsy, having convulsions, or having trouble breathing, call 911 or an emergency ambulance.

Swallowed Poisons. Any nonfood substance is a potential poison. Call the Poison Center (a phone number that you should have readily available) immediately. Do not induce vomiting except on professional advice. The Poison Center will give you instructions for use of syrup of ipecac (a bottle of this should be kept on hand at all times).

Fumes, Gases, or Smoke. Protect yourself first. Get the victim into fresh air. Call 911 or the fire department. If the victim is not breathing, start mouth-to-mouth resuscitation or CPR as appropriate, and continue until help arrives.

Skin Exposure. If acids, lye, pesticides, or any potentially poisonous substance comes in contact with a victim's skin, brush off dry material gently. Wash skin with large quantities of water and soap. Remove contaminated clothing. Wear rubber gloves if possible. Call Poison Center for further advice.

Eye Exposure. If any substance is splashed in the eye, flush with water for at least fifteen minutes (see previous section on eye injuries). Call the Poison Center for further advice.

Bites and Stings

Snake Bites. Call the Poison Center. Do not apply ice. Take the victim to the emergency room. For a snake bite on the arm or leg, if you cannot get medical advice within the hour, LOOSELY apply a WIDE band of cloth between the bite and the victim's heart. Do not make it too tight.

Stinging Insects. Remove the stinger with the scraping motion of a fingernail. Do NOT pull the stinger out. Put a cold compress on the bite to relieve pain. If hives, pallor, weakness, nausea, vomiting, tightness in the chest, breathing difficulty, or collapse occur, call 911.

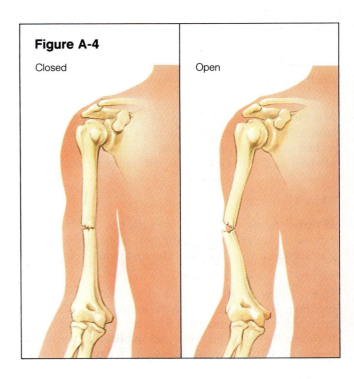

Figure A-4

Closed Open

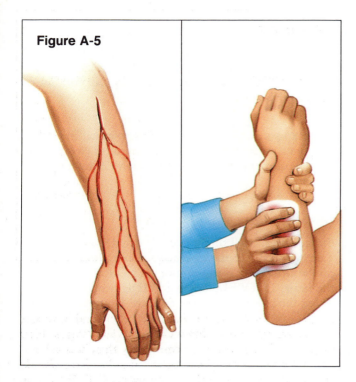

Figure A-5

Ticks. Place tweezers close to the head of the tick and pull the tick away from the point of attachment. Call your doctor if the head remains attached.

Animal Bites. Wash the wound thoroughly with soap and water. If the animal is a bat, racoon, skunk, fox, or unprovoked cat or dog, it may have rabies. Call your doctor.

Marine Animals. For sting ray, lionfish, catfish, and stonefish stings, submerge the sting area in warm water to inactivate the toxin. For other marine stings, flush the affected area with clean water and call your doctor.

Skin Wounds

Bruises. Apply cold compresses for one-half hour. For extensive bruises, crushing injuries, or bicycle-spoke injuries, consult your doctor or the emergency department.

Cuts. Apply pressure with a clean cloth to stop the bleeding. If the wound is on the arm or leg, elevate the extremity while maintaining pressure (see Figure A–5). If the cut is large and deep, call for help and maintain pressure until help arrives. If bleeding cannot be stopped using direct pressure, application of pressure at pressure points, as shown in Figure A–6, may be helpful. For minor cuts, wash with soap and water and cover with a dressing. Tourniquets should not be used without professional training. They are used only in life-threatening situations when the affected limb must be sacrificed to save the victim's life.

Scrapes. Wash the scrape with soap and water. Cover it with a nonstick dressing.

Splinters. Wash the area with soap and water. Remove small splinters with tweezers. If the splinter is not easily removed, call your doctor.

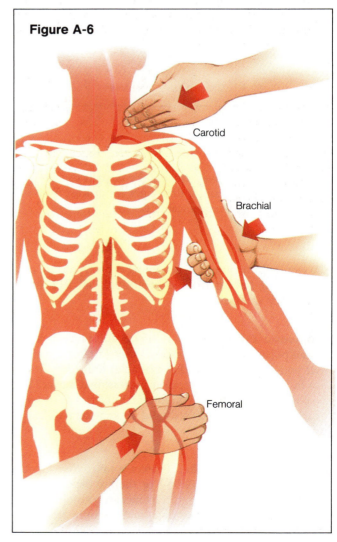

Figure A-6

Puncture Wounds. Do NOT remove large objects such as knives or sticks; call your doctor or 911. For minor puncture wounds, wash with soap and water and call your doctor. The victim may need a tetanus booster.

Shock

Many injured people will show signs and symptoms of shock. Sometimes even an uninjured person will suffer from shock after an accident or other mishap. Shock is a serious condition and may result in death, even if the victim's injuries are not severe.

The most significant symptom of shock is weakness. Victims may be nauseous and vomit. Their skin will be pale, cold, and clammy, and they may sweat profusely. The pulse is usually weak and rapid. Victims of shock should be kept lying down with their feet elevated (see Fig. A–7). Blankets should be used to help maintain normal body heat. Nothing, not even water, should be given to a victim by mouth.

Heat Exhaustion and Heat Stroke

The signs and symptoms of heat exhaustion are similar to those of shock. Rapid, shallow breathing may also occur. Victims of heat exhaustion should be moved to a cool location, such as the shade of a tree. Excess clothing should be removed. The victim should be lying down with feet elevated, as in the treatment of shock. Cooling of the body should be gradual.

In contrast, heat stroke victims have hot, flushed, dry skin (see Fig. A–8). The pupils are dilated, and body

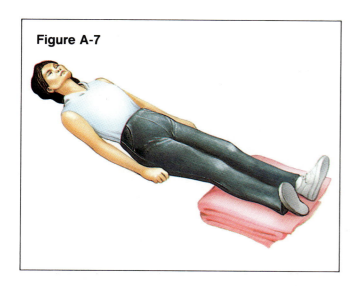

Figure A-7

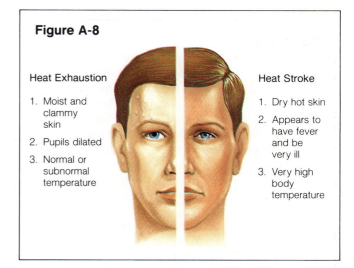

Figure A-8

Heat Exhaustion
1. Moist and clammy skin
2. Pupils dilated
3. Normal or subnormal temperature

Heat Stroke
1. Dry hot skin
2. Appears to have fever and be very ill
3. Very high body temperature

temperature is abnormally high. Breathing and heart rate may be strong initially but weak in the later stages. Heat stroke is a far more serious emergency than heat exhaustion. Clothing should be removed and the victim should be cooled with wet cloths or ice packs. Call 911 for an ambulance or transport the victim to an emergency room as soon as possible.

Heart Attack

The major symptom of a heart attack is pain originating in the center of the chest below the breastbone and radiating to the left arm, jaw, or back. Patients usually describe the pain with phrases such as "it felt like someone was sitting on my chest." Generally, the pain is continuous and is not relieved by changing position. Victims often have difficulty breathing, sweat profusely, and may complain of nausea.

Call 911 for an ambulance if you suspect a heart attack. While waiting, keep the victim calm. It is very important that you also remain calm. Allow the victim to find a comfortable position. Usually, he or she will find sitting to be the most comfortable. Be prepared to do mouth-to-mouth resuscitation or CPR if it becomes necessary.

Choking

Begin the following if the victim is choking and is unable to breathe. If the victim is coughing, crying, or speaking, DO NOT do any of the following, but call your doctor for further advice.

FOR INFANTS UNDER ONE YEAR OLD (A):

- Call for emergency services or 911.
- Place infant face down over your arm with head lower than the trunk. Rest your forearm on your thigh.
- Deliver four blows with the heel of the hand, striking high between the infant's shoulder blades.
- If blockage is not relieved, roll the infant over. Lay the child down, face up, on a firm surface. Give four rapid chest compressions over the breastbone using two fingers.
- If the above measures have not removed the blockage, open the mouth with thumb over tongue and fingers wrapped around lower jaw.
- If you can see the foreign body, remove it with a sideways sweep of a finger. (Never poke your finger straight into the throat.) Be careful, though, because finger sweeps may push the object further down the airway.
- If blockage is not relieved and the child cannot breathe, begin the technique of pulmonary support (D), outlined below in (D).
- Rapid transport to a medical facility is urgent if these emergency first aid measures fail.

FOR ADULTS AND CHILDREN OVER ONE YEAR OLD:

- Call for emergency services or 911.
- Place victim on his back. Kneel at the victim's feet. Put the heel of one hand on the victim's abdomen in the midline between the navel and rib cage. Place the second hand on top of the first. (B)
- The older, larger child or adult can be treated in a sitting, standing, or recumbent position. (C)
- Press firmly, but gently, into the abdomen with a rapid inward and upward thrust. Repeat six to ten times. These abdominal thrusts—called the Heimlich maneuver—should be applied until the foreign body is expelled.
- If the above measures have not removed the blockage, open mouth with thumb over tongue and fingers wrapped around lower jaw.
- If you can see the foreign body, remove it with a sideways sweep of a finger. (Never poke your finger straight into the throat.) Be careful, though, because finger sweeps may push the object further down the airway.
- If blockage is not relieved and the victim cannot breathe, begin the technique of pulmonary support as illustrated in (D) following.
- Rapid transport to a medical facility is urgent if these emergency first aid measures fail.

Cardiopulmonary Resuscitation (CPR)

To be used in situations such as drowning, electric shock and smoke inhalation or when breathing or heartbeat stops.

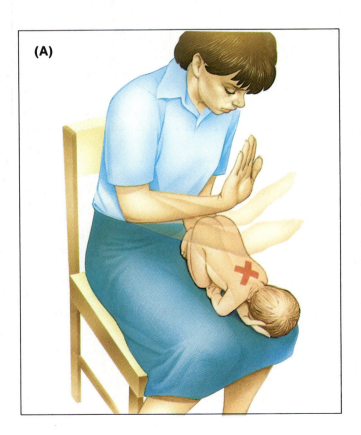

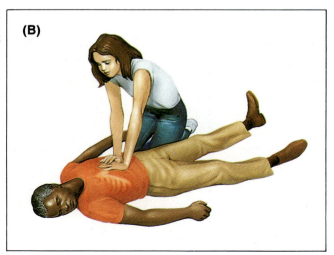

APPENDIX A ■ FIRST AID 553

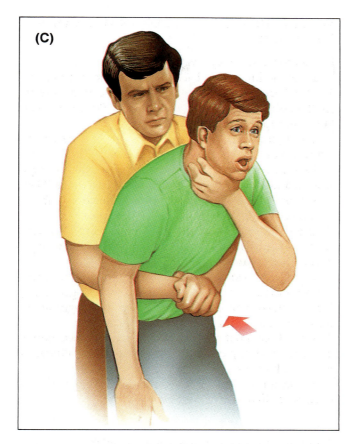

- Give slow steady breaths into infant's nose and mouth and into larger child's and adult's mouth with nostrils pinched closed.
- Breathe at 20 breaths per minute for infants and 15 breaths per minute for children and adults, using only enough air to move chest up and down

TECHNIQUE OF CARDIAC SUPPORT (E) (F):
Begin the following if the victim has no heartbeat:

- Place victim on firm surface.
- In the infant, using 2 fingers depress breastbone ½" to 1" at a level of one finger's breadth below nipples. (**E**) Compress at 100 times/minute.
- In the child and adult, depress lower ⅓ of breastbone with heel of hand at 80 compressions/minute. There should be five compressions to one respiration. (**F**)

(Some of the information in this appendix was prepared with permission of the American Academy of Pediatrics as adapted for adults.)

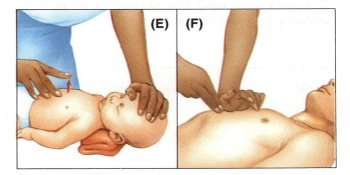

TECHNIQUE OF PULMONARY SUPPORT (D):
Begin the following if the victim is not breathing:

- Place victim on back.
- Straighten neck (unless neck injury is suspected) and lift jaw.

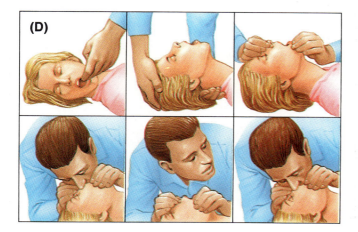

APPENDIX B

Classification of Mental Disorders and Illness

Simplified DSM-III-R Classifications of Mental Disorders

- Disorders usually first evident in infancy, childhood, or adolescence
  Developmental disorders (includes mental retardation, autism, and other learning disabilities)
  Disruptive behavior disorders
  Anxiety disorders of childhood or adolescence
  Eating disorders
  Gender identity disorders
  Tic disorders
  Elimination disorders
  Speech disorders
- Organic mental disorders
  Dementias
  Psychoactive substance-induced disorders
- Psychoactive substance-use disorders
- Schizophrenia
- Delusional (paranoid) disorder (such as unwarranted feelings of persecution, jealousy, or grandiosity)
- Psychotic disorders not elsewhere classified
- Mood disorders
- Anxiety disorders (excessive fears or phobias and avoidance behaviors)
- Somatoform disorders (physical symptoms with no organic basis)
- Dissociative disorders (upset of identity, memory, and consciousness)
- Sexual disorders
  Sexual dysfunctions
  Paraphilias
- Sleep disorders
- Factitious disorders (intentionally feigned physical or psychological symptoms)
- Impulse-control disorders not elsewhere classified
- Adjustment disorder (maladaptive reaction to stress)
- Psychological factors affecting physical condition
- Personality disorders
- Conditions not attributable to a mental disorder (includes such things as academic problems, antisocial behavior, malingering, marital problems, occupational problems, and other interpersonal and family problems)

Discussion

Although mental disorders are classified, it is not assumed that each is a clearly discrete entity with sharp boundaries or that everyone diagnosed as having a particular mental disorder displays all of the same characteristics. Caution should be used not to view people as if they were inanimate objects or as if their conditions were unchangeable. Just because someone has a particular mental disorder doesn't mean that the person *is* the disorder. It should be remembered that he or she is a human being who happens to have a particular mental problem. One final warning—do not attach labels to yourself just because you may occasionally exhibit some characteristics of a mental disorder.

The American Psychiatric Association has devised an extensive system of classifying mental disorders, which is published in the *Diagnostic and Statistical Manual,* third edition, revised, or DSM-III-R. This classification is summarized in the preceding outline. Rather than explain all of these categories here, only the major types of emotional and behavioral disorders will be discussed.

Actually, the most common and usually least severe type of mental disorder, which most of us have experienced to one degree or another, has been omitted from the DSM-III-R. That is *neurosis,* the inability to cope effectively with anxiety, which in turn causes conflict and distress within the individual. People with neurotic disorders experience symptoms that are upsetting, and they recognize them as being unacceptable, necessitating change. There are no grossly deviant behaviors, however, and perception of reality is intact. Still, the condition will usually endure unless attention is paid to changing it, either through a self-help plan of action or with the aid of a counselor, psychologist, or psychiatrist.

Psychosis is a more serious disorder that interferes with a person's ability to function fully and normally. Someone with a psychosis may be extremely disoriented and disorganized in his or her thoughts and feelings, and therefore may be unable to behave realistically much of the time. A psychosis may be of organic origin or it can be triggered by a chemically toxic substance, such as alcohol. It may also be functional (in other words, although the person's behavior is abnormal, the brain appears to be physiologically normal).

Most *schizophrenia,* a psychosis in which there is a split with reality, is functional, although recent research has implicated chemical changes in the brain. Schizophrenia may be acute, appearing rapidly and perhaps brought on by a traumatic experience, or it may take years to develop. Although schizophrenia may occur in successive generations in a family, the disorder itself does not appear to be inherited.

When an individual has difficulty relating appropriately and fully to others in a social situation, the whole array of behavior patterns is called a *personality disorder*. Such a disorder usually represents a long-standing behavioral style. The individual's behavior is usually not overly out of touch with reality nor does it cause the person great direct internal discomfort, but it does interfere with that person's ability to function effectively in social and vocational aspects of living. Because people with severe personality disorders "march to a different drummer," they often have social and legal troubles.

People with *mood disorders* (also called affective disorders) are affected by mood swings that are out of their conscious control. An example is manic-depression, in which feelings of unhappiness and elation are so extreme that they become unrealistic and debilitating. It is said that manic-depression is like riding a roller coaster of extremely high peaks and low valleys. During the lowest states, depression becomes severe and life threatening, sometimes triggering attempted suicide. In such instances, the individual experiencing the depression unrealistically believes it to be never ending. Self esteem is extremely low, and it is often hard for the individual to reestablish his or her true self-worth.

Glossary

abortion: spontaneous or medical termination of pregnancy before the fetus can survive outside the uterus.
accident prone: the tendency or likelihood of being involved in more accidents than is usual.
acidosis: a rise in the level of uric acid in the blood.
action therapy: the psychotherapeutic techniques aimed directly at alleviating psychological distress.
active euthanasia: a compassionate, overt act that leads directly to the death of someone in order to alleviate pain. Sometimes called *mercy killing*.
actual failure rate: the rate of failures of a contraceptive method that are due to both failure of the method and failure of people to use it correctly.
adenocarcinoma: a malignancy arising from mucous glands in epithelial tissue.
adipose tissue: connective tissue containing fat cells.
adrenal glands: two endocrine glands, one of which is located above each kidney.
adulterated: the addition of impure substances to a pure substance, thereby reducing its strength and effectiveness.
aflatoxin: a poisonous substance that may be present in peanuts and peanut products contaminated with Aspergillus molds.
afterbirth: the expulsion of the placenta and the rest of the umbilical cord shortly after the birth of a baby.
ageism: a form of discrimination on the basis of age.
aging: a physiologic process that continues from birth to death.
alienation: a feeling of hostility or separation from another person or group.
alkaloid: the chemical form in which certain drugs occur in plants.
Alzheimer's disease: a neurologic disease that causes the degeneration of certain brain cells.
amino acids: the chief structural material of protein.
amnioscentesis: a procedure for examining amniotic fluid and used to detect certain genetic diseases.
amniotic sac: a fluid-filled membrane which surrounds and protects the fetus.
amphetamine: a chemical substance which stimulates the central nervous system.
analgesic: a drug that relieves pain.
androsperm: sperm carrying a Y chromosome.

anesthetic: substance that leads to the loss of sensation.
angina pectoris: chest pains associated with inadequate supply of oxygen to heart muscle tissue.
anorexia nervosa: a severe self-imposed limitation of food intake.
antibiotic: drugs used to treat infection by either preventing the growth of infectious organisims or by destroying them.
antibodies: substances produced by the body in response to the presence of foreign substances (antigens).
anticipatory crisis: a reaction to what one perceives as a crisis situation before the crisis actually occurs.
antigen: substance that stimulates the body to produce antibodies.
antihistamine: an agent that dries up excessive secretions in the body.
anti-inflammatory: an agent that counteracts inflammation.
antitoxin: a naturally produced substance capable of counteracting a biological toxin.
aphrodisiac: a drug or chemical that causes an increase in sexual desire.
arthropod vector: an organism belonging to the phylum arthropoda such as fleas and ticks and capable of transmitting disease from one animal to another.
assigned gender: the state of being male or female.
asymptomatic: not having symptoms.
autoimmunity: destruction of the body by its own protective immune system.
autonomic nervous system: the portion of the nervous system which involuntarily controls internal tissues essential for normal functioning.

B-lymphocyte: a type of white blood cell.
basal metabolic rate: refers to the number of calories required to maintain all the cellular activities that are necessary to sustain life.
benzocaine: a local anesthetic used topically.
bereavement: the loss of a loved one.
binging: unrestrained indulgence.
bioaccumulate: when certain chemicals and radioactive materials concentrate in particular parts of the body and

are stored there for long periods of time, such as the pesticide DDT in fat tissues and strontium 90 in bone.
bioavailability: refers to how available a drug is to the body for its intended purpose once it is taken.
biodegrade: to decay naturally in the environment.
biological age: age that is based on the physical changes that occur as a person becomes older.
biological death: the permanent cessation of the functioning of body organs.
biopsy: surgical removal of a sample of tissue which can then be examined for malignant cells.
birth control: a technique, drug, or device used to prevent conception, implantation, or birth.
bisexuality: being sexually attracted to members of both sexes.
blastocyst: a hollow spherical mass of cells produced soon after conception by the cleavage of the fertilized egg.
bloody show: a bloody vaginal discharge that appears prior to labor.
body composition: the component parts of the body.
body fat: consists of both essential fat and storage fat present in the human body.
brand name: the manufacturer's name for a given drug product.
bran: the outer coat of the grain which is an excellent source of fiber.
buffered aspirin: aspirin to which a substance has been added to offset its acidic effects.
bulimia: an eating disorder characterized by compulsive binging and purging.
bulk producers: indigestible, noncaloric substances that absorb water during digestion and supposedly trick the brain into thinking that the stomach is full.

caesarean section: the surgical delivery of a baby through an incision in the abdominal wall.
calorie: a unit in which energy is measured.
carbohydrates: a group of chemical substances that contain carbon, hydrogen and oxygen and are the most important energy sources available.
carcinogens: substances or agents that induce or incite cancer.
cardiovascular disease: any disease associated with the heart or blood vessels.
cataracts: an eye condition characterized by a white cloudiness that covers the eye's lens, causing objects to appear blurred.
celibacy: choosing not to share sexual activity with others.

cervical cap: a thimble-shaped device that fits tightly over the cervix to prevent sperm from entering into the uterus.
cervix: the lower end of the uterus that extends into the vagina.
chancre: the lesion associated with primary syphilis.
chlorofluorocarbons: chemicals that are made up of carbon, fluorine and chlorine.
cholesterol: the chief sterol in the body found in all tissues, especially the brain, nerves, adrenal cortex, and liver.
chromosomes: the strands of nucleic acids in the nucleus of each cell which contain the genetic material.
circumcision: the surgical removal of the foreskin that covers the glans of the penis.
climacteric: that period that marks the lessening of sexual activity in the male.
clinical death: the permanent cessation of vital body functions including respiration, circulation, and nervous system activity.
clinical psychologist: human behavior specialists who help patients cope with problems of living.
clitoris: highly sensitive erectile tissue located just below the point where the labia minora converge at the top of the vulva.
cloning: making an exact genetic replica of a living being.
clue cells: epithelial (skin) cells covered with the bacteria indicative of bacterial vaginosis.
cognitive ability: the perception, understanding and utilization of information and knowledge.
coinsurance: a cost-sharing stipulation found in many insurance policies stating that medical expenses are proportionately divided between the insurance company and the individual.
coitus interruptus: removal of the penis from the vagina before ejaculation occurs.
collagen: a cushiony protein that gives fullness to the body.
collective unconscious: deep unconscious thought, shared by all, which cannot be brought to a conscious level of awareness.
combined oral contraceptive: a pill containing both estrogen and progestin taken by a woman to prevent pregnancy.
complementary protein combination: the process of combining incomplete proteins to form a complete protein.
complete proteins: foods that contain sufficient amounts of all the essential amino acids.
complex carbohydrates: a term used to describe foods high in starch.

condom: a sheath that is placed over an erect penis for prevention of pregnancy and protection from certain sexually transmitted diseases.
congeners: by-products of the fermentation and manufacture of alcoholic beverages.
contraception: a technique, drug, or device used to prevent conception.
contraindicated: specific circumstances under which a normal course of treatment would not be appropriate.
controlled substances: those drugs that, because of their potential for abuse, require legal control.
copayment: a cost-sharing stipulation found in many insurance policies stating the amount of money that the insured individual will pay toward each medical charge before the insurance company assumes the remaining charges.
Cowper's glands: two pea-sized glands located on each side of the urethra just beneath the prostate gland.
cremate: to burn a dead body until only ashes and unburnable bone fragments are left.
crisis: a time of acute danger often necessitating outside assistance.
cross tolerance: tolerance to one substance that also causes tolerance to other similar substances.
cruciferous: vegetables of the mustard family such as cabbage, cauliflower, broccoli, Brussel sprouts, and kohlrabi.
cryogenics: the practice of freezing a body for the purpose of bringing it back to life in the future.
cyst: a benign growth containing either solid or liquid material and surrounded by a wall or membrane.
cytoplasm: cell material outside the nucleus.

decongestant: an agent that reduces congestion.
deductible: a cost-sharing stipulation found in many insurance policies stating a fixed sum of money that the insured individual must pay each year before the insurance coverage becomes effective.
dehydration: a condition resulting from excessive loss of body fluid.
dementia: a condition of deteriorating mental functions.
deoxyribonucleic acid (DNA): the carrier of genetic information present in chromosomes of the nuclei of cells.
dermatitis: inflammation of the skin.
diaphragm: a dome-shaped rubber or latex device inserted inside the vagina and placed over the cervix to prevent sperm from entering into the uterus.
diethylstilbestrol (DES): a highly potent estrogen.

dilation and curettage (D&C): dilation of the cervix followed by scraping of the uterine lining.
dilation and evacuation (D&E): an abortion method generally used in the second trimester, where an instrument is used to break and then extract the contents of the uterus.
disability benefits: a type of insurance coverage that offers protection from loss of income resulting from illness or accident.
disaccharides: two simple sugar molecules linked together.
disequilibrium: a state of unbalance between body systems.
distress: damaging effects on the body caused by various stressors.
diuretic: an agent which increases the secretion of urine.
douche: cleansing of the vagina.
dying trajectory: the pattern that people follow in moving through the dying process.
dysplasia: the abnormal development of body tissue.

ectomorph: an individual with a long and slender body frame and has a lesser capacity for storing fat.
ectopic pregnancy: implantation of a fertilized ovum (egg) in a place other than the uterus.
ejaculate: the milky white, alkaline fluid containing sperm.
ejaculatory ducts: two ducts that enter the prostate gland and lead to the urethra.
ejaculatory inevitability: the uncontrollable occurrence of ejaculation.
electolytes: particles that become electrically charged when in the body fluids.
electro-convulsive therapy: the use of electrical brain stimulation to treat severe mental disorders.
electron microscope: a device used to examine objects too small to be seen with an ordinary light microscope.
embryo: the term used for the unborn from the second to the eighth week of pregnancy.
emetic: an agent that induces vomiting.
encephalitis: inflammation of the brain.
endocrine glands: ductless glands that deliver their hormones directly into the bloodstream.
endometrium: the inner lining of the uterus.
endomorph: an individual with a short and broad body frame and has a greater capacity for storing fat.
endosperm: the soft inside portion of the grain which contains starch and proteins.
enrichment: the addition of vitamins and minerals, specifically thiamin, riboflavin, niacin, and iron, to processed

cereal and grain products to restore the amount lost in processing.
enzyme: a protein capable of inducing or speeding up various chemical changes in the body.
epidemiologist: a person who studies the relationships leading to the spread of disease.
epidemiology: the study of the incidence, distribution, and control of disease in a community.
epidermis: the skin's outer layer.
epididymis: a tightly coiled tube located at the top of each testis.
episiotomy: an incision made from the bottom of the entrance to the vagina down toward the anus to prevent anal and vaginal tissues from being injured during childbirth.
erotic love: an intense form of love usually characterized by a strong desire for physical, emotional, and sexual intimacy with another person.
essential amino acids: amino acids that cannot be produced by the body and must be obtained from food.
essential fat: fat in the body that is necessary in the structure of various cells and also for protection of some internal organs.
estrogen: a general name for feminizing sex hormones.
euphoria: a feeling of well-being.
eustress: a condition whereby stressors encountered increase the level of human wellness.
expected date of confinement: the predicted date of birth.
expectorant: an agent that loosens and facilitates the removal of mucous from the respiratory tract.

fallopian tube: the tube that transports the egg from the ovary to the uterus.
fasting: voluntary starvation.
fat: a group of compounds that include both fats and oils.
fat-soluble vitamins: vitamins that can be stored in body fat until needed.
fermentation: a chemical process involving the action of enzymes from a yeast or mold and resulting in the breakdown of a complex substance into simpler substances.
fertility awareness techniques: any of several timing techniques that can identify a woman's fertile days.
fertilization: the union of sperm and egg.
fetus: the term used for the unborn from the ninth week of pregnancy to birth.
fiber: a general term which describes the indigestible portions of plant foods.
fibrocystic breasts: a condition in which fibrocysts, a certain type of benign tumor, develop in the breasts.
fimbriae: the long, finger-like projections attached to each fallopian tube at the ovarian end.
follicle: the tissue capsule in the ovary that contains an egg.
follicle-stimulating hormone (FSH): a hormone secreted by the pituitary gland that stimulates the production of sperm in males and follicle and ovum development in females.
follicular phase: that phase in the menstrual cycle when several follicles ripen and mature within an ovary.
fomite: inanimate objects that transmit disease.
force field analysis: understanding a situation by analyzing enabling and restricting factors.
foreskin: a loosely fitting fold of skin covering the glans of the penis. Also referred to as the prepuce.
fructose: a monosaccharide known also as fruit sugar.

galactose: a monosaccharide.
ganglion: groups of nerve tissue located outside the central nervous system.
gangrene: death of normal tissue.
gender: the state of being male or female.
gender identity: the feeling that one is a male or a female.
gender role: the traits and behaviors expected of males versus females in a given culture.
gender role identification: the way in which a person incorporates into his/her personality the behaviors expected of males and females in his/her culture.
generic name: the common name for a given drug product.
genetic gender: the presence of either an XX or XY chromosome configuration.
genital gender: the presence of either female external genitalia or male external genitalia.
germ: the nutrient-rich part of the grain responsible for reproduction.
gerontologists: individuals who study aging and the aged.
glans: the enlarged head of the penis.
glaucoma: an eye disease related to an increase in pressure within the eye.
globulins: protein substances derived from blood serum and containing antibodies against disease.
glucose: a monosaccharide, often called blood sugar, because it is the principal carbohydrate found in mammalian blood.
gonadal gender: the presence of either ovaries or testes.
gonadotropins: hormones that affect only the testes and ovaries.
gonads: a general name for the sex organs.

Grafenberg spot: a theoretical area located on the upper front wall of the vagina that, in some women, is highly sensitive to erotic stimulation.
grief: the emotional pain accompanying the loss of a loved one.
gynecologist: a physician who specializes in diseases of the female reproductive tract.
gynosperm: sperm carrying an X chromosome.

health: a state of spiritual, social, mental and physical fitness which enables one to live life to the fullest.
hemoglobin: the iron-containing pigment of the red blood cells whose function is to carry oxygen from the lungs to the tissues.
hemophiliac: an individual with a blood disease in which the blood does not properly clot.
hemorrhoid: the result of dilation of certain veins in the area of the rectum.
heterosexuality: being sexually attracted to persons of the opposite sex.
holistic health: the synergistic functioning of the total self including the mental, physical, social and spiritual dimensions.
homeostasis: the ability to keep bodily processes in a state of equilibrium or balance.
homophobia: fear of homosexuals.
homosexuality: being sexually attracted to persons of the same sex.
hormonal gender: the presence of either high levels of estrogen or testosterone.
hormones: the internal secretions of the endocrine glands that are released directly into the blood stream.
hospice: a humanistic program of care for dying people and their families.
host: an organism on which another organism is a parasite.
human chorionic gonadotropin: a hormone produced by the placenta.
hymen: a connective membrane that partially covers the vaginal entrance of most women from birth until after first sexual intercourse.
hyperlipidemia: the presence of excess fat in the blood.
hypertension: high blood pressure, generally involving a systolic pressure of 140 or greater and/or a diastolic pressure of 90 or greater.
hypothalamus: the primary controlling mechanism, located in the brain, that triggers the production and secretion of sex hormones.
hysterectomy: surgical removal of the uterus through the vagina or abdominal wall.
hysterotomy: an infrequent procedure for late abortion where an abdominal incision is made and the fetus is removed from the uterus.

immune system: the body system which provides active protection from disease.
immunity: resistance to disease usually due to the presence of antibodies from a previous exposure or vaccination.
immunization: the administration of a vaccine, usually by injection, to generate immunity against a specific disease.
implantation: the attachment of the blastocyst to the lining of the uterus.
incomplete proteins: foods that are deficient in one or more of the essential amino acids.
insight therapy: the psychotherapeutic techniques whereby the therapist and patient come to an understanding of why the patient feels and behaves the way he or she does.
insoluble fiber: fiber which speeds up the movement of food through the intestines and promotes regularity.
interment: putting a dead body in the ground or in a tomb.
interpersonal: the relationship that exists between two individuals.
intima: the inner lining of an artery or vein.
intraamniotic injection: an abortion method generally used in the second trimester, where amniotic fluid is replaced with either saline solution or prostaglandins.
intrapersonal: that which exists within an individual.
intrauterine device: small plastic device inserted into the uterus in order to prevent pregnancy.
intravenous: administration of a drug or fluid through a vein.

jaundice: yellowing of the skin and mucous membranes due to an accumulation of bile pigment resulting from excess bilirubin in the blood.

K-Y jelly: a water soluble lubricant that can be used on a condom.
ketosis: the accumulation of ketone acids in the body resulting from the incomplete metabolism of fatty acids.
kilocalorie: a unit of measure of the amount of heat a food substance will release when completely burned.

labia majora: two large folds of skin that enclose and protect the female external genitalia.
labia minora: thin, hairless folds of skin lying within the labia majora.

labor: the process of childbirth.
lactating: producing milk.
lacto-ovo-vegetarian: a vegetarian who excludes animal flesh from the diet, but eats such animal products as milk and eggs.
lanugo: fine downy hair covering the body.
laparoscope: a long, hollow instrument that permits viewing the inside of the abdominal cavity.
laparoscopy: a form of female sterilization where the fallopian tubes are cut and then the ends are either tied or cauterized.
lean body mass: consists of those tissues other than body fat, such as muscle, heart, liver, kidneys, and other organs.
legal death: the condition when a body has no responsivity, no respiration, no reflexes, and no measurable brain waves.
legumes: edible seeds, such as dried peas and beans.
length of life (longevity): the average number of years lived, usually limited to persons in a particular group.
lesion: any type of wound, injury, or change in tissue.
lethargy: a condition in which a person may be sluggish or exceedingly tired.
leukemia: cancer of the blood forming tissues.
life expectancy: the average remaining years for people at any specific age.
life span: the greatest number of years that a human being can live.
limerence: love that is marked by obsession and preoccupation with the loved one.
linoleic acid: the most common dietary polyunsaturated fatty acid.
lipid: a fat-like substance.
lipoprotein: a molecule consisting of protein and fat responsible for transporting fat from place to place in the body.
living-dying interval: the time span from when a person is aware that he or she is dying until the death actually occurs.
living will: a signed statement declaring the circumstances under which someone wishes life-sustaining medical procedures to be withheld.
longevity: see length of life.
luteal phase: that phase in the menstrual cycle when the empty follicle, called the corpus luteum, secretes high levels of progesterone in preparation for the implantation of a fertilized egg.
luteinizing hormone (LH): a hormone secreted by the pituitary gland that stimulates the production of testosterone in males and ovulation in females.
lymphoma: cancer in the lymph system.
lymph nodes: a capsule of lymphatic tissue found at various points in the lymph system.
lymph system: a system of vessels in which flows a usually clear, colorless fluid.

macrominerals: minerals needed in amounts greater than 100 milligrams a day.
major medical: a type of insurance coverage designed to supplement basic health benefits by providing protection against the high costs of prolonged illnesses or serious accidents.
mammogram: an x-ray picture of the breast used to detect cancer.
mantra: an object of focus used to facilitate a meditative response.
meatus: the opening into the penis.
melanin: the dark pigment found in the skin and hair roots.
melanocytes: the cells that manufacture melanin.
menarche: the first occurrence of menstruation.
menopause: the natural cessation of menstruation.
menstrual extraction: removal of menstrual blood and tissue from the uterus.
menstrual synchrony: a phenomenon in which the menstrual cycles of females living or working together begin to occur at the same time.
menstruation: that phase in the menstrual cycle when the uterine lining degenerates and blood, mucus, and dead cells are discharged.
mesomorph: an individual with a muscular body frame and tends to be less likely to have a weight problem.
metastasize: the movement of malignant cells from the original site of a tumor to sites often far removed in the body.
minerals: inorganic compounds that serve the body in a structural, functional or regulatory capacity.
mole: an area on the surface of the skin usually darker in color than surrounding tissue.
monocyte: a large white blood cell having a single nucleus.
monosaccharides: a unit of simple sugar.
monounsaturated fat: a fatty acid that lacks two hydrogen atoms and has one double bond between carbons.
mons veneris: the area over the female's pubic bone consisting of fatty tissue covered by skin and pubic hair.
mood disorder: having extreme and/or unrealistic feelings of sadness and elation.
morning-after-pill: a highly potent estrogen given to a woman within seventy two hours of unprotected intercourse in order to prevent pregnancy.
mourning: the expression of grief following the loss of a loved one.

mutation: any type of permanent change in characteristics from one generation to the next.
myocardial infarction: damage to heart muscle resulting from obstruction of a coronary artery and subsequent lack of oxygen to the tissue.
myometrium: the middle layer of the uterus.

natural foods: refers to those foods that have undergone minimal processing and do not contain artificial ingredients.
neuroendocrine system: that portion of the nervous and glandular system which controls the secretion of hormones.
neurological: of or relating to the nerves or nervous system.
neurosis: the inability to adequately cope, causing psychological distress.
neurosurgery: treating neurological disorders with surgical techniques.
neurotransmitter: a chemical responsible for transmission of nerve impulses across synapses.
nonessential amino acids: amino acids that can be produced by the body and are not required in the diet.
nonoxynol-9: the active ingredient found in many spermicides.
normality: the range of usual or expected behavior.
nucleus: the central body of a cell.
nutrients: substances found in foods that meet the body's needs for energy, growth and good health.

obese: an excessive accumulation of body fat; usually reserved for those individuals who are 20–25 percent or greater above the recommended weight for their size.
oleic acid: the most common dietary monounsaturated fatty acid.
organic foods: foods grown without chemical fertilizers and pesticides.
osteoporosis: a bone condition characterized by decreased bone mass and an increased susceptibility to fractures.
ovaries: the female sex organs.
ova: the female reproductive cells.
over-the-counter drug (OTC): a drug that can be purchased without a prescription.
overweight: implies a quantity of heaviness; an individual's body weight is greater than that which is recommended for one's size.
ovulation: the release of a mature egg from the ovary into the fallopian tube.
ozone: a form of oxygen in the atmosphere.

pap smear: a test used to detect cancer of the uterine cervix.
paranoia: a psychological or mental disorder characterized by a feeling of persecution.
parasympathetic nervous system: that part of the autonomic nervous system which inhibits body functions such as heartbeat and breathing.
Parkinson's disease: chronic nervous disease characterized by muscular weakness, fine tremors, and a shuffling gait.
passive euthanasia: an act of omission of lifesaving procedures that enables a person to die.
pathogen: a disease causing microorganism.
pathology: the study of organic disease.
pelvic inflammatory disease: swelling and inflammation of the uterus, fallopian tubes, and sometimes the ovaries due to infection by various microorganisms.
penis: the male organ through which both urine and semen pass.
perimetrium: the outer layer of the uterus.
peripheral resistance: the pressure exerted in the arteries during diastole and responsible for diastolic pressure.
peristalsis: involuntary, wavelike movements of the intestines and other specific organs that aid the movement of material through the gastrointestinal tract.
personality disorder: the inability to relate fully and appropriately to others.
personal unconscious: information stored at the unconscious level of thought which can be brought to a conscious level of awareness.
pharmacology: the study of the effects of drugs on animals.
phenylpropanolamine: a nasal decongestant and the active ingredient found in many over-the-counter diet pills.
pheromones: chemical substances externally secreted through the skin and other body openings.
physiological dependence: the mental and physical state of being dependent on a substance that usually results in withdrawal symptoms upon discontinuation.
pituitary gland: an endocrine gland attached to the base of the brain that is responsible for secreting a number of hormones that regulate bodily processes.
placenta: an organ that attaches to the uterine wall and exchanges nutrients and waste products between the mother and the fetus.
platelets: particles found in the blood of certain animals which adhere to each other and play an important role in the clotting of blood.
polyp: a benign growth often found in the nose or rectum.
polysaccharides: long molecular chains of simple sugar units linked together.

polyunsaturated fat: a fatty acid that lacks four or more hydrogen atoms and has two or more double bonds between carbons.
preexisting condition clause: refusal by an insurance company to cover an individual for any illness or condition that exists, or had existed in the past, at the time the policy is purchased.
pregnancy: the condition of carrying a developing embryo in the uterus.
premenstrual syndrome (PMS): the intense feelings that some women experience prior to menstruation.
prenatally: before birth.
presbycusis: permanent hearing loss.
primary stressor: a stimulus which results directly in a stress response.
progesterone: a feminizing sex hormone.
progestin-only pill: a pill containing just progestin taken by a woman to prevent pregnancy.
prognosis: the possible or probable future outcome of a disease.
proof: a measure of the concentration of an alcoholic beverage.
prostaglandins: hormones that stimulate contraction of smooth muscle tissue, such as the uterus.
prostate gland: a gland found only in the male that surrounds the urethra and is located directly beneath the bladder.
prostatitis: inflammation of the prostate gland.
psychiatric social worker: a credentialled specialist who provides help to emotionally disturbed people and families.
psychiatrist: a medical doctor who specializes in treating emotional disorders.
psychological age: age that is based on how a person thinks and feels as he or she becomes older.
psychological death: the inability to recognize the outer world even though one's vital organs are functioning, such as when a person is in a comatose state.
psychological dependence: dependence resulting from the incorporation of a particular activity or substance into a person's lifestyle.
psychosexually: relating to mental or emotional attitudes about sexual activity.
psychosis: any major mental disorder leading to the inability to function normally.
psychotherapy: the treatment of emotional disorders by psychological techniques.
puberty: the period of accelerated growth and development culminating in a sexually mature person.
puffery: an advertising technique, frequently used to sell a product, in which the characteristics or value of a product is magnified or exaggerated.

purging: to rid the body of an unwanted substance.
purulent: containing pus.

quickening: the sensation of movement of the developing fetus by the mother usually from around the end of the fourth month of pregnancy.

receptor site: a location where a particular drug or chemical attaches to produce its specific effect.
refractory period: a period of time when an individual is unresponsive to specific stimuli.
reinforcement: any reward or punishment applied to an individual which tends to strengthen or weaken a behavior.
relationship: a bonding between two or more people.
retinoblastoma: a cancer found in the eye and usually occurring in children.
retrovirus: a group of viruses that replicate in a way opposite to that of most other viruses.
reuptake: the reabsorption of a neurotransmitter back into the vesicles from which it was initially released.
ribonucleic acid (RNA): the nucleic acid that directs the formation of proteins within the body.

salutogenesis: the development of good health.
saturated fat: a fatty acid that has all its chemical bonds filled with hydrogen atoms.
schizophrenia: a mental disorder in which there is a split between reality and the way in which it is interpreted.
scrotum: a pouch of skin, located under the penis, that houses the testes.
secondary stressor: stress which is created as a result of the initial stress reaction.
self-concept: the perception people have of who they are.
semen: a grayish-white, alkaline fluid that is secreted at the time of male ejaculation.
seminal vesicles: the saclike glands located on each side of the male's bladder.
senility: physiological degeneration in the brain.
sense of coherence: having a sense of fitting into one's environment.
sexual preference: erotic attraction toward persons of the same gender, the opposite gender, or both genders.
sexual response: the series of changes that take place in the body as men and women become progressively more sexually aroused.
sex flush: patches of darker coloring on the skin associated with sexual arousal.
sigmoidoscope: an instrument used to examine the colon.

significant others: those individuals who someone is closest to emotionally.
simple carbohydrates: a term used to describe foods high in sugar.
social age: age that is based on how a person behaves as he or she becomes older.
social death: when a person is not recognized by others as existing.
social network: a set of relationships which exist among a group of people.
social support: any person or persons who provide assistance in meeting one's basic needs.
soluble fiber: fiber which appears to help lower blood cholesterol levels and help stabilize blood sugar levels.
spermatozoa: the male reproductive cells.
spermicides: chemicals that kill or immobilize sperm.
spirochete: a corkscrew shaped bacteria such as that causing syphilis.
spore: a reproductive cell formed by certain bacteria, fungi, and protozoa.
storage fat: fat that accumulates and is stored in the adipose tissue.
stress: the nonspecific response of the body to any demand made upon it.
sympathomimetic: a drug that mimics the effects of the sympathetic nervous system.
synergism: the combination of two or more drugs resulting in a multiplication of effect.
synesthesia: the sensation of having one sensory impulse being converted to another such as "hearing smells" or "feeling sounds".

T lymphocyte: a type of lymphocyte (white blood cell) that is passed through the thymus gland where it becomes able to provide cellular immunity.
teratogen: any substance or condition that can adversely affect a developing fetus.
testes or testicles: the male sex organs.
testosterone: the principal male sex hormone.
thanatologist: a person who specializes in the study of death and dying.
theoretical failure rate: the failure rate of a contraceptive method when it is used consistently and correctly.
tolerance: resistance to the effects of a drug due to repeated exposure to it.
toxic shock syndrome (TSS): a bacterial infection characterized by fever, vomiting, diarrhea, and rash and often associated with the use of super-absorbent tampons.
toxin: a poisonous substance.
toxoid: a toxin that has been treated so as to prevent it from causing illness yet still able to induce antibody production upon injection.
trace minerals: minerals needed in amounts less than 100 milligrams a day.
transpersonal: that which goes beyond the physical being of an individual.
transsexuality: the condition of believing that one is trapped in the body of the wrong sex.
triglycerides: a compound composed of carbon, hydrogen and oxygen arranged as a molecule of glycerol with three fatty acids attached to it.
tubal ligation: female sterilization involving cutting or tying of the fallopian tubes.
tubal pregnancy: an ectopic pregnancy in which the embryo is implanted in the fallopian tube.

ulceration: an open sore, usually on the skin or a mucous membrane.
ulcerative colitis: inflammation of the colon involving the formation of ulcerations.
umbilical cord: the cord that connects the fetus to the placenta.
umbilication: a depression or dimpling.
underweight: an individual's body weight is less than that which is recommended for one's size.
unitive experience: an experience which brings one to a state of feeling at one with the universe.
urethra: a tube that transports urine out of the body. In the male, its function is also to transport semen out of the body.
urethritis: inflammation of the urethra.
uterus: a hollow, pear-shaped organ located in the female reproductive tract.

vaccine: a preparation made from an infectious agent that, when introduced into an animal, stimulates the production of antibodies.
vacuum aspiration: the removal of the contents of the uterus through use of a suction machine.
vagina: a hollow, muscular organ located in the female reproductive tract.
vaginal sponge: a small sponge-like device, containing spermicide, inserted inside the vagina and placed over the cervix to prevent sperm from entering into the uterus.
vaginal suppository: a solid substance, containing a spermicide, that when inserted into the vagina dissolves and becomes a contraceptive foam or gel.
vaginitis: inflammation of the vagina.
varicose veins: distended, swollen, or twisted superficial veins.

vasectomy: male sterilization involving cutting or tying of the vas deferens.

vasocongestion: narrowing of the blood vessels resulting in the accumulation of blood.

vas deferens: two slender ducts through which sperm are transported.

vegan: a vegetarian who excludes all animal flesh and animal products from the diet, eating only plant foods.

vegetarian: one whose food is of vegetable or plant origin.

vesicle: any small sac containing fluid.

vestibule: the area located between the labia minora.

vitamins: organic compounds that are found in small amounts in most foods.

vulva: the collective name for the female external genitalia.

wart: a type of growth on the skin or mucous membrane caused by a virus.

wasting metabolism: the process that occurs when there is food deprivation and the body starts drawing on its stored food reserves.

water-soluble vitamins: vitamins that dissolve in water and cannot be stored in the body.

wellness: the optimal functioning of each individual at the present time.

withdrawal: the sudden stopping of a drug resulting in symptoms associated with the specific drug.

zygote: the single celled organism which results from the union of sperm and egg.

INDEX

A

A. H. Robins Co., 234
Ability, cognitive, 18
Abortion:
  defined, 246
  first-trimester methods of, 248
  pill for, 249
  postcoital methods of, 247–248
  procedures for, 246–249
Abscence (*petit mal*) seizure, 435
Absorption, of alcohol, 305–306
Acceptance:
  of dying, 535
  of others, mental wellness and, 32, 41
Accident prone, 495
Accidents, 494–499
  analyzing, 495–496
  epidemiology of, 496
  fires, 497–499
  motor-vehicle, 496–497
  nonmotor-vehicle, 497
Acetylcholine, 279
Acid:
  amino, 96
  barbituric, 328
  linoleic, 99
  oleic, 100
Acid rain, 480
Acidosis, 133
Acquired immunodeficiency syndrome (AIDS), 383–388
  diseases associated with, 385–386
  incidence of, 384
  origin of, 384
  prevention of, 386
  as public health issue, 383–384
  testing for, 387–388
  treatment of, 386
Action therapy, 50
Active euthanasia, 537
Active immunity, 360–361
Activities:
  choosing exercise, 159–169
  during pregnancy, 266
Activity levels of exercise, 153–155, 158
Actual failure rates, 226
Acute grief syndrome, 542
Acyclovir, 389
Adam. *See* MDMA

Addiction Research Center, 282
Adenocarcinoma, 417
Adipocytes, 122
Adipose tissue, 122
Adopt a Smoker program, 289, 291
Adrenal glands, 205
Adult Children of Alcoholics (A.C.A.), 323, 324
Adulterated drugs, 333
Advertising:
  deceptive, 445
  health and, 445–448
Aerobic exercise, 159–164
  defined, 159
  high-impact versus low-impact, 162–163
  high-impact, 160–162
  low-impact, 162
  setpoint level and, 130
  video exercise programs for, 163
  See also Exercise; Physical fitness
Aerobics (Cooper), 154
Affatoxin, 111
Afterbirth, 269–270
Age:
  biological, 506–507
  cancer and, 419
  cardiovascular disease and, 406
  psychological, 507
  social, 507
Ageism, 509–510
Aging, 506–524
  ageism and, 509–510
  Alzheimer's disease and, 518–520
  being old versus, 506–507
  bone changes and, 517–518
  caregiving and, 521–524
  defined, 506
  "error-induced," 508
  free-radical, 508
  hair changes and, 515
  hearing and, 516–517
  overcoming stereotypes of, 510–514
  physiological changes of, 514–518
  process of, 507
  sexuality and, 520–521
  smoking and, 288–290
  successful retirement and, 521
  theories of, 508–509
  vision changes and, 515–516
  wrinkles and, 514

Agriculture, Department of, 87, 491
AIDS. *See* Acquired immunodeficiency syndrome
Air, toxic chemicals in, 487–488
Airborne transmission of disease, 356
Al-Anon, 321, 323
Alarm reaction, 59
Alateen, 321, 323, 324
Alcohol, 303–326
  absorption of, 305–306
  amount of, in selected beverages, 305
  basic facts about, 303–305
  blood circulation and, 311
  breath readings and effects of, 307
  butyl, 304
  cancer and, 311
  deaths related to, 282
  dependence on, 309
  disease and, 311–312
  drinking age and, 312
  driving and, 312–316
  elimination of, 305–306
  ethyl (ethanol), 304
  guidelines for responsible use of, 319
  isopropyl, 304
  legislation concerning, 312–316
  methyl, 304
  nutrition and, 311
  pharmacology of, 305–311
  physiological effects of, 307–308
  propyl, 304
  psychological effects of, 311
  reasons for drinking, 318
  smoking and, 281
  synergism and, 309–311
  teenagers and, 318
  tolerance of, 308–309
  vitamin deficiency and, 311
Alcoholic hepatitis, 311
Alcoholics Anonymous (A.A.), 320, 322–324
Alcoholism, 318–324
  Alcoholics Anonymous (A.A.) and, 320, 322–324
  coping with another's, 321, 323
  gender and, 319–320
  self-inventory for, 320
  theories explaining, 319–320
Alienation, 45
Alkaloids, 331

Allergy preparations, 462–463
Alzheimer's disease, aging and, 518–520
Alzheimer's Disease and Related Disorders Association, 520
American Cancer Society, 111, 285, 290, 294, 416, 420, 421, 422, 426
   recommendations for cancer detection issued by, 416–417
American College of Sports Medicine (ACSM), 152, 153, 155
American College of Surgeons (A.C.S.), 453
American Council on Science and Health, 282
American Dietetic Association, 110
American Heart Association, 101, 134, 294
American Journal of Health Promotion, 36
American Lung Association, 290, 294, 295, 297, 491
American Medical Directory, The, 452
American Psychiatric Association, 138
American Society of Plastic and Reconstructive Surgeons, 135
American Way of Death, The (Mitford), 540
Amino acids:
   essential, 96
   nonessential, 96
Amniocentesis, 436
Amniotic sac, 266–267
Amotivational syndrome, 339–340
Amphetamines, 335, 340–341
   defined, 134
   dextroamphetamine, 335
   long-term use of, 335
   MDA, 341
   MDEA, 341
   MDMA, 340–341
   methamphetamine, 335
   overdose of, 335
   STP (DOM), 341
   TMA, 341
   tolerance of, 335
   weight reduction and, 134
Anaerobic exercise, 164–166
Analgesics, 331, 460–462
Analingus, 208
Analysis:
   force-field, 20
   transactional, 51
Anatomy, sexual, 198–205
Androgens, 260–261
Anemia, sickle-cell, 435–436
Anesthetic, cocaine as, 332–333
Angel dust. *See* PCP
Anger, 44
   during dying process, 534
Angina pectoris, 408
Ankylosing spondylitis (Marie Strumpel disease), 431
Anorexia nervosa, 138
Anti-inflammatory drug, 461

Antibiotics, 352
Antibodies, 358
Antidiabetic medications, alcohol and, 311
Antigen, 358
Antihistamine, 462
Antitoxins, 354
Antonovsky, Aaron, 70
Anxiety, 45
Aphrodisiac, 341
Arteries:
   hardening of. *See* Arteriosclerosis
   hypertension in, *illustrated*, 407
Arterioles, 403
Arteriosclerosis:
   angina pectoris and, 408
   congestive heart failure and, 408
   defined, 407
   myocardial infarction and, 408
   stroke (cerebrovascular accident) and, 409
   transient ischemic attack and, 408–409
Arthritis, 428–432
   ankylosing spondylitis, 431
   defined, 428
   gout, 431
   juvenile, 430
   osteoarthritis, 430–431
   quackery and, 432
   rheumatoid, 428–430
   systemic lupus erythematosus (SLE), 431–432
   warning signs of, 429
Arthritis Foundation, 430
Arthropod vectors, 354
Artificial sweeteners, setpoint level and, 131
Aspirin, 461
   alcohol combined with, 311
   buffered, 462
   deteriorated, 462
Assigned gender, 270
Asthma, 434
   age and, 434
Asymptomatic, 364
Atherosclerosis, 410–412
   early and late, *illustrated*, 410
Athletic training, 169–171
   carbohydrate loading and, 170
   concepts of, 169–170
   overload concept and, 169–170
   progression in, 170
   specificity of, 169
   steroids and, 170–171
   See also Exercise programs
Aura, 435
Autocroticism, 208
Autoimmune theory of aging, 509
Autoimmunity, 509
Autonomic nervous system (ANS), 278
   defined, 59
   parasympathetic, 278
   sympathetic, 278

Awareness:
   behavioral change and, 23
   spiritual, 36–40
Axon, of neuron, 279
Azidothymidine (AZT), 386
Aztecs, 337

B

Bacilli, 353
Bacteria, 353–354
   antibiotics and, 354
   bacilli, 353
   cocci, 353
   diseases caused by, 353
   spirilla (spirochetes), 353
Bacterial diseases, 367–369
   chancroid, 382
   chlamydia infection, 380
   gonorrhea, 379
   granuloma inguinale, 382
   lymphogranuloma venereum, 382–383
   nongonococcal urethritis (NGU), 380
   nonspecific urethritis (NSU), 380
   pelvic inflammatory disease, 380–381
   syphilis, 376–378
   tetanus, 368
   tuberculosis (TB), 368–369
   vaginosis, 381
   whooping cough (pertussis), 367–368
Bacterial toxins, 354
Baeyer, Adolph von, 328
Baller, Seth, exercise video by, 164
Ballistic stretching, 166
Banks, Rebecca, 36
Barbital, 330
Barbiturates, 328–330
   synergism and, 309, 329
Barbituric acid, 328
Bargaining, during dying process, 534–535
Bartholin's glands, 202
Basal body temperature (BBT):
   birth control and, 244–246
   new device for measuring, 250–251
Basal cell carcinoma, 421
Basal metabolic rate (BMR):
   caffeine and, 344
   defined, 90
   weight loss and, 123–124
Base-line mammogram, 424
Basic food groups, 86–87
Baulieu, Etienne, 249
Beall, Robert, 436
Behavior:
   eating. *See* Eating behavior
   exploitive, 181–182
   impulsive, sexually transmitted disease and, 374–375
   as learned trait, 18–19

normal, 33
personal perceptions of health and, 18–19
sexual, 207–208, 222–223
See also Health behavior
Behavioral change:
analyzing problem solutions and, 20–22
awareness and, 23
commitment and, 22
evaluation and, 23
problem solving and, 19–20
restructuring of environment and, 23
self-management and, 22–23
strategies for, 19–26
Behavioral-change contract, 23–26
illustrated, 23
outline for, 26
Behavioral psychology, 51
Belongingness needs, 17
Benign neoplasm, 416
versus malignant, 418
Benzedrine, 335
Benzocaine, 135
Benzodiazepines, 330
Bereavement, 541
Berne, Eric, 51
Beta carotene, 290
Better Business Bureau (BBB), 450
National Advertising Division (NAD) of, 451
Beverly Hills Diet, 134
Beverly Hills Diet, The (Mazel), 134
Bhopal, India, catastrophe, 475, 486
Biking, video exercise program for, 164
Bingeing, 139–140
Bioaccumulate, 475
Bioavailability, 467
Biodegrade, 494
Biological age, 506–507
Biological death, 530
Biology, health and wellness and, 11
Biopsy, 421
Birth control, 223–246
cervical cap, 241
coitus interruptus and, 243–244
condoms and, 234–236
contraception versus, 223
defined, 223
diaphragm and, 237–239
failure rates of methods used for, 226
fertility-awareness techniques of, 244–246
future trends in, 250–251
intrauterine devices (IUDs) and, 233–234
methods of, 223–246
oral contraceptives, 229–231
self-inventory of attitude toward, 224–225
sexually transmitted disease and, 374
smoking and, 406
tubal ligation and, 226–228
vaginal sponge and, 239–240

vasectomy and, 228–229
Birth, stages of, *illustrated*, 269
Bisexuality, 207
Blackmun, Harry A., 247
Blastocyst, 259
Blood alcohol concentration (BAC), 313
Blood alcohol content (BAC), 497
Blood alcohol level (BAL), 307, 313
Blood circulation:
alcohol and, 311
collateral, 150
exercise and, 149
illustrated, 404
Blood pressure:
diastolic, 403
exercise and, 149
high. *See* Hypertension
low, *See* Hypotension
measurement of, 403
normal, 403, 405
peripheral resistance and, 403
systolic, 403
Bloody show, 268
Blue Cross/Blue Shield, 456
Body, defense mechanisms of, 358–359
Body composition, 121–122
Body dynamics, 83–174
Body fat, 121–122
Body lice, 392
Body weight, 120–121
ideal, 120
Bones, aging and, 517–518
Brain hypothesis of aging, 509
Brain imaging, 49
Bran, 94
Brand identity, 446
Brand-name drugs, 464–465
Breast, fibrocystic disease of, 343
Breast cancer, 422–425
incidence of in U.S. compared to Japan, 420
treatment for, 424–425
Breast self examination (BSE), 423–424
illustrated, 424
Brody, Elaine, 524
Bronchodilators, 335, 344
Brown fat, 129–130
Buffered aspirin, 462
Bulimia, 139–141
Bulk producers, 135
Bureau of Census, U.S., 506
Burroughs Wellcome Co., 386
Butyl alcohol, 304

C

Caesarean section, 389
Caffeine, 342–344
basal metabolic rate and, 344

high doses of, 344
setpoint level and, 131
Caffeinism, 343–344
Calendar method of birth control, 244–246
Califano, Joseph A., 4
California Medical Association, 287
Calories:
awareness of, 90–91, 123–124
defined, 90
expenditure of, through exercise, 150, 151
food labels and, 126
Cambridge diet, 133
Camus, Albert, 37
Cancer, 416–428
age and, 419
alcohol and, 311
breast, 420, 422–425
carcinogenic substances and, 419
colorectal, 425
cures for, 420–421
deaths by, 416
detection of, 417, 418, 421
diet and, 95, 112–113, 419–420
endometrial, 427–428
general information about, 416
guidelines for reducing risk of, 420
heredity and, 418
incidence of, 416
leukemia, 428
lung, 285, 422
lymphoma, 428
ovarian, 428
prostate, 425
seven warning signals of, 418
sex and, 420
signs and symptoms of, 417, 421
skin, 421–422
smoking and, 285, 286
socioeconomic and geographic factors and, 420
terminology of, 416–418
testicular, 426
types of, 420–428
of uterine cervix, 426–427
Candida albicans (Monilia), 391–392
Cannabis americana, 338
Cannabis indica, 338
Cannabis sativa, 338
Capillaries, 403
Carbohydrate loading, 170
Carbohydrates, 91–95
complex, 91, 93, 131
defined, 91
diets low in, 133
fibers, 94–95
simple, 91, 92, 130–131
Carbon monoxide, 284–285
Carcinogenic, *defined*, 419
Carcinogenic substances (carcinogens), 285, 419

occupational, 479–480, 481
tars, 285
Carcinoma:
    basal cell, 421
    defined, 417
    squamous cell, 421
    See also Cancer
Cardiovascular disease, 403–412
    arteriosclerosis, 407–410
    atherosclerosis, 410
    defined, 403
    diet and, 95
    exercise and, 149
    guidelines for reducing, 408
    hypertension and, 403–407
    physiology of, 403
    self-inventory of risk for, 411
    smoking and, 286–287, 297, 406
    sodium intake and, 406
    stress and, 406
Cardiovascular fitness, 159–166
    aerobics and, 159–160
    anaerobic exercise and, 164–166
    determining target heart rate and, 161
    high-impact aerobics and, 160–162
    high-impact versus low-impact aerobics and, 162–163
    low-impact aerobics and, 162
Caring:
    for elderly parent, 521–524
    and social contact, 188
Carlyon, William, 12
Carotid pulse, how to take, *illustrated,* 161
Cataracts, 516
Caveat emptor, 444
Caveat venditor, 444
Celibacy, 207
Cell body of neuron, 279
Cells, fat-storing, 122
Centers for Disease Control, 281, 282, 368, 384, 390
Central nervous system (CNS), 278
Cerebrovascular accident (stroke), 409
Cervical cap, 241
Cervix, 204
    uterine, 426–427
Challenger, 486
Chancroid, 382
Change:
    behavioral, *See* Behavioral change
    stress and, 61, 62, 64–66
Chapman, Larry, 36
Chemical industry, hazardous waste and, 475
Chernobyl nuclear explosion, 486
Chewing tobacco, 296–297
Chicken pox (varicella):
    herpes zoster and, 362
    vaccine for, 362
Childbirth, 268–270
    labor and, 268–270

China White, 341
Chlamydia, 352, 380, 381
Chlorofluorocarbons (CFCs), 480
Cholesterol, 100–101
Chromosomes, 418
    defined, 258
    sex-determining, 258, 260
Chronic bronchitis, 434
Chronic diseases, 416–437
    arthritis, 428–432
    cancer, 416–428
    chronic obstructive pulmonary disease, 434–435
    cystic fibrosis, 436
    diabetes mellitus, 432–434
    epilepsy, 435
    genetic disorders, 435–437
    phenylketonuria (PKU), 437
    risk factors and, 400–402
    sickle-cell anemia, 435–436
    Tay-Sachs disease, 436–437
Chronic obstructive pulmonary disease (COPD), 434–435
    asthma, 434
    chronic bronchitis, 434
    emphysema, 434
Cigarettes, 282
    clove, 297
    constituents of smoke created by, 282
    substitutes for, 290
    U.S. per capita consumption of, 281
    See also Nicotine, Smoking: Tobacco
Cilia, as defense mechanism, 358
Circulation, blood. *See* Blood circulation
Circumcision, 199
Cirrhosis, 311
Class, social, health behavior and, 16
Clean Water Act, 475
Cleo Wrap, 492
Climacteric, 520–521
Clinical death, 530
Clinical psychologists, 51
Clitoris, 202
Cloning, 533
Clove cigarettes, 297
Clue cells, 381
Coca Cola, cocaine in, 332
Cocaine, 332–335
    adulterated, 333
    as anesthetic, 332–333
    "crack," 334
    deaths related to, 282
    drug-induced psychosis from, 333
    long-term use of, 333
    overdose of, 333
    "rock," 334
    users of, 332
    withdrawal from, 333
Cocaine hotline, 334
Cocci, 353
    diplococci, 353

staphylococci, 353
streptococci, 353
Codeine, 331
Coffee, decaffeinated versus caffeinated, 343
Cognitive ability, 18
Cognitive dissonance, 16
Cognitive therapy, 51
Coherence, sense of, 70
Coinsurance, 457–458
Coitus interruptus, 243–244
Cold, common, 365–366
Cold preparations, 462–463
Colitis, ulcerative, 425
Collagen, 514
Collective unconscious, 35
College students:
    stress and, 66
    Social Readjustment Rating Scale for, 64–65
Colorectal cancer, 425
Colostomy, 425
Columbus, Christopher, 376
Commitment, behavioral change and, 22
Common cold, 365–366
    preparations for, 462–463
Commoner, Barry, 492
Communicable diseases, 349–397
    acquired immunodeficiency syndrome (AIDS), 352
    antibiotics and, 352
    bacterial, 367–369, 376–383
    body's defense mechanisms and, 358–359
    guidelines for maintaining immunity to, 391
    guidelines for reducing exposure to, 360
    guidelines for recovery from, 366
    immunity to, 352, 359–362
    incubation period of common, 357
    influenza, 352
    organisms causing. *See* Pathogenic organisms
    prevention of, 358–361
    sexually transmitted. *See* Sexually transmitted diseases
    smallpox, 352
    stages of, 357–358
    transmission of, 356–357
    tuberculosis, 352
    viral, 361–367, 383–391
Communication, 41
    effective, 186–189
Community right-to-know programs, 490
Companionate love, 185
Companionship, social networks and, 77
Complaint, letter of, 450
Complementary protein combination, 97
Complete Book of Running, The (Fixx), 158
Complete fasting diet, 132–133
Complete proteins, 96–97
Complex carbohydrates, 93
    defined, 91

setpoint level and, 131
Comprehensive Drug Abuse Prevention and Control Act of 1970, 469
Condoms, 234–236
   application of, *illustrated*, 235
   for females, 250
Condra, Michael, 287
Confidence:
   self inventory of, 192–193
   and social contact, 188
Conflict, intrapersonal, 61
Congenital immunity, 362
Congestive heart failure (CHF), 408
Congressional Budget Office, 478
Connolly, Gregory, 282
Consideration, and social contact, 188
Constitution, U.S., abortion and, 246–247
Consumer Bill of Rights, 444
Consumer Product Safety Commission, 491
Consumer Protection and Environmental Health Service, 444
Consumer protection agencies, 444–445
Consumer protection movement, 444
Consumer protection skills, 448–451
Consumers:
   advertising and, 445–448
   health information and, 451–452
   health insurance and, 456–460
   over-the-counter drugs and, 460–463
Contact, guidelines for good, 188
Contraception:
   birth control versus, 223
   defined, 223
   guidelines for effective, 228
   responsible sexual behavior and, 222–223
Contraceptive sponge, 239–240
   placement of, *illustrated*, 239
Contraceptives:
   development of safer, 250
   oral, 229–231
Contract, behavioral-change. *See* Behavioral-change contract
Contraindicated drug, 461
Controlled substances, 469
   five schedules of, 469
   legal classification of, 468
Convalescence stage, 358
Cooper, Kenneth H., 154, 159
Copayment, 457
Copper T-380A IUD, 234
Corpus luteum, 212
Cosmopolitan Magazine, 139
Cosmos, perception of, and spiritual well-being, 37
Counselors, grief, 539
County District Attorney, 491
County Health Department, 491
County/Regional Air Quality Board, 491
County/Regional Water Quality Board, 491
Cowper's glands, 198, 201
"Crack" (cocaine), 334

Creativity, and social contact, 188
Cremains, 539
Cremated, 539
Crises:
   defined, 66
   managing, 66–69
Cross tolerance:
   to alcohol, 309
   to barbiturates, 329
Cross-linkage theory of aging, 508–509
Cross-training workouts, 163
Cruciferous, 112
Cryogenics, 532
Culture, health behavior and, 16
Cunnilingus, 208
Cycle:
   menstrual, 210–212
   sexual response, 208–210
Cyclevision Tours (video), 164
Cystic fibrosis, 436, 536
Cystic Fibrosis Foundation, 436
Cysts, 417
Cytoplasm, 418

D

D-lysergic acid diethylamide. *See* LSD
Dalkon Shield IUD, 234
Date of confinement, expected (EDC), 264
Date rape, 181
DBCP. *See* Dibromochloropropane
DDT, 475, 480, 486, 492
de Varona, Donna, exercise video by, 164
Death, 528–542
   biological, 530
   causes of, in U.S., 400–402
   certificate of, *illustrated*, 529
   chances of, in next ten years, 401–402
   clinical, 530
   concepts of, 530–531
   fears of, 531–533
   funeral arrangements after, 539–540
   handling grief and, 541–542
   leading causes of, 4, 5
   legal, 530
   lifestyle and causes of, 12
   psychological, 530
   role of, in life, 528–530
   self-inventory of attitude toward, 535
   social, 530
   See also Dying
Death, Grief, and Caring Relationships (Kalish), 541
Decongestant, 462
Deductible, 457
Defense mechanisms, 358–359
   cilia, 358
   interferon, 358
   tears, 358
   white blood cells, 358

Defervescence stage, 358
Dehydrating agent, 307
Dehydration, 107
Deliriants:
   poppers, 328
   volatile solvents, 328
Dementia, 518
Dendrites of neuron, 279
Denial:
   during dying process, 534
   of sexually transmitted disease, 375
Deoxyribonucleic acid (DNA), 507
Dependence:
   on alcohol, 309, 319–320
   on barbiturates, 329
   on cocaine, 333
   on LSD, 336
   physiological, 309, 329, 331, 336
   psychological, 331, 333
Depo-Provera, 250
Depressants, 328–332
   barbiturates, 328–330
   minor tranquilizers, 330
   opiates, 331–332
Depression, 43
   during dying process, 535
   number of Americans suffering from, 43
Dermatitis, 393
Designer drugs, 340–344
   China White, 341
   MDA, 341
   MDEA, 341
   MDMA 340–341
   MPPP, 341
   STP (DOM), 341
   TMA, 341
Desoxyn, 335
Dexedrine, 335
Dextroamphetamine, 335
Diabetes mellitus, 432–434
   control of, 434
   symptoms of, 433
   Type I, 432–433
   Type II, 432–434
Diaphragm, 237–239
   insertion of, *illustrated*, 238
Diastole, 403
Diastolic blood pressure, 403
Diastolic hypertension, 405
Dibromochloropropane (DBCP), 486–491
   sterility and, 487, 490
Diet:
   amphetamines and, 134
   anti-cancer, 95, 112–113
   Beverly Hills, 134
   Cambridge, 133
   cancer and, 419–420
   complete fasting, 132–133
   Fit for Life, 134
   healthy-heart, 95
   low-carbohydrate, 133

over-the-counter (OTC) preparations for, 134–135
pregnancy and, 264–265
protein-supplemented modified fast, 133
rice, 134
See also Eating behavior; Nutrition; Weight control
Dietary Goals for the United States, 93–94
Dietary guidelines, 87
Diethylstilbestrol (DES), 247–248
Dignity, dying with, 537–538
Dilatation and curettage (D&C), 249
Diplococci, 353
Direct contact, and disease transmission, 356
Director of Medical Specialties, The, 452
Disaccharides, 91
Disease(s):
  alcohol and, 311–312
  Alzheimer's, 518–520
  chronic, 400–402
  communicable. *See* Communicable diseases; Sexually transmitted diseases
  contagious. *See* Communicable diseases
  fibrocystic breast, 343
  genetic, 435–437
  infectious. *See* Communicable diseases
  Marie Strumpel (ankylosing spondylitis), 431
  occupational. *See* Occupational diseases
  Parkinson's, 341
  prevention of, exercise and, 149
  sexually transmitted. *See* Sexually transmitted diseases
  Tay-Sachs, 436–437
Disequilibrium, 66
Dispositional tolerance, 308
Distress, 58
Diuresis, caffeine and, 344
Diuretics, 107, 406
Divorce, 190–191
DNA. *See* Deoxyribonucleic acid
Dolophine, 331
DOM (STP), 341
Dopamine, 279
Down's Syndrome, 317
DPT (diphtheria, pertussis, and tetanus) series, 368
Drinking age, 312
Drinking water, toxic chemicals in, 487–488
Driving, drinking and, 312–316
Drowning, 497
Drug-induced psychosis:
  from cocaine, 333
  from PCP, 338
Drugs, 275–347
  alcohol, 282, 303–326
  antidiabetic, 311
  anti-inflammatory, 461
  antihistamines, 462

barbiturates, 309, 328–330
benzodiazepines, 330
bioavailability of, 467
brand-name, 464–465
bronchodilators, 335
cocaine, 282
contraindicated, 461
controlled substances, 469
decongestants, 462
deliriants, 328
dependence on. *See* Dependence
depressants, 328–332
designer, 340–344
diuretics, 406
effects of combining. *See* Drugs, synergism and
expectorants, 463
Food and Drug Administration and, 444
generic, 464–467
guidelines for healthy attitude toward, 341
hallucinogens, 335–338, 340–341
marijuana, 309, 311, 338–340
minor tranquilizers, 330
nervous system and, 278–279
nicotine, 277–301
nonsteroidal anti-inflammatory (NSAIDs), 429–430
opiates, 331–332
over-the-counter, 460–463
prescription (legend), 464–469
psychoactive, 327–347
sedative-hypnotics, 328–330
self-inventory for responsible use of, 343
smokeless tobacco, 296–297
stimulants, 332–335, 343–344
sympathomimetics, 463
synergism and, 310–311, 329, 331
understanding prescriptions for, 464, 465
vasodilators, 406
withdrawal from, 282, 329, 331, 333
Ducts:
  ejaculatory, 200
  genital, 200
Duesberg, Peter H., 388
Duration of exercise, 153
Dying, 528–542
  concepts of, 530–531
  with dignity, 537–538
  fears of, 531–533
  handling grief and, 541–542
  See also Death
Dying process, 533–537
  acceptance of, 535
  anger at, 534
  bargaining and, 534–535
  denial of, 534
  depression and, 535
  guidelines helping friend or relative during, 536
Dying trajectory, 534

Dysplasia, 285

E

E. I. DuPont de Nemours & Co., 494
Eating behavior, 119–143
  assessment of, 124–125
  healthy, self-inventory for, 114
  setpoint level and, 131
  See also Diet; Nutrition; Weight control
Eating disorders, 138–141
  anorexia nervosa, 138
  bulimia, 139–141
"Ecstasy." *See* MDMA
Ectomorph, 128, 129
Ectopic pregnancy, 259, 380
EEG. *See* Electroencephalogram
Ehrlich, Paul, 483
Eighty/twenty (80:20) theory, 495
Einstein, Albert, 482
Ejaculate, 258
Ejaculatory ducts, 200
Elderly:
  caring for the, 521–524
  self-inventory of attitudes toward, 511
Electroconvulsive (electroshock) therapy, 51
Electroencephalogram (EEG), 530
Electrolytes, 106–107
Electron microscope, 352
Elimination, of alcohol, 305–306
ELISA test, 386
Embryo, 267
Emotional responses, chain of, 42
Emotions:
  anger, 44
  anxiety and fear, 45
  depression and, 42–43
  expressing, 41–46
  guilt, 44–45
  joy/sadness, 42
  loneliness, 45–46
  mental health and, 32, 41–46
Empathy, 41
Emphysema, 434
Encephalitis, 435
Endocrine glands, 205
Endometrium, 204
  cancer of, 427–428
Endomorph, 128, 129
Endosperm, 94
Endotoxins, 354
Endurance, muscular, 147
Energy nutrients, 90
Enrichment, 94
Entamoeba histolytica, 355
Environment:
  abuse of, and stress, 62
  acid rain and, 480
  behavioral change and, 23

INDEX

chlorofluorocarbons (CFCs) and, 480
greenhouse effect and, 480
hazardous substances in. *See* Hazardous substances
health and wellness and, 11, 474–499
risks from, 474–499
See also Occupational diseases
Environmental Protection Agency (EPA), 444, 476, 480, 488, 491
Enzymes, 308
Epidemiological triangle, 495
Epidemiologists, 374
Epidemiology of accidents, 496
Epidermis, 514
Epididymis, 200
Epididymitis, 380
Epilepsy, 435
Epinephrine, 59
Episiotomy, 269
Epstein-Barr virus, 366
Equilibrium, 58
Error hypothesis of aging, 508
Erythroxylon coca, 332
Essential amino acids, 96
Essential fat, 122
Essential hypertension, 405
risk factors for, 405–406
Esteem needs, 18. *See also* Self-esteem
Estrogen, 207, 260–261
birth control and, 229–231
Ethanol, 304
Ethyl alcohol, 304
Euphoria, 328
Eustress, 58
Euthanasia:
active, 537
passive, 537
Events, stress and, 61, 64–66
Excitement phase of sexual response cycle, 208, 209, 210
Executive Office of the President, 445
Exercise:
aerobic, 130, 159–164
anaerobic, 164–166
benefits of, 148–152
disease prevention and, 149
goals of, 147–148
guidelines for selecting shoes for, 162
heart disease and, 149
percentage of U.S. population undertaking, 146
physiological benefits of, 149–151
psychological benefits of, 151–152
See also Physical fitness
Exercise programs:
cardiovascular fitness and, 159–164
choosing activities for, 159–167
controversy over activity level and, 153
designing, 167
developing, 158–169

duration of exercise and, 153
flexibility and, 166–167
frequency of exercise and, 152
goal definition and, 159
guidelines for planning, 155
high-activity, 154
intensity of exercise and, 153
low-activity, 154–155, 158
moderate-activity, 154
muscular fitness and, 165–166
overload concept and, 169–170
principles of, 152–158
progression in, 170
specificity of, 169
sports and, 167
time pattern for ideal, 160
video, comparison of, 163–164
See also Athletic training
Exhaustion, stage of, 59
Existential psychotherapy, 51
Exotoxins, 354
Expected date of confinement (EDC), 264
Expectorant, 463
Exploitive behavior, 181–182
External genitals:
female, 201–202
male, 198–200

F

Fallopian tubes, 204–205
Falls, accidental, 497
Family, stress and, 61
Family and Medical Leave Act, 523
Family planning, 222–255. *See also* Birth control
Family psychotherapy, 50, 51
Fast food, nutrition and, 98
Fastigium stage, 358
Fasting, 132
weight-reduction diets and, 132–133
Fat(s), 98–101
body, 121
brown, 129–130
cholesterol, 100–101
essential, 122
food labels and, 126
storage, 122
triglycerides, 99–100
white, 129–130
Fat-cell theory of weight control, 129
Fat-soluble vitamins, 101
Fear:
of death and dying, 531–533
mental wellness and, 45
Federal legend, 469
Federal Superfund. *See* Superfund
Federal Trade Commission (FTC), 444, 445
Federal Trade Commission Act, Wheeler-Lea Amendment to (of 1938), 451

Fellatio, 208
Fellow of the American College of Surgeons (F.A.C.S.), 453
Female, sexual anatomy and physiology of, 201–205
Femshield, 250
Fermentation, 304
Fertility, smoking and, 287
Fertility-awareness contraceptive techniques, 244–246
Fertilization:
defined, 258
illustrated, 259
process of, 258–259
Festinger, Leon, 16
Fetal alcohol syndrome (FAS), 316–317
Fetus:
defined, 267
development of, 267–268
effect of smoking on, 287–288
illustrated, 266
See also Pregnancy
Fibers, 94–95
guidelines for increasing intake of, 95
Fibroadenomas, 423
Fibrocystic breast disease, 343, 423
Fibrosis, cystic, 436
Fimbriae, 204–205
Firearms, suicides and, 48
Fires, 497–499
guidelines for extinguishing, 498
First trimester:
abortion during, 248
fetal development during, 267–268
Fisk, Carlton, 296
Fit for Life, 134
Fit for Life diet, 134
Fitness:
cardiovascular. *See* Cardiovascular fitness
muscular. *See* Muscular fitness
physical. *See* Physical fitness
programs for. *See* Exercise programs
Fixx, James, 158
Flagyl, 381
Flatworms, 355
Fleming, Alexander, 376
Flexibility, 166–167
exercises to improve, 166
injury prevention and, 167
Fluid-producing glands, 200–201
Foams, contraceptive, 242
Follicle, 258
Follicle-stimulating hormone (FSH), 205–206, 212
Follicular phase of menstrual cycle, 212
Fonda, Jane, 154
exercise video by, 163
Food(s):
fast, nutrition and, 98
toxic chemicals in, 487–488

health, 111–112
high-fat, 130
imitation, 126
labeling of, 125–126
light or lite, 126
low-calorie, 126
low-fat, 126
natural, 126
naturally sweetened, 126
organic, 111, 126
reduced-sodium, 126
sodium-free, 126
sugar-free or sugarless, 126
Food, Drug, and Cosmetic Act of 1938, 444
Food and Drug Administration (FDA), 110, 112, 215, 240, 241, 248, 250, 340, 386, 389, 390, 444, 461, 467, 491
food-labeling regulations of, 125
Force-field analysis, 20–21
Foreskin, 199
Four Basic Food Groups, 86–87
Fourteenth Amendment, abortion and, 246–247
Frame size, 121
Frankl, Victor, 51
Fraud, mail, 445
Free radical theory of aging, 508
Freebasing, 334
Frequency of exercise, 152
Freud, Sigmund, 51
Friedman, Meyer, 406
Fructose, 91
Funeral directors, 539
Funerals, 539–540
Fungi, 355

G

G-spot. *See* Grafenberg Spot
G. D. Searle and Co., 234
Galactose, 91
Ganglia, 362
Gangrene, 407
Garner, Donald, 281
Gender:
assigned, 270
genetic, 260
genital, 261
gonadal, 260
hormonal, 260–261
See also Sex
Gender differentiation:
postnatal, 270–271
prenatal, 260–261
Gender identity, 270
Gender role, 270
Gender role identification, 270
General adaptation syndrome (GAS), 59
Generic drugs, 464–467
cost of, 467
Generic name, 464

Genetic disorders, 435–437
cystic fibrosis, 436
phenylketonuria (PKU), 437
sickle-cell anemia, 435–436
Tay-Sachs disease, 436–437
Genetic gender, 260
Genetic limit theory, 508
Genetic predisposition theory of weight control, 128–129
Genital ducts, 200
Genital gender, 261
Genitals:
female, 201–202
male, 198–201
Geographic factors, cancer and, 420
Germ, 94
German measles (rubella), 364
localization of rash of, illustrated, 364
Gerontologists, 521
Glands:
adrenal, 205
Bartholin's, 202
Cowper's, 198, 201
endocrine, 205
fluid-producing, 200–201
pituitary, 205
prostate, 201
Skene's, 202
Glans (of penis), 198
Glaucoma, 516
Global instability, stress and, 62
Glover, Elbert, 297
Glucagon, 433
Glucose, 91
Glutethimide, 330
Goals, exercise, 159
Gold, Mark, 334
Gonadal gender, 260
Gonadotropin-releasing factor (GnRF), 205
Gonads:
defined, 260
female (ovaries), 205
male (testes), 200
Gonorrhea, 352, 379
babies of mothers with, 379
treatment for, 379
Gore, Albert, 494
Gossypol, 251
Gout, 431
treatment of, 431
Grafenberg Spot (G-spot), 203
illustrated, 203
Grain alcohol, 304
Grand mal (tonic-clonic) seizure, 435
Granuloma inguinale, 382
Gratification, mental wellness and, 32
Great American Smokeout, 289, 290
Greenhouse effect, 480
Grief:
defined, 541
handling, 541–542
Grief counselors, 539

Grief syndrome, acute, 542
Growths, benign versus malignant, 419. *See also* Neoplasms
Guilt, 44–45
Guinness Book of World Records, 14
Gum disease, smoking and, 287
Gynecologist, 264

H

Hackett, Thomas, 151
Haemophilus vaginalis, 381
Hair, aging and, 515
Hallucinogens, 335–338, 340–341
defined, 335
LSD, 336
mescaline, 337
ololiuqui, 337
PCP (phencyclidine), 337–338
peyote, 336–337
psilocybin, 337
"Shrooms," 337
Handbook of Nonprescription Drugs, The (American Pharmaceutical Association), 460
Hardening, of arteries. *See* Arteriosclerosis
Hardt death attitude scale, 535
Harmony House, 332
Harvard University Medical School, 530
Hashish, 338–339
Hayflick, Leonard, 508
Hazard Communication Law, 490
Hazard Evaluation Service and Information System (HESIS), 490
Hazardous (toxic) substances, 475
community protection against, 491–494
guidelines to avoid injury from 484
health effects of, 478–482
lack of information concerning, 476
occupational exposure to, 479–480, 481, 484–486
persons affected by, 484–486
Hazardous (toxic) waste, 478
chemical industry and, 475
community protection against, 491–494
disposal sites for, 474
distribution of industrial, 478
at end of WWII, 478
household, 475–476
management techniques for, 493
Hazardous Waste in America (Gore), 494
Head lice, 392
Health:
Canadian concept of determinants of, 10
community programs to protect, 491–494
consumer, 444–469
continuum of levels of, 13
defined, 5
dimensions of, 6–10
drug abuse and. *See* Alcohol; Psychoactive drugs; Tobacco

INDEX

effects of hazardous substances on, 478–482
environment and, 11, 474–499
factors affecting, 10–15
fitness components related to, 147
health-care organizations and, 12–13, 452–455
holistic, 10
human biology and, 11
information concerning, accuracy of, 451–452
lifestyle and, 12
nutrition and. *See* Diet; Eating behaviors; Nutrition
occupational and environmental risks to, 474–499
personal perceptions of, 18–19
social support and, 76–77
stress and, 62
See also Mental health
Health, Education, and Welfare, Department of, 444, 445
Health and Human Services, Department of, 4, 87, 294, 444, 491
Health behavior:
cultural and class background and, 16
motivation and, 15–18
significant others and, 16–17
See also Behavior; Behavioral change
Health Belief Model, 18–19
illustrated, 19
Health care, 12–13, 452–455
Health Consequences of Involuntary Smoking, The (Surgeon General's report, 1986), 295
Health Consequences of Smoking (Surgeon General's report, 1971), 288
Health Consequences of Smoking: Nicotine Addiction, The (Surgeon General's report, 1988), 282
Health foods, 111–112
Health insurance, traditional 456–458
coinsurance clauses and, 457–458
copayment for, 457
deductible for, 457
disability, 457
major medical, 457
preexisting condition clauses and, 458
Health maintenance organizations (HMOs), 458–460
Health products, advertising and, 445–448
Health Tips (California Medical Association), 287, 289
Healthiest couple, The (Carlyon), 12, 13
Hearing, aging and, 516–517
Heart attack. *See* Myocardial infarction
Heart disease. *See* Cardiovascular disease
Heart rate, target (THR), 153, 154
determining, 161
Heberdon's nodes, 431
Height, 120–121
Height and weight tables, 120

Hemoglobin, 107, 285, 435
Hemophiliacs, 385
Hemorrhoids, 425
Hepatitis:
alcoholic, 311
A, 367
B (serum hepatitis), 367
B immune globulin (HBIG), 390
vaccine for, 390
Heredity, cancer and, 418
Heroin, 331
Herpes:
simplex, 388–389
zoster (shingles), 362
Heterosexuality, 207
Hierarchy of needs, Maslow's 17–18
High-density lipoproteins (HDLs), 311, 411–412
High-fat foods, setpoint level and, 130
High-impact aerobics, 160–162
Hippocrates, 146
Hiroshima, 482
Hoffman, Albert, 336
Holistic health, 10
Holmes, Sherlock, 332
Holmes, Thomas, 61, 64
Homeostasis, 509
Homophobia, 388
Homosexuality, 208
Honesty with others, 41
Hong Kong virus, 366
Hooker Chemical Co., 474
Hormonal gender, 260–261
Hormones:
androgens, 260–261
defined, 205
endocrine glands and, 205
epinephrine, 59
estrogen, 207, 229–231, 260–261
follicle-stimulating (FSH), 205–206, 212
gender differentiation and, 260–261
gonadotropin-releasing factor (GnRF), 205
luteinizing (LH), 205–206, 212
progesterone, 207, 260
sex and sexual functioning and, 205–207, 261
testosterone, 200, 206–207, 260
Horowitz, David, 451
Hospice program, 537–538
Host organism, 353
Hotline, cocaine, 334
Household toxic chemicals, 475–476
alternatives to, *listed*, 477
"Hug drug." *See* MDMA
Human chorionic gonadotropin (HCB), 264
Human papilloma virus (HPV) (venereal warts), 390
Humanistic psychology, 51
Hydrocodone, 331
Hymen, 203
Hyperlipidemia, 127

Hypertension, 403–407
in an artery, *illustrated*, 407
being a good listener and, 44
causes of, 403
defined, 405
diastolic, 405
essential, 405
hostile individuals and, 44
idiopathic, 405
primary, 405
risk factors for, 405–406
secondary, 405
treatment of, 406
Hypotension, 405
Hypothalamus, 59, 205
Hysterectomy, 249
pelvic inflammatory disease and, 380

I

Ibuprofen, 461
Identity, gender, 270
Idiopathic hypertension, 405
Ignorance, sexually transmitted disease and, 375
Ignorance, sexually transmitted disease and, 375
Illness, mental, 49–52
Imitation foods, 126
Immune system:
defined, 59
guidelines for maintaining a strong, 391
Immunity, 360
active, 360–361
congenital, 362
passive, 361–362
Immunizations, 352, 359–361
childhood, 360
Implantation, 259
Impulsive behavior, sexually transmitted disease and, 374–375
Incomplete proteins, 97
Incubation period, 357
of common diseases, *listed*, 357
Indirect contact, and disease transmission, 356
Individual psychotherapy, 50
Infectious mononucleosis, 366–367
Influenza, 366
Influenza viruses, 366
Information:
health, 451–452
social networks and, 77
Injuries:
accidental, 494–499
occupational, 479
prevention of, exercise and, 167
Insight therapy, 50
Insoluble, 94
Insulin, 432
nasal spray form of, 434

Insurance. *See* Health insurance
Intensity of exercise, 153
Interferon, 358
Interment, 539
Interpersonal factors, 34
Interpersonal relationships, stress and, 61
Intestinal bypass surgery, 135
Intima, 410
Intimacy, physical, 182–183
Intraamniotic injection, 249
Intrapersonal conflict, stress and, 61
Intrapersonal factors, 34
Intrauterine device (IUD), 233–234
    Copper T-380A, 234
    Dalkon Shield, 234
    postcoital insertion of, 248
    Progestasert, 234
    "tail-less," 250
Intrusion speech pattern, 519
Involuntary (passive) smoking, 295–296
    guidelines for preventing, 296
Iron, 107–109
Irresponsibility, sexually transmitted disease and, 375
Isokinetic programs, 166
Isometric programs, 166
Isopropyl alcohol, 304
Isotonic programs, 166

J

Jane Fonda's Low-Impact Aerobic Workout! (video), 163
Japan, low incidence of cancer in, 420
Jarvik, Murray, 290
Jaundice, 367
Jaw, wiring of, 135
Jellies, contraceptive, 242
Johnson, Virginia E., 208
Journal of Clinical Gastroenterology, The, 287
Journal of Clinical Periodontology, 287
Journal of the American Medical Association, 285, 421
Journal:
    keeping a, stress management and, 74–75
    suggested themes for entries in, 75
Joy, 42
Jung, Carl, 35
Juvenile arthritis, 430

K

Kaiser Foundation Health Plan, 458
Kalish, Richard, 541
Kennedy, John F., 444
Ketosis:
    defined, 91
    fasting and, 133

Khaw, Kay-Tee, 288
Kilocalorie, *defined*, 90
Kimball, Bruce, 496, 497
Koop, C. Everett, 282
Koplik's spots, 362
Kubler-Ross, Elizabeth, 534, 535

L

Labels, food, 125–126
Labia majora, 201
Labia minora, 202
Labor:
    defined, 268
    first stage of, 268–269
    second stage of, 269
    third stage of, 269–270
Lacto-ovo vegetarian, 97
LaLonde, Marc, 10
Lancet, 154
Lanugo, 138
Laparoscopy, 228
Law(s):
    alcohol and, 312–316
    tobacco and, 297–298
    drug, 467–469
Lean body mass, 121, 122
Legal death, 530
Legend drugs. *See* Drugs, prescription
Legumes, 93
Length of life (longevity), 14–15
Lesion, 376
Lethargy, 362
Letter of complaint, how to write, 450
Leukemia, 428
Leukoplakia, 297
Lice:
    body, 392
    head, 392
    pubic, 392–393
Life:
    length of (longevity), 14–15
    meaning and purpose in, 32, 37
    stressful changes and events in, 61, 64–66
Life After Life (Moody), 531
Life Change Units (LCUs), 61
Life expectancy, 14, 14–15
    according to race and sex, 15
    in poorest countries, 15
    smoking and, 290
Life span, 14
    longest recorded, 508
Lifestyle:
    health and wellness and, 12
    healthful, self-inventory of, 24–25
Light or lite foods, 126
Limerence, 184
Linoleic acid, 99
Lipid, 98
Lipoproteins, 410–412
    high-density (HDL), 411–412

    low-density (LDL), 411–412
    very-low-density (VLDL), 411
Liposuction, 135
Listening, 41
Liver, alcohol and, 311
Living will, 537
    illustrated, 538
Living-dying interval, 534
Logotherapy, 51
Loneliness and Love (Moustakis), 541
Loneliness, 45–46
    shyness and, 46
Longevity, 14–15
Los Angeles Times, 282, 494
Loss of loved one. *See* Death; Dying
Love:
    being in, 184
    being out of, 186
    companionate, 185
    falling in, 184
    falling out of, 185
    healthy versus unhealthy, 180
    mental wellness and, 32
    need for, 17
    physical intimacy and, 182–183
    readiness for, 184
    romantic, 183–186
    spiritual well-being and, 37, 40
    transitional, 185
Love Canal, 474, 484, 490, 491
Low-calorie foods, 126
Low-carbohydrate diets, 133
Low-density lipoproteins (LDL), 411–412
Low-fat foods, 126
Low-impact aerobics, 162
LSD (d-lysergic acid diethylamide), 336, 469
    psychotic reactions to, 336
    tolerance to, 336
Lumpectomy, 424
Lung cancer, 285, 422
    smoking and, 422
Lupus erythematosus, systemic, 431–432
Luteal phase of menstrual cycle, 212
Luteinizing hormone (LH), 205–206, 212
Lymph nodes, 364
Lymph system, 417
Lymphogranuloma venereum, 382–383
Lymphoma, 428

M

Macrominerals, 104
Mail fraud, 445
Major medical, 457
Make Today Count (self-help group), 533
Malanin, 514
Male, sexual anatomy and physiology of, 198–201
Malignant neoplasm, 416
    versus benign, 418

Mammogram, 424
  base-line, 424
Mantra, 73
March of Dimes, 288
Marie Strumpel disease (ankylosing spondylitis), 431
Marijuana, 338–340
  synergism and, 309, 311, 340
Marmor, Judd, 183
Marriage(s), 189–190
  median age of, 189–190
  number and rate of, 191
Marsee, Sean, 297
Martina Navratilova Fitness and Conditioning Workout Program (video), 163
Maryland Institute for Emergency Medical Services, 313
Maslow, Abraham, 17
Maslow's hierarchy of needs, 17–18
Mass, lean body, 121
Mastectomy, 425
Masters, William H., 208
Masturbation, 208
  mutual, 208
Material support, social networks and, 77
Mazel, Judy, 134
MDA, 341
MDMA, 340–341
MDEA, 341
Meadows, Donella H., 494
Meaning in life, spiritual well-being and, 37
Measles:
  rubella (German), 364
  rubeola, 362–363
Meatus, 200
Medicaid, 456
Medical record, *illustrated*, 8–9
Medical specialties and subspecialties, *listed*, 453
Medicare, 456
Meditation, 72–74
  methods, of, *illustrated*, 72
Melanocytes, 514
Melanoma, 421
Menarche, 210
Menopause, 520
Menstrual cycle, 210–212
  follicular phase of, 212
  illustrated, 211
  luteal phase of, 212
  menstruation phase of, 212
  ovulation phase of, 212
Menstrual extraction, 248
Menstrual synchrony, 213
Menstruation, 212
  defined, 212
  etymology of, 210
  exercise and, 154
  myths about, 213–214
Mental health, 31–56
  emotions and, 41–46
  issues in, 52

  practitioners of, 50–52
  self-inventory of, 47
  See also Mental well-being
Mental illness, 49–52
  caring for, 49–52
  groups vulnerable to, 52
  psychotherapies for, 50
Mental well-being, 7
  components of, 32–33
  enhancing, 40–41
  normality and, 33
  self-esteem and, 33–35
  See also Mental health
Meperidine, 331
Mescaline, 337
Mesomorph, 128, 129
Metabolism:
  of alcohol, 306
  basal. *See* Basal metabolic rate
  wasting, 132
Metastases, 417
Metastasis, 417
Methadone, 331–332
Methamphetamine, 335
Methaqualone, 330, 331
  withdrawal from, 331
Methedrine, 335
Methyl alcohol, 304
Methylprylon (Noludar), 330
Metronidazole, alcohol combined with, 311
Metropolitan Life Insurance Co., 120
Microscope, electron, 352
Mifepristone, 249
Miller, Henry S., 154
Minamata Bay, Japan, poisoning of, 484
Minerals, 104–110
  defined, 104
  electrolytes, 106–107
  iron, 107–109
  macrominerals, 104
  setpoint level and, 131
  trace, 104
Minor tranquilizers, 330
Mitford, Jessica, 540
Model, Health Belief, 18–19
Moles, 417
Molluscum contagiosum, 391
Money, stress and, 62
Monilia (Candida albicans), 391–392
Mononucleosis, infectious, 366–367
Monosaccharides, *defined*, 91
Monounsaturated triglycerides (fats), 99–100
Mons veneris (mons pubis), 201
Moody, Raymond, 531
Moral principles, spiritual well-being and, 37
Morbidity:
  defined, 4
  social support and, 76–77
Morbidity and Mortality Weekly Report, 374
Morning-after pills, 247–248
Morphine, 331

Mortality:
  defined, 4
  social support and, 76–77
  rates for, in U.S., 400–402
Motivation:
  general principles of, 16–17
  health behavior and, 15–18
Motor vehicle accidents, 496–497
Mourning, 541
Moustakis, Clark, 541
MPPP, 341
Mucous method of birth control, 244–246
Mumps (parotitis), 364–365
  effect of, on body systems, 365
Muscular endurance, 147, 165
Muscular fitness, 147, 165–166
  isokinetic programs and, 166
  isometric programs and, 166
  isotonic programs and, 166
Muscular strength, 147, 165
Mutations, 418
Mutual masturbation, 208
Myocardial infarction (MI), 408
  illustrated, 409
  symptoms of, 410
Myometrium, of uterus, 204

N

Nagasaki, 482
Narcosis, 331
Narcotics, 331
National Academy of Sciences, 88–89, 107, 476
National Advertising Division (NAD) of Better Business Bureau, 451
National Cancer Institute, 294
National Injury Prevention Foundation, 161
National Institute of Child Health and Development, 317
National Institute of Occupational Safety and Health (NIOSH), 479
National Institute on Alcohol Abuse, 320
National Institute on Drug Abuse, 296, 332
National Interagency Council on Smoking and Health, 294
National Research Council, 89, 101, 288, 295
Natural foods, 111, 126
Naturally sweetened foods, 126
Navratilova, Martina, exercise video by, 163
Near-death experiences, 531
Needs:
  belongingness and love, 17
  esteem, 18
  Maslow's hierarchy of, 17–18
  physiological, 17
  safety, 17
  self-actualization, 18
Nei Ching (The Yellow Emperor's Classic of Internal Medicine), 70

Neisseria gonorrhea, 379, 381
Neoplasm, 416
  benign, 416
  benign versus malignant, 418
  malignant, 416
Nervous system, 278–279
  autonomic (ANS), 59, 278
  central (CNS), 278
  organization of, *illustrated*, 278
  parasympathetic, 73, 278
  peripheral (PNS), 278
  somatic (SNS), 278
  sympathetic, 278
Networks, social, 76
Neuroendocrine system, *defined*, 59
Neuron, 278
  axon of, 279
  cell body of, 279
  dendrites of, 279
  terminals of, 279
Neurosurgery, 51
Neurotransmitters, 278–279
  effect of drugs on, 279
New Jersey virus, 366
New Yorker, 492
Nicorette, 290
Nicotine, 284
  addition to, 282
  cardiovascular effects of, 297
  gum containing (Nicorette), 290
  substitutes for, 290
  withdrawal from, 282
  See also Cigarettes; Smoking; Tobacco
Nodes, lymph, 364
Noludar (methyprylon), 330
Nonessential amino acids, *defined*, 96
Nongonococcal urethritis, 380
Nonoxynol-9, 242
Nonsteroidal anti-inflammatory drugs (NSAIDs), 429–430
Norepinephrine, 279
Normality, 33
Nuclear war, 482–483
Nuclear winter, 483
Nucleii, 418
Nutrients, 88–89
  defined, 88
  energy, 90
Nutrition, 86–117
  alcohol and, 311
  calorie awareness and, 90–91
  cancer prevention and, 112–113
  carbohydrates and, 91–95
  dietary guidelines and, 88
  fats and, 98–101
  health foods and, 111–112
  minerals and, 104–110
  nutrients and, 88–89
  protein and, 95–98
  vitamins and minerals and, 101–103, 109–110

water and, 110–111
  See also Diet; Eating behavior
Nutrition, Weight Control, and Exercise (Katch and McCardle), 163

O

OA. *See* Overeaters Anonymous
Obituary, sample form for, 530
Occupation:
  carcinogens and, 479–480, 481
  diseases related to, 479–480, 481, 484–491
  exposure to hazardous substances and, 484–491
  health and, 474–499
  injuries related to, 479
  risks related to, 474–499
Occupational Safety and Health Administration (OSHA), 487, 488
Office of Consumer Affairs, 444, 445, 450
Office of Technology Assessment, 282
Oleic acid, 100
Ololiuqui, 337
Openness with others, 41
Opiates, 331–332
  synergism and, 331
Opium, 331
Oral contraceptives, 229–231
  development of safer, 250
  guidelines for using, 231
  for males, 251
Organic foods, 111, 126
Organisms:
  host, 353
  pathogenic. *See* Pathogenic organisms
Orgasm, 208, 209, 210
Osteoarthritis, 430–431
  symptoms of, 430
  treatment of, 431
Osteoporosis, 289–517
  exercise and, 154
Ova, 258
  fertilization of, 258–259
Ovaries, 205
  cancer of, 428
  effects of hormones on, 205–206
Over-the-counter (OTC) diet preparations, 134–135
  benzocaine, 135
  bulk producers, 135
  phenylpropanolamine, 134
Over-the-counter drugs, 460–463
  analgesics, 460–462
  cold and allergy preparations, 462–463
Overeaters Anonymous (OA), 136
Overload concept, in fitness programs, 169–170
Ovral, 247–248
Ovulation, 212, 258
Oxycodone, 331

P

Paffenberger, Ralph, 154, 155, 158
Papanicolau (Pap) smear, 389, 427
Paranoia, cocaine use and, 333
Parasitic worms, 355–356
  flatworms, 355
  pinworms, 355
  Trichinella, 355–356
Parasympathetic nervous system, 73, 278
Parenthood, question of, 262–264
Parest, 330
Parke-Davis, 337
Parkes, C. M., 542
Parkinson's disease, 341
Parotitis (mumps), 364–365
  effect of, the body systems, 365
Partial (psychomotor) seizure, 435
Passive euthanasia, 537
Passive immunity, 361–362
Passive smoking, 295–296
Pathogen, 352
Pathogenic organisms, 352–356
  bacteria, 353–354
  fungi, 355
  listed, 352
  parasitic worms, 355–356
  protozoa, 354–355
  rickettsia, 354
  transmission of, 356–357
  viruses, 352–353
Pathology, 52
PCBs, 486, 492
PCP (phencyclidine), 337–338, 469
  drug-induced psychosis from, 338
  long-term use of, 338
  overdose of, 338
PDR (Physician's Desk Reference) for Nonprescription Drugs, The (U.S. Pharmacopeial Convention), 460
Peace of mind, exercise and, 151–152
Pelvic inflammatory disease, 233, 380–381
Penis, 198–200
  glans of, 198
Peptide-T, 386
Performance-related fitness components, 147–148
Perimetrium, of uterus, 204
Peripheral nervous system (PNS), 278
Peripheral resistance, 403
Peristalsis, 331
Personal unconscious, 35
Pertussis (whooping cough), 367–368
Petit mal (absence) seizure, 435
Peyote, 336–337
Pharmacodynamic tolerance, 308
Pharmacology:
  of alcohol, 305–311
  defined, 340
Phenacetin, 461

Phencyclidine. *See* PCP
Phenobarbital, 329
Phenylketonuria (PKU), 437
Phenylpropanolamine, 134
Pheromones, 213
Philadelphia Geriatric Center, 524
Phoenix House, 332
Physical fitness, 146–171
   athletic training and. *See* Athletic training
   components of, 147–148
   contract for, 169
   defined, 146–147
   developing program for. *See* Exercise programs
   evaluation of, 158–159
   exercise and. *See* Exercise
   health-related components of, 147
   performance-related components of, 147–148
   reviewing resources for, 167
   self-inventory of, 156–157
Physical intimacy, love and, 182–183
Physical well-being, 6–7
Physicians, number of women, 455
Physiological benefits of exercise, 149–151
Physiological dependence, 309
    on barbiturates, 329
    on LSD, 336
    on opiates, 331
Physiological needs, 17
Physiology, sexual, 198–205
Pinworms, 355
Pituitary gland, 59, 205
Placenta, 205, 266, 267
Planning, family. *See* Family planning
Plateau phase of sexual response cycle, 208, 209, 210
Platelets, 286
Poison Control Center, 491
Polyps, 417
Polyunsaturated triglycerides (fats), 99
Poppers, 328
Population:
   elderly. *See* Elderly
   projections of, 506
Porter, Cole, 332
Positive thinking, steps in nurturing, 71
Postcoital methods of abortion, 247–248
Preexisting condition clause, 458
Preferences, sexual, 207–208
Pregnancy, 264–266
   activity and, 266
   alcohol and, 316–317
   average length of human, 264
   beginning of, 259
   childbirth and, 268–270
   determining child's sex during, 261–262
   diet and, 264–265
   ectopic, 259, 380
   fetal development during, 267–268
   gender differentiation during, 260–261

   smoking and, 287–288
   syphilis and, 378
   teenage, 222
   testing for, 264
   tubal, 259
Premenstrual syndrome (PMS), 214–215, 343
Presbycusis, 516
Prescriptions:
   commonly used abbreviations in, 465
   understanding, 464, 465
   See also Drugs, prescription
President's Council on Physical Fitness, 146
   definition of physical fitness by, 146
Pressure, blood. *See* Blood pressure
Prevention:
   of communicable disease, 358–361
   of disease, exercise and, 149
Primary hypertension, 405
Primary stressor, 61
Problem solving:
   analyzing solutions and, 20–21
   as behavior-change strategy, 19–20
Prodromal stage, 357
Progestasert IUD, 234
Progesterone, 207, 260
Progestin implants, subdermal, 250
Progestin injections, long-acting, 250
Prognosis, 420
Progression, in exercise program, 170
Progressive resistance, 170
Proof (alcohol), 304
Propyl alcohol, 304
Prostaglandinq, 201
   intraamniotic injection of, 249
Prostate cancer, 425
Prostate gland, 201
Protein, 95–98
   complete, 96–97
   defined, 95
   incomplete, 97
   for the vegetarian, 97–98
Protein-supplemented modified fast diet, 133
Protozoa, 354–355
   diseases caused by, 355
Psilocin, 337
Psilocybin, 337
Psychiatric illness, sexual abuse and, 52
Psychiatric social workers, 51
Psychiatrists, 50–51
Psychoactive drugs, 327–347
   deliriants, 328
   depressants, 328–332
Psychoanalysis, 51
Psychological age, 507
Psychological benefits of exercise, 151–152
Psychological death, 530
Psychological dependence:
   on cocaine, 333
   on opiates, 331
Psychological effects of alcohol, 311

Psychologists, clinical, 51
Psychology:
   behavioral, 51
   humanistic, 51
   transpersonal, 51
Psychomotor (partial) seizure, 435
Psychosexual attraction, 208
Psychosis, drug-induced. *See* Drug-induced psychosis
Psychotherapy:
   action, 50
   characteristics of, 51
   cognitive, 51
   defined, 50
   existential, 51
   family, 50, 51
   individual, 50
   insight, 50
   logotherapy, 51
   person-centered, 51
   reality, 51
   types of, 50
Puberty, 258
Pubic lice, 392–393
   treatment of, 393
Public interest consumer/environmental/ toxics group, 491
Puffery, 446, 451
Pulmonary disease, chronic obstruction, 434–435
Pusle, how to take, *illustrated*, 161
Purging, 139–140
Purpose in life:
   mental wellness and, 32
   spiritual well-being and, 37
Pursuit of Loneliness, The (Slater), 45
Purulent, 379

Q

Quaalude, 330
Quality of life, 13–15
   indicators of, 14
   quantity of life and, 13–15
Quantity of life, 13–15
   quality of life and, 13–15
Queens University (Ontario), 287
Quickening, 268

R

R. J. Reynolds Tobacco Co., 290
Race, cardiovascular disease and, 406
Radial pulse, taking your, *illustrated*, 161
Radiation therapy, for breast cancer, 425
Radon, 486
Rahe, Richard, 61, 64
Rape, 181
   date, 181
   guidelines for helping victim of, 181

Reaction, alarm, 59
Reality therapy, 51
Recommendation Dietary Allowances (RDAs), 88–89
Reduced-sodium foods, 126
Refractory period, 186
Rehabilitation, from shock of loss, 542
Reinforcements, *defined*, 24
Relationship(s), 178–196
   communication in, 188–189
   defined, 178
   divorce and, 190–191
   exploitive behavior in, 181–182
   foundations for a healthy, 178–180
   healthy versus unhealthy love in, 180
   loss of, 190–193. *See also* Death; Dying
   love and physical intimacy in, 182–183
   marriage and, 189–190, 191
   romantic love cycle and, 183–186
   interpersonal, 61
Relaxation, methods of, 72–74
   illustrated, 72
Renewal of normal life style, after loss, 542
Resistance:
   progressive, 170
   stage of, 59
Resolution phase of sexual response cycle, 208, 209, 210
Resources, physical fitness, 167
Respiratory system:
   exercise and, 150
   smoking and, 285–286
Responsibility, social, 32
Resuscitation, from shock of loss, 542
Retinoblastoma, 419
Retirement, successful, 521
Retrovir, 386
Retrovirus, 423
Reuptake, 333
Reye's syndrome, 362, 461
Reynolds, Patrick, 290
"Reynolds Stop Smoking Program," 290
Reynolds, R. J., 290
Rheumatoid arthritis, 428–430
   causes of, 429
   treatment of, 429–430
Ribonucleic acid (RNA), 507
Rice diet, 134
Rickettsia, 354
   antibiotics and, 354
   diseases caused by, 354
Right to know (of exposure to toxic chemicals), 490–491
Risk factors:
   for cancer, 418–421
   chronic disease and, 400–402
   occupational and environmental, 474–499
RNA. *See* Ribonucleic acid
Robinson, Don, 532
"Rock" (cocaine), 334
Roe v. Wade, 246–247

Rogers, Carl, 51
Role, gender, 270
Role identification, gender, 270
Romantic love cycle, 183–186
Rosenman, Ray, 406
Roussel-Uclaf, 249
Rowing, video exercise program for, 164
Rowing Machine Companion (video), 164
RU 486 (abortion pill), 249
Rubella (German measles), 364
   localization of rash of, *illustrated*, 364
Rubeola (measles), 362–363
Runner's World, 148
Running, 158
   injuries related to, 162
   video exercise program for, 163
Running Great with Grete Waitz (video), 164

S

Sadness, 42
   depression and, 42
Safety belts, 497
Safety needs, 17
Sagan, Carl, 483
Saline, intraamniotic injection of, 249
Salutogenesis, 70
Sarcoma, 417. *See also* Cancer
Saturated triglycerides (fats), 99
Scabies, 393–394
Schedules of controlled substances, 469
Schick Laboratories, 294
School, stress and, 62
Second opinion, 455
Second trimester, fetal development during, 268
Second-hand smoke, *See* Involuntary smoking
Secondary hypertension, 405
Secondary stressor, 61
Seizure:
   grand mal (tonic-clonic), 435
   petit mal (abscence), 435
Self-acceptance, mental wellness and, 32
Self-actualization needs, 18
Self-actualized individuals, characteristics of, 18
Self-concept, 34–35
Self-control, achieving, 21
Self-esteem, 33–35
   social networks and, 77
Self-help groups, weight reduction and, 136
Self-management, as behavior-change strategy, 22–23
Self-perception, 33–35
Self-potential, checklist for fulfilling, 34
Self-responsibility, achieving, 7
Selflessness, spiritual well-being and, 37
Selye, Hans, 58, 60

Semen, 200
Seminal vesicles, 201
Senility, 512
Serotonin, 279
Serum hepatitis, 367
Setpoint level:
   aerobic exercise and, 130
   artificial sweetners and, 131
   caffeine and, 131
   eating behavior and, 131
   high-fat foods and, 130
   mineral intake and, 131
   simple carbohydrates and, 130–131
   stress and, 131
Setpoint theory:
   of weight control, 130–131
   aerobic exercise and, 150–151
Seventh Day Adventist Church, 294
Sex:
   cancer and, 420
   cardiovascular disease and, 406
   determining child's, 261–262
   hormones and, 206–207, 261
   See also Gender
Sexual abuse, psychiatric illness and, 52
Sexual anatomy and physiology:
   female, 201–205
   male, 198–201
Sexual behavior, responsible, 222–223
Sexual bodyworks, 197–210
Sexual functioning, hormones and, 205–206
Sexual preferences:
   behaviors and, 207–208
   defined, 207
Sexual response, 208
Sexual response cycle, 208–210
   female responses during, *listed*, 210
   male responses during, *listed*, 209
Sexuality:
   aging and, 520–521
   understanding, 175–273
Sexually transmitted diseases, 373–397
   acquired immunodeficiency syndrome (AIDS), 383–388
   asymptomatic victims of, 376
   bacterial, 376–383
   birth control pills and, 374
   candida albicans (Monilia), 391–392
   chancroid, 382
   chlamydia infection, 352, 380
   defined, 374
   denial and, 375
   factors affecting transmission of, 374
   gonorrhea, 352, 379
   granuloma inguinale, 382
   guidelines for prevention of, 383
   guidelines for reducing risk of complications from, 393
   herpes simplex, 388–389
   human papilloma virus (HPV)(venereal warts), 390

ignorance and, 375
impulsive behavior and, 374–375
incidence of, 374, 375
irresponsibility and, 375
lack of reporting of, 375–376
lack of vaccines for, 376
lymphogranuloma venereum, 382–383
molluscum contagiosum, 391
nongonococcal urethritis (NSU), 380
nonspecific urethritis (NSU), 380
pelvic inflammatory disease, 380–381
prevention of, 394
pubic lice, 392–393
reporting card for, *illustrated*, 377
scabies, 393–394
syphilis, 376–378
trichomonas vaginalis, 392
vaginosis, 381
viral, 383–391
Shakespeare, William, 37
Shoes, exercise, 162
Shopping behavior, self-inventory of, 449.
  See also Advertising; Consumer protection skills
"Shrooms," 337
Shyness, 46
Sickle-cell anemia, 435–436
Sigmoidoscope, 425
Significant others, 16–17
Simon, Harvey, 155
Simple carbohydrates, 92
  defined, 91
  setpoint level and, 130–131
Skene's glands, 202
Skin cancer, 421–422
  basal cell carcinoma, 421
  melanoma, 421
  squamous cell carcinoma, 421
  ultraviolet radiation and, 422
Skin tests, 368
Slater, Philip, 45
Smith, Charlie, 14
Smog standards, cities in violation of federal, 482
SmokeEnders, 294
Smokeless tobacco, 296–297
  cancer and, 296–297
Smoking:
  aging and, 288–290
  alcohol and, 281
  Alzheimer's disease and, 287
  basic facts about, 279–282
  benefits of quitting, 295
  birth control pills and, 406
  cancer and, 285, 286
  cardiovascular disease and, 286–287, 406
  children and, 280–281, 295
  deaths related to, 282
  effects of, on body, 280
  ethnic differences and, 281
  fertility and, 287

gum disease and, 287
health and, 285–290
health guidelines concerning, 289
incidence of, 280
involuntary (passive), 295–296
life expectancy and, 290
life-style and, 279–280
osteoporosis and, 289
pregnancy and, 287–288
productivity and health care costs of, 282
quitting, 290, 292–295
respiratory disease and, 285–286
self-inventory of reasons for, 283
sterility and, 287
ulcers and, 287
See also Cigarettes; Nicotine; Tobacco
Snuff, 296–297
Social age, 507
Social companionship, social networks and, 77
Social deaths, 530
Social networks:
  defined, 76
  specific functions served by, 77–78
Social Readjustment Rating Scale, 63
  for college students, 64–65
Social responsibility, mental wellness and, 32
Social Security, 522
Social support:
  buffering effect of, 77
  defined, 76
  direct effect of, 77
  health and, 76–77
  social well-being and, 76
Social well-being, 7
  stress and, 75–78
Social workers, psychiatric, 51
Socioeconomic factors, cancer and, 420
Sodium:
  food labels and, 126
  cardiovascular disease and, 406
Sodium-free foods, 126
Soluble 94
Somatic nervous system (SNS), 278
Sopor, 330
Specificity, of exercise program, 169
Spermatozoa (sperm), production of, 258
Spermicides, 242–243
  application of, *illustrated*, 242
  with cervical cap, 241
  with diaphragm, 237–239
Spirilla (spirochetes), 353
Spiritual awareness, 36–40
Spiritual issues, stress and, 62
Spiritual well-being, 7, 10, 36–40
  love and, 37, 40
  meaning and purpose in life and, 37
  moral principles and, 37
  perception of cosmos and, 37
  selflessness and, 37
  self-inventory of, 38–39

Spirochete, 376
Spirochetes (spirilla), 353
Sponge, vaginal, 239–240
Sports, physical fitness and, 167
Squamous cell carcinoma, 421
Stage:
  of exhaustion, 59
  of resistance, 59
Staphylococci, 214, 353
Static stretching, 166
Status, social networks and, 77
Sterility:
  dibromochloropropane and, 487, 490
  sexually transmitted diseases and, 352
  smoking and, 287
  temporary, 251
Sterilization. *See* Tubal ligation; Vasectomy
Steroids, athletic training and, 170–171
Stimulants, 332–335
  amphetamines, 335
  caffeine, 343–344
  cocaine, 332–335
Stomach-reduction surgery, 135
Storage fat, 122
STP (DOM), 341
Strength, muscular, 147
Streptococci, 353
Stress:
  cardiovascular disease and, 406
  defined, 58
  general adaptation syndrome (GAS) and, 59
  management of, 57–81
  managing crises and, 66–69
  manifestations of, 69–70
  mental wellness and, 32
  patterns of, 59–60
  physiology of, 59
  setpoint level and, 131
  short- and long-term responses to, 59–60
  social well-being and, 75–78
  sources of, 61–62, 64–66
Stress management, 70–72
  coping strategies and, 70–75
  keeping a journal and, 74–75
  positive thinking and, 71
  relaxation techniques and, 72–74
Stressful event, 67, 68
Stressor:
  primary, 61
  secondary, 61
Stretching:
  ballistic, 166
  for exercise, 166, 168
  static, 166
Stroke (cerebrovascular accident), 409
Students Against Driving Drunk (SADD), 313
  "Contract for Life" of, *illustrated*, 314
Subdermal progestin implants, 250
Substances, carcinogenic, 419

Sudden infant death syndrome (SIDS), 287
Sugar, guidelines for minimizing intake of, 93. *See also* Carbohydrates
Sugar-free or sugarless foods, 126
Suicides, 46, 48–49
   barbiturates and, 329
   firearms and, 48
Superfund, 474
Support:
   material, 77
   unconditional, 41
Suppositories, vaginal, 242
Supreme Court, U.S., abortion and, 246–247
Surgeon General of the United States, 146–422
   1979 report of, 422
   1971 report of, 288
   1986 report of, 295
   1988 report of, 282
Surgery:
   getting second opinion for, 455
   for weight-loss purposes, 135
Sweeteners, artificial, 131
Swimming, video exercise program for, 164
Swimming for Fitness (video), 164
Syanon, 332
Sympathetic nervous system, 278
Sympathomimetics, 463
Synapse, 278
Syndrome:
   acute grief, 542
   amotivational, 339–340
   Down's, 317
   fetal alcohol, 316–317
   premenstrual (PMS), 214–215, 343
   Reye's, 362, 461
   toxic shock, 214
Synergism:
   alcohol and, 309–311
   barbiturates and, 329
   defined, 10
   marijuana and, 340
   opiates and, 331
Synovial membrane, 429
Syphilis, 376–378
   late stage of, 378
   latent stage of, 378
   pregnancy and, 378
   primary stage of, 376–377
   secondary stage of, 377–378
   treatment for, 378
Systemic lupus erythematosus (SLE), 431–432
Systole, 403
Systolic blood pressure, 403

T

T lymphocyte, 385
Take Off Pounds Sensibly (TOPS), 136

Tampons:
   guidelines for using, 215
   toxic shock syndrome and, 214
Tapeworms, 355
Target heart rate (THR), 153, 154
   determining, 161
Tars, 285
Taste, sense of, aging and, 514
Tay-Sachs disease, 436–437
Tears, as defense mechanism, 358
Technology, stress and, 62
Teenagers:
   alcohol and, 318
   cocaine use among, 332
Tennov, Dorothy, 184
Teratogenic, 343
Terminals, of neuron, 279
Test:
   ELISA, 386
   pregnancy, 264
   skin, 368
   Western Blot, 387
Testes, testicles, 200
   effects of hormones on, 205–206
   cancer of, 426
   self examination of, 426
Testosterone, 200, 206–207, 260
Tetanus, 368
Tetrahydrocannabinol (THC), 311, 338–339
   tolerance to, 340
Thanatologist, 541
Theophylline, 344
Theoretical failure rates, 226
Therapeutic communities, 332
Therapy, electroconvulsive (electroshock), 51. *See also* Psychotherapy
Third trimester, fetal development during, 268
Thoresen, Carl, 22
Time pressure, stress and, 62
Tissue, adipose, 122
TMA, 341
Tobacco, 277–301
   economics of, 281–282
   legislation concerning, 297–298
   smokeless, 296–297
   substitutes for, 290
Tolerance:
   to alcohol, 308–309
   to amphetamines, 335
   to barbiturates, 329
   cross, 309, 329
   dispositional, 308
   to opiates, 331
   pharmacodynamic, 308
Tonic-clonic (*grand mal*) seizure, 435
TOPS. *See* Take Off Pounds Sensibly
Toxic shock syndrome (TSS), 214
Toxic substances. *See* Hazardous substances
Toxic waste. *See* Hazardous waste
Toxins, 353–354, 480

Trace minerals, 104
Traffic accidents. *See* Motor vehicle accidents
Traffic fatalities, alcohol-related, 316, 317
Training, athletic. *See* Athletic training
Transactional analysis, 51
Transient ischemic attack (TIA), 408–409
Transition, love in, 185
Transmission of disease, 356–357
Transpersonal psychology, 51
Transsexuality, 208
Trichinella, 355–356
Trichinosis, 356
Trichomonas vaginalis, 392
Triglycerides, 99–100
   monounsaturated, 99–100
   polyunsaturated, 99
   saturated, 99
Trimester:
   first, 267–268
   second, 268
   third, 268
Tubal ligation, 226–228
   illustrated, 227
Tubal pregnancy, 259
Tuberculosis (TB), 368–369
Tufts University Diet and Nutrition Letter, 125
Tumors, 416. *See also* Neoplasms
Tylenol, 460–461
Type A personality, 406
Type B personality, 406

U

Ulceration, 382
Ulcerative colitis, 425
Ulcers, smoking and, 287
Ultraviolet radiation, skin cancer and, 422
Umbilical cord, 266, 267
Umbilication, 391
Unconscious:
   collective, 35
   personal, 35
Undertakers, 539
Underweight, 126
United States Postal Service (USPS), 444
Urethra, 200
Urethritis, 380
   nongonococal (NGU), 380
   nonspecific (NSU), 380
Urology, 287
Uterine cervix, cancer of, 426–427
Uterus, 204
   endometrium, of, 204
   myometrium of, 204
   perimetrium of, 204

V

Vaccines, birth control and, 251
Vacuum-aspiration, 248

Vagina, 202–203
Vaginal Contraceptive Film (VCF), 242
Vaginal ring, 250
Vaginal shield, 250
Vaginal sponge, 239–240
  placement of, *illustrated*, 239
Vaginal suppositories, 242
Vaginosis, 381
Van Camp, Steven, 155
Varicella. *See* Chicken pox
Vas deferens, 200
Vasectomy, 228–229
Vasocongestion, 208
Vasodilators, 406
Vegan, 97
Vegetables, cruciferous, 112
Vegetarian:
  defined, 97
  lacto-ovo, 97
  protein for the, 97–98
  vegan, 97
Venereal warts, 390
Venules, 403
Veronal, 330
Very-low-density lipoproteins (VLDLs), 411
Vesicles, seminal, 201
Vestibule, 202
Victoria virus, 366
Video exercise programs:
  for aerobics, 163
  for biking, 164
  comparison of, 163–164
  for rowing, 164
  for running, 164
  for swimming, 164
Viral diseases, 361–367
  acquired immunodeficiency syndrome (AIDS), 383–388
  chicken pox (varicella), 361–362
  common cold, 365–366
  German measles (rubella), 364
  hepatitis A, 367
  herpes simplex, 388–389
  human papilloma virus (HPV) (venereal warts), 390
  infectious mononucleosis, 366–367
  influenza, 365–366
  measles (rubeola), 362–363
  molluscum contagiosum, 391–392
  mumps (parotitis), 364–365
  human immunodeficiency, 383
Viruses, 352–353
  antibiotics and, 353
  diseases caused by, 353
  influenza, 366

Vision, aging and, 515–516
Vitamins, 101–103, 109–110
  deficiency of, alcohol and, 311
  defined, 101
  fat-soluble, 101
  thirteen essential, 102–103
  water-soluble, 101
Volatile solvents, 328
Vulva, 201

W

Waitz, Grete, exercise video by, 164
War, nuclear. *See* Nuclear war
Warts, 417
  venereal, 390
Water:
  nutrition and, 110–111
  toxic chemicals in, 487–488
Water-soluble vitamins, 101
Webster v. Reproductive Health Services, 246, 247
Weight, body, 120–121
Weight control:
  assessment of eating habits and, 124–125
  calorie awareness and, 123–124
  eating disorders and, 138–141
  fat-cell theory of, 129
  gaining weight and, 126–127
  genetic predisposition theory of, 128–129
  losing weight and, 122–126
  self-inventory for, 137
  setpoint theory of, 130–131
  theories of, 127–131
  understanding food labels and, 125–126
  white fat versus brown fat activity theory of, 129–130
  See also Diet; Eating behavior; Nutrition
Weight reduction, 131–136
  popular diets for, 132–134
  self-help groups and, 136
  surgical procedures for, 135
Weight-regulating mechanism (WRM), 130
Weight Watchers, 136
Well-being:
  mental, 7. *See also* Mental health; Mental wellness
  physical, 6–7
  social, 7, 75
  spiritual, 7, 10, 36–40
Wellness:
  defined, 5–6
  dimensions of, 6–10

environment and, 11
  factors affecting, 10–15
  health actions and, 3–29
  health-care organizations and, 12–13
  human biology and, 11
  lifestyle and, 12
  mental. *see* Mental wellness
Western Blot test, 387
Wheeler-Lea Amendment of 1938, 451
White blood cells:
  B lymphocytes, 358
  as defense mechanism, 358
  macrophages, 358
  T lymphocytes, 358
White fat versus brown fat activity theory of weight control, 129–130
Whooping cough (pertussis), 367–368
Will, living. *See* Living will
Withdrawal:
  from barbiturates, 329
  from cocaine, 333
  from methaqualone, 331
  from nicotine, 282
Work:
  stress and, 62
  toxic substances and. *See* Occupation
Worker Right-to-Know Law, 490
World Health Organization, 280, 384
World War II, atomic bomb and, 482
Worms, parasitic, 355–356
Worth Health Organization, 282
Wrinkles, aging and, 514

X

X androsperm, 258
X gynosperm, 258
XTC. *See* MDMA

Y

Years of potential life lost (YPLL), 400, 401, 495
Yellow Emperor's Classic of Internal Medicine, The (Nei Ching), 70

Z

Zygote, 259

Photo Credits

ii Burton McNeely, Image Bank; x Obremski, Image Bank; xii Russ Kinne, Comstock; xiv Russ Kinne, Comstock; xv S. Murphy, Comstock; 1 Comstock; 3 Milton Feinberg, Stock, Boston; 5 Barth Falkenberg, Stock, Boston; 11(t) Peter Menzel, Stock, Boston; 11(b) Eric Neurath, Stock, Boston; 14 Abel Kiviat, Gamma-Liaison; 17 Joe Traver, Gamma-Liaison; 20 Gerard Champlong, Image Bank; 31 Bryce Flynn, Stock, Boston; 35 Cary Wolinsky, Stock, Boston; 40 Alvis Upitis, Image Bank; 41 ©Kashi; 43 Mel Digiacomo, Image Bank; 45 Comstock; 50 ©Kashi; 57 ©Paul Markow, FPG; 69 ©Daemmrich, Stock, Boston; 70 Werner Dietrich, Image Bank; 76 Peter Vandermark, Stock, Boston; 83 Comstock; 85 FPG; 87 Frank Siteman, Taurus; 91 Comstock; 92 Comstock; 96 Derek Murray Photography, Inc., Image Bank; 108 P. Pfander, Image Bank; 109 Philip Jon Bailey, Taurus; 112 Obremski, Image Bank; 119 Frank Whitney, Image Bank; 125 ©Kashi; 136 Marilyn Ferguson, PhotoEdit; 139 Russ Kinne, Comstock; 145 David Madison, Focus on Sports; 148 Jerry Wachter, Focus on Sports; 150 John P. Kelly, Image Bank; 153 Jim Harrison, Stock, Boston; 155 Norman R. Thompson, Taurus; 161 Scott Ransom, Taurus; 165 Comstock; 175 Al Satterwhite, Image Bank; 177 Larry Gatz, Image Bank; 178 Robert Brenner, PhotoEdit; 183 Tony Freeman, PhotoEdit; 185 Janeart, Ltd., Image Bank; 186 Marlleen Ferguson, PhotoEdit; 189 Cary Wolinsky, Stock, Boston; 197 Comstock; 221 Jean-Francois Podevin, Image Bank; 230 ©Tony Freeman, PhotoEdit; 236 Gamma Liaison; 240 Murray Alcosser, Image Bank; 257 Comstock; 262 ©Kashi; 266 Nancy Brown, Image Bank; 268 Larry Dale Gordon, Image Bank; 270 Russ Kinne, Comstock; 275 Comstock; Michael Melford, Image Bank; Comstock; 277 Hallinan, FPG; 280 Mieke Maas, Image Bank; 284 Martin M. Rotker, Taurus Photo; 289 Nick Pavloff, Image Bank; 290 James Stevenson/Science Photo Library; 303 Richard Hutchings, PhotoEdit; 312 ©Tony Freeman, PhotoEdit; 318 Bob Daemmrich, Stock, Boston; 327 A. Gescheidt, Image Bank; 328 ©Tony Freeman, PhotoEdit; 331 Matthew Naythons, Stock, Boston; 331 Lawrence Migdale, Stock, Boston; 334 Lawrence Migdale, Stock, Boston; 335 Taurus Photo; 338 Barbara Alper, Stock, Boston; 344 Comstock; 349 ©Stuart Cohen, Comstock; 351 ©Alec Duncan, Taurus Photo; 355 Biophoto Associates/Science Source; 361 Michael Melford, Image Bank; 362 Jim Holland, Stock, Boston; 373 Medical, Uniphoto; 377 U. S. Centers for Disease Control; 378 U. S. Centers for Disease Control; 385 Lawrence Migdale, Stock, Boston; 387(t) Mark Green, Gamma-Liaison; 387 Rob Crandall, Stock, Boston; 389 Rotker, Taurus Photos; 394 Rhoda Sidney, Stock, Boston; 399 Michel Tcherevkoff, Image Bank; 403 Mike & Carol Werner, Comstock; 406 Comstock; 415 William Johnson, Stock, Boston; 421 Courtesy American Academy of Dermatology; 422 Courtesy American Academy of Dermatology; 423 Russ Kinne, Comstock; 432 Martin M. Rotker, Taurus Photos; 435 Science Photo Library, Taurus Photos; 441 ©Kashi; 443 Comstock; 445 Roger Miller, Image Bank; 447 Charles Gupton, Stock, Boston; 458 Comstock; 461 ©Tony Freeman, PhotoEdit; 462 Robert Houser, Comstock; 466 ©Daemmrich, Stock, Boston; 473 Richard Pasley, Stock, Boston; 474 Elaine Wicks, Taurus; 476 Robert Houser, Comstock; 483 Gamma Liaison; 484 Russ Kinne, Comstock; 488 ©Kashi; 489 Jim Howard, FPG; 492 William Wright, Taurus; 498 Russ Kinne, Comstock; 503 Comstock; 505 Dale O'Dell, Comstock; 507 ©Eric Kroll, Taurus; 510 Michael Hayman, Stock, Boston; 512 Suzanne L. Murphy, FPG; 514 ©Townsend P. Dickinson, Comstock; 515 Richard Pasley, Stock, Boston; 519 Rick Brady, Uniphoto; 521 Frank Siteman, Taurus; 527 Comstock; 537 Ellis Herwig, Stock, Boston; 539 Mark Mittelman, Taurus; 541 John Coletti, Stock Boston.